D0571122

Blood and Marrow Stem Cell Transplantation

Principles, Practice, and Nursing Insights

THIRD EDITION

Susan Ezzone, MS, RN, CNP

Nurse Practitioner
Blood and Marrow Transplant Program
The Ohio State University Medical Center
Arthur G. James Cancer Hospital and Solove Research Institute
Columbus, Ohio

Kim Schmit-Pokorny, RN, MSN, OCN®

Manager/Case Manager
Blood and Marrow Transplant Program
University of Nebraska Medical Center
Omaha, Nebraska

JONES AND BARTLETT PUBLISHERS

Sudbury, Massachusetts

BOSTON   TORONTO   LONDON   SINGAPORE

World Headquarters
Jones and Bartlett Publishers
40 Tall Pine Drive
Sudbury, MA 01776
978-443-5000
info@jbpub.com
www.jbpub.com

Jones and Bartlett Publishers Canada
6339 Ormindale Way
Mississauga, Ontario L5V 1J2
CANADA

Jones and Bartlett Publishers
International
Barb House, Barb Mews
London W6 7PA
UK

Jones and Bartlett's books and products are available through most bookstores and online booksellers. To contact Jones and Bartlett Publishers directly, call 800-832-0034, fax 978-443-8000, or visit our website, www.jbpub.com.

Substantial discounts on bulk quantities of Jones and Bartlett's publications are available to corporations, professional associations, and other qualified organizations. For details and specific discount information, contact the special sales department at Jones and Bartlett via the above contact information or send an email to specialsales@jbpub.com.

Library of Congress Cataloging-in-Publication Data
Blood and marrow stem cell transplantation : principles, practice, and nursing insights.— 3rd ed. / [edited by] Susan Ezzone and Kim Schmit-Pokorny.
   p. ; cm.
Includes bibliographical references.
ISBN 0-7637-4719-X (casebound)

   [DNLM: 1.   Hematopoietic Stem Cell Transplantation—Nurses' Instruction. 2.   Bone Marrow Transplantation—Nurses' Instruction.   WH 380 B6545 2006] I. Ezzone, Susan. II. Schmit-Pokorny, Kim.
   RD123.5.B56 1997
   617.4'410592—dc22

2005012146

6048

Production Credits
Acquisitions Editor: Kevin Sullivan
Production Director: Amy Rose
Associate Editor: Amy Sibley
Associate Production Editor: Alison Meier
Marketing Associate: Serena Ciampa
Manufacturing Buyer: Amy Bacus
Composition: Auburn Associates, Inc.
Cover Design: Kristin E. Ohlin
Cover Image: © Photos.com
Printing and Binding: Malloy, Inc.
Cover Printing: Malloy, Inc.

The authors, editor, and publisher have made every effort to provide accurate information. However, they are not responsible for errors, omissions, or for any outcomes related to the use of the contents of this book and take no responsibility for the use of the products described. Treatments and side effects described in this book may not be applicable to all patients; likewise, some patients may require a dose or experience a side effect that is not described herein. The reader should confer with his or her own physician regarding specific treatments and side effects. Drugs and medical devices are discussed that may have limited availability controlled by the Food and Drug Administration (FDA) for use only in a research study or clinical trial. The drug information presented has been derived from reference sources, recently published data, and pharmaceutical research data. Research, clinical practice, and government regulations often change the accepted standard in this field. When consideration is being given to use of any drug in the clinical setting, the health care provider or reader is responsible for determining FDA status of the drug, reading the package insert, reviewing prescribing information for the most up-to-date recommendations on dose, precautions, and contraindications, and determining the appropriate usage for the product. This is especially important in the case of drugs that are new or seldom used.

Printed in the United States of America
10 09 08 07 06   10 9 8 7 6 5 4 3 2 1

Contents

Chapter 1: Bone Marrow to Blood Stem Cells Past, Present, Future 1

John Wingard, MD

Chapter 2: Understanding Hematopoiesis 29

Melinda S. Chouinard, RN, BSN, OCN®
Kathleen T. Finn, RN, NP, AOCN®

Chapter 3: Hematopoietic Stem Cell Transplant Immunology 59

Boglarka Gyurkocza, MD
Melinda S. Chouinard, RN, BSN, OCN®

Chapter 4: Blood and Marrow Transplantation: Indications, Procedure, Process 75

Kim Schmit-Pokorny, RN, MSN, OCN®

Chapter 5: Conditioning Regimens in Hematopoietic Stem Cell Transplantation 109

Cathleen M. Poliquin, MS, APRN-BC, AOCN®

Chapter 6: Graft-Versus-Host Disease: Complex Sequelae of Stem Cell Transplantation 147

Viki Anders, RN, MSN, CRNP
Margaret Barton-Burke, PhD, RN, AOCN®

Chapter 7: Hematologic Effects of Transplantation 183

Shelley Burcat, RN, MSN
Francis McAdams, RN, MSN, AOCN®

Chapter 8: Gastrointestinal Effects 207

Elizabeth Warnick, RN, MSN, CRNP, BC

Chapter 15: Hematopoietic Cell Transplantation: The Trajectory of Quality of Life 391

Liz Cooke, RN, MN, ANP, AOCN®
Marcia Grant, RN, DNSc, FAAN
Deborah Eldredge, PhD, RN

Chapter 16: Models of Care Delivery for Hematopoietic Stem Cell Transplant Patients 423

Theresa Franco, RN, MSN
Rosemary C. Ford, RN, BSN, OCN®

Chapter 17: Transplant Networks and Standards of Care: International Perspectives 441

Susan Ezzone, MS, RN, CNP
Monica Fliedner, MSN
Jan Sirilla, MSN, RN, OCN®

Chapter 18: The Bone Marrow and Blood Stem Cell Transplant Marketplace 463

Rita Potter, RHIA

Chapter 19: Nursing Research in Blood Cell and Marrow Transplantation 479

Mel Haberman, PhD, RN, FAAN

Chapter 20: Patients' Perspectives *491*

Susan Stewart

Preface

It is overwhelming to reflect on the advancements that have occurred in the field of hematopoietic stem cell transplant over the past three or more decades. The first edition of this book then titled *Bone Marrow Transplantation: Principles, Practice, and Nursing Insights*, edited by Marie Whedon, in 1991, was a long awaited significant contribution to the nursing literature on transplantation. The second edition published in 1997, titled *Blood and Marrow Stem Cell Transplantation: Principles, Practice and Nursing Insights, Second Edition*, edited by Marie Whedon and Debra Wujcik, further described changes occurring in the field of transplantation and remains a valuable resource for nurses. When we were approached to become editors of the third edition of the book, we humbly accepted. It is an honor and privilege to follow the lead of the previous editors and attempt to update this book providing new insights into the ever-changing field of hematopoietic stem cell transplantation (HSCT).

When reflecting back through the years, there have been many changes in the field of HSCT, but many practice strategies remain the same. The third edition of this book follows the tradition of previous editions and attempts to provide an updated review of the current practice of HSCT. Transplantation continues to be considered standard therapy for many hematologic diseases, and new clinical trials offer additional treatment options for many diseases. An updated review of the history of HSCT is presented in Chapter 1, providing insight related to the past, present, and future of transplantation. Since an understanding of hematopoiesis and HLA typing has become more complex, chapters have also been updated to provide information regarding current knowledge. The indications for transplant have expanded, and the overall process is described. The purpose and types of preparative regimens used for autologous, allogeneic and non-myeloablative allogeneic HSCT have become more diverse and are reviewed in detail. Although acute and late effects of transplantation remain the same, new understanding offers insights that have an impact on the medical and nursing management of each complication. Complications of transplantation that are presented include graft versus host disease, hematologic, gastrointestinal, pulmonary, cardiac, renal, hepatic, neurologic, and delayed effects. Other issues that remain important to the management of the patient during the transplant process are presented. These include family issues, psychosocial effects, ethical issues, financial issues, and quality of life. In addition, models of care across all sites of care delivery, transplant networks and standards of care, and past and present nursing research initiatives are reviewed. Finally, patient perspectives on the transplant process are offered.

As editors, we hope this book will continue to be a valuable resource for nurses and others working in the field of HSCT. It has been challenging and rewarding to work with all of the contributors in developing content that will continue to offer new insights for nurses caring for persons undergoing HSCT.

Acknowledgments

The authors would like to acknowledge the contributions of all of the authors and thank them for their expertise and diligent efforts during completion of the book. We also thank the behind-the-scenes help of many persons who assisted through secretarial support, library assistance, and employers who understood the need to achieve completion of each component of individual chapters. Thanks also to the staff of Jones and Bartlett Publishers for their continued persistence and patience during the final steps of completion of the book.

I would like to thank my family, husband Jay, and children Nathan and Sara, for their patience and support over the past years during completion of the book.

—SE

I would like to thank my husband, Kevin, and children, Christopher and Megan, for their love and encouragement that supported me throughout this project.

—KSP

Contributors

Viki Anders, RN, MSN, CRNP
BMT Nurse Practitioner
GVHD Clinic Coordinator
The Sidney Kimmel Comprehensive Cancer Center
     at Johns Hopkins
Baltimore, Maryland

Margaret Barton-Burke, PhD, RN, AOCN®
Oncology Nurse Specialist
University of Massachusetts Medical Center
Assistant Professor of Nursing
University of Massachusetts School of Nursing
Amherst, Massachusetts

Ann Breen, RN, MN, APRN, OCN®
Patient and Family Education Coordinator
Transition Coordinator
Seattle Cancer Care Alliance
Seattle, Washington

Shelley Burcat, RN, MSN
Clinical Nurse Specialist
Bone Marrow Transplant Unit
Thomas Jefferson University Hospital
Philadelphia, Pennsylvania

Mary Reilly Burgunder, MS, BSN, RN, OCN®
Infusion/Oncology Specialty Clinician
University of Pittsburgh Medical Center
South Hills Health System Home Health, LP
Pittsburgh, Pennsylvania

Melinda S. Chouinard, RN, BSN, OCN®
Seattle Cancer Care Alliance
Seattle, Washington

Liz Cooke, RN, MN, ANP, AOCN®
Research Specialist
City of Hope Medical Center
Duarte, California

Tracy T. Douglas, RN, MSN, OCN®
BMT Clinical Nurse Specialist
The Sidney Kimmel Comprehensive Cancer Center
     at Johns Hopkins
Baltimore, Maryland

June Eilers, PhD, APRN, BC
Clinical Nurse Specialist
Clinical Nurse Researcher
The Nebraska Medical Center
Omaha, Nebraska

Deborah Eldredge, PhD, RN
Assistant Professor
School of Nursing
Oregon Health and Science University
Portland, Oregon

Susan Ezzone, MS, RN, CNP
Nurse Practitioner
Blood and Marrow Transplant Program
The Ohio State University Medical Center
Arthur G. James Cancer Hospital and Solove
    Research Institute
Columbus, Ohio

Kathleen T. Finn, RN, NP, AOCN®
Boston University Medical Center
Cancer Research Center
Boston, Massachusetts

Monica Fliedner, MSN
Advanced Nurse Practitioner
Clinical Nurse Specialist Oncology
University Hospital
Bern, Switzerland

Rosemary C. Ford, RN, BSN, OCN®
Nurse Manager
Transplant Clinic
Seattle Cancer Care Alliance
Seattle, Washington

Theresa Franco, RN, MSN
Executive Director—Cancer Care Service Line
The Nebraska Medical Center
Omaha, Nebraska

Marcia Grant, RN, DNSc, FAAN
Director, Nursing Research and Education
City of Hope Medical Center
Duarte, California

Boglarka Gyurkocza, MD
Hematology/Oncology Fellow
Department of Hematology/Oncology
University of Massachusetts Memorial Medical
    Center
Worcester, Massachusetts

Mel Haberman, PhD, RN, FAAN
Associate Dean for Research and Professor
Intercollegiate College of Nursing
Washington State University
Spokane, Washington

Francis McAdams, RN, MSN, AOCN®
Clinical Director
Oncology Program
Temple University Hospital
Philadelphia, Pennsylvania

Joyce L. Neumann, RN, MS, AOCN®
Program Director, BMT
Advanced Practice Nurse
Department of Blood and Marrow Transplantation
The University of Texas MD Anderson Cancer
    Center
Houston, Texas

Cathleen M. Poliquin, MS, APRN-BC, AOCN®
Nurse Practitioner
Bone Marrow Transplant Program
Massachusetts General Hospital
Boston, Massachusetts

Rita Potter, RHIA
Director of Managed Care
The Nebraska Medical Center
Omaha, Nebraska

Kathy Ruble, RN, MSN, CPNP, AOCN®
Coordinator, Long Term Follow-up Program
Johns Hopkins University
Baltimore, Maryland

Deborah Rust, RN, MSN, CRNP, AOCN®
Clinical Coordinator Genentech BioOncology
Adjunct Instructor
University of Pittsburgh Nurse Practitioner
    Program
Pittsburgh, Pennsylvania

Kim Schmit-Pokorny, RN, MSN, OCN®
Manager/Case Manager
Blood and Marrow Transplant Program
University of Nebraska Medical Center
Omaha, Nebraska

Brenda K. Shelton, MS, RN, CCRN, AOCN®
Clinical Nurse Specialist
The Sidney Kimmel Comprehensive Cancer
  Center at Johns Hopkins
Baltimore, Maryland

Jan Sirilla, MSN, RN, OCN®
Administrative Director, BMT Program
The Ohio State University
Arthur G. James Cancer Hospital and Solove
  Research Institute
Columbus, Ohio

Susan Stewart
Editor
BMT Newsletter
Highland Park, Illinois

Elizabeth Warnick, RN, MSN, CRNP, BC
Nurse Practitioner, Shadyside Hospital
University of Pittsburgh Cancer Institute
Pittsburgh, Pennsylvania

John Wingard, MD
Professor and Director BMT Program
College of Medicine
University of Florida
Gainesville, Florida

Chapter 1

Bone Marrow to Blood Stem Cells Past, Present, Future

John Wingard, MD

The mythical figure of the chimera has often been used to symbolize the field of bone marrow transplantation (BMT). The chimera was a fire-spouting monster with a lion's head, a goat's body, and a serpent's tail. This creature was feared because it killed many animals and people. The monster was eventually killed with the consent of the gods, with the hope that the earth would be freed of this scourge.

In the field of BMT, the term *chimera* was first used by Ford and colleagues in 1956 to describe animals lethally irradiated and then given bone marrow from another animal: This maneuver resulted in the recipient's carrying a foreign hematopoietic system derived from the other animal. It is somewhat ironic that this creature, which originally evoked fear and revulsion and represented a cruel perversion of nature, now symbolizes a medical therapy offered with hope and concern and represents one of modern medicine's successful attempts to correct a number of nature's ailments afflicting human beings.

Evolution of BMT as a Treatment of Human Disease

Human bone marrow administration as a treatment for disease has been attempted sporadically since the late 19th century. Many of the early applications involved feeding or injecting bone marrow or spleen extracts into patients who had a variety of ailments, such as several kinds of anemia, including the "anemia of rapid growth, overwork and underfeeding," leukemia, and chlorosis (Quine, 1896). Sometimes, arsenic and iron were given adjunctively. Although some benefits were ascribed to the bone marrow treatments, the reason for improvement was unclear, and these efforts now seem quaint and unscientific.

In the modern era, human bone marrow transplantation began in 1957 when French and Yugoslav physicians treated several laboratory workers who had been exposed to radiation during the Vinca nuclear reactor accident (Mathe et al., 1959). One patient received fetal spleen and liver cells but died from hemorrhage. Four patients were given allogeneic bone marrow cells and all recovered marrow function. However, although there was some evidence of temporary engraftment, whether the bone marrow transplant conveyed any lasting benefit was uncertain (van Bekkum and de Vries, 1967).

Almost three decades later, in 1986, at Chernobyl, a nuclear reactor accident of significantly larger proportions in Russia hospitalized hundreds of individuals and led to the employment of marrow transplants once again to attempt to reverse the hematologic toxicity from accidental exposure to radiation (Baranov et al., 1989). Of the 33 persons estimated to have received more than 600 cGy, half had severe nonhematologic toxicity (mainly burns), which made survival unlikely. Thirteen received marrow transplants and one was given fetal liver because no histocompatible donor was available. Of the marrow transplants, 10 were from siblings (five HLA identical, the remainder one-haplotype identical). Although transient hematologic recovery occurred in most patients, there were only two long-term survivors. Most of the deaths were due to burns and other non-hematologic radiation injury. Thus, even three decades later than the Vinca incident, despite a wealth of new knowledge and advances in supportive care, we are reminded of the limitations of BMT and other treatment modalities used to deal with radiation accidents—the mortality related to the nonhematologic toxic effects of radiation, such as burns, gastrointestinal, pulmonary, or central nervous system injuries, is not affected. However, although BMT has not proved a useful tool for treating the devastating effects of accidental irradiation,

enormous utility has been found in a variety of medical applications.

During the early years of human BMT, attention was directed to determining the optimal source of bone marrow cells and methods of preserving the cells, achieving safe techniques for administering marrow intravenously to avoid pulmonary emboli, estimating the number of cells needed, and defining the types of illnesses to which BMT could be applied (Thomas et al., 1957; Thomas and Storb, 1970).

In 1970, a review of the reported human bone marrow transplant experience indicated that approximately 200 transplants had been performed during the preceding decade (see Table 1-1) (Bortin, 1970). The early results did not bode well. More than half of the patients had failed to engraft; three fourths had died. There was evidence of chimerism in only a few of the cases in which there were markers of donor cells, and only three chimeric patients were alive at the time of reporting. Of the patients with aplastic anemia treated by allogeneic marrow, none engrafted, but five of seven patients given syngeneic marrow transplants recovered.

Because of this very disappointing early experience, the number of marrow transplants performed during the early 1960s declined (see Figure 1-1). Improvements in the results of BMT awaited developments in several ancillary fields: supportive care (especially transfusion support and antibiotics), histocompatibility testing, conditioning regimens, and control of graft-versus-host disease (GVHD).

As a result of the advances in these related fields, a resurgence of interest in bone marrow transplantation took place in the late 1960s. At this time, human tissue typing permitted intentionally matched marrow transplants, which were applied to the treatment of genetic immunode-

Table 1-1 RESULTS OF THE FIRST 203 REPORTED HUMAN BONE MARROW
TRANSPLANTS (BEFORE 1970),

Disease	Number of Patients	Number with No Engraftment	Number with Secondary Disease**	Number of Allogeneic Diseases
Aplastic anemia	73	66	5	0
Leukemia	84	33	32	3
Malignant disease	31	23	1	1
Immune deficiency	15	3	11	7
Total	203	125	49	11*

*Three alive at the time of this report.
**Graft-versus-host disease.
Source: M.M. Bortin, A compendium of reported human bone marrow transplants, *Transplantation* 9(6):571–587, © Williams &
Wilkins, 1970. Reprinted with permission.

ficiency syndromes. These disorders are rare but have provided important biologic insights.

The wider application of BMT in the 1970s occurred initially in the therapy of severe aplastic anemia, or acute leukemia, for which other treatment had failed. Improved results were reported in 1975 (Thomas et al., 1975) (see **Figure 1-2**). As supportive care of patients

Figure 1-1 Reported human bone marrow transplants.

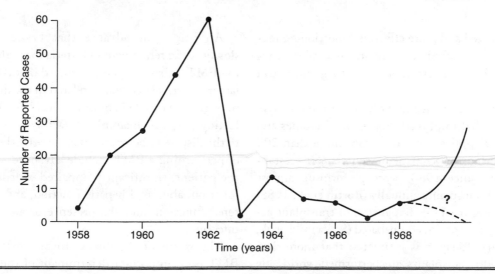

Source: M.M. Bortin, A compendium of reported human bone marrow transplants, *Transplantation* 9(6):571–587, © Williams &
Wilkins, 1970. Reprinted with permission.

Figure 1-2 Survival curves in 70 patients with acute leukemia given a marrow graft from a major-histocompatibility-complex-matched sibling.

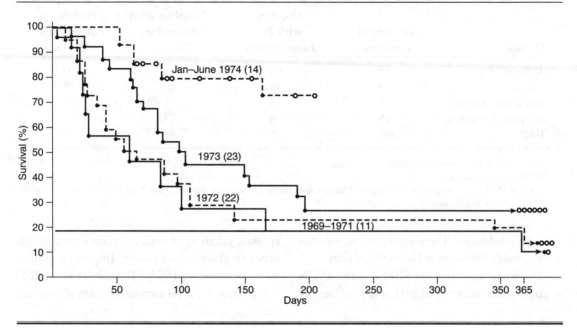

Note: Open circles indicate living patients.
Source: Reprinted by permission of the *New England Journal of Medicine* 292:841, 1975.

improved and more effective conditioning regimens were applied, 6-month survival rates increased from less than 20% to greater than 70%.

Since then, steady increases in interest have paralleled improved long-term outcomes and wider applications. By 1986, more than 200 bone marrow transplant centers (60% established since 1980) were performing almost 5000 transplants annually (Bortin et al., 1988) (see **Figure 1-3**). Expansion of transplant activity has continued unabated (Sobocinski et al., 1994). Today it is estimated that more than 50,000 transplants are performed worldwide annually (Goldman and Horowitz, 2002).

An important advance that has evolved slowly is the refinement of criteria for performing BMT. It has become recognized that certain factors (both related and unrelated to the disease to be treated by BMT) must be considered in selecting patients. Examples of factors unrelated to the disease to be treated that increase the risk of performing a BMT include advanced age of the patient, significantly impaired ventilatory function, abnormal hepatic function, abnormal renal function, and the presence of an active infection.

The status of the disease to be treated by BMT is an important determinant of the outcome for the patient. When BMT was performed

Figure 1-3 Annual number of patients receiving allogeneic bone marrow transplants and annual number of new transplant teams formed.

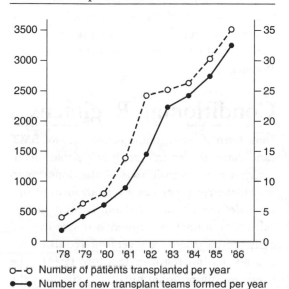

o–o Number of patients transplanted per year
●–● Number of new transplant teams formed per year

Source: M.M. Bortin, Current status of BMT in humans: report from the International Bone Marrow Transplant Registry. *Nat Immun Cell Growth Regul* 7:339, © S. Karger A.G., Basel. Used with permission.

in patients with acute leukemia in full relapse, long-term, disease-free survival rates of approximately 15% were seen. In contrast, when BMT was done in patients in chemotherapy-induced remission, the mortality rate fell dramatically, due to both a lower relapse rate and a decreased rate of transplant-associated mortality. Similarly, the earlier in the course of the disease the transplant is performed the better: The risk of relapse is lower and the likelihood of toxicity from the conditioning regimen is less than if the transplant is performed after multiple relapses or multiple courses of therapy.

By adopting patient selection criteria, one can minimize the risk of failure from toxicity. By performing the transplant at the appropriate time in the course of an individual's disease, one can optimize the likelihood of control of the underlying disease.

During the 1980s, the capability to cryopreserve hematopoietic progenitor cells was developed, initially using glycerol as a cryopreservative, but subsequently dimethylsulfoxide (DMSO) (Barnes and Loutit, 1955). Numerous animal models demonstrated that cryopreserved marrow could reconstitute hematopoiesis following lethal irradiation. The first attempts in humans in the late 1950s to exploit this in autologous BMT (ABMT) were disappointing (Kurnick et al., 1958). However, a number of clinical trials conducted since 1975 have been more promising. Because of potential contamination by tumor cells, especially for lymphohematopoietic malignancies, attempts to define effective purging methods have been made. The role for ex vivo purging using either pharmacologic or antibody-mediated means remains uncertain.

During the 1980s the frequency of autologous transplantation increased tremendously (Applebaum, 1996). The use of autologous peripheral blood progenitor cells during the early 1980s demonstrated the capacity for hematologic reconstitution (Goldman et al., 1980; Juttner et al., 1985). Hematopoietic growth factors or the combination of cytotoxic agents plus growth factors can increase the number of hematopoietic progenitor cells in the circulating blood and permit collection by apheresis of "enriched" progenitor cells capable of speedy engraftment. Not only has autologous BMT become more common than allogeneic BMT, but peripheral blood is now more commonly used than marrow as a source of progenitor cells to effect engraftment following marrow-lethal cytoreductive therapies. Now, the term *stem cell transplant (SCT)* has largely replaced BMT when referring to autologous transplants.

Autologous SCT was initially a treatment modality mostly for lymphopoietic malignancies as salvage treatment. In the past 10 years, however, the use of autologous SCT expanded to new applications in the therapy of solid tumors such as neuroblastoma, breast cancer, testicular cancer, and ovarian cancer. Although initial studies in patients with breast cancer suggested superior outcomes with SCT over conventional chemotherapy regimens, subsequent randomized trials did not. In contrast, randomized trials have clearly shown improved survival with SCT for multiple myeloma (Attal et al., 1996; Hahn et al., 2003). Recent studies demonstrated double autologous SCT for multiple myeloma offered an even greater benefit than a single SCT (Attal et al., 2003). The potential of autologous SCT is also being explored as a potent immunomodulatory treatment for severe autoimmune diseases such as scleroderma, systemic lupus erythematosis, rheumatoid arthritis, Crohn's disease, and multiple sclerosis (Burt et al., 2003).

The majority of patients who could benefit from an allogeneic BMT do not have suitably matched family members to serve as donors. The 1986 development of the National Bone Marrow Transplant Donor Registry in the United States and similar donor registries in other countries throughout the world have made it possible for patients without family donors who would otherwise not be candidates for BMT to undergo this treatment.

As with autologous SCT, peripheral blood is being evaluated as a source of hematopoietic cells in allogeneic transplantation, from both siblings and unrelated donors (Bensinger and Storb, 2001). Early results suggest a benefit in terms of greater graft versus tumor effects but at a cost: greater chronic GVHD. Cord blood, a tissue ordinarily discarded at birth, is a source of stem cells that have become yet another resource for allogeneic transplantation (Barker and Wagner, 2003).

Conditioning Regimens

Some form of conditioning is necessary for BMT candidates, except in certain rare situations in which a monozygotic twin is the donor or in which the recipient has a certain form of immunodeficiency and the donor is HLA identical. From animal experiments, it was learned early on that there are several prerequisites for a conditioning regimen (Santos, 1974). The conditioning regimen must first suppress the recipient's immunity to prevent graft rejection. Second, it must create "space" for the donor marrow—not physical space, but rather an effect (still poorly understood) on the marrow microenvironment that permits the establishment and growth of hematopoietic progenitors. A third requirement for patients to receive transplants for malignant disease is an antitumor effect, to eradicate residual tumor cells.

Total body irradiation (TBI), cyclophosphamide, or a combination of the two, were the first conditioning regimens. Both agents possess all three properties desirable in conditioning agents.

Experiments in mammals (reviewed by van Bekkum and de Vries, 1967) had demonstrated three types of syndromes after exposure to irradiation. Animals exposed to lethal TBI up to 1200 cGy die 8–14 days later from the effects of marrow aplasia (the so-called hematopoietic syndrome). Mice given 1200–12,000 cGy die 4–5 days later due to the sequelae from gut damage (the gastrointestinal syndrome). Animals subjected to more than 12,000 cGy die within hours or 1–2 days after exposure due to toxicity to the central nervous system (the cerebral syndrome). Infusions of syngeneic bone marrow will reverse the hematopoietic syndrome, but have no effect on the other two syndromes. In animals subjected to less than lethal irradiation, the frequency and persistence of engraftment after marrow transplant was found to be related to the TBI dose. In general, supra lethal TBI doses were necessary for long-lasting chimerism.

Aside from the extensive experience with TBI in animals, there were several other reasons TBI was a good choice as a preparative regimen. Irradiation was known to be effective in killing leukemic cells. It was able to bypass supposed sanctuary sites, such as the testes and central nervous system, to eliminate any occult contaminating tumor cells. One of its major organ toxicities, bone marrow, is not a concern when it is to be replaced by donor marrow. Initially, TBI doses of 800–1000 cGy were given at a rate of 3–6 cGy/min as a single dose. This was successful in achieving engraftment, but was not very effective in eradicating leukemia.

Experience with cyclophosphamide in animals (Santos et al., 1970) similarly led to its use in humans. The combination of cyclophosphamide and total body irradiation (CyTBI) was introduced very early and has since become a common conditioning regimen in the treatment of malignant disease (Thomas et al., 1977). During the 1970s, it was recognized that the risk for another major nonhematologic toxicity, interstitial pneumonitis, could be reduced by fractionation of the TBI, rather than administration in a single dose (Meyers et al., 1983). Another regimen, busulfan plus cyclophosphamide (BuCy), was developed as an alternative preparative regimen to CyTBI. Busulfan has very little immunosuppressive potency, but it has excellent antitumor and space-making properties. The combination regimen of BuCy has been shown to be at least as effective as CyTBI in the treatment of acute nonlymphocytic leukemia (ANLL) (Santos et al., 1983). In recent years, it has also been found to be effective as a conditioning regimen for chronic myelogenous leukemia (CML), Hodgkin's disease, non-Hodgkin's lymphoma, and beta thalassemia.

Other agents have also been introduced into preparative regimens to try to improve the antitumor efficacy. One agent used increasingly is etoposide, which has excellent antitumor activity, as well as some immunosuppressive activity—although not as much as cyclophosphamide (Gassman et al., 1988). Caution must be exercised in allogeneic transplantation to avoid agents with little or no immunosuppressive properties, especially in situations where there is an increased risk of graft rejection such as with a nonsibling donor, a mismatched donor, or a marrow graft manipulated ex vivo to remove T lymphocytes. In recent years, the addition of antithymocyte globulin or thiotepa to the preparative regimen has been explored to reduce the risk of graft rejection in high-risk transplants.

With autologous SCT, there is no such concern for graft rejection or the need for immunosuppression, and thus a panoply of preparative regimens have been and continue to be explored. The major objective is to develop combinations of drugs and/or radiotherapy with additive or synergistic antitumor activity and toxicities that do not overlap or are associated with minimal nonhematologic toxicities.

With respect to severe aplastic anemia, there is no necessity for antitumor activity, but the risk of graft rejection is substantive, and immunosuppression of the host is the paramount consideration in choosing a conditioning regimen. Of the first 66 patients transplanted with allogeneic marrow for aplastic anemia, none benefitted, and none demonstrated chimerism (Bortin, 1970). This was due, in large measure, to the fact that none received vigorous immunosuppressive pretreatment. Santos developed the use of high-dose cyclophosphamide alone as a conditioning regimen for patients with aplastic anemia (Santos, 1974). This continues to be the most common preparative regimen for allogeneic BMT for aplastic anemia. For patients who have been sensitized to the donor through blood transfusions or prior pregnancy (by exposure to fetal alloantigens), one of the major difficulties to overcome was graft rejection. It was learned that by increasing the immunosuppression in the conditioning regimen, rejection could be reduced. Initially, this was done by adding TBI to cyclophosphamide; the rejection rate decreased, but there was no increase in survival due to the sequelae of the irradiation toxicity. Subsequently, the use of cyclosporin or total lymphoid irradiation has provided better immunosuppression without the added mortality from toxicity.

In recent years, reduced intensity conditioning regimens have been developed in an attempt to allow allogeneic transplantation to individuals who, because of co-morbidities or advanced age, would not be considered for conventional conditioning regimens (Slavin et al., 2002; Mielcarek and Storb, 2003). This has been made possible because of the introduction of new, potent immunosuppressive agents including purine analogues (e.g., fludarabine or cladribine) and anti-T cell antibody preparations (e.g., antithymocyte globulin preparations) which provide as potent immunosuppression as intensive chemoradiotherapy. Further, recognition of the importance of the donor immunity mediating much of the antitumor effects of allogeneic transplantation has led to new insights: Perhaps the curative potential of BMT can be achieved more safely with less toxicity by using reduced intensity regimens. Such transplants are generally known as *nonmyeloablative stem cell transplants (NST)*. NST seems to work best for situations where the tumor burden is low, whereas relapse rates are high if the tumor burden is high. One approach being explored is to combine the excellent cytotoxicity achieved with autologous SCT with the graft-versus-tumor effects mediated by NST by using tandem autologous SCT followed by allogeneic NST (Maloney et al., 2003).

Developments in Tissue Typing

Dausset (1954, 1958) first presented evidence of leukoantibodies in patients receiving multiple transfusions. Initially thought to be autoantibodies, they were later shown to be alloantibodies to antigens expressed on the leukocytes. Family studies showed human leukocyte antigens (HLA) to be genetically determined. These antigens are the gene products of the HLA (or major histocompatibility) complex, which is a series of genes located on human chromosome 6. Although initially thought to be leukocyte specific, the HLA antigens subsequently were found to be broadly distributed tissue antigens.

The HLA system plays a critical role in the cellular interactions that occur as part of immune reactions to viruses and other foreign antigens in that T lymphocytes only recognize foreign antigens when they are physically associated with HLA gene products, HLA gene products have been recognized as important determinants of allograft rejection.

In 1964, Terasaki and McClelland introduced the microlymphocytotoxicity assay, which continues to be a major procedure to perform HLA typing. During the 1960s, two serologically defined loci (the A and B loci) were identified, and in 1970 the C locus was defined. These now are grouped as class I loci. The D region was initially assessed by the mixed lymphocyte reaction. It has subsequently been learned that there are several loci within the region, some of which can be defined serologically (such as DR and DQ). The D loci are grouped as class II loci.

The dismal results of the initial human bone marrow transplantation experience were, in large measure, due to the lack of tissue typing in the selection of donors. In the compilation of early human BMT experience by Bortin (1970), matched donors (using the mixed leukocyte culture test) were used in only three cases, and all three lived; only two of the 200 patients who received transplants without histocompatibility matching survived.

Beatty and colleagues (1985) have shown the importance of HLA identity between the host and the donor in determining the outcome of the allogeneic BMT. As the number of HLA antigens not shared by both donor and recipient increases, the rate and severity of GVHD increase, the risk for delayed engraftment or nonengraftment increases, and the rate of survival decreases. Attempts to improve the potential success for transplantation using donors who are unrelated or who are only partially matched are in the developmental stages in the field of BMT, and the

issues involved are discussed in subsequent chapters. The development of new DNA techniques to more precisely define the class II alleles permits the selection of more closely matched unrelated donors (Schreuder et al., 1991; Mickelsen, Petersdorf, and Hansen, 2002).

Developments in Supportive Care

Blood Banking

The presence of different blood groups has been known since the early part of the 20th century. Initially, the major ABO groups were defined in the first decade of that century, and in 1940, the Rh system was described. Subsequently, more than 200 blood group systems have been discovered. Blood preservation and anticoagulation were also developed in the first half of the 20th century. The first blood banks were organized in the 1930s, and during the 1940s, blood transfusion was available in many U.S. hospitals. The introduction of plastic equipment in the late 1940s facilitated wider applications of transfusion. Refrigeration, improved preservative solutions, automated equipment for separating and processing blood, and serologic testing for viruses have all led to improved utilization and safety of blood components.

In the 1960s, the introduction of component therapy, in which whole blood could be divided into red cells, plasma, platelets, and other components, enabled the targeted use of blood products to replace specific needed elements and avoid unnecessary components. This led to improved safety and efficacy and has allowed better utilization of donor supplies because a larger number of therapeutic units are derived from each donation.

The advances of BMT have depended heavily on the availability of blood component support. In the early 1960s, platelet transfusions were available only at some large hospitals with cancer treatment programs. The use of platelets has subsequently grown meteorically. For example, the American Red Cross Blood Services distributed 196,000 units in 1972, but now more than 4 million platelet tranfusions are given annually in the United States. This increase is attributable to the development of standardized criteria for the use of these products, the increasing use of aplasia-producing cytotoxic therapy in the treatment of malignant diseases, and improved technology with the advent of differential centrifugation increasing the availability of these products. In 1963, the relationship between the number of circulating platelets and the risk for hemorrhage was described (Gaydos et al., 1962). The incidence of spontaneous hemorrhage was found not to significantly increase until the count fell below 20,000/μl. The risk of hemorrhage also was shown to be reduced by transfusion (Freireich et al., 1963). Using these data, in many centers, the general practice has evolved to prophylactically transfuse patients at counts less than 10,000–20,000/μl in chemotherapy-treated patients. Platelets can be obtained either by concentration of pooled multiple-donor components or by single-donor platelets obtained by plateletpheresis. Both techniques are used widely, but the latter is preferred because it exposes the patient to fewer different HLA antigens, reduces the chance for alloimmunization, and lessens the risk of exposure to infectious agents in the product.

Neutropenic patients were found to be at greater risk for infection, especially at neutrophil counts less than 500/μl. The initial attempts to correct neutropenia used transfusions from patients with chronic myelogenous leukemia (CML) with high circulating neutrophil counts. During the early 1970s, the source of neutrophils shifted from CML patients to normal donors with a yield of only 10% of that used in early studies. One early technique to obtain neutrophils was removal of cells from donors by leukopheresis and passage of the cells over nylon wool columns to which neutrophils selectively adhered. This provided an excellent yield, but some damage to the neutrophils impaired their functional capacity; most important, donors occasionally suffered potentially serious toxicities such as activation of complement, and signs and symptoms of leukostasis. Accordingly, this technique was abandoned and the technique of flow centrifugation has become prominent with the use of an erythrocyte sedimenting agent, such as hydroxymethyl starch, to facilitate the separation. Sometimes, corticosteroids are also used to elevate the donor's neutrophil count and improve the yield. Generally, 1×10^9 to 1.5×10^9 cells are obtained. Neutrophil transfusions have been shown to be efficacious in the treatment of bacterial sepsis. Trials in which neutrophil transfusions are given prophylactically during neutropenia have generally shown a reduction in infections but no reduction in deaths.

During the late 1970s, several BMT studies (Winston et al., 1980) demonstrated that the risk of death from infection by cytomegalovirus (CMV), which is transmitted via blood products, was significantly increased in BMT patients who were given neutrophil transfusions. Subsequently, the routine use of neutrophil transfusions has largely been abandoned in the management of aplasia soon after BMT, due to the concern of exposure to CMV. In recent years, the use of hematopoietic growth factors has permitted the collection of even larger numbers of granulocytes. These enriched granulocytes are being evaluated as adjunctive therapy in life-threatening fungal and antibiotic-resistant bacterial infections.

There are several unique challenges in the area of transfusion support in BMT. In the setting of profound immunosuppression present shortly after BMT, donor lymphocytes in blood transfusions can transiently engraft and produce GVHD. Transfusions of all types of cellular blood products have been shown to cause GVHD. Therefore, all cellular blood products should be irradiated with 1500–3000 cGy to eliminate the proliferative potential of lymphocytes.

As mentioned, infection with CMV is a major cause of morbidity and death after BMT (Meyers et al., 1983). Seropositive patients can reactivate latent endogenous virus, and to date, there is no effective preventive strategy. However, seronegative patients can acquire the virus through the marrow graft (if the donor is seropositive) or through blood transfusions, because the majority of adult Americans who constitute the donor pool are seropositive. One possible way to avoid acquisition of CMV is through the use of blood products screened to eliminate CMV-positive donors; this approach has been found to eliminate CMV primary infection (Bowden et al., 1986). It is applicable to only the situation in which both donor and recipient are seronegative, however. Fortunately, the risk of CMV disease in such patients is low even without CMV screening (Wingard et al., 1990). Also, the use of CMV-screened blood products in syngeneic and autologous BMT patients does not appear necessary since studies have shown the risk of CMV disease to be low

(Wingard et al., 1988), although some advocate its use in this setting (Rowe et al., 1994).

Filtration of blood products is an area of interest in recent years, offering the potential for reducing transmission of viral pathogens such as CMV that reside mostly within leukocytes, reduction of alloimmunization, and reduction of febrile and other transfusion reactions. High-efficiency leukocyte filters are currently available for erythrocyte and platelet products and several studies suggest a benefit (De Witte et al., 1990). An alternative strategy is to filter the products as they are collected, which may reduce the level of cytokines in the product during storage, which may mediate some of the reactions.

The genes controlling the major blood groups are located on chromosome 9, not chromosome 6, where the HLA complex resides. Thus, it is possible for a patient and donor to be HLA identical, yet ABO mismatched. Because red cells make up a substantial part of the marrow product, techniques had to be developed to avoid major hemolytic transfusion reactions when the patients were infused. One early technique was intensive plasma exchange of the recipient to remove anti-A and/or anti-B isohemagglutinins. With the advent of cell separators, the most common technique now is to differentially centrifuge the marrow product using hydroxymethyl starch to remove the donor erythrocytes and resuspend the marrow in recipient-type erythrocytes (Braine et al., 1982). The recipient is also given copious fluids and monitored closely to minimize the hazard for an ABO-incompatible transfusion reaction.

Antimicrobial Therapy

As previously mentioned, life-threatening infection has been a major obstacle to advances in BMT (Winston et al., 1979). Infection was the most common cause of death in the early history not only of BMT, but also the chemotherapy of leukemia (Hersh et al., 1965; Levine et al., 1974).

One of the first advances in this area was the recognition of the association between neutropenia and the risk for infection (Bodey et al., 1966). The incidence of any type of infection has been found to increase as the number of circulating neutrophils falls below 500/μl; the incidence of serious infection was noted to be particularly high at neutrophil counts below 100/μl. The duration of neutropenia also was found to be significantly correlated with the risk of infection. The major type of infection in neutropenia was due to enteric gram-negative bacteria. During the second or third week of neutropenia, fungi, especially *Candida* and *Aspergillus*, emerged as important pathogens. In recent years, with the routine use of indwelling venous catheters, gram-positive bacteria have become increasingly important pathogens during neutropenia.

An equally important advance in the control of infection was the recognition that fever during neutropenia was usually caused by infection, and that the use of empiric broad-spectrum antibiotics was much more effective in treating the infection than waiting until the infection was documented by blood culture or some other diagnostic test. Initially, various combinations of a semisynthetic penicillin plus an aminoglycoside were used, but more recently, single-agent therapy with cafepime, ceftazidime, imipenem, and several other agents has been found to be effective (Hughes et al., 2002).

A variety of antimicrobial agents have been used over the years to prevent infections. Combinations of nonabsorbable agents (such as orally administered vancomycin, gentamicin,

and nystatin) and absorbable agents (such as trimethoprim-sulfamethoxazole) have been studied in multiple centers but have not been found to be consistently useful. In recent years, the advent of the quinolone family of antibiotics has provided a group of agents that can be administered orally and have a wide antibacterial spectrum, including *Pseudomonas*. Ciprofloxacin and other quinolorals are effective in BMT patients (Lew et al., 1995). With the emergence of gram-positive bacterial pathogens, many of which are resistant to methicillin, some clinicians advocate the use of intravenous vancomycin prophylactically (Karp et al., 1986). Because of the emergence of vancomycin-resistant enterococci, vancomycin prophylaxis is no longer deemed advisable and caution needs to be exercised by limiting the use of vancomycin to situations in which the need is great and alternatives are not possible. New antibiotics, such as linezolid, quinupristin-dalfopristin, and daptomycin, offer new choices for vancomycin-resistant isolates.

The most elaborate strategy to prevent infections is isolation of the patient in a laminar air flow (LAF) room, along with the use of topical and oral antibiotics and sterile food. This has been shown to be effective, but is very expensive. It also exacts an emotional toll on the patient because of the isolation from human contact. In addition, several studies showed no increase in survival (Armstrong, 1984; Bodey, 1984). One study showed a reduced rate of GVHD in patients with aplastic anemia who received transplants in LAF (Storb et al., 1983). However, in the absence of a substantial benefit of LAF, and with its high cost, most BMT units do not use LAF. Moreover, with the introduction of a panoply of safe and effective antibiotics with a wide spectrum of activity, death from bacterial infections has diminished. Many BMT units use simple reverse isolation, with patients placed in single rooms or rooms equipped with high-efficiency particulate air (HEPA) filters.

As the control of bacterial infections has been refined, attention has turned to the more problematic fungal infections, which are the most common cause of death from infection before engraftment. Because of the difficulty in early diagnosis and the poor success rate when therapy is delayed, efforts to prevent *Candida* infection have been numerous. Orally administered non-absorbable agents have not been consistently effective, in part because of poor tolerance of oral medications after chemotherapy. Two strategies (empiric therapy and systemic prophylaxis) have been found to be effective (Leather and Wingard, 2002). Amphotericin B given intravenously, started empirically 3 to 7 days after the start of the antibacterial empiric regimen in persistently febrile patients reduces fungal infections (Pizzo et al., 1982; EORTC, 1989). Lipid formulations of amphotericin B are much better tolerated in BMT patients and are generally used in place of amphotericin B. Fluconazole, an azole, has been shown to be highly efficacious given prophylactically (Goodman et al., 1992) and is widely used; it may offer a survival advantage (Slavin et al., 1995). Unfortunately, fluconazole, which is less toxic than amphotericin B, is not effective against *Aspergillus*. In the past, *Aspergillus* infections were uniformly fatal, despite the use of amphotericin B. In recent years, however, use of the CT scan to detect early distinctive pulmonary lesions, coupled with the use of early, high-dose amphotericin B has improved control rates (Burch et al., 1987; Kuhlman et al., 1987). Although itraconazole offers a less toxic alternative to amphotericin B with good activity against *Aspergillus*, its bioavailability is variable soon after BMT. One study found itraconazole to offer greater protection against invasive fungal infections than fluconazole (Winston et al., 2003), but because of the small numbers and concerns about toxicity, further study is needed. A recently introduced antifungal agent, voriconazole, has been shown to be more effective than amphotericin B for treatment of aspergillosis (Herbrecht et al., 2002).

Over the years, the major postengraftment infectious complication has been CMV pneumonitis; indeed, this has represented one of the most common causes of death after BMT. Until recently, there was no effective therapy. Thus, over the past decade, efforts have focused on prevention through the use of CMV-negative blood products, anti-CMV immunoglobulin, and high-dose acyclovir. However, even in the absence of such measures, the incidence of CMV pneumonia in some centers has decreased in recent years, without any change in the rates of CMV infection. This may be due to the adoption of cyclosporin as anti-GVHD prophylaxis and to improved control of GVHD. Several studies have shown the combination of ganciclovir plus intravenous immunoglobulin to be an effective therapy for CMV pneumonitis, with 50–70% survival rates (Reed et al., 1988). Ganciclovir prophylaxis or preemptive therapy initiated at the first detection of active infection have been shown to prevent illness from CMV infection (Goodrich et al., 1991; Goodrich et al., 1993; Winston et al., 1993). Acyclovir prophylaxis has similarly been shown to reduce the risk for CMV disease (Prentice et al., 1994).

The availability of the CMV antigen test (or PCR assays) to readily detect virus in the blood has led to the widespread use of preemptive ganciclovir. These approaches have led to a dramatic reduction in the risk for CMV disease shortly after BMT; an unexpected downside is the emergence of late-onset disease for which new strategies are being tested (Boeckh et al., 2003).

Various infection control measures can have an important role in optimizing BMT outcomes. Guidelines to minimize infectious complications after BMT have been jointly developed by the American Society of Blood and Marrow Transplantation, the Centers for Disease Control and Prevention, and the Infectious Disease Society of America (Guidelines for Preventing Opportunistic Infections, 2000).

Hematopoietic Growth Factors

A variety of glycoprotein cytokines that have important roles in the regulation of the proliferation and maturation of bone marrow progenitor cells of all lineages have been identified. With the recombinant DNA technology, erythropoietin and several myeloid growth factors have become commercially available. Erythropoietin has been shown to be beneficial in the anemia associated with chronic renal failure and in some cases of anemia associated with cancer. Studies have suggested promise in some BMT situations (Link et al., 1994), but the determination of its optimal role after BMT has yet to be elucidated.

Both granulocyte-colony stimulating factor (G-CSF) and granulocyte-macrophage-CSF (GM-CSF) have been shown in controlled randomized trials to have significant shortening of time to neutrophil recovery after both autologous and allogeneic BMT. In addition, these myeloid growth factors have been found to be extremely effective in mobilizing primitive hematopoietic progenitor cells from the bone marrow compartment to the peripheral blood. Collection of large numbers of stem cells are now possible by pheresis, and a number of uncontrolled trials have suggested more rapid recovery of neutrophil and platelet function through the use of these enriched stem cell products. Although durable engraftment was an initial concern, it is now clear that stable engraftment after myeloablative regimens occurs. Thus, an enriched peripheral blood stem cell product collected after mobilization of hematopoietic growth factors (HGF) or chemotherapy represents a viable alternative to bone marrow and its use in autologous transplantation is well established; it is also effective for allogeneic transplantation (Bensinger and Storb, 2001). HGF have had less substantial benefit in the reduction of infectious morbidity, but shortening of duration of antibiotics, duration of hospitalization, and the interval of fever have frequently been noted. A reduction in the use of health-care resources and costs also have been a welcome accompaniment.

Nutritional Considerations

The gastrointestinal side effects of the chemoradiotherapy in the conditioning regimen include anorexia, nausea, vomiting, and diarrhea. Additionally, graft-versus-host disease and enteric viruses can cause severe, prolonged diarrhea. Up to half of BMT patients have enteritis severe enough to cause a protein-losing enteropathy (Weisdorf et al., 1983). Mucositis often makes oral intake of fluid and nutrients difficult. In summary, loss of nitrogen results from reduced intake of nutrients, enteral loss in diarrhea, and the direct catabolic effect of the cytotoxic therapy, infection, graft-versus-host disease and corticosteroids, and immobilization.

Early in the history of BMT, when patients referred for BMT often had residual leukemia, malnutrition was frequently present. Animal studies demonstrated that hematopoietic recovery without adequate nutrition was compromised (Stuart and Sensenbrenner, 1979). Thus, many BMT centers routinely used total parenteral nutritional (TPN) support to replete nutrition and ensure marrow engraftment. In recent years, the character of transplant patients has changed. Patients are frequently in remission at time of transplant and are well nourished. Thus, the goal has changed from nutritional repletion to maintenance. Many studies of well-nourished patients undergoing chemotherapy and radiotherapy have shown no benefits from total parenteral nutrition (Koretz, 1984), although some have noted more rapid hematologic recovery (Hays et al., 1983). One randomized trial in BMT patients compared patients given TPN to those given maintenance IV fluids plus enteral feedings as tolerated (Weisdorf et al., 1987). Patients who received TPN had improved overall survival and disease-free survival rates. In contrast, another study of BMT patients compared TPN and an enteral feeding program in a randomized trial (Szeluga et al., 1987). The Weisdorf study began the trial during cytoreductive therapy; the Szeluga study started the nutritional program just before marrow infusion (after completion of the conditioning regimen). Both studies found that patients were unable to achieve maintenance nutritional status with an enteral feeding program. The Szeluga study, however, found no long-term benefit in survival or disease-free survival. Szeluga and colleagues (1987) speculate that TPN may have potentiated the effects of the antineoplastic therapy rather than supported marrow recovery; thus, an effect might

be seen when given during chemotherapy, but in the absence of a gross nutritional deficiency, TPN would not offer a benefit.

A survey of BMT centers in 1987 indicated that various methods were being used to provide oral nutritional support (Dezenhall et al., 1987). Sterile food was rarely used due to cost and poor acceptance by patients. Most commonly used were either a reduced-bacterial diet or a house diet without fresh vegetables or fruit. Frequently, patients have prolonged poor oral intake after marrow engraftment. In the past, this necessitated delays in hospital discharge. Now, with the availability of home IV therapy, many patients can be discharged and continue to receive TPN without compromising their nutrition (Lenssen et al., 1983).

Severe oral mucositis is one of the major impediments to adequate nutrition during the first several weeks after BMT. Recently, palifermin, keratinocyte growth factor, a member of the fibroblast growth factor family, was licensed due to its ability to reduce severe oral mucositis in intensively treated patients with hematologic malignancies (Spielberger et al., 2004). This has the potential not only for ameliorating the painful manifestations of mucositis, but also enhancing adequate nutrition.

BMT *in the Outpatient Setting*

Several developments have led to the performance of transplant care in the outpatient setting that was traditionally done in the hospital setting. The availability of home health services has permitted the delivery of infusional therapies in an outpatient residential setting. This has been facilitated by the availability of programmable portable infusion pumps, computerized informational services, and skilled nursing professionals with both infusional expertise and knowledge of oncologic principles. The creation of "day" hospitals has permitted timely skilled clinical and laboratory assessments; the administration of fluids, electrolytes, antibiotic infusions, and blood products; and the delivery of a variety of supportive care measures (Peters et al., 1994). The introduction of oral antibiotics with broad-spectrum activity and the demonstration that antibiotic prophylaxis and once-daily infusional antibiotic for neutropenic fever are effective has made feasible the therapy of neutropenic fever in the outpatient setting (Gilbert et al., 1994; Hughes et al., 2002). Careful analyses of neutropenic fever have led to the recognition of low-risk and high-risk cases so patients can be grouped according to which treatment in the outpatient setting is likely to be successful and which may be too risky (Hughes et al., 2002). NST procedures are clearly amenable to the outpatient setting since neutropenia typically is very short and infectious complications are less frequent.

These advances in medical technology have arrived at a time when the public is demanding lower-cost health care. These initiatives are likely to lower the cost of transplantation at a time when the application of transplantation is growing in volume. Finally, many patients want greater autonomy and a larger role in their own care.

For these activities to be successfully performed in the outpatient setting, communication between the patient and the health-care team is vital to ensure that important clinical events are recognized by the patient and brought to the attention of the health-care team. Moreover, in the event of a complication requiring immediate care by health professionals, prompt access to a full range of inpatient services is needed. Generally, it is desirable that a partner be available to the patient to assist in the provision of care. The initial efforts of outpatient transplants have been performed in solid tumor autotransplants. Regimens causing little gastrointestinal toxicity have been particularly appropriate for the outpatient setting. Moreover, the preparative regimens have been less intensive than some of the regimens for allogeneic transplantation or those for leukemia. This is also gaining acceptance for allogeneic transplantation using reduced-intensity conditioning regimes.

Developments in the Control of GVHD

Once techniques to ensure engraftment by adequate conditioning were developed, it became clear that GVHD was a major obstacle for allogeneic BMT. From animal studies, it was recognized that GVHD was caused by donor T lymphocytes. It was learned that the frequency and severity of GVHD depended on the degree of HLA compatibility and the dose of lymphocytes. Although GVHD had harmful effects, being one of the major causes of death, it was found to also have beneficial effects associated with an antileukemic effect (Weiden et al., 1979). Thus, the goal of prevention and treatment of GVHD was moderation of its severity without complete elimination.

Based on studies in dogs, methotrexate was employed as a prophylaxis against GVHD in some centers, and based on studies in rodents, cyclophosphamide was used in other centers. In randomized trials, cyclosporin was found to be a more effective preventive measure and has been substituted as the preferred GVHD prophylaxis by many centers (Santos et al., 1987;

Deeg et al., 1985; Storb et al., 1992). Other studies demonstrated a combination of methotrexate and cyclosporin to be more effective (Storb et al., 1986a, 1986b). Tacrolimus plus methotrexate was found to be even more effective than cyclosporin plus methotrexate (Ratanatharathorn et al., 1998). Incorporation of several new immunosuppressive agents into immunosuppressive regimens is being evaluated.

High doses of corticosteroids have been the mainstay of treatment of GVHD over the years. In cases of refractory GVHD, antithymocyte globulin (ATG) has sometimes been useful. Another prophylaxis strategy investigated in the past decade is the removal of the T lymphocytes from the donor marrow. A variety of techniques have been used: anti-T cell monoclonal antibodies, corticosteroids, lectins, and counterflow centrifugal elutriation. These have been shown to reduce GVHD in a variety of studies. Unfortunately, these techniques have also been associated with increased rates of relapse (Goldman et al., 1988), apparently eliminating the graft-versus-leukemia (GVL) effect seen with allogeneic BMT (reviewed in Wingard et al., 1992a). Techniques to deplete selected cell subpopulations to preserve the GVL effect while diminishing GVHD are being explored (Champlin et al., 1996).

For chronic GVHD, combination therapy with steroids plus azathioprine was the preferred treatment for many years (Sullivan, 1983). A study comparing prednisone plus azathioprine versus prednisone showed prednisone alone to be as effective and to be associated with fewer infectious complications (Sullivan et al., 1988b). For high-risk patients, the combination of steroids plus cyclosporin is more effective (Sullivan et al., 1988a, 1988b). In recent years, prednisone alone appears to offer advantages over combination therapy (Koc et al., 2002). However, because a sizeable proportion of patients have poor control of chronic GVHD, new combination regimens, new immunosuppressive agents, and the use of extracorporeal photopheresis are being explored.

Nursing Care

As the field of bone marrow transplantation has evolved, so, too, has BMT nursing, which has become one of the most challenging nursing specialties. Its roles have become more complex and have expanded enormously in recent years.

The traditional major concern of attending to the acute care needs of patients has become increasingly difficult. BMT patients are generally young, but span the age range from infancy to the sixties and seventies; skill in managing pediatric, adolescent, and adult concerns are prerequisites. BMT nurses are frequently called upon to provide the highly technical critical care services needed to manage the problems of nutritional support, electrolyte and fluid management, aplasia, sepsis, severe graft-versus-host disease, transfusion management, and vital organ failure (O'Quin and Moravec, 1988). Knowledge of general oncologic principles, transplant knowledge, and a detailed understanding of an array of chemotherapeutic agents is fundamental. The introduction of computerized information systems to the clinical setting have required mastery of automated data systems. Within the Oncology Nursing Society (ONS) a special interest group (SIG) has developed, focusing solely on the concerns of BMT nurses. These concerns include efforts to develop national standards of BMT nursing care, especially with respect to management of mucositis, skin care, indwelling venous catheter care, and isolation procedures.

The role of nursing in patient and family education has also expanded. Patients and their families require orientation to the treatment modalities and to the specific objectives in the plan of care. Although many patients have been under the care of an oncology treatment team before referral, few have a good understanding of what is to be undertaken. Specific issues that require emphasis in patient orientation include a prolonged hospitalization with some type of isolation, the attendant loss of control associated with the restrictions of a hospital environment, the unique problems of graft-versus-host disease, and the need for avoidance of crowds for several months after recovery of marrow function to avoid contagious illness until the slower recovery of cellular immunity occurs. Teaching self-care tasks, especially with respect to exercise, nutrition, and indwelling catheters, and to encourage the patient to exercise as much control over his or her care as possible is very important. For patients newly referred to the transplant center, orientation to the inpatient and outpatient units enables them to best use the center's resources.

A greater emphasis on the psychosocial needs of patients and families has also emerged (Haberman, 1988). Nurses play a pivotal role in the recognition of patients' psychosocial needs and are called on to ensure that appropriate resources are directed to dealing with them. Patients who do not reside in the same community as the transplant center are especially in need of psychosocial resources since their network of family and friends is unable to be physically present during much of the BMT experience. Changes in family roles are universal concerns for patients and significant others. The primary nurse or case manager must be adept at engaging the services of social workers, psychiatric liaison nurses, child life specialists, occupational therapists, and so forth. Passage between inpatient and outpatient units must be accomplished seamlessly because more care is being delivered in the outpatient setting; communication, assessment of patient and family resources, and support to both the patient and his or her nonprofessional caregivers are crucial to assess continuity of care, to allay stress, and to encourage confidence in success.

Follow-up care is becoming increasingly important because there are more and more long-term survivors (Nims and Strom, 1988). During the first year after transplant, the patient and primary care team must be vigilant for the possible occurrence of chronic graft-versus-host disease, infections, obstructive airway disease, and recurrence (if transplanted for malignancy). Ovarian failure, which requires hormonal replacement, is a concern for adult women. Issues regarding sexuality are frequent concerns for both men and women (Wingard et al., 1992b). For children, growth and development must be monitored to detect pituitary, thyroid, or adrenal insufficiency (Sanders et al., 1988). Resumption of employment and former family social roles emerges as a task for patients as the acute illness recedes into the background (Baker et al., 1994). Recognition of these "late" concerns, and assisting patients and families in dealing with these issues of survivorship, have become important roles for nursing.

Considerations for the Future

In the first half century of human bone marrow transplantation, enormous strides have occurred in the treatment of human disease. Currently, success rates in severe aplastic anemia exceed 70%, in acute nonlymphoblastic leukemia in first remission 55%, in relapsed Hodgkin's or non-Hodgkin's lymphoma 50%, and chronic myelogenous leukemia 50–70%. There is a variety of other less common diseases for which success rates exceed 50%. In recognition of the importance of this medical discipline and the singular contributions of E. Donnall Thomas, the 1990 Nobel prize in medicine was awarded to Dr. Thomas for his pioneering work in bone marrow transplantation. There remains a variety of limitations to the greater application of BMT, which require further improvements. The major causes of failure are graft-versus-host disease, immunodeficiency and infection, toxicities from the preparative regimen, and relapse. Further, only one third of patients have an HLA-identical sibling as a potential donor.

One strategy to address the lack of a compatible donor is the further development of the National Bone Marrow Donor Registry. The growth of cord blood tissue banks and cord blood registries are allowing increased use of this source of alternative stem cells, particularly for children. This is addressed in a subsequent chapter. The use of related donors who are haploidentical is another alternative, but that alternative remains limited as an option at present until better techniques are developed to control graft-versus-host disease.

With ex vivo purging of T cells from the donor graft, serious GVHD can be prevented. Unfortunately, this and other measures successful in preventing GVHD have generally resulted in an increased relapse rate, by abrogation of the graft-versus-leukemia effect. There is some experimental evidence that the cell populations that mediate the GVL effect differ from the lymphocytes that mediate GVHD, although other data do not support this (reviewed in Wingard,

1992a; Fassas et al., 2002). In the future, there will certainly be attempts to identify, characterize, and grow cells that mediate GVL and not GVHD. If successful, the marrow graft can be engineered to contain enriched populations of GVL cells and depleted of cells that mediate GVHD. Attempts to enrich the marrow with natural killer (NK) cells or lymphokine-activated killer (LAK) cells to enhance the antileukemic potential are also likely in the near future (Imamura and Tanaka, 2003; Riddell et al., 2003; Voutsadakis, 2003).

Recent studies suggest that the graft-versus-leukemia effect is much more potent than previously appreciated. Infusions of donor buffy coat cells in relatively small numbers in patients with early relapse after allogeneic transplant have been shown to reestablish durable remissions (Kolb et al., 1990; Drobyski et al., 1992). One current shortcoming of this approach is a substantial risk of graft-versus-host disease or aplasia. With improved understanding of the effector cells responsible for this antitumor activity, infusions of selected populations may provide the beneficial antitumor effect without the deleterious complications. Using cell culture techniques now available, large numbers of cloned cytotoxic T lymphocytes with desired specificity can be administered to the transplant recipient. Clinical trials are exploring the use of donor cytotoxic T cells to treat CMV and Epstein Barr Virus (EBV) disease in the transplant setting (Papadopopoulos et al., 1994; Riddell et al., 1994; Riddell and Greenberg, 2000). Patients at high risk for relapse may benefit from staged infusions of these effector cells at intervals after the transplant to prevent relapse. Indeed, preemptive infusions of donor lymphocytes may lower the risk of relapse after T cell depletion (Baron and Beguin, 2002).

Posttransplant infusions of donor lymphocytes still contain the potential to cause harmful

GVHD. So-called "suicide" genes are inserted into the cells so that they can be eliminated if severe GVHD develops (Ciceri and Bordignon, 2002; Kramm, 2003; Kolb et al., 2004). Gene therapy may offer the potential to induce or enhance antitumor responses in a variety of other ways as well (Schmidt-Wolf and Schmidt-Wolf, 2003).

Identification of novel antigens that are tumor specific or tumor associated offer the potential to select, clone, and expand populations of cytotoxic immune cells that target tumor cells, yet spare recipients the dangers of GVHD. Minor histocompatibility antigens have received the most interest to date. Those that are preferentially expressed on hematopoietic cells and poorly expressed on non-hematopoietic tissues are particularly of interest (Falkenburg et al., 2002; Riddell et al., 2002; Mutis, 2003).

Another exciting opportunity to develop potential antitumor immunotherapy and to circumvent the problem of lack of matched donors is to perform stringent T cell depletion of haploidentical donors in which the donor and recipient are mismatched at killer Ig-like receptors (KIRs). KIRs are a group of receptors expressed on the surface of natural killer (NK) cells. Mismatching at KIRs has been found to be associated with potent antileukemic responses (Martelli et al., 2002; Ruggeri et al., 2002; Parham and McQueen, 2003; Cook et al., 2004).

Yet another new frontier is the use of immunomodulatory cytokines to enhance immune reconstitution. Interleukin 7 has been shown to enhance thymic output of newly developed T cells and improve T cell reconstitution after BMT (Alpdogan et al., 2003; Broers et al., 2003). Keratinocyte growth factor, recently

evaluated for amelioration of mucositis, has been shown to provide protection from thymic epithelial cell injury after BMT and to improve efficiency of production of thymocytes (Min et al., 2002; Rossi et al., 2002). These offer the potential to reduce infectious complications after BMT.

The use of nonablative conditioning regimens, which are better tolerated, are allowing the exploration of allogeneic BMT for solid tumors. The best studied to date is renal cell carcinoma, with gratifying results even in patients with disseminated disease (Slavin et al., 2003; Srinivasan et al., 2004).

An alternative way to avoid the limitations of GVHD and unavailability of a donor is with the use of autologous BMT. Results with autologous SCT have been improving in recent years, especially with lymphomas and acute nonlymphocytic leukemia (Santos et al., 1989; Blume, 2001). With the absence of GVHD, the early posttransplant mortality is lower than after allogeneic BMT. However, the relapse rate is generally substantially higher, due to contamination of the marrow graft with occult tumor cells and also due to the absence of any GVL effect. Efforts to improve elimination of contaminating tumor cells are under development. Unfortunately, efforts to purge tumor cells from stem cell grafts and efforts to select stem cells with immunoabsorbant columns have failed to substantially reduce relapse rates. The role of various biologic response modifiers to reduce the risk for relapse after autologous BMT will be more fully explored. Administration of an antibody (by itself or linked with a cellular toxin or radioisotope) specific for tumor antigens, or the administration of immunomodulatory cytokines such as IL-2, IL-4, or IL-12 can be performed after transplant. Tumor vaccines or tumor antigen-loaded dendritic cell infusions are being explored. Such immunoadjuvant therapeutics would be expected to be most effective at a time of minimal residual disease, shortly after transplant.

The infusion of donor lymphocytes in patients with relapsed chronic myelogenous leukemia was shown to effect high rates of durable disease control and cure in many (Kolb et al., 1990). Similar responses have been observed with other hematologic diseases at time of relapse but at lower rates. The mechanism of this phenomenon is being explored in several research laboratories with the goal to identify the specific cell populations that mediate this effect, as well as strategies to augment it. As knowledge of the complex immune system improves, the ability to augment desired immune responses will grow.

With the delivery of transplant care in the outpatient setting, the utility of multiple tandem transplants with dose-intensive therapy is possible. Each course is followed by an infusion of stem cells to provide a tolerable, multicourse, dose-intensive treatment regimen. This might be particularly attractive for epithelial tumors for which multiple treatments may be more efficacious than a single-dose treatment. Recently, double transplants were found to be more effective for multiple myelomas than single transplants (Attal et al., 2003).

Techniques to select hematopoietic stem cells (HSC) by immunophenotypic differences from tumor cells and other cells not necessary for engraftment permit the exploration of transplantation of small numbers of pluripotent HSC to effect engraftment and to provide a product free of contaminating tumor cells. This is being explored in transplantation for lymphoma, multiple myeloma, and breast cancer.

Highly purified stem cell populations also permit the exploration of techniques to expand the numbers of cells ex vivo through incubation of small numbers of cells with cocktails of growth factors. Thus, one might be able to perform BMT through the use of very few donor cells that will enhance the acceptability of volunteer stem cell donations (Brugger et al., 1995). Again, the hope is to make stem cell donation more palatable. An area of active investigation is the insertion of genes into hematopoietic stem cells to correct a genetic deficiency, to provide resistance to chemotherapeutic drugs, or to convey resistance to certain viral pathogens, such as human immunodeficiency virus (HIV). The use of gene insertion techniques might broaden the applicability of BMT to other disease processes (Schmidt-Wolf and Schmidt-Wolf, 2003).

One concern increasing in emphasis in recent years is the quality of life of survivors of various cancer treatments. Several small studies suggest that outcomes are similar to survivors of other types of cancer (Andrykowski et al., 1989a, 1989b), but impairments in physical and mental health outcomes are present compared to healthy individuals (Andrykowski et al., 2005).

Survivors have reported both positive and negative changes in plans and activities, relationships, physical status, and existential concerns, but positive changes often exceeded the negative changes (Bishop et al., 2003), except in physical status (Baker et al., 1991; Wingard et al., 1991; Curbow et al., 1993a, 1993b). Life satisfaction has been rated favorably by most (Baker et al., 1994, Bishop and Wingard 2004). High levels of function and excellent health have been reported by many patients. Most survivors have returned to work or school. Twenty to thirty percent reported improved family relations, greater compassion, redirected life goals, and existential recovery, and 36% reported psychological gains after recovery from the transplant. Although most appear to have been successful in reintegrating their lives, some reported significant losses: 16% reported their health to be ill or bad, 9% said social function was limited "a good bit," and 13% reported moderate to severe pain (Baker et al., 1994). The role of the family has been recognized as an important predictor of posttransplant emotional distress (Syrjala et al., 1993). A variety of challenges need to be addressed and studied in further psychosocial research of BMT survivors (Wingard, 1994).

In summary, the historical developments of BMT have occurred because of the dedication and perseverance of specialists in many fields. Advances in the biological sciences, supportive care, and nursing care have resulted in improved outcomes for patients undergoing BMT and other types of cancer therapy as well. These developments bode well for the future of BMT as an important treatment modality with expanding applications.

References

Alpdogan, O., Muriglan, S.J., Eng, J.M., et al. 2003. IL-7 enhances peripheral T cell reconstitution after allogeneic hematopoietic stem cell transplantation. *J Clin Invest* 112:1095–1107.

Andrykowski, M.A., Bishop, M.M., Hahn, E.A., Cella, D.F., Beaumont, J.L., Brady, M.J., et al. 2005. Long-term health-related quality of life, growth, and spiritual well-being after hematopoietic stem-cell transplantation. *J Clin Oncol* 23:599–608.

Andrykowski, M.A., Henslee, P.J., Barnett, R.L. 1989a. Longitudinal assessment of psychosocial functioning of adult survivors of allogeneic bone marrow transplantation. *Bone Marrow Transplantation* 4:505–509.

Andrykowski, M.A., Henslee, P.J., Farrall, M.G. 1989b. Physical and psychosocial functioning of adult survivors of allogeneic bone marrow transplantation. *Bone Marrow Transplantation* 4:75–81.

Applebaum, F.R. 1996. The use of bone marrow and peripheral blood stem cell transplantation in the treatment of cancer. *CA-Canc J Clinicians* 46(3):42–164.

Armstrong, D. 1984. Protected environments are discomforting and expensive and do not offer meaningful protection. *Am J Med* 76:685–689.

Attal, M., Harousseau, J.L., Facon, T., et al. 2003. Single versus double autologous stem-cell transplantation for multiple myeloma. *N Engl J Med* 349:2495–2502.

Attal, M., Harousseau, J.L., Stoppa, A.M., Sotto, J.J., Fuzibet, J.G., Rossi, J.F., et al. 1996. A prospective, randomized trial of autologous bone marrow transplantation and chemotherapy in multiple myeloma. Intergroupe Francais du Myelome. *N Engl J Med* 335:91–97.

Baker, F., et al. 1994. Quality of life of bone marrow transplant long-term survivors. *Bone Marrow Transplantation* 13:589–596.

Baker, F., Curbow, B., Wingard, J.R. 1991. Role retention and quality of life of bone marrow transplant survivors. *Soc Sci Med* 32:697–704.

Baranov, A., et al. 1989. Bone marrow transplantation after the Chernobyl nuclear accident. *N Engl J Med* 321: 205–212.

Barker, J.N., Wagner, J.E. 2003. Umbilical-cord blood transplantation for the treatment of cancer. *Nat Rev Cancer* 3:526–532.

Barnes, D.W.H., Loutit, J.F. 1955. The radiation recovery factor: preservation by the Polge-Smith-Parkes technique. *J Natl Cancer Inst* 15:901.

Baron, F., Beguin, Y. 2002. Preemptive cellular immunotherapy after T-cell-depleted allogeneic hematopoietic stem cell transplantation. *Biol Blood Marrow Transplant* 8:351–359.

Beatty, P.G., et al. 1985. Marrow transplantation from related donor other than HLA-identical siblings. *N Engl J Med* 313:765–771.

Bensinger, W.I., Storb, R. 2001. Allogeneic peripheral blood stem cell transplantation. *Rev Clin Exp Hematol* 5:67–86.

Bishop, M.M., Brady, M.J., Beaumont, J.L., et al. 2003. Post-traumatic growth: a late effect of stem cell transplantation. *Biol Blood Marrow Transplant* 9:70 [Abstract #23].

Bishop, M.M., Wingard, J.R. 2004. Thriving after hematopoietic stem cell transplant: a focus on positive changes in quality of life. *Expert Rev Pharmacoeconomics Outcomes Res* 4(1):99–110.

Blume, K.G. 2001. Improve the outcome of autologous hematopoietic cell transplantation! *Biol Blood Marrow Transplant* 7:527–531.

Bodey, G.P. 1984. Current status of prophylaxis of infection with protected environments. *Am J Med* 76: 678–684.

Bodey, G.P., et al. 1966. Quantitative relationships between circulating leukocytes and infection in patients with acute leukemia. *Ann Intern Med* 64:328–340.

Boeckh, M., Nichols, W.G., Papanicolaou, G., et al. 2003. Cytomegalovirus in hematopoietic stem cell transplant recipients: current status, known challenges, and future strategies. *Biol Blood Marrow Transplant* 9:543–558.

Bortin, M.M. 1970. A compendium of reported human bone marrow transplants. *Transplantation* 9:571–587.

Bortin, M.M., Horowitz, M.M., Gale, R.P. 1988. Current status of bone marrow transplantation in humans: report from the International Bone Marrow Transplant Registry. *Nat Immun Cell Growth Regul* 7:334–350.

Bowden, R.A., et al. 1986. Cytomegalovirus immune globulin and seronegative blood products to prevent primary cytomegalovirus infection after marrow transplantation. *N Engl J Med* 314:1006–1010.

Braine, H.G., et al. 1982. Bone marrow transplantation with major ABO blood group incompatibility using erythrocyte depletion of marrow prior to infusion. *Blood* 60:420–425.

Broers, A.E., Posthumus-van Sluijs, S.G., Spits, H., et al. 2003. Interleukin-7 improves T-cell recovery after experimental T-cell-depleted bone marrow transplantation in T-cell-deficient mice by strong expansion of recent thymic emigrants. *Blood* 102:1534–1540.

Brugger, W., Heimfeld, S., Berenson, R.J., et al. 1995. Reconstitution of hematopoiesis after high-dose chemotherapy by autologous progenitor cells generated ex vivo. *N Engl J Med* 333:283–287.

Burch, P.A., et al. 1987. Favorable outcome of invasive aspergillosis in patients with acute leukemia. *J Clin Oncol* 5:1985–1993.

Burt, R.K., Arnold, R., Emmons, R., et al. 2003. Stem cell therapy for autoimmune disease: overview of concepts from the Snowbird 2002 tolerance and tissue regeneration meeting. *Bone Marrow Transplant* 32(Suppl 1): S3–S5.

Champlin, R., Giralt, S., Gajewski, J. 1996. T cells, graft-versus-host disease and graft-versus-leukemia: innovative approaches for blood and marrow transplantation. *Acta Hematol* 95(3–4):157–163.

Ciceri, F., Bordignon, C. 2002. Suicide-gene-transduced donor T-cells for controlled graft-versus-host disease and graft-versus-tumor. *Int J Hematol* 76:305–309.

Cook, M.A., Milligan, D.W., Fegan, C.D., et al. 2004. The impact of donor KIR and patient HLA-C genotypes on outcome following HLA-identical sibling hematopoietic stem cell transplantation for myeloid leukemia. *Blood* 103:1521–1526.

Curbow, B., Baker, F., Somerfield, M.R., et al. 1993a. Personal changes, dispositional optimism and psychological adjustment to bone marrow transplantation. *J Behav Med* 16:423–443.

Curbow, B., Legro, M.W., Baker, F., et al, 1993b. Loss and recovery themes of long-term survivors of bone marrow transplants. *J Psychosoc Oncol* 10:1–20.

Dausset, J. 1954. Leukoagglutinins. IV. Leukoagglutinins and blood transfusions. *Vox Sang* 4:190.

Dausset, J. 1958. Iso-leuco-anticorps. *Acta Haematol* (Basel) 20:156–166.

Deeg, H.J., Storb, R., Thomas, E.D., Flournoy, N., Kennedy, M.S., Banaji, M. et al. 1985. Cyclosporine as prophylaxis for graft-versus-host disease: a randomized study in patients undergoing marrow transplantation for acute nonlymphoblastic leukemia. *Blood* 65:1325–1334.

De Witte, T., et al. 1990. Prevention of primary cytomegalovirus infection after allogeneic bone marrow transplantation by using leukocyte-poor random blood products from cytomegalovirus-unscreened blood-bank donors. *Transplantation* 50:964.

Dezenhall, A., et al. 1987. Food and nutrition services in bone marrow transplant centers. *J Am Dietetic Assoc* 87:1351–1353.

Drobyski, W.R., Roth, R.S., Thibodeau, S.N., et al. 1992. Molecular remission occurring after donor leukocyte infusions for the treatment of relapsed chronic myelogenous leukemia after allogeneic bone marrow transplantation. *Bone Marrow Transplantation* 10: 301–304.

EORTC International Antimicrobial Therapy Cooperative Group. 1989. Empiric antifungal therapy in febrile granulocytopenic patients. *Am J Med* 86:668–672.

Falkenburg, J.H., Marijt, W.A., Heemskerk, M.H., Willemze, R. 2002. Minor histocompatibility antigens as targets of graft-versus-leukemia reactions. *Curr Opin Hematol* 9:497–502.

Fassas, A.B., Morris, C., Badros, A., et al. 2002. Separating graft-versus-tumor from graft-versus-host reactions. *Leuk Lymphoma* 43:725–733.

Ford, C.E., Hamerton, J.L., Barnes, D.W.H., Loutit, J.F. 1956. Cytological identification of radiation-chimaeras. *Nature* 177:452–454.

Freireich, E.J., et al. 1963. Response to repeated platelet transfusions from the same donor. *Ann Intern Med* 59:277–287.

Gassmann, W., et al. 1988. Comparison of cyclophosphamide, cytarabine, and etoposide as immunosuppressive agents before allogeneic bone marrow transplantation. *Blood* 72:1574–1579.

Gaydos, L.A., Freireich, E.J., Mantel, N. 1962. The quantitative relation between platelet count and hemorrhage in patients with acute leukemia. *N Engl J Med* 266:905–909.

Gilbert, C., et al. 1994. Sequential prophylactic oral and empiric once-daily parenteral antibiotics for neutropenia and fever after high-dose chemotherapy and autologous bone marrow support. *J Clin Oncol* 12: 1005–1011.

Goldman, J.M., Horowitz, M.M. 2002. The international bone marrow transplant registry. *Int J Hematol* 76(suppl 1):393–397.

Goldman, J.M., et al. 1980. Haematological reconstitution after autografting for chronic granulocytic leukaemia in transformation: the influence of previous splenomegaly. *Br J Haematol* 45:223.

Goldman, J.M., et al. 1988. Bone marrow transplantation for chronic myelogenous leukemia in chronic phase: increased risk of relapse associated with T cell depletion. *Ann Intern Med* 108:806–814.

Goodman, J.L., et al. 1992. A controlled trial of fluconazole to prevent fungal infections in patients undergoing bone marrow transplantation. *N Engl J Med* 326:845–851.

Goodrich, J.M., Bowden, R.A., Fisher, L., et al. 1993. Ganciclovir prophylaxis to prevent cytomegalovirus disease after allogeneic marrow transplant. *Ann Intern Med* 118:173–178.

Goodrich, J.M., Mori, M., Gleaves, C.A., et al. 1991. Early treatment with ganciclovir to prevent cytomegalovirus disease after allogeneic bone marrow transplant. *N Engl J Med* 325:1601–1607.

Guidelines for Preventing Opportunistic Infections Among Hematopoietic Stem Cell Transplant Recipients. 2000. Recommendations of CDC, Infectious Diseases Society of America, and American Society of Blood & Marrow Transplantation. *Biol Blood Marrow Transplant* 6(6a):659–734.

Haberman, M.R., 1988. Psychosocial aspects of bone marrow transplantation. *Sem Oncol Nurs* 4:55–59.

Hahn, T., Wingard, J.R., Anderson, K.C., Bensinger, W.I., Berenson, J.R., Brozeit, G., et al. 2003. The role of cytotoxic therapy with hematopoietic stem cell transplantation in the therapy of multiple myeloma: an evidence-based review. *Biol Blood Marrow Transplant* 9: 4–37.

Hays, D.M., et al. 1983. Effect of total parenteral nutrition on marrow recovery during induction therapy for acute nonlymphocytic leukemia in childhood. *Med Pediatr Oncol* 11:134–140.

Herbrecht, R., Denning, D.W., Patterson, T.F., et al. 2002. Voriconazole versus amphotericin B for primary therapy of invasive aspergillosis. *N Eng J Med* 347: 408–415.

Hersh, E.M., et al. 1965. Causes of death in acute leukemia. *JAMA* 193:99–103.

Hughes, W.T., Armstrong, D., Bodey, G.P., et al. 2002. 2002 guidelines for the use of antimicrobial agents in neutropenic patients with cancer. *Clin Infect Dis* 34: 730–751.

Imamura, M., Tanaka, J. 2003. Immunoregulatory cells for transplantation tolerance and graft-versus-leukemia effect. *Int J Hematol* 78:188–194.

Juttner, C.A., et al. 1985. Circulating autologous stem cells collected in very early remission from acute non-lymphoblastic leukemia produce prompt but incomplete haemapoietic reconstitution after high dose melphalan or supralethal chemoradiotherapy. *Br J Haematol* 61:739.

Karp, J.E., et al. 1986. Empiric use of vancomycin during prolonged treatment-induced granulocytopenia: randomized, double-blind, placebo-controlled clinical trial in patients with acute leukemia. *Am J Med* 106:1–7.

Koc, S., Leisenring, W., Flowers, M.E., Anasetti, C., Deeg, H.J., Nash, R.A., et al. 2002. Therapy for chronic graft-versus-host disease: a randomized trial comparing cyclosporine plus prednisone versus prednisone alone. *Blood* 100:48–51.

Kolb, H.J., et al. 1990. Donor leukocyte transfusions for treatment of recurrent chronic myelogenous leukemia in marrow transplant patients. *Blood* 76:2462–2465.

Kolb, H.J., Schmid, C., Barrett, A.J., Schendel, D.J. 2004. Graft-versus-leukemia reactions in allogeneic chimeras. *Blood* 103:767–776.

Koretz, R.L. 1984. Parenteral nutrition. Is it oncologically logical? *J Clin Oncol* 2:534–538.

Kramm, C.M. 2003. Alternative concepts of suicide gene therapy for graft-versus-host disease after adoptive immunotherapy. *Acta Haematol* 110:132–138.

Kuhlman, J.E., et al. 1987. Invasive pulmonary aspergillosis in acute leukemia. *Chest* 92:95–99.

Kurnick, N.B., et al. 1958. Preliminary observations and treatment of post irradiation haematolopoietic depression in man by the infusion of stored autogenous bone marrow. *Ann Intern Med* 49:969.

Leather, H.L., Wingard, J.R. 2002. Prophylaxis, empirical therapy, or pre-emptive therapy of fungal infections in immunocompromised patients: which is better for whom? *Curr Opin Infect Dis* 15:369–375.

Lenssen, P., et al. 1983. Parenteral nutrition in marrow transplant recipients after discharge from the hospital. *Exp Hematol* 11:974–981.

Levine, A.S., et al. 1974. Hematologic malignancies and other marrow failure states: progress in the management of complicating infections. *Semin Hematol* 11:141–202.

Lew, M.A., et al. 1995. Ciprofloxacin versus trimethoprim/sulfamethoxazole for prophylaxis of bacterial infections in bone marrow transplant recipients: a randomized, controlled trial. *J Clin Oncol* 13:239–250.

Link, H., et al. 1994. A controlled trial of recombinant human erythropoietin after bone marrow transplant. *Blood* 84:3327–3335.

Maloney, D.G., Molina, A.J., Sahebi, F., et al. 2003. Allografting with non-myeloablative conditioning following cytoreductive autografts for the treatment of patients with multiple myeloma. *Blood* 102:3447–3484 (Prepublished online 7/10/03).

Martelli, M.F., Aversa, F., Bachar-Lustig, E., et al. 2002. Transplants across human leukocyte antigen barriers. *Semin Hematol* 39:48–56.

Mathe, G., et al. 1959. Transfusions et greffes de moeille osseuse homologue chez les humains irradiés à hautes doses accidentellement. *Rev Fr Etud Clin Biol* 4:238.

Meyers, J.D., et al. 1983. Biology of interstitial pneumonia after marrow transplantation. In Gale, R.P. (Ed.) *Recent Advances in Bone Marrow Transplantation*. New York: A.R. Liss, 405–423.

Mickelson, E.M., Petersdorf, E.W., Hansen, J.A. 2002. HLA matching and hematopoietic cell transplant outcome. *Clin Transpl*: 263–271.

Mielcarek, M., Storb, R. 2003. Non-myeloablative hematopoietic cell transplantation as immunotherapy for hematologic malignancies. *Cancer Treat Rev* 29:283–290.

Min, D., Taylor, P.A., Panoskaltsis-Mortari, A., et al. 2002. Protection from thymic epithelial cell injury by keratinocyte growth factor: a new approach to improve thymic and peripheral T-cell reconstitu-tion after bone marrow transplantation. *Blood* 99:4592–4600.

Mutis, T. 2003. Targeting alloreactive donor T-cells to hematopoietic system-restricted minor histocompatibility antigens to dissect graft-versus-leukemia effects from graft-versus-host disease after allogeneic stem cell transplantation. *Int J Hematol* 78:208–212.

Nims, J.W., Strom, S. 1988. Late complications of bone marrow transplant recipients: nursing care issues. *Semin Oncol Nurs* 4:47–54.

O'Quin, T., Moravec, C. 1988. The critically ill bone marrow transplant patient. *Semin Oncol Nurs* 4:25–30.

Papadopopoulos, E.B., et al. 1994. Infusions of donor leukocytes to treat Epstein-Barr virus-associated lymphoproliferative disorders after allogeneic bone marrow transplantation. *N Engl J Med* 330:1185–1191.

Parham, P., McQueen, K.L. 2003. Alloreactive killer cells: hindrance and help for haematopoietic transplants. *Nat Rev Immunol* 3:108–122.

Peters, W.P., et al. 1994. The use of intensive clinic support to permit outpatient autologous bone marrow transplantation for breast cancer. *Semin Oncol* 21:25–31.

Pizzo, P.A., et al. 1982. Empiric antibiotic and antifungal therapy for cancer patients with prolonged fever and granulocytopenia. *Am J Med* 72:101–111.

Prentice, H.G., et al. 1994. Impact of long-term acyclovir on cytomegalovirus infection and survival after allogeneic bone marrow transplantation. *Lancet* 343:749.

Quine, W.E. 1896. The remedial application of bone marrow. *JAMA* 26:1012–1013.

Ratanatharathorn, V., Nash, R.A., Przepiorka, D., Devine, S.M., Klein, J.L., Weisdorf, D., et al. 1998. Phase III study comparing methotrexate and tacrolimus (prograf, FK506) with methotrexate and cyclosporine for graft-versus-host disease prophylaxis after HLA-identical sibling bone marrow transplantation. *Blood* 92:2303–2314.

Reed, E.C., et al. 1988. Treatment of cytomegalovirus pneumonia with ganciclovir and intravenous cytomegalovirus immunoglobulin in patients with bone marrow transplant. *Ann Intern Med* 109: 783–788.

Riddell, S.R., Berger, C., Murata, M., et al. 2003. The graft versus leukemia response after allogeneic hematopoietic stem cell transplantation. *Blood Rev* 17:153–162.

Riddell, S.R., Greenberg, P.D. 2000. T-cell therapy of cytomegalovirus and human immunodeficiency virus infection. *J Antimicrob Chemother* 45(Suppl T3): 35–43.

Riddell, S.R., Murata, M., Bryant, S., Warren, E.H. 2002. Minor histocompatibility antigens—targets of graft versus leukemia responses. *Int J Hematol* 76(Suppl 2):155–161.

Riddell, S.R., Walter, B.A., Gilbert, M.J., Greenberg, P.D. 1994. Selective reconstitution of CD8+ cytotoxic T lymphocyte responses in immunodeficient bone marrow transplant recipients by the adoptive transfer of T cell clones. *Bone Marrow Transplantation* 14:S78–S84.

Rossi, S., Blazar, B.R., Farrell, C.L., et al. 2002. Keratinocyte growth factor preserves normal thymopoiesis and thymic microenvironment during experimental graft-versus-host disease. *Blood* 100:682–691.

Rowe, J.M., et al. 1994. Recommended guidelines for the management of autologous and allogeneic bone marrow transplanation: a report from the Eastern Cooperative Oncology Group (ECOG). *Ann Intern Med* 120:143–158.

Ruggeri, L., Capanni, M., Urbani, E., et al. 2002. Effectiveness of donor natural killer cell alloreactivity in mismatched hematopoietic transplants. *Science* 295: 2097–2100.

Sanders, J.E., et al. 1988. Growth and development of children after bone marrow transplantation. *Horm Res* 30:92–97.

Santos, G.W. 1974. Immunosuppression for clinical marrow transplantation. *Semin Hematol* 11:341–351.

Santos, G.W., et al. 1970. Rationale for the use of cyclophosphamide as immunosuppression for marrow transplants in man. In Bertelli, A., Monoco, A.P. (Eds.) *International Symposium on Pharmacological Treatment in Organ and Tissue Transplantation*. Amsterdam: Experta Medical Found., 24.

Santos, G.W., et al. 1983. Marrow transplantation for acute nonlymphocytic leukemia after treatment with busulfan and cyclophosphamide. *N Engl J Med* 309: 1347–1353.

Santos, G.W., et al. 1987. Cyclosporin plus methylprednisolone versus cyclophosphamide plus methylprednisolone as prophylaxis for graft-versus-host disease: a randomized, double-blind study, in patients undergoing allogeneic marrow transplantation. *Clin Transpl* 1:21–28.

Santos, G.W., Yeager A.M., Jones R.J. 1989. Autologous bone marrow transplantation. *Ann Rev Med* 40: 99–112.

Schmidt-Wolf, G.D., Schmidt-Wolf, I.G. 2003. Gene therapy for hematological malignancies. *Clin Exp Med* 3:4–14.

Schreuder, G.M.T.H., et al. 1991. Increasing complexity of HLA-DR2 as detected by serology and oligonucleotide typing. *Hum Immunol* 32:141–149.

Slavin, M.A., et al. 1995. Efficacy and safety of fluconazole prophylaxis for fungal infections after marrow transplantation: a prospective, randomized, double-blind study. *J Infect Dis* 171:1545–1552.

Slavin, S., Aker, M., Shapira, M.Y., et al. 2002. Nonmyeloablative stem cell transplantation for the treatment of cancer and life-threatening non-malignant disorders; past accomplishments and future goals. *Transfus Apheresis Sci* 27:159–166.

Slavin, S. Morecki, S., Weiss, L., Or, R. 2003. Immunotherapy of hematologic malignancies and metastatic solid tumors in experimental animals and man. *Crit Rev Oncol Hematol* 46:139–163.

Sobocinski, K.A., et al. 1994. Bone marrow transplantation–1994: a report from the International Bone Marrow Transplant Registry and the North American Autologous Bone Marrow Transplant Registry. *J Hematother* 3:95–102.

Spielberger, R.P., Stiff, W., Bensinger, T., Gentile, D., Weisdorf, T., Kewalramani, T., et al. 2004. Palifermin for oral mucositis after intensive therapy for hematologic cancers. *N Engl J Med* 351:2590–2598.

Srinivasan, R., Barrett, J., Childs, R. 2004. Allogeneic stem cell transplantation as immunotherapy for nonhematological cancers. *Semin Oncol* 31:47–55.

Storb, R., et al. 1983. Graft-versus-host disease and survival in patients with aplastic anemia treated by marrow grafts from HLA-identical siblings: beneficial effect of a protective environment. *N Engl J Med* 308:302–307.

Storb, R., Deeg, H.J., Farewell, V., Doney, K., Appelbaum, F., Beatty, P., et al. 1986a. Marrow transplantation for severe aplastic anemia: methotrexate alone compared with a combination of methotrexate and cyclosporine for prevention of acute graft-versus-host disease. *Blood* 68:119–125.

Storb, R., Deeg, H.J., Whitehead, J., Appelbaum, F., Beatty, P., Bensinger, W., et al. 1986b. Methotrexate and cyclosporine compared with cyclosporine alone for prophylaxis of acute graft versus host disease after marrow transplantation for leukemia. *N Engl J Med* 314: 729–735.

Storb, R., Martin, P., Deeg, H.J., et al. 1992. Long-term follow-up of three controlled trials comparing cyclosporine versus methotrexate for graft-versus-host disease prevention in patients given marrow grafts for leukemia. *Blood* 79:3091–3092.

Stuart, R.K., Sensenbrenner, L.L. 1979. Adverse nutritional deprivation of transplanted hematopoietic cells. *Exp Hematol* 7:435–442.

Sullivan, K.M. 1983. Graft-versus-host disease. In Blume, K.G., Petz, L.D. (Eds.) *Clinical Bone Marrow Transplantation.* New York: Churchill Livingston, 91–130.

Sullivan, K.M., et al. 1988a. Alternating-day cyclosporin and prednisone for treatment of high-risk chronic graft-v-host disease. *Blood* 72:555–561.

Sullivan, K.M., et al. 1988b. Prednisone and azathioprine compared with prednisone and placebo for treatment of chronic graft-versus-host disease: prognostic influence of prolonged thrombocytopenia after allogeneic marrow transplantation. *Blood* 72:546–554.

Syrjala, K.L., Chapko, M.K., Vitaliano, P.P., et al. 1993. Recovery after allogeneic marrow transplantation: prospective study of predictors of long-term physical and psychosocial functioning. *Bone Marrow Transplantation* 11:319–327.

Szeluga, D.J., et al. 1987. Nutritional support of bone marrow transplant recipients: a prospective, randomized clinical trial comparing total parenteral nutrition to an enteral feeding program. *Cancer Res* 47: 3309–3316.

Terasaki, P.I., McClelland, J.D. 1964. Microdroplet assay of human serum cytotoxins. *Nature* 204:998–1000.

Thomas, E.D., et al. 1957. Intravenous infusion of bone marrow in patients receiving radiation and chemotherapy. *N Engl J Med* 257:491–496.

Thomas, E.D., et al. 1975. Bone marrow transplantation. *N Engl J Med* 292:832–843, 895–902.

Thomas, E.D., et al. 1977. One hundred patients with acute leukemia treated by chemotherapy, total body irradiation and allogeneic marrow transplantation. *Blood* 49:511–533.

Thomas, E.D., Storb, R. 1970. Techniques for human marrow grafting. *Blood* 36:507–515.

van Bekkum, D.W., de Vries, J.J. 1967. *Radiation Chimeras.* London: Logos.

Voutsadakis, I.A. 2003. NK cells in allogeneic bone marrow transplantation. *Cancer Immunol Immunother* 52: 525–534.

Weiden, P.L., Flournoy, N., Thomas, E.D. 1979. Antileukemic effect of graft-versus-host disease in human recipients of allogeneic marrow grafts. *N Engl J Med* 300:1068–1073.

Weisdorf, S.A., et al. 1983. Graft-versus-host disease of the intestine: a protein losing enteropathy characterized by fecal alpha-I-antitrypsin. *Gastroenterology* 85: 1076–1081.

Weisdorf, S.A., et al. 1987. Positive effect of prophylactic total parenteral nutrition on long-term outcome of bone marrow transplantation. *Transplantation* 43: 833–838.

Wingard, J.R. 1994. Functional ability and quality of life of patients after allogeneic marrow transplantation: factors affecting social and occupational functions: strategies to improve social and job reintegration. *Bone Marrow Transplantation* 14:S29–S33.

Wingard, J.R., et al. 1988. Cytomegalovirus infection after autologous bone marrow transplantation with comparison to infection after allogeneic bone marrow transplantation. *Blood* 71:1432–1437.

Wingard, J.R., et al. 1990. Cytomegalovirus infections in patients treated by intensive cytoreductive therapy with marrow transplant. *Rev Infect Dis* 12(suppl 7): 805–810.

Wingard, J.R., et al. 1991. Health, functional status, and employment of long-term survivors after bone marrow transplantation. *Ann Intern Med* 114:113–118.

Wingard, J.R., et al. 1992a. Bone marrow transplantation: a form of adoptive immunotherapy. In Mitchell, M.D. (Ed.) *Biological Approaches to Cancer Treatment: Biomodulation.* New York: McGraw-Hill, 554–573.

Wingard, J.R., Curbow B, Baker F, et al. 1992b. Sexual satisfaction in survivors of bone marrow transplantation. *Bone Marrow Transplantation* 9:185–190.

Winston, D.J., et al. 1979. Infectious complications of human bone marrow transplantation. *Medicine* 58: 1–31.

Winston, D.J. et al. 1980. Cytomegalovirus infections associated with leukocyte transfusions. *Ann Intern Med* 93:671–675.

Winston, D.J., et al. 1993. Ganciclovir prophylaxis of cytomegalovirus infection and disease in allogeneic bone marrow transplant recipients. *Ann Intern Med* 118: 179–184.

Winston, D.J., Maziarz, R.T., Chandrasekar, P.H., et al. 2003. Intravenous and oral itraconazole versus intravenous and oral fluconazole for long-term antifungal prophylaxis in allogeneic hematopoietic stem-cell transplant recipients. A multicenter, randomized trial. *Ann Intern Med* 138:705–713.

Chapter 2

Understanding Hematopoiesis

Melinda S. Chouinard, RN, BSN, OCN®

Kathleen T. Finn, RN, NP, AOCN®

Introduction

Hematopoiesis, or blood cell formation, is a multifaceted, multistep process necessary for the production, regulation, and maintenance of all human blood cells. Initial hematopoiesis takes place during early embryogenesis at approximately 3 to 4 weeks postfertilization with fetal development (Brunstein and Verfailie, 2004). By week 20 of fetal development, human bone marrow is producing all cells of the eight major cell lines of hematopoiesis (Metcalf, 1998). Hematopoiesis represents an intricate, organized, and migratory process, which initiates in the yolk sac, where hematopoietic cells have been noted as early as 8 days gestation (Sutherland, 2000), and continues through fetal development into adulthood. All variants of human cells initiate as the pluripotent stem cell (Wujcik, 1997). This cell is unique in its ability to self-replicate and produce multilineage cells, and it is highly prolific. Thus, the basic premise of hematopoiesis purports that cells, once growth is initiated, commit to being either myeloid or lymphoid. It is a stratification system that allows for the production of massive cell numbers from just a few pluripotent stem cells (Metcalf, 1998).

Hematopoietic stem cell transplantation (HSCT) is a treatment modality indicated for treatment of malignant and nonmalignant diseases. Myeloablative doses of chemotherapy and/or total body irradiation are given to eradicate disease and prepare the bone marrow to receive the transplanted cells. Recent refinements of conditioning regimens and a better understanding of the bone marrow microenvironment and chimerism have led to the relatively new and less toxic nonmyeloablative hematopoietic stem cell transplant (NMHSCT). Whether a traditional HSCT or the newer NMHSCT, basic knowledge of hematopoiesis is critical for nurses managing these patients. This chapter will review the structure and function of the bone marrow, major cells that constitute myeloid and lymphoid cell lines, hematopoietic growth factors (HGFs), cell markers, and the sources of stem cells used in transplantation.

Hematopoiesis: Structure and Processs

Hematopoiesis is the general term for the formation and development of the various blood cells from the pluripotent stem cell. This process includes proliferation, differentiation, and maturation of cells. Proliferation is simply the division of the cells to form two daughter cells. Differentiation consists of acquiring specialized functions and characteristics different from the immature cell. Maturation refers to the cell developing into a functionally active cell.

The classic depiction of blood cell growth is a treelike cascade with orderly progression from immature to fully mature cells (see **Figure 2-1**). As more has been understood about hematopoiesis, additional cells and the proteins that direct this growth have been identified (Wujcik, 1997; Emerson, et al., 2000; Munker et al., 2000).

Blood-Forming Organs

Bone Marrow

The blood-forming organs include the bone marrow, spleen, and liver (Widmaier et al., 2004). The bone marrow, one of the largest organs in the body, has three basic functions: hematopoiesis, phagocytosis, and antibody production. The bone marrow milieu is a delicate balance of cells in various stages of development and sinusoidal spaces surrounded by the bone marrow stroma, a framework of supportive tissue. The bone marrow contains endothelial cells, fibroblasts, adipocytes, and macrophages and it produces collagen and adhesive proteins. The immature cells adhere to the collagen and proteins while maturation and development occur. The growth and proliferation of the bone marrow cells are influenced by hematopoiesis growth factor (HGF).

Hematopoiesis occurs in the flat bones, including the sternum, ribs, skull, pelvis, shoulders, vertebrae, and inominates. The marrow capable of producing cells, or red marrow, is found in the distal ends. With aging, inactive marrow can again become active red marrow.

The bone marrow microenvironment can be damaged by chemotherapy and radiation. Successful engraftment of transplanted stem cells depends on the quality and quantity of stem cells and the integrity of the marrow's microenvironment (Charbord, 1994; Kessinger, 2003; Brunstein and Verfaillie, 2004).

Spleen

The spleen is the largest lymphoid organ. It is the site of B and T cell proliferation and an important component of the reticuloendothelial system. The spleen has many functions that support hematopoiesis (Griffin, 1986). These include removing old and dead red blood cells (RBCs) and platelets, culling activity (removing particles that form RBCs without injuring the cell), platelet storage, antigen filtration, and preparation of antigens for phagocytosis (Wujcik, 1997).

Liver

The liver contributes to hematopoiesis through production of fibrinogen, prothrombin, and other procoagulant and anticoagulant factors. The liver destroys old RBCs and, if needed, can contribute to production of RBCs (Widmaier et al., 2004).

Blood Cell Types

Blood cell production is a complex and intricate series of cellular divisions. At each step in maturation, different colony-forming units are produced, sending signals for further maturation and cellular development to occur. The following

Figure 2-1 Hematopoiesis chart.

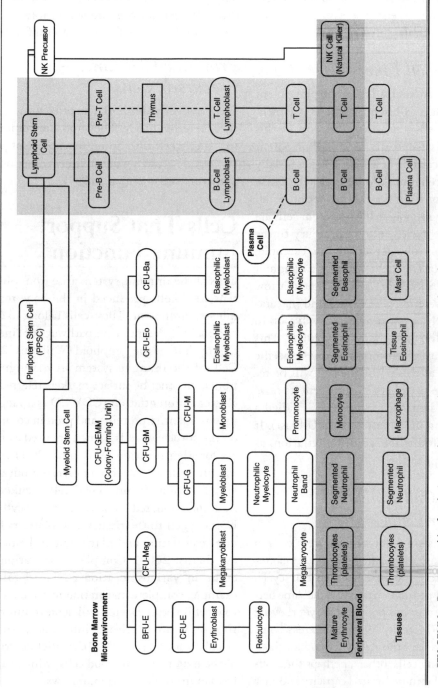

CFU-GEMM = Precursor capable of producing granulocytes, erythrocytes, monocytes, and megakaryocytes.

CFU-GM = colony-forming unit–granulocyte, macrophage.

The most primitive cells have the greatest self-renewal capability and are responsible for long-term engraftment. Multipotent CD34+ progenitor cells include cells giving rise to mixed granulocyte/erythrocyte/macrophage/megakaryocytic colonies (CFU-GEMM or CFU-Mix) and to long-term engrafment cells.

Source: Adapted from Wujcik, D. (1997). Hematopoiesis. In Whedon, M.B. (Ed.). *Blood and marrow stem cell transplantation: Principles, practice, and nursing insights.* 2nd ed. Sudbury, MA: Jones and Bartlett Publishers, p. 26.

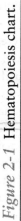

represents a brief description of both primitive and mature immune cells. These cells are further summarized in **Table 2-1**.

Primitive Cell Lines—Stem Cells

All blood cells are derived from the pluripotent stem cell. In fact, all hematopoiesis is dependent on the cell-generating capacity of this subset of cells (Metcalf, 1998). Pluripotent stem cells are capable of a complex, potentially life-long self-renewal (Williams, 2004). These cells are responsible for the formation of all myeloid and lymphoid cell lines. Stem cells are in a nonactive cycle. Following injury to the marrow or marrow depletion, for example, after myeloablative chemotherapy, a daughter cell will leave its resting space in the marrow and undergo a series of divisions and maturations. Typically, a pathway can involve up to five cellular divisions (Williams, 2004). This results in a mature cell committed to a specific cell line. It is at this point the cell will be released into the periphery to complete its task. The earliest identifiable stem cell is called a colony-forming unit-blast cell (CFU-blast). It is capable of multilineage differentiation, as well as self-replication.

Primitive Cell Lines—Progenitor Cells

Progenitor cells are different from stem cells in that they are larger, undifferentiated, mononuclear cells. Most are in an active cell cycle. Progenitor cell populations exhibit the same heterogenicity as stem cell populations, yet they are quite unique (Metcalf, 1998). Whereas some progenitor cells have the ability to produce thousands of offspring cells, others, perhaps these offspring, have a far more limited capacity and may only produce cells numbering in the low hundreds. Progenitor cells are irreversibly committed to single lineage function (Metcalf, 1998).

Primitive Cell Lines—Precursor Cells

Precursor cells are similar to progenitor cells in their heterogenicity. They, too, are committed to a single cell line. Some are capable of proliferative cell growth whereas others function only as mature cells (Wujcik, 1997).

Cells That Support Immune Function

Cells of the immune system arise from pluripotent stem cells produced in the bone marrow microenvironment. These cells belong to one of two main differentiation pathways or lineages, the myeloid or the lymphoid (Williams, 2004). Cells of the immune system are distinguished from each other by surface markers referred to as cluster differentiation (CD). CD is a language used to identify proteins and protein complexes on the surface of cells, which are used as markers for identification (Williams, 2004). Fully mature cells are capable of carrying out a specific function. White blood cells (leukocytes) fight infection, red blood cells (erythrocytes) deliver oxygen to the tissues, and platelets facilitate coagulation and play a role in hemostasis (Williams, 2004). Complete maturation may occur in various locations. Neutrophils, for example, complete maturation in the bone marrow, while erythrocytes will achieve full maturity only after release into the peripheral circulation (Wujcik, 1997). A brief description of the major mature blood cells, which support human immune function, follows.

Table 2-1 BLOOD CELLS OF THE IMMUNE SYSTEM.

Name of Blood Cell	Normal Cell Count in cell/mm³	Percentage of Complete Blood Count	Lifespan	Function
Neutrophil	3000–6000	50–90%	7–12 hours	• Phagocytizes bacteria • Most abundant of all varieties of leukocytes
Eosinophil	150–300	2–5%	About 8 hours	• Phagocytizes parasites and fungus • Involved in allergic response • Elevated in asthma and allergies
Basophil	0–100	0.05%		
Monocyte/macrophage	300–600	6–8%	Several months to years	• Defense against fungal, protozoan, and parasitic infections
B lymphocyte	200–1200	9%		• Provides humoral immunity • Involved in antibody production
T lymphocyte helper/inducer cytotoxic suppressor	800–3600			• Provides cellular immunity • Recognizes and binds to antigens • Inhibits B and T lymphocyte function
T memory				• Produces memory effect
Erythrocyte Male Female	4.6–6.2 million 4.1–5.4 million		90–140 days	• Transport oxygen for tissue oxygenation
Thrombocyte (platelet)	150,000–350,000		7–8 days	• Facilitates clotting • Assists with hemostasis

Sources: Adapted from Wujcik, D. (1997). Hematopoiesis. In Whedon, M.B. (Ed.), *Blood and marrow stem cell transplantation: Principles, practice, and nursing insights.* 2nd ed. Sudbury, MA: Jones and Bartlett Publishers, p. 28 and Bauer, Susan M. (2000). Immunology. In Yarbro, et al. (Eds.), *Cancer nursing principles and practice.* 5th ed. Sudbury, MA: Jones and Bartlett Publishers, p. 28.

Erythrocytes—Red Blood Cells (RBCs)

The burst-forming unit-erythrocyte (BFU-e) serves as the progenitor for all red blood cells, or erythrocytes. The precursor proerythroblast and erythroblast continue cellular division. The ability to proliferate and divide is lost once the cell matures into a normoblast. Reticulocytes (immature erythrocytes) are released into the periphery where final maturation occurs. This process takes 1 to 2 days. The primary role of the mature erythrocyte is to carry oxygen to the tissues and eliminate carbon dioxide via hemoglobin (see Table 2-1).

Thrombocytes—Platelets

The thrombocytic progenitor for platelets is colony-forming unit-megakaryocyte (CFU-MEG), as well as precursor cells called megakaryoblasts and megakaryocytes. Once mature, thrombocytes shed platelets. They are responsible for maintaining hemostasis, control of bleeding through release of platelets, and initiation of the clotting cascade by conversion of fibrinogen into fibrin. The mature thrombocyte is relatively vital, with a lifespan of 4 to 7 days (Williams, 2004).

Leukocytes—White Blood Cells (WBCs)

Although there are two lineages of WBCs, their primary function is the same: to provide immediate protection from invaders that are potentially harmful to the body. WBC production is stimulated primarily by initiation of an immune-mediated response, either inflammation or infection (Williams, 2004).

Granulocytes (Neutrophils, Eosinophils, and Basophils)

The most abundant of all granulocytes (mature WBCs) are neutrophils. Neutrophils compromise 50–90% of circulating polymorphs (Bauer, 2000). Maturation occurs in the bone marrow over a period of approximately 10 days. Under healthy conditions, there are 10–20% mature neutrophils stored within the marrow as reserve available for rapid mobilization when needed as defense against invaders (Williams, 2004). In the first 4 to 5 days of the maturation process, cellular division occurs as the myeloblast morphs into a promyelocyte, then a myelocyte, and finally a metomyelocyte. At this stage, the cell's ability to divide is lost, but maturation continues until the fully mature neutrophil is released into the periphery (Wujcik, 1997). Neutrophils constitute the immune system's first line of defense against invaders. Their chief role is phagocytosis of bacteria and other foreign organisms. Depletion of neutrophils or neutropenia after chemotherapy, radiation therapy, and/or marrow and stem cell transplant places patients at significant risk for infection.

Eosinophils represent another weapon in the immune system's arsenal and are a type of granulocyte responsible for fighting infectious organisms. Eosinophils comprise 2.5% of the total white blood cell count. Development and maturation includes the committed colony-forming unit-eosinophil, the precursor cells, eosinophil myeloblast, promyelocyte, and myelocyte. The role of the eosinophils is to migrate into the tissues and ingest bacteria; as such, they are short lived in the periphery. Additionally, eosinophils play a specific role in the immune response to parasites, including certain worms (Bauer, 2000). Moreover, eospinophils play a role in allergy response by activating mediators released by mast cells during allergic reaction (Wujcik, 1997).

Basophils represent the last of the granulocytes. Cellular division and maturation of basophils is similar to that of other granulocytes; with the progenitor (cell colony-forming unit-basophil), precursors (basophilic myeloblast), and finally, a mature basophil (Wujcik, 1997). Basophils comprise less than 0.2–0.5% of circulating granulocytes (Bauer, 2000). Mast cells and basophils are almost indistinguishable, though mast cells are found only in body tissues. Both play key roles in allergic and hypersensitivity response. With exposure to an environmental allergen, basophils are released, thus playing a role in human allergic response (Williams, 2004).

Monocytes/Macrophages

Monocytes and macrophages make up what was formerly referred to as the reticuloendothelial system. Monocytes are circulating leukocytes. They give rise to cells, which make up the mononuclear phagocyte system. Produced by the colony-forming unit granulocyte-macrophage (CFU-GM), its earliest precursor is the monoblast, followed by the promonocyte and finally the monocyte. Released by the marrow prior to complete maturation, monocytes are capable of limited phagocytosis. Monocytes comprise 6–8% of the circulating WBCs. Once monocytes migrate to the tissues, maturation is complete and the cells become macrophages. In a healthy state, approximately 95% of cells are macrophages while only 2% are circulating monocytes. It is clear from this that macrophages represent

a significant weapon against infection. Macrophages are also very hearty cells capable of survival for several months to years (Ellerhorst-Ryan, 2000). Additionally, these cells play an important role in both innate and adaptive immunity. Examples include Kupffer cells, spleen sinus macrophages, and lymph node sinus macrophages. Their two main functions include their roles as: 1) phagocytic macrophages' removal of particulate antigens and 2) antigen-presenting cells, which present antigens to the lymphocytes (Bauer, 2000).

Lymphocytes

"The lymphocytes are the workhorses of the immune system" (Sutherland, 2000, p. 2.7). These cells are responsible for both humoral and cellular immunity and constitute 25–30% of the overall WBC count (Ellerhorst-Ryan, 2000). A more thorough review of immunology appears later in this chapter. What follows next is a brief description of the role B and T lymphocytes/cells play in immune response. A more detailed description of these vital cells will follow with the discussion on humoral and cell-mediated immunity.

B lymphocytes secrete antibodies into body fluids such as blood or lymph known as humors; hence they are responsible for humoral immunity. In contrast to T cells, B cells are programmed with specificity for one antigen and produce antibodies appropriate to that antigen (Sutherland, 2000). These antibodies identify foreign proteins and neutralize or destroy them via phagocytosis (Ellerhorst-Ryan, 2000; Sutherland, 2000). It is important to note that these antibodies serve only as antigen markers and are not capable of cell kill on their own (Sutherland, 2000).

T lymphocytes/cells have a more direct effect on antigens than their B lymphocyte counterparts and are responsible for cellular immunity (Sutherland, 2000). T cells initiate a variety of direct and indirect activities resulting in eradication of dangerous microorganisms (Ellerhorst-Ryan, 2000). T cells are responsible for protection against fungi and viruses in particular. There are five subsets of T cells, each with its own unique function within the immune system. Memory cells recognize those antigens where prior exposure has occurred. Cytotoxic T cells directly attack antigens and will destroy any cells bearing foreign antigens. They also play an important role in rejection of transplanted tissues and organs. Helper and suppressor T cells serve as chief regulators of immune function via secretion of protein mediators known as cytokines. Lastly, memory T cells are produced by T cells that have been exposed to a specific antigen. These cells are capable of delivering rapid response to an exposure of a previously seen antigen. Memory T cells are also known for their remarkable life span (Sutherland, 2000).

Homeostasis

Homeostasis is the balance between cellular growth and death; it is critical for normal bone marrow and immune function. Apoptosis, or programmed cellular death, is the mechanism by which homeostasis is achieved (Williams, 2004). Under normal conditions, the bone marrow is capable of producing WBCs, RBCs, and platelets numbering in the billions per day (see Table 2-1). As new cells are developed, other cells within the same lineage die, thereby maintaining the appropriate number of cells per line within the body at any given time (Williams, 2004). The rate of production increases five- to tenfold under such stressful conditions as in-

fection, hemorrhage, or injury to the bone marrow (Wujcik, 1997). Maintaining this balance between what exits and what is required is just another example of the amazing work done by the human bone marrow.

Hematopoietic Growth Factors

The establishment of pluripotent stem cells as paramount to hematopoiesis is well documented. However, as important as these cells may be, it is now being recognized that it is only through 1) a complex and ordered series of interactions within the stromal microenvironment; 2) contact with matrix proteins; and 3) exposure to soluble proteins with growth stimulatory and inhibitory properties, such as human growth factors, that stem cells are able to function as they do. Hematopoietic growth factors (HGFs) are a group of glycoproteins that facilitate regulation, differentiation, growth, and function of all hematopoietic cell lines (Bagby and Heinrich, 1999). These proteins are released during inflammatory and other immune-mediated responses (Wujcik, 1997).

The past two decades have seen a plethora of research into the field of identification and ex vivo production of HGFs (Kutler and Beagley, 2002). The original molecules were described as colony-stimulating factors (CSFs). Early in the study of CSFs, it was theorized that they could only be isolated in humans, but the development of recombinant DNA techniques has led to mass production of CSFs. Additionally, it has opened the field wide for further study and application of other HGFs (Buchsel et al., 2002). The research and development of HGFs has revolutionized the management of patients receiving chemotherapy, mobilization therapy for stem cell donation, and marrow and stem cell transplantation. A summary of FDA-approved recombinant HGFs can be found in **Table 2-2**.

The list of HGFs is complex and expanded to include the interleukins (ILs), which influence hematopoiesis. A summary of the ILs and their roles in hematopoiesis can be found in **Table 2-3**. Growth factors can be classified as either specific or multilineage, depending on the type of mature cells that grow in lineage-specific colonies in response to growth factors. HGFs that inspire growth and production with specificity for a single cell line are lineage-specific. Examples of lineage-specific HGFs include erythropoietin and granulocyte colony-stimulating factor (G-CSF). In contrast, multilineage HGFs have the capacity to affect multiple cell lines simultaneously. Granulocyte macrophage colony-stimulating factor (GM-CSF), for example, stimulates the production of granulocytes, dendritic cells, and macrophages (Buchsel et al., 2002).

Erythropoietin

Erythropoietin (EPO) was the first of the endogenous growth factors to be identified and made available via recombinant technology (Finke and Mertelsmann, 2004). EPO acts on erythroid progenitor cells in response to decreased oxygen in the tissues of the kidneys. It then stimulates the production of mature erythrocytes. Anemia is seen in as many as 15–90% of all cancer patients (Littlewood et al., 2003). Symptomatic anemia in the HSCT patient continues to be a significant cause of morbidity (Finke and Mertelsmann, 2004). Additionally, numerous studies have shown a direct correlation between anemia and de-

creased quality of life (Littlewood et al., 2003). Multiple factors contribute to anemia in the HSCT population including myeloablative chemotherapy, total body irradiation (TBI), and immunosuppressive agents used in the prophylaxis and treatment of GVHD such as cyclosporine. Currently, there are two recombinant erythropoiesis-stimulating agents with Food and Drug Administration (FDA) approval. Epoetin alfa has been shown to increase hemoglobin levels and decrease the need for transfusions. One limitation of epoetin alfa is the dosing/administration route. Due to the short half-life of epoetin alfa, patients may require daily subcutaneous (SQ) injections to achieve the desired outcome. However, the novel approach of pegylation has led to a new generation of EPO growth factors, which achieve the same outcome with a decreased number of injections. Darbepoietin alfa is an example of such engineering. Darbepoietin alfa is a glycoprotein similar to epoetin alfa in its ability to stimulate erythropoiesis. It differs in that two additional carbohydrate chains have been added. These additional chains increase the molecular weight, and desirable outcomes can be achieved with less frequent (weekly) administration (Vance, 2003).

Granulocyte Colony-Stimulating Factor (G-CSF)

G-CSF is a potent myeloid growth and differentiation factor and is produced by multiple cell types including monocyte-macrophages, endothelial cells and fibroblasts (Finke and Mertelsmann, 2004). G-CSF is responsible for growth and differentiation of neutrophils. Similar to epoetin alfa, G-CSF has been cultivated in the lab via recombinant technology. Filgrastim received FDA approval in 1992. It is

Table 2-2 FDA-APPROVED HEMATOPOIETIC GROWTH FACTORS.

Name	Indications	Dosing (HSCT-specific where available)	FDA Approval Date
Epoetin alfa	• Indicated for treatment of anemia in patients with nonmyeloid malignancies and/or to decrease the need for transfusions in patients receiving chemotherapy courses concurrently for > 2 months.	• Dosing may be institution specific; normal dose range = 50–150 units/kg. • If no increase in HCT in 8 weeks, increase dose by 25–50. units/kg/dose to max of 300 units/kg.	July 1999
Darbepoetin alfa	• Indicated for treatment of anemia in patients with nonmyeloid malignancies receiving concurrently administered courses of chemotherapy.	• Initial = 2.25 mcg/kg IV or SQ weekly. • Dosages should be targeted to not exceed a Hgb of 12 g/dl. • If Hgb > 12, decrease dose by 35%.	July 2002
Filgrastim	• Indicated to reduce the risk/length of neutropenia and related complications in patients with nonmyeloid malignancies receiving myelosuppressive chemotherapy regimens. • To reduce neutropenia in patients following HSCT. • To reduce time to neutrophil recovery in patients receiving consolidation therapy for AML. • Used in combination with chemotherapy for mobilization therapy for apheresis stem cell collection.	• Recommended initial dose = 10 g/kg/day SQ. • Doses may be increased by 5 mcg/kg/day.	February 1991

Pegfilgrastim	• Indicated to decrease the incidence of neutropenia-related infection in patients with nonmyeloid leukemia receiving myelosuppressive chemotherapy.	• 6 mg SQ once per chemo cycle.	January 2002
Oprelvekin	• Stimulates megakaryocytopoiesis and thrombopoiesis by direct stimulation of IL-11. • Is indicated for prevention of severe thrombocytopenia and reduction of need for platelet transfusions in patients receiving myelosuppressive chemotherapy.	• 50 mcg/kg per day SQ.	September 2003
Sargramostim	• Accelerates myeloid recovery in selected patients undergoing HSCT. • Known to stimulate production of dendritic cells, which participate in tumor kill	• 250 mcg/m^2 IV over 2–4 hours. • Dose is same for indications for post-HSCT, mobilization, and postchemotherapy.	November 1996

Sources: FDA Web site. *Listing of approved oncology drugs with approved indications.* Retrieved February 23, 2004, from http://www.fda.gov/cder/cancer/druglistframe.htm Roman-Unfer, S., & Shpall, E.J. (1999). The use of cytokines to enhance collection of stem cells and blood for transplantation. In Wingard, J.R., & Demetri, G.R. (Eds.), *Clinical applications of cytokines and growth factors* (pp. 369–380). Norwell, MA: Kluwer Academic Publishers. Wilkes, G.M., Ingwerson, K., and Barton-Burke, M. (2003). *2003 oncology nursing drug handbook.* Boston: Jones and Bartlett Publishers, pp. 317–362.

Table 2-3 INTERLEUKINS AND HEMATOPOIETIC FUNCTION.

Name	Source	Hematopoietic Function
IL-1	Macrophages, monocytes, endothelial cells, fibroblasts, neurons, keratinocytes, and epithelial cells	• Induces proliferation of T cells and macrophages • Enhances NK cells • Released as part of inflammatory response
IL-2	Activated T cells	• Induces proliferation and activation of T and B lymphocytes and NK cells • Induces expression of IL-1 in macrophages and monocytes
IL-3	T cells, thymic epithelium, keratinocytes, neurons, mast cells	• Responsible for stimulation of multilineage colony growth factors • Stimulates primitive hematopoietic stem cell lines with multilineage potential, e.g., CFU-GEMM
IL-4	CD4+ cells. Activated mast cells, basophils, and some CD8+ cells	• Induces prolific production of activated B and T cells, fibroblasts, and macrophages
IL-5	CD4+ cells, activated mast cells	• Implicated in eosinophil production and activation • Activation of cytotoxic T cells
IL-6	T cells, endothelial cells, monocytes, and fibroblasts	• Responsible in part for immunoglobulin secretion • Differentiates myeloid cells, B cells, and plasma cells • Maturation of megakaryocytes
IL-7	Stromal cells, including bone marrow, thymus, spleen, and kidney	• Supports growth of B cells • Has marked activity on mature and immature T cells
IL-8	Monocytes, endothelial cells, T cells, fibroblasts, neutrophils, keratinocytes, hepatocytes, chondrocytes, and NK cells	• Enhances IL-3 and GM-CSF by production of activated T cells • Modulates neutrophil production • Stimulates angiogenesis
IL-9	Certain CD4+ cells	• Stimulates proliferation of preactivated T cell and helper T cell lines
IL-10	T and B cells, activated macrophages	• Suppresses helper T cells • Costimulator of B cell proliferation
IL-11	Stromal fibroblasts, neurons, gut epithelium, alveolar and bronchial epithelium	• Increases number and cycling activity of committed progenitor cell • Increases peripheral platelet and neutrophil counts

IL-12	Dendritic cells, B cells, macrophages	• Increases differentiation of helper T cells • Augments functional activity of NK cells
IL-13	Activated T cells, basophils, and mast cells	• Similar in effect to IL-4 • Has influence on T cells
IL-14	T cells	• Stimulates the production of pre-B cell acute lymphocytic leukemia (ALL) and hairy cell leukemic cells
IL-15	Activated monocytes and macrophages, bone marrow stromal cells	• Stimulates production of immunoglobulin by activated T cells • Induces proliferation and activation of T cells, B cells, and natural killer cells
IL-16	Mast cells, CD8+ cells, and T cells	• Stimulates mass cell production • Acts as growth factor for CD4+ T cells
IL-17	T cells, particularly activated CD4+ cells	• Induces IL-2 functional receptors on CD4+ T cells • Induces secretion of IL-6, IL-8, PGE2 and G-CSF from stromal cells in bone marrow
IL-18	Osteoblasts	• Augments NK activity • Inhibits IL-10 production by T cells • Induces granulocyte-macrophage colony stimulating factor production from T cells

Sources: Adapted from Wujcik, D. (1997). Hematopoiesis. In Whedon, M.B. (Ed.), *Blood and marrow stem cell transplantation: Principles, practice, and nursing insights* (pp. 25–42). Sudbury, MA: Jones & Bartlett Publishers; Roman-Unfer, S., & Shpall, E.J. (1999). The use of cytokines to enhance collection of stem cells and blood for transplantation. In Wingard, J.R., & Demetri, G.R. (Eds.), *Clinical applications of cytokines and growth factors* (pp. 369–380). Norwell, MA: Kluwer Academic Publishers; and Bagby, G.C., & Heinrich, M.C. (1999). Cytokines, growth factors, and hematopoiesis. In Wingard, G.R., & Demetri, G.R. (Eds.), *Clinical applications of cytokines and growth factors* (pp. 2–55). Norwell, MA: Kluwer Academic Publishers.

indicated for patients with neutropenia related to chemotherapy, radiation, and HSCT. Filgrastim is administered daily by SQ injection. Patients may require clinic visits or may be taught to administer the injection themselves. Either option represents inconvenience and trauma for the patient. Undesirable side effects include bone pain, irritation at injection site, and fever; a potential for multiple clinic visits also exists. Pegylation also has been applied to filgrastim to attempt to lengthen the half-life, thus decreasing injection frequency while achieving durable neutrophil counts. Pegfilgrastim received FDA approval in 2003. Pegfilgrastim stimulates the production of myeloid precursors and rapid maturation and differentiation of neutrophils. Initial clinical trial results demonstrate that a single dose of pegfilgrastim supported neutrophil production from nadir to complete neutrophil recovery (Crawford, 2003).

The use of recombinant G-CSF in the HSCT population is well studied in both the autologous and peripheral blood cell transplant populations. Results of these large, randomized studies confirm a marked increase in neutrophil recovery when used in this setting (Finke and Mertelsmann, 2004). However, use in the allogeneic population elicits concerns secondary to potential stimulation of myeloid or lymphoid malignancies, as well as the potential to exacerbate GVHD. Several studies have looked at these concerns. In one, 54 patients were randomly assigned to filgrastim versus placebo. Patients in the filgrastim arm achieved durable neutrophil recovery on day +11 post-transplant versus day +15 for the placebo arm. There was no significant increase of GVHD noted in the filgrastim arm at day +100. Further studies are needed to determine the significance of these and other concerns (Finke and Mertelsmann, 2004).

Granulocyte Macrophage Colony-Stimulating Factor (GM-CSF)

GM-CSF stimulates the division and maturation of multilineage colonies, including granulocytes and monocytes (Finke and Mertlesmann, 2004; Wilkes et al., 2003). Mature neutrophils and macrophages serve multiple functions, including tumoricidal activity, antibody-dependent cell-mediated cytotoxicity, and phagocytosis, to name a few (Finke and Mertelsmann, 2004). Sargramostim is a recombinant preparation of the endogenous HGF. In clinical trials, it has proven to be less efficacious than filgrastim in terms of time to neutrophil engraftment in the autologous HSCT population (Finke and Mertelsmann, 2004). In similar trials in the allogeneic population, patients were randomly given sargramostim versus sequentially given sargramostim followed by filgrastim. Neutrophil recovery was similar in both arms of the study. Thus, it would appear that further study is needed to determine primary efficacy of sargramostim for neutrophil engraftment in the post-HSCT setting.

Any discussion of GM-CSF would be remiss if it did not include its stimulatory effects on dendritic cells (DC). DCs originate in the bone marrow and serve as sentinels of immune response. They constantly survey the immune landscape for antigens in the form of microbes, allergens, viruses, and tumor cells. Various processes allow the DC to capture antigens and facilitate destruction. Current clinical trials involving DCs include those aimed at enhancing the functional effects of tumor vaccines on DCs (Buchsel et al., 2002). DC vaccines are being developed in several ways, including the isolation and preservation of cluster differentiation-34 (CD34+) progenitor cells. Once cells are thawed for use, sargramostim and other cytokines are added to cultivate DCs. These enhanced cells are then exposed to a specific tumor antigen. The intent is to develop a general cancer vaccine that can be primed with cells of the patient's own tumor. Determining the implications of dendritic cells and their role in cancer vaccines will require additional research (Buchsel et al., 2002).

Growth Factor Mobilization of Peripheral Blood Hematopoietic Cells (PBHC)

An additional role for the recombinant growth factors is in the mobilization of peripheral blood hematopoietic cells (PBHC). These agents have been used in mobilization therapy for the last decade. Multiple studies have described the pros and cons of single-agent mobilization versus mobilization with an HGF in combination with chemotherapy. Initial studies in the late 1980s showed that mobilization with recombinant human granulocyte macrophage colony-stimulating factor (rhGM-CSF) alone increased the number of peripheral HPCs 18 times (Schmit-Pokorny, 2004). Additional studies have looked at optimal dosing regimens. In these studies, higher doses of filgrastim yielded far superior CD34+ cell counts (Ng-Cashin and Shea, 2004). Given these results, additional studies have been done to determine optimal dosing and frequency (once daily 5 mcg/kg versus twice daily 10 mcg/kg). The twice-daily dosing achieved higher CD34+ yields. Still more studies looked at even higher dosing between 10 and 16 mcg/kg/day. Although more research is indicated, it is clear that higher doses of HGFs produced significantly higher CD34+ cell counts and

shorter procedure times for donors (Ng-Cashin and Shea, 2004).

Thrombopoietin and Interleukin-11 (IL-11)

Thrombopoietin (TPO) stimulates the differentiation and maturation of megakaryocyte progenitors to increase platelet production. Moreover, TPO acts in synergy with other HGFs to enhance primitive hematopoietic cells committed to erythroid and monomyelocyte lines (Gajewski et al., 2002). Thrombocytopenia is a major clinical issue for patients receiving dose-intensive chemotherapy, radiation, and/or HSCT. Platelet therapy is currently the only treatment for severe, symptomatic thrombocytopenia. Although they provide temporary efficacy, platelet transfusions are associated with a number of negative outcomes including transfusion reactions, potential for transfer of infectious organisms, alloimmunization, and platelet refractoriness (Kutler and Beagley, 2002). Multiple clinical trials have studied the usefulness of recombinant TPO, both in the solid tumor setting and HSCT. IN HSCT, the bulk of patients received recombinant human TPO (rhTPO) in combination with filgrastim to support myeloid recovery. Study results have not been overwhelmingly positive. The role of rhTPO requires additional study. In addition, reports of adverse events including development of neutralizing antibodies and thrombophilia have led to a delay in approval by the FDA (Finke and Mertelsmann, 2004).

Another thrombopoiesis-inducing cytokine is interleukin-11 (IL-11). IL-11 is produced by fibroblasts in bone marrow stromal cells. IL-11 has a stimulatory role in megakaryopoiesis. Oprelvekin received FDA approval in 1997, and is licensed for use in prevention of severe thrombocytopenia and to decrease need for supplemental platelet transfusions. Although oprelvekin has shown modest success in decreasing the overall number of platelet transfusions, as well as time from platelet nadir to recovery, its use in HSCT is controversial. The toxicity profile of oprelvekin includes acute hypersensitivity reaction, massive fluid retention, and edema. As such, its use in HSCT is not recommended (Finke and Mertelsmann, 2004).

In summary, the role of recombinant growth factors in HSCT has been defined in several situations. Its success in mobilization of CD34+ cells is clearly documented. Furthermore, there is strong clinical evidence to support use in the post-HSCT setting, especially when graft failure or rejection is present. However, determining future indications will require additional clinical study.

Immunity

Immunity is characterized as a series of events that protect the body against foreign substances. It is composed of many different types of cells that work together. To be effective, the immune system must be intact and have the ability to recognize and destroy invading microorganisms such as proteins, viruses, bacteria, and parasites that are not part of the body's normal environment (Griffin, 1986; Caudell and Whedon, 1991; Shames and Kishiyama, 2003; Widmaier et al., 2004). A great deal of immunity is acquired in childhood. By the time a child enters school, he or she has a mature immune system with the ability to protect against infection, preserve the internal environment through removal of dead and damaged cells, and destroy malignant cells that arise in the body by a function known as *immune surveillance*.

The immune system consists of nonspecific (natural) and specific (acquired) immunity, both of which interact with each other and have overlapping functions. White blood cells (leukocytes) are the cells that provide immunity. Granuloctyes (neutrophils, eosinophils, and basophils), monocytes, and their tissue complements provide *nonspecific immunity*. Lymphocytes are the essential cells responsible for *specific immunity*. The two main types of lymphocytes are B lymphocytes (B cells) and T lymphocytes (T cells), both of which circulate in the blood and lymph system.

Both nonspecific and specific immunity are negatively altered by the effects of conditioning chemotherapy and total body irradiation. These treatments alter all normal defenses against infection for months to several years (Wujcik, 1997).

Nonspecific Immune Defense (Natural Immunity)

Nonspecific or natural immunity, also referred to as "innate immunity," matures over a lifetime of exposure to antigens. Nonspecific defenses do not distinguish one infectious agent from another and provide both external and internal protective barriers. The body's first line of nonspecific defense is external and consists of the skin, mucous membranes, and secretions they produce. The body's second line of nonspecific defense is internal and involves the phagocytic white blood cells, the secretion of antimicrobial proteins, the inflammatory response, and the inhibition of viral replication by interferons (Rieger, 1999; Widmaier et al., 2004).

Skin and Mucous Membrane Defenses

Under normal circumstances, the intact skin is the first line of defense; however, even the smallest abrasions can allow passage of bacteria or viruses. The epithelial lining of the digestive, respiratory, and genitourinary tracts contain protective antimicrobial proteins secreted by the mucous membranes. The salivary glands and lacrimal glands also inhibit microbial colonization by the secretion of antimicrobial proteins from saliva and tears. The high acidity of the stomach destroys most microbes present in food or water before they enter the intestinal tract; however, some pathogens such as the hepatitis A virus can survive the gastric acidity and invade the digestive tract (Widmaier et al., 2004).

Inflammatory Response and Phagocytosis

Inflammation is a series of sequential changes in the tissues in response to injury. The injury causes release of chemical mediators such as histamine, bradykinin, and serotonin. Tissue spaces are walled off as lymphatics are blocked due to fibrinogen clots. This delays the spread of bacteria or toxins. Next, the neutrophils leave the bloodstream and flow along the vessel to the site of inflammation. The cells then begin to adhere to the surface of endothelial cells (*margination*). The neutrophils, which are very loose and flexible, begin to penetrate between the cells into tissue (*diapedesis*). By following the chemical signals, the cells migrate to the site of infection (*chemotaxis*). Neutrophils begin invading organisms, killing them with intracellular peroxide superoxide. The neutrophil continues to ingest and digest the organisms, until toxic substances released during the digestive process kill the neutrophil or deplete it of essential enzymes. This is usually after each neutrophil has engulfed from 5 to 25 bacteria.

Neutrophils accumulate at the site of injury or infection. They are quickly replaced by monocytes called *macrophages* residing in the tissue. These macrophages are found as histiocytes in subcutaneous tissue, alveolar tissue in lungs, Kupffer cells in liver, and glial cells in brain. They are the cells able to respond during the first hour of injury.

The monocytic response to infection is a slower, but longer, continuing process. Monocytes migrate to the site and in 8 to 12 hours swell and mature into macrophages. The macrophages then phagocytose and digest the dead neutrophils. After several days, a cavity is formed in the inflamed tissue. The cavity contains necrotic tissue, dead neutrophils, and macrophages, and it causes pus to form. The monocytes process the antigen they phagocytose and present it to the other WBCs such as lymphocytes. This processed antigen can stimulate specific immunity. Monocytes bridge the gap between nonspecific and specific immunity. If the nonspecific immunity fails, the specific defense (acquired immunity) is enlisted.

Interferons

Interferons (cytokines) are also nonspecific messengers that provide instructions against viruses. When a virus is encountered by the body, interferons are produced and secreted into the extracellular fluid, triggering the production of other antiviral proteins. The job of the antiviral proteins is then to stop viral replication (Widmaier et al., 2004).

Specific Immune Defenses (Acquired Immunity)

Specific immunity requires recognition of foreign substances (antigens) and a memory response. To be effective, this system must also identify and tolerate its own cells and their products. An antigen (also termed *immunogen*) is any foreign molecule capable of stimulating a specific immune response. Examples of antigens include viruses, cancer cells, transplanted cells, and toxins. Lymphocytes, the essential cells responsible for recognizing antigens and inducing specific host defenses, have surface molecules called *cluster differentiation (CD) antigens.* These CD markers allow identification of subtypes and function of specific lymphocytes (e.g., CD4 for helper T subset and CD34 for hematopoietic progenitors) (Munker et al., 2000; Widmaier et al., 2004).

The lymphocytes are produced in lymphoid organs. There are two classifications of lymphoid organs, called primary and secondary. The bone marrow and thymus make up the primary lymphoid organs, and the lymph nodes, spleen, and tonsils make up the secondary lymphoid organs. The three main lymphocytes considered to be the powerhouses of the immune system and providing the specific defenses are the B, T, and NK (natural killer) cells (Widmaier et al., 2004).

Humoral (Antibody-Mediated) Immunity

B Cells (B Lymphocytes)

B cells mature in the bone marrow (primary lymphoid organ) before migrating to the secondary lymphoid organs to divide and make more B cells. Upon activation, B cells differentiate into plasma cells to make and secrete antibodies (immunoglobulins) into the extracellular fluids. Plasma cells are formed when groups of antigen-specific B lymphocytes or clones respond to the presence of antigens. Antigen specificity is determined by the B cell plasma membrane receptors. Each plasma cell produces only one *specific* type of antibody (immunoglobulin), which matches up to a specific antigen and its binding site. Other activated B lymphocytes remain quiescent and turn into memory cells (Widmaier et al., 2004).

The primary antibody-mediated response to the antigen takes days. The first antibody formed is immunoglobulin M (IgM). As the response continues, IgM matures and ultimately produces IgG. The secondary response is also called the memory response and is much faster, with antibodies produced within 1 to 2 days and the antibody titer increased up to 50 times that of the primary response (Wujcik, 1997).

Antigen-Antibody Reactions and Complement

Humoral immunity is also provided through antigen-antibody (Ag-Ab) reactions and the complement system. The antigen-antibody response causes death of the antigens through one or more processes. The first is precipitation. The insoluble antibodies, in combination with the soluble antigens, lead to precipitation of the complex. A clump is formed and is quickly destroyed through phagocytosis. *Agglutination* is the process whereby an antigen attaches itself to particulate matter and the antigen-antibody complexes form clumps. This is the process during a transfusion reaction when the antigen-antibody response reaction causes RBCs to clump. Neutralization occurs where the antibody neutralizes bacterial toxins. Finally, *opsonization* is the reaction between antigen and antibody that causes the antigens to become sticky, which makes it easier for phagocytes to engulf them.

The complement system is a series of enzymatic reactions resulting in antigen destruction by lysis. Complement is an encompassing term for 20 serum proteins circulating in inactive forms. The complement protein recognizes and binds with a specific antibody. The antigen is coated with immunoglobulin, which complement recognizes as a red flag. The antibody destroys any cell marked with the immunoglobulin. The complement response hinges in the ability to recognize self. Once the body identifies self as foreign, the complement system mechanism can be catastrophic. For example, in graft-versus-host disease (GVHD), this process can be life-threatening. The complement system serves to bridge the two interdependent processes, cellular and humoral immunity (Rieger, 1999; Widmaier et al., 2004).

Cell-Mediated Immunity

T Cells (T Lymphocytes)

T cells are the moderators of the entire immune system and are involved in the elimination of intracellular pathogens, infected cells, tumor cells, and foreign grafts. As previously stated, T cells are formed in the bone marrow but leave early in development and mature in the thymus before migrating to the secondary organs to divide and make new T cells. Like B cells, the T cells' plasma-membrane receptors (TCR) have specific antigen-binding sites but do not secrete

immunoglobulins. They recognize antigens in the context of self or major histocompatibility complex (MHC), also known as human leukocyte antigens (HLA). T cells respond in two ways: Their response is either turned on or it is turned off in response to the foreign antigen. There are two main classes of T lymphocytes circulating in the blood: *cytotoxic T cells (CD8+)*, which are capable of killing virus-infected cells independently of antibodies, and *helper T cells (CD4+)*, which stimulate B cells (antibody production) and moderate the entire immune response. The secretion of cytokines is responsible for this type of cell communication.

NK (Natural Killer) Cells

NK cells morphologically look like large lymphocytes; however, they are not considered T cells or B cells. NK cells are antigen independent and are capable of killing some tumor cells and virus-infected cells by natural immunity (Munker et al., 2000; Widmaier et al., 2004).

In summary, the nonspecific and specific immune responses work together to make up the very complex immune system. If pathogens are able to get past the first group of nonspecific defenses (external defenses), they encounter a second group of nonspecific defenses (internal defenses) acting at a more cellular level. If the foreign invaders are still not destroyed by the nonspecific defenses, then the more advanced specific defenses become elicited, provided the immune system is intact. Patients receiving marrow-ablative treatments for their disease are at risk for developing infection, anemia, and bleeding. The longer the immune system is compromised, the higher the risk for opportunistic infections and life-threatening complications. Myeloid engraftment takes approximately 2 to 3 weeks to occur, and lymphoid engraftment takes even longer even when the WBC count appears normal (Rieger, 1999; Witherspoon, 2000; Widmaier et al., 2004).

Impact of Transplantation on Hematopoiesis and Immunologic Recovery

Pluripotent hematopoietic stem cells (HSC), the most primitive cells in the bone marrow (BM), are responsible for production and differentiation of blood cells and homeostasis of the bone marrow milieu. In order to maintain a constant pool of stem cells, some must divide and differentiate into specific blood cells, and some divide and differentiate into more stem cells. The production and differentiation of blood cells becomes accelerated when the body is stressed; the bone marrow has the capability to work on supply and demand and the actual process is ongoing. The myeloid cell lineages increase to meet the body's demand for extra cells by producing white cells (neutropoiesis) every 8 hours, platelets (thrombopoiesis) every 7 days, and red cells (erythropoiesis) approximately every 4 months. Other cells that are not derived from stem cells but play a role in homeostasis of the bone marrow milieu are stromal cells, which assist with growth and differentiation of stem cells. The stroma (hematopoietic microenvironment) maintains hematopoiesis by producing mobile monocytes, T lymphocytes, and NK cells (Emerson et al., 2000). High-dose chemotherapy, with or without total body irradiation (myeloablative therapy), causes an intentional, temporary, and lethal disruption to the cells in the bone marrow and its milieu with the purpose of controlling or curing disease. Hematologic and immunologic recovery from this therapy is as important as treating the disease itself.

The two major sources of hematopoietic stem cells for long-term reconstitution of hematopoiesis after myeloablative therapy are the bone marrow and the peripheral blood. Over the past 30 years, important strides have been made in the delivery, safety, and effectiveness of this therapy; however, acute and chronic effects from therapy still exist. Recovery of hematologic function is the first critical factor of concern. The longer it takes for hematologic recovery (return of white blood cells and platelet cells), the higher the risk of infection. The longer it takes for immune function recovery (B cells and T cells), the greater the impact on long-term survival and quality of life. The rate of hematologic and immune recovery is believed to be influenced by the type of transplant. Peripheral blood cells have more T cells and more natural killer cells, and immune function is more rapid than with autologous marrow transplantation (Kessinger, 2003). However, because hematopoietic stem cells move constantly between extracellular marrow spaces and peripheral blood, the quality of stem cells from either BM or peripheral blood (PB) is the same (Korbling and Anderlini, 2001).

Hematologic Recovery (Engraftment)

Following myeloablative therapy, peripheral blood counts usually reach their nadir approximately 5 to 7 days posttransplant. As described earlier in this chapter, the body's immune system responds to infection with migration of specific cells for protection and repair. Similarly, once myeloablative therapy is administered and stem cells are infused back into the host, a migration of cells also occurs with homing and reengraftment of circulating hematopoietic stem cells. The rate of hematologic recovery can depend on the source of stem cells, the conditioning/preparative regimen, posttransplant growth factors, infections, and GVHD. A consistent rise in the WBC count is the most promising indication of hematopoietic recovery. Once the WBC count increases, the lymphocyte count decreases and the neutrophil counts increase. Hematopoietic recovery following peripheral blood stem cell transplant (PBSCT) is more rapid than recovery after bone marrow transplant with a shorter nadir period. Although it is not completely known why recovery differs, there are some explanations, one being hematopoietic growth factor support during stem cell mobilization and posttransplant. Normally, hematopoietic stem cells circulate in the peripheral blood in low concentrations. When hematopoietic growth factors (G-CSF or GM-CSF) are administered prior to stem cell collection, the WBC count increases significantly, forcing hematopoietic progenitor cells (CD34+) out of the bone marrow and into the peripheral blood, allowing easy access to high numbers of CD34+ cells to be collected by apheresis. In the autologous peripheral blood stem cell (PBSC) setting, transplantation of >2.5 × 10^6 CD34+ cells per kilogram leads to engraftment of granulocytes to 500/μl by day 12 and platelets to 20,000/μl by day 14. This is more rapid than with autologous marrow, and subsequently shows few cases of morbidity from transplantation. If marrow is the source of stem cells, recovery of neutrophils to 500/μl occurs by day 22. Thus the use of G-CSF-mobilized peripheral blood stem cells speeds the rate of recovery by approximately 1 week when compared to mar-

row (Mechanic et al., 2003). Use of G-CSF or GM-CSF posttransplant can further accelerate recovery by 3 to 5 days, while use of methotrexate to prevent GVHD delays engraftment by a similar period in the allogeneic setting (Korbling and Anderlini, 2001).

In a study by Bensinger and colleagues (2001), 172 patients with hematologic malignancies were randomized between allogeneic bone marrow and allogeneic mobilized peripheral blood stem cells. The objective was to compare rates of engraftment and incidence of GVHD. It was found that the time to > 500 neutrophils/mm^3 was 16 days for peripheral blood and 21 days for bone marrow ($p < 0.001$), and time to > 20,000 platelets/mm^3 was 13 days for peripheral blood and 19 days for bone marrow ($p < 0.001$). GVHD was slightly higher in the peripheral blood stem cells group; however, the 2-year disease-free survival was significantly improved, as compared to bone marrow transplant group (65% versus 45%, $p = 0.03$). This study concluded that mobilized allogeneic peripheral stem cells have faster engraftment rates, similar incidences of GVHD, and a significant improvement in rates of disease control compared to stem cells harvested from bone marrow (Bensinger et al., 2001).

Another source of hematopoietic stem cells for use after myeloablative therapy is umbilical cord blood (UCB). Umbilical cord blood contains a high concentration of hematopoietic progenitor cells, but engraftment is slower than with marrow. GVHD is less frequent because of the lower number of T cells in cord blood. A disadvantage of UCB as a source of hematopoietic stem cells is the myelosuppression (approximately 28 days for neutrophils and 60 days for platelets), which is lengthier than for peripheral blood and bone marrow. Another disadvantage is that the number of CD34+ cells collected from a single donor is not adequate to transplant to an adult (Gluckman et al., 2000; Rocha et al., 2001).

Graft Failure

Graft failure after autologous transplant is not common, but it can occur. Causes of graft failure include inadequate numbers of stem cells being transplanted, damage of stem cells during ex vivo treatment or during the freezing and storage process, use of myelotoxic drugs posttransplant, or infections with cytomegalovirus (CMV) or human herpes virus type 6. After allogeneic transplantation, rejection may occur because of immunologic rejection of the stem cell product by immune-competent host cells. This is more common when patients receive T cell-depleted stem cells or cells from HLA-mismatched donors.

Immune Recovery

The literature comparing immune reconstitution after allogeneic PBSCT or BMT is limited because of the potential for further immunosuppression and myelosupression from treatment for GVHD and antifungal and antiviral infections (Korbling and Anderlini, 2001). The two determinants of immunologic recovery after allogeneic BMT are time after transplant and chronic GVHD (Parkman and Weinberg, 2004). The short-term consequence of severe immunosuppression occurring after myeloablative therapy is the susceptibility to bacterial, fungal, and viral infections. Even though the granulocyte count may appear normal after transplant, it is expected that during the first 4 months, the newly generated granulocytes will function on a suboptimal level. B and T cells may reach normal levels 3 to 4 months after

BMT. To date, no studies have clearly shown a difference in either B cell or T cell recovery after allogeneic PBSC transplantation compared to BM transplantation (Cottler-Fox et al., 2003).

Immune recovery after umbilical cord blood hematopoietic cell transplant (UCBHCT) is similar or slightly less superior to BMT. NK cell activity is similar for both BMT and UCB (Johnston and Blume, 2000).

B Cell Reconstitution

As previously stated, the number of mature B cells (CD19 and CD20), are decreased during the first 3 months after autologous hematopoietic stem cell transplant (AHSCT) and increase gradually, taking up to 18 months to normalize. (Porrata et al., 2001). For both allogeneic and autologous stem cell transplant, B cell production of immunoglobulins is also delayed. Normal serum levels of IgM may take up to 6 months to return and those of IgG may take 12 to 18 months but can take longer.

This causes the antibody response to recall antigens such as tetanus toxoid, diphtheria toxoid, or measles virus to be delayed for a year or longer (Porrata et al., 2001).

T Cell Reconstitution

When stem cells are harvested by apheresis, there are 10 times more T cells present than in a bone marrow harvest. Levels of CD3+ T lymphocytes (CD3+ signifies mature T cells) can remain low for 1 year or longer. CD8+ cells (T suppressor cells) increase and return sooner than CD4+ cells (T helper cells), which are decreased, causing in an inverted CD4/CD8 ratio for up to 1 year (Witherspoon, 2000).

NK cells recover normal levels within one month of transplant and recover faster for patients who have had an autologous BMT versus allogeneic BMT. However, 80 to 100 days posttransplant, both autologous BMT and autologous peripheral blood stem cell transplantation showed the same percentage of NK cells.

Even when it appears that hematologic recovery has occurred, and neutrophils and platelets appear normal, recovery of normal humoral and cellular immunity can take up to 1 year. In order for immunizations with vaccine to be effective, long-term, adequate T lymphocyte immune competence must be established (Parkman and Weinberg, 2004). Guidelines are in place by the Centers for Disease Control and Prevention (CDC) for reimmunizing patients after HSCT (CDC, 2000).

The quality and rate of immunologic recovery is thought to be influenced by specific cell populations present in the bone marrow or blood stem cell product at the time of transplantation. PBSCs contain more T cells and more NK cells than bone marrow cells. This results in a more rapid return of cellular immune function, evidenced by in vitro assays; however, little information is available comparing the infection rates among autologous PBSC and marrow recipients after hematopoietic recovery (Kessinger, 2000, 2003).

In summary, mobilized peripheral blood stem cells show a more rapid engraftment time for both neutrophils and platelets as compared to bone marrow stem cells and umbilical cord blood stem cells. UCB transplants have the slowest rate of engraftment overall. Source of stem cells, conditioning/preparative regimen, inadequate number of CD34+ stem cells, myelosuppressive drugs used posttransplant, infections, and chronic GVHD all have the ability to interfere with hematopoietic and immunologic recovery.

The longer it takes for hematopoietic and immunologic recovery to occur, the higher the risk for morbidity and mortality. Research is ongoing to find less toxic ways of controlling diseases of the bone marrow by manipulating the bone marrow cells and bone marrow environment without causing devastating side effects to bone marrow.

Identification of Cells for Transplantation

All hematopoietic cells derived from the pluripotent stem cells have the capacity for long-term, self-repopulation into all hematopoietic cell lineages. One stem cell can produce 10^6 mature hematopoietic cells, and a healthy adult can produce more than 10^{12} hematopoietic cells in a day. Progenitor cells, are more mature than hematopoietic stem cells in that they are committed to a certain cell lineage, i.e., neutrophil or platelet (see Figure 2-1). Physical properties distinguish stem cells needed for transplantation from others contained in the marrow and blood. A number of quantitative assays are used to identify and isolate these primitive hematopoietic cells based on their physical characteristics (Donahue and Carter, 1995; Munker et al., 2000).

Evaluation of Pluripotent Stem Cells for Transplantation

In vitro assays are used to determine the presence and number of primitive and lineage-committed hematopoietic stem cells. The first method to measure the number of pluripotent stem cells in the marrow was the spleen colony assay. In the early 1960s, McCulloch and Till (1960) described the ability of injected bone marrow cells to form colonies in the spleens of mice that had received lethal doses of irradiation. For the next 30 years, this colony-forming unit-spleen (CFU-S) assay was used as an indicator of stem cell frequency in infused cell suspensions. These cells do not have long-term repopulating ability and are not the cells responsible for long-term engraftment. Thus the CFU-S does not identify the true stem cell (McNiece and Briddell, 1994; Sekhsaria et al., 1995).

From this beginning, a number of other systems have been developed to identify the various subpopulations of hematopoietic cells. Cell culture assays were developed in animal models and adapted for human cells (Messner and McCullough, 1994). Semisolid culture mediums are used to identify clones of progenitor cells at levels of differentiation (McNiece and Briddell, 1994). The most immature population of cells that can be identified by this method is denoted colony-forming unit-blast (CFU-blast) cells, which, if left to grow in culture, develop into megakaryocytes, erythrocytes, and granulocytes in 6 to 8 weeks. These cells can be cloned to form exact colonies, but they do not have the same indefinite self-renewal ability (McNiece and Briddell, 1994; Sekhsaria et al., 1995). Long-term culture-initiating cells (LTC-IC) are cells in colonies that give rise to mature cells after an interval of 5 to 8 weeks in marrow culture systems (Orlic and Bodine, 1994). The LTC-ICs can be used with both marrow and blood stem cells, and they are also called long-term marrow culture (LTMC); however, these culture assays are time-consuming and costly and take several weeks to obtain results (Meagher, 2003). High-proliferative potential cultures (HPPCs) measure cells between LTC-IC and assays for CFU-GM, colony-forming unit-erythroid (CFU-E), and CFU-GEMM. They are considered to be very primitive cells (Charbord, 1994). Stem cell factor was described using HPPC assays.

CD34-Positive Cells

Another method to distinguish cell populations relies on staining cell surface molecules with a monoclonal antibody linked to fluorescent dyes. These cluster differentiation (CD) antigens and the monoclonal antibodies that attach to them are assigned CD numbers. For example, CD5 marks both T and B lymphocytes; CD1, CD3, and CD7 are markers only for T lymphocytes; CD21, CD22, CD37, and CD40 are associated only with B lymphocytes; and CD34 marks the hematopoietic stem and progenitor cells (Munker et al., 2000).

The CD34 assay is the most common way to identify stem cells for engraftment (Bensinger, 1994; Cottler-Fox et al., 2003). The stem cells are found in the mononuclear fraction of the marrow suspension, and their morphology resembles blast cells. The CD34 marker was identified when a monoclonal antibody was developed against a leukemia cell line, separating cells that could give rise to all hematopoietic colonies.

Within the CD34+ cells there is a subpopulation that has the property of self-renewal (Berenstein et al., 1991). It is estimated that the actual number of true stem cells ranges from 1×10^4 to 2×10^5 cells. Efforts continue to separate the rich subpopulations such as lineage-negative cells (lin-cells), cells in G0 phase (resting phase of cell cycle), and others that are present in fetal cord blood and in low concentrations in normal peripheral blood (Bender et al., 1994). In addition to using CD34 assays to identify cells for a transplant, these cells are being manipulated ex vivo to increase their numbers. Expansion of small populations of cells could decrease the number of phereses required, or it could make specific cells available for therapeutic gene transfer (Brugger et al., 1993).

CD34 antigens are not found on breast tumors, neuroblastoma, lymphoma, and multiple myeloma cells (Shpall et al., 1994). In theory, stem cell isolates from these patients should be free of tumor contamination. In other words, CD34 + selection should deplete cancer cells from the marrow or peripheral blood (Berenson, 1993). However, the purity of the cells is not complete. For example, one third of the cells collected using the common system, the avidin-biotin system, are neither stem cells nor progenitors (Bensinger, 1994). In addition, the CD34 antigen is also expressed in certain types of leukemia cells. Efforts continue to identify ways to purify marrow and blood cells from patients with leukemia (Berenson, 1993).

In summary, stem cells continue to be best identified by the expression of the CD34 antigen by flow cytometry. Most stem cells express CD34. A small amount of CD34 cells are pluripotent cells, capable of self-renewal and differentiating into all blood cell lineages. The majority of CD34+ cells are progenitor cells already committed to a certain cell lineage. Thus, for marrow transplantation to be complete and sustained, a sufficient number of stem cells must be transplanted. The number of stem cells collected for transplantation varies between centers but usually falls between 2 and 5×10^6 CD34+ cells/kg (Munker et al., 2000; Cottler-Fox et al., 2003). Specifics concerning stem cell infusions and the amounts used are discussed in another chapter of this book.

Sources of Stem Cells for Transplantation

Hematopoietic stem cell transplantation is a well-established treatment modality and has been used for more than three decades to treat an expanding list of malignant and nonmalignant disease processes. Sadly, this life-saving treatment is not available for all who seek it due to lack of a suitable donor. Although the primary source of hematopoietic cells (HCs) has traditionally been the bone marrow (BM), noteworthy clinical research has expanded the graft employed by marrow-derived HCs to include peripheral blood (PB) and umbilical cord blood (UCB) (Warkentin et al., 2004). A short description of the sources of HCs available to patients today follows. A more detailed description will be provided in Chapter 4.

Bone Marrow

Harvested from the iliac crest, BM can be obtained from related, unrelated, HLA-matched, and mis-matched donors. The amount required to achieve hematopoiesis is 10–15 ml/kg of recipient body weight. The marrow is processed and filtered to remove fat and bone chips, is heparinized to prevent coagulation, and is otherwise manipulated to achieve any additional supportive effects to minimize posttransplant complications, for example T cell depletion to minimize GVHD (Wujcik, 1997). The final product, although rich in stem cells, also contains a fair amount of RBCs, which accounts for its deep, red color. Because of its large final volume and precise infusion parameters, BM can take between 4 to 12 hours to infuse. Care must be taken to ensure accurate documentation of completion of BM, since this correlates with the designation of day 0, transplant day status. This milestone is important for the initiation of GVHD prophylaxis. Of particular note with the sources of stem cell products is the time to engraftment. Time to engraftment varies based on stem cell source. For related or unrelated BM, engraftment occurs around +21 post-HSCT (Schmitz, 2004).

Peripheral Blood Hematopoietic Cells (PBHC)

In 1909, Alexander Maxinov first hypothesized the presence of hematopoietic progenitor cells (HPCs) in the peripheral blood (Schmitz, 2004). PBHC was first introduced as a viable stem cell source in 1981 (Korbling and Anderlini, 2001). Research into this hypothesis continued for decades, but it wasn't until the advent of recombinant growth factors in the mobilization of CD34+ progenitor cells that autologous, then allogeneic PBHC transplants emerged in the clinical arena. With filgrastim, collection of CD34+ cell counts ranging from 2–20 × 10^6/kg body weight were achieved (Schmitz, 2004). This was a remarkable enhancement to a newly established treatment modality.

There are many differences in the harvested products of BM versus PBHC beyond the obvious decreased volume. PBHC harvests contain 10 times more T cells than does BM. Remarkably, this increased number of T cells does not correlate with an increase in acute GVHD. Acute GVHD, grades II–IV, was similarly experienced by PBHC patients as by BM patients. One disadvantage was an increase in chronic GVHD seen in the PBHC patients. Furthermore, a remarkably higher number of CD14+ cells, dendritic cells, and natural killer cells have also been documented. Engraftment occurs much faster in PBHC transplant. On average, initial signs of engraftment are seen 2 to 6 days earlier than in the BM population, often as early as day +11 with an average of day +16. The longest time to engraftment was noted at day +29.

Umbilical Cord Blood (UCB)

Despite successful transplantation of BM and PBHC, suitable HLA-matched donors are not available for all patients in need of transplant. National Marrow Donor Program (NMDP) statistics indicate that fewer than 80% of Caucasians and approximately 50% of African-American donors have a suitably matched unrelated donor (Wadlow and Porter, 2002). In the last decade, expansive research has been conducted in the area of umbilical cord blood as a cell source for transplantation (Broxmeyer and Smith, 2004). The first cord blood transplant was performed in 1988 in France on a 5-year-old Fanconi's anemia patient. Its success ushered in a new era in transplant medicine and provided yet another readily available source of stem cells. It also led to the development of the UCB banking system in use today (Broxmeyer and Smith, 2004; Wadlow and Porter, 2002).

There are both advantages and disadvantages to the use of UCB. UCB is a rich source of hematopoietic cells (Warkentin et al., 2004). It is also readily available and places donors at no apparent risk (Broxmeyer and Smith, 2004). Because the fetal immune system is not fully mature at the time of birth, T cells within the final product are also very immature (Wadlow and Porter, 2002). These immunologically immature T cells allow for cord blood to be transplanted in mismatched donors without the significant risk of acute and chronic GVHD (Broxmeyer and Smith, 2004). However, the disadvantages associated with UCB transplant are significant. There is ample evidence to support delayed neutrophil and platelet recovery, placing the patient at increased risk for morbidity and mortality secondary to infection and bleeding. This is due, in part, to the fact that cord blood units have only one tenth as many nucleated cells and CD34+ cells as BM or PBHC (Wadlow and Porter, 2002). Because of this, and the lack of determination of appropriate volume to infuse, numerous ex vivo expansion techniques are being explored. Such manipulation places the patient at increased risk for hypersensitivity reaction and poor tolerance of product infusion. Finally, long-term data associated with unrelated UCB transplants is limited, and little is known about the transference of undetected genetic abnormalities (Broxmeyer and Smith, 2004). The true advantages and disadvantages of UCB transplantation are still being explored. Moreover, there are multiple ethical, legal, and financial considerations in cord blood banking yet to be explored. Ex vivo expansion techniques and managing the issues related to latent neutrophil and platelet recovery all require additional research (Broxmeyer and Smith, 2004).

Conclusion

The past 30 years have provided a wealth of new information and insight into the miraculous process of human hematopoiesis. Such learning has enabled researchers to hone the treatment of marrow and stem cell transplantation. Increased knowledge of human growth factor has facilitated the development of recombinant drugs supporting mobilization therapy and symptom management, giving way to quicker and more durable grafts. The advent of nonmyeloablative stem cell transplant has expanded this life-saving treatment option to a new patient population, and hematopoiesis is at the core of this modality. It is this commitment to the science and technology of transplant medicine that focuses and guides the future of this fascinating field of medicine.

Dedication

Kathleen Finn and I would like to dedicate this chapter to the many patients and families who have helped give face to our understanding of human hematopoiesis. Their willingness to walk the stem cell transplant journey has opened a world of understanding to this subject and transplant in general. It is for them that we continually strive to learn more, work harder, and be better!

I would personally like to dedicate my work on this chapter to my wonderful family, who have supported me throughout my transplant career, never tiring of my endless stories or fascination with the science and research that is stem cell transplant. To my brother, David John, whose battle with acute lymphocytic leukemia ended in 1968, when transplant was in its infancy, thank you for inspiring me every day.

Melinda S. Chouinard, RN, BSN, OCN®

References

Bagby, G.C., & Heinrich, M.C. (1999). Cytokines, growth factors, and hematopoiesis. In Wingard, J.R. & Demetri, G.R. (Eds.), *Clinical applications of cytokines and growth factors* (pp. 2–55). Norwell, MA: Kluwer Academic Publishers.

Bauer, S. (2000). Immunology. In Yarbro, C.H., Frogee, M.H., Goodman, M., & Groenwald, S.L. (Eds.), *Cancer nursing principles and practice* (5th ed., pp. 35–48). Boston: Jones & Bartlett.

Bender, J.G., Unverzagt, K., Walker, D.E., Lee, W., Smith, S., Williams, S., et al. (1994). Phenotypic analysis and characterization of CD34-positive cells from normal human bone marrow, cord blood, peripheral blood, and mobilized peripheral blood from patients undergoing autologous stem cell transplantation. *Clin Immunopathol, 70*(1), 10–18.

Bensinger, W. (1994). Isolating stem and progenitor cells. In Gale, R.P., Juttner, C.A., & Henon, P. (Eds.), *Blood* stem cell transplants (pp. 32–42). New York: Cambridge University Press.

Bensinger, W.I., Martin, P.J., Storer, B., Clift, R., Forman, S.J., Negrin, R., et al. (2001). Transplantation of bone marrow as compared with peripheral blood cells from HLA-identical relatives in patients with hematologic cancers. N Engl J Med, 344, 175.

Berenson, R. (1993). Human stem cell transplantation (review). Leukemia & Lymphoma, 11(suppl. 2), 137–139.

Berenstein, I.D., Andrews, R.G., & Zsebo, K.M. (1991). Recombinant human stem cell factor enhances the formation of colonies by CD34-positive and CD34 positive lin-cells, and the generation of colony-forming progeny from CD34-positive lin-cells cultured with interleukin-3 (IL-3), granulocyte-macrophage colony-stimulating factor (GM-CSF). Blood, 77, 2316–2321.

Broxmeyer, H.E., & Smith, F.O. (2004). Cord blood hematopoietic cell transplantation. In Foreman, S., Blume, K., & Appelbaum, F. (Eds.), Thomas's hematopoietic cell transplantation (4th ed., pp. 550–564). Malden, MA: Blackwell Publishing.

Brugger, W., Mocklin, W., Heimfeld, S., Berenson, R.J., Mertelsmann, R., & Kantz, L. (1993). Ex vivo expansion of enriched peripheral blood CD34 positive progenitor cells by stem cell factor, interleukin-1 beta (IL-1beta), IL-6, IL-3, interferon-gamma, and erythropoietin. Blood, 81(10), 2579–2584.

Brunstein, C., & Verfaillie, C.M. (2004). The hematopoietic microenvironment. In Foreman, S., Blume, K., & Appelbaum, F. (Eds.), Thomas's hematopoietic cell transplantation (3rd ed., pp. 53–61). Malden, MA: Blackwell Publishing.

Buchsel, P.C., Forgey, A., Browning Grape, F., & Hamann, S.S. (2002). Granulocyte macrophage colony-stimulating factor: Current practice and novel approaches. Clin J Oncol Nurs, 6(4). Retrieved June 11, 2005, from http://www.ons.org/ publication/journals/CJON/volume6/Issue4/0604198-asp

Caudell, K.A., & Whedon, M.B. (1991). Hematopoietic complications. In Whedon, M.B. (Ed.), Bone marrow transplantation: Principles, practice, and nursing insights (pp. 135–159). Boston: Jones & Bartlett.

Centers for Disease Control and Prevention. (2000). Guidelines for preventing opportunistic infections among hematopoietic stem cell transplant recipients: Recommendations of CDC, the Infectious Disease Society of America, and the American Society of Blood and Marrow Transplantation. MMWR, 49(No. RR-10), 52–53.

Charbord, P. (1994). Hematopoietic stem cells: Analysis of some parameters critical for engraftment. Stem Cells, 12, 545–562.

Cottler-Fox, M.H., Lapidot, T., Petit, I., Kellet, O., DiPersio, J.F., & Link, D. (2003). Stem cell mobilization. In Berliner, N., Larson, R.A., Leung, L.L., & Bajus, J.L. (Eds.), Hematology: American Society of Hematology. Education program book. (pp. 419–437).

Crawford, J. (2003). Pegfilgrastim: The promise of pegylation fulfilled. Ann Oncol, 14, 6–7.

Donahue, R.E., & Carter, B.S. (1995). In Brecher, M.E., Lasky, L.C., Sacher, R.A., & Issitt, L.A. (Eds.), Hematopoietic progenitor cells: Processing, standards and practice (pp. 41–57). Bethesda, MD: American Association of Blood Banks.

Ellerhorst-Ryan, J.M. (2000). Infection. In Yarbro, C.H., Frogee, M.H., Goodman, M., & Groenwald, S.L. (Eds.), Cancer nursing principles and practice (5th ed., pp. 691–708). Boston: Jones & Bartlett.

Emerson, G., Adams, S., & Taichman, R. (2000). The hematopoietic microenvironment. In Armitage, J.O., & Antman, K.H. (Eds.), High-dose cancer therapy: Pharmacology, hematopoietins, stem cells (3rd ed., pp. 185–192). Philadelphia: Lippincott Williams & Wilkins.

Finke, H., & Mertelsmann, R. (2004). Recombinant growth factors after hematopoietic cell transplantation. In Foreman, S., Blume, K.G., & Appelbaum, F. (Eds.), Thomas's hematopoietic cell transplantation (4th ed., pp. 613–623). Malden, MA: Blackwell Publishing.

Gajewski, J. (2002). Use of thrombopoietin in combination with chemotherapy and granulocyte colony-stimulating factor for peripheral blood progenitor cell mobilization. Biol Blood Marrow Transplantation, 8, 550–556.

Gluckman, E., Rocha, V., & Chastang, C. (2000). Allogeneic cord blood hematopoietic stem cell transplants in malignancies. In Armitage, J.O., & Antman, K.H. (Eds.), High-dose cancer therapy: Pharmacology, hematopoietins, stem cells (3rd ed., pp. 211–220). Philadelphia: Lippincott Williams & Wilkins.

Griffin, J.P. (1986). Immunity. In Griffin, J.P. (Ed.), Hematology and immunology for nurses (pp. 41–54). Norwalk, CT: Appleton-Century-Crofts.

Johnston, C., & Blume, K. (2000). Hematologic reconstitution after allogeneic hematopoietic cell transplantation. In Armitage, J.O. & Antman, K. H. (Eds.), High-dose cancer therapy: Pharmacology, hematopoietins, *stem cells* (3rd ed., pp. 193–209). Philadelphia: Lippincott Williams & Wilkins.

Kessinger, A. (2003). Clinical features of autologous and allogeneic peripheral blood progenitor cell transplantation. In McLeod, B.C. (Ed.), *Apheresis: Principles and practice* (2nd ed., pp. 493–502). Bethesda, MD: AABB Press.

Kessinger, A. (2000). Reestablishing hematopoiesis with peripheral stem cells. In Armitage, J.O., & Antman, K.H. (Eds.), *High-dose cancer therapy: Pharmacology, hematopoietins, stem cells* (3rd ed., pp. 272–273. Philadelphia: Lippincott Williams & Wilkins.

Korbling, M., & Anderlini, P. (2001). Peripheral blood stem cell versus bone marrow allotransplantation: Does the source of hematopoietic stem cell matter? *Blood, 98*(10), 2900–2908.

Kutler, D.J., & Beagley, S.G. (2002). Recombinant human thrombopoietin: Basic biology and evaluation of clinical studies. *Blood, 15*(100), 3457–3469.

Littlewood, T.J., Nortier, J., Rapoport, B., Pawlicki, M., deWalsch, G., Vercammen, E., et al. (2003). Epoetin alfa corrects anemia and improves quality of life in patients with hematologic malignancies receiving non-platinum based chemotherapy. *Hematol Oncol, 21,* 169–180.

McCulloch, E.A., & Till, J.E, (1960). The radiation sensitivity of normal mouse bone marrow cells, determined by quantitative marrow transplantation into irradiated mice. *Radiat Res, 13,* 115–125.

McNiece, I.K., & Briddell, R.A. (1994). Primitive hematopoietic colony-forming cells with high proliferative potential. In Freshney, R.I., Pragnell, I.B., & Freshney, M.G. (Eds.), *Culture of hematopoietic cells* (pp. 23–29). New York: Wiley.

Meagher, R.C. (2003). Peripheral blood progenitor cell graft engineering. In McLeod, B.C. (Ed.), *Apheresis: Principles and practice* (2nd ed., pp. 545–556). Bethesda, MD: AABB Press.

Mechanic, S.A., Krause, D., Proytcheva, M.A., & Snyder, E.L. (2003). Mobilization and collection of peripheral blood progenitor cells. In McLeod, B.C. (Ed.), *Apheresis: Principles and practice* (2nd ed., pp. 503–530). Bethesda, MD: AABB Press.

Messner, H.A., & McCullough, E.A. (1994). Mechanisms of human hematopoiesis. In Forman, S.J., Blume, K.G., & Thomas, E.D. (Eds.), *Bone marrow transplantation* (pp. 41–54). Boston: Blackwell Scientific.

Metcalf, D. (1998). Mechanism of human hematopoiesis. In Thomas, E.D., Blume, K.G., & Foreman, S.J. (Eds.), *Hematopoietic cell transplantation* (pp. 48–87). Boston: Blackwell Scientific.

Munker, R., Hiller, E., & Paquette, R. (2000). *Modern hematology: Biology and clinical management* (pp. 1–18, 341–346). Totowa, NJ: Humana Press.

Ng-Cashin, J., & Shea, T. (2004). Mobilization of autologous peripheral blood hematopoietic cells in support of high dose cancer therapy. In Foreman, S., Blume, K., & Appelbaum, F. (Eds.), *Thomas's hematopoietic stem cell transplantation* (pp. 576–586). Malden, MA: Blackwell Publishing.

Orlic, D., & Bodine, D.M. (1994). What defines a pluripotent stem cell (PHSC): Will the real PHSC please stand up! *J Am Soc Hematol, 84*(12), 3991–3994.

Parkman, R., & Weinberg, K.I. (2004). Peripheral blood hematopoietic cells for allogeneic transplantation. In Foreman, S., Blume, K., & Appelbaum, F. (Eds.), *Thomas's hematopoietic cell transplantation* (4th ed., pp. 588–598). Malden, MA: Blackwell Publishing.

Porrata, L.F., Litzow, M.R., & Markovic, S.N. (2001). Immune reconstitution after autologous hematopoietic stem cell transplant. *Mayo Clinc Proc, 76,* 407–412.

Rieger, P.T. (1999). The immune system. In Vis, G., & Ames, L. (Eds.). *Clinical handbook for biotherapy* (pp. 22–46). Boston: Jones & Bartlett.

Rocha, V., Cornish, J., Sievers, E.L., Filipovich, A., Locatelli, F., & Peters, C. (2001). Comparison of outcomes of unrelated bone marrow and umbilical cord blood transplants in children with acute leukemia. *Blood, 97,* 2962.

Schmit-Pokorny, K. (2004). Stem cell collection. In Ezzone, S. (Ed.), *Hematopoietic stem cell transplantation: A manual for nursing practice* (pp. 23–42). Pittsburgh, PA: ONS Publishing.

Schmitz, N. (2004). Peripheral blood hematopoietic cells for allogeneic transplantation. In Foreman, S., Blume, K., & Appelbaum, F. (Eds.), *Thomas's hematopoietic cell transplantation* (4th ed., pp. 588–598). Malden, MA: Blackwell Publishing.

Sekhsaria, S., Sacher, R.A., Malech, H.L., & Fleisher, T.A. (1995). Flow cytometric characterization of umbilical cord blood progenitor cells. In Brecher, M.E., Lasky, L.C., Sacher, R.A., & Issitt, L.A. (Eds.), *Hematopoietic progenitor cells: Processing, standards and practice* (pp. 19–35). Bethesda, MD: American Association of Blood Banks.

Shames, R.S., & Kishiyama, J.L. (2003). Disorders of the immune system. In McPhee, S., Lingappa, V.R., Ganong, W. & Lange (Eds.). *Pathophysiology of disease* (4th ed., pp. 37–57). New York: McGraw-Hill.

Shpall, E.J., Jones, R.B., Bearman, S.I., Franklin, W.A., Archer, P.G., Curiel, T., et al. (1994). Transplantation of enriched CD34-positive autologous marrow into breast cancer patients following high-dose chemotherapy: Influence of CD34-positive peripheral blood progenitors and growth factors on engraftment. *J Clin Oncol, 12*(1), 28–36.

Sutherland, C.W. (2000). The immunology of peripheral blood stem cell transplantation. In Buchsel, P., & Kapustay, P.M. (Eds.), *Stem cell transplant: A clinical textbook* (pp. 2.03–2.24). Pittsburgh, PA: Oncology Nursing Society Press.

Vance, R. (2003). Darbopoetin alfa. *Clin J Oncol Nursing,* 7(5), 599–600.

Wadlow, R.C., & Porter, D.L. (2002). Umbilical cord blood transplantation: Where do we stand? *Biol Blood Marrow Transplantation, 8,* 637–647.

Warkentin, P.L., Lewis, N., & Shpall, E. (2004). Hematopoietic cell procurement, processing and transplantation: Regulation and accreditation. In Foreman, S., Blume, K., & Appelbaum, F. (Eds.), *Thomas's hematopoietic cell transplantation* (4th ed., pp. 531–537). Malden, MA: Blackwell Publishing.

Widmaier, E.P., Hershel, R., & Strang, K.T. (2004). In Vander, A.J., Sherman, J., & Luciano, D.S. (Eds.), *Human physiology: The mechanisms of body function* (9th ed., pp. 695–730). New York: McGraw-Hill.

Wilkes, G.M., Ingwerson, K., & Barton-Burke, M. (2003). *2003 oncology nursing drug handbook* (pp. 317–363). Boston: Jones & Bartlett.

Williams, L. (2004). Comprehensive review of hematopoiesis and immunology: Implications for hematopoietic stem cell transplant recipients. In Ezzone, S. (Ed.), *Hematopoietic stem cell transplantation: A manual for nursing practice* (pp. 1–12). Pittsburgh, PA: ONS Publishing.

Witherspoon, R.P. (2000). Immunologic reconstitution after high-dose chemoradiotherapy and allogeneic or autologous bone marrow or peripheral blood hematopoietic stem cell transplant. In Armitage, J.D., & Antman, K.H. (Eds.), *High-dose cancer therapy: pharmacology, hematopoietins, stem cells* (3rd ed., pp. 283–300). Philadelphia: Lippincott Williams & Wilkins.

Wujcik, D. (1997). Hematopoiesis. In Whedon, M.B. (Ed.), *Blood and marrow stem cell transplantation: Principles, practice, and nursing insights* (pp. 25–42). Sudbury, MA: Jones & Bartlett.

Chapter 3

Hematopoietic Stem Cell Transplant Immunology

Boglarka
Gyurkocza, MD

Melinda S.
Chouinard, RN,
BSN, OCN®

"Blut ist ein ganz besond'rer Saft."
(Blood is a quite particular fluid)
—*Mephisto in Goethe's* Faust

"When mice are given an otherwise lethal dose of X rays to the whole body they can recover if injected intravenously with homologous {allogeneic} myeloid cells. . . . This suggests that leukemia of the mouse might be successfully treated. On the one hand, the dose of X rays which is sufficiently lethal to normal cells of the bone marrow and lymphatic tissue to cause death of the animal might well be completely lethal to leukemic cells. . . . On the other hand, if the dose of X rays sufficient to kill the animal is not 100% lethal to leukemic cells, the malignant condition would in these circumstances recur by growth from these surviving cells, since neither host nor graft has the ability to resist; but, if homologous bone marrow from a different strain of mouse were given, the colonizing cells might retain the capacity of the donor to destroy by the reaction of immunity these residual leukemic cells—and perhaps also the host."

Barnes et al., 1956

The double-edged sword, like the nature of the immunologic reactions following allogeneic stem cell transplantation, was recognized as early as five decades ago. Since then, our understanding of these reactions became more sophisticated, and a molecular-level description of alloimmune interactions and the process of immune recovery leading to tolerance has emerged. However, we are still unable to optimally utilize the therapeutic effects of these immunologic phenomena without imposing mortality and significant morbidity on our patients.

During allogeneic stem cell transplantation, the establishment of the donor's immune system in an antigenically distinct recipient may provide a therapeutic graft-versus-malignancy effect, but at the same time, it causes graft-versus-host disease (GVHD) and prolonged immune dysfunction. In this chapter, new developments of understanding alloresponses and strategies to control immune reconstitution will be discussed.

The curative effect of allogeneic stem cell transplantation is attributed, at least partially, to an allogeneic immune response: the graft-versus-leukemia (or graft-versus-tumor) effect.

For the last two decades or so, our understanding of the graft-versus-leukemia (GVL) phenomenon has changed dramatically.

In the late 1970s, as teams around the world began performing allogeneic transplantations for leukemia patients, some patients were noted to have a remarkable response. In 1978, a published case discussed a patient whose leukemia was recurring following an allogeneic transplant (Odom et al., 1978). This patient then developed GVHD and, coincidentally, achieved hematologic remission. A year later, the clinical experience of the Seattle transplant team was summarized (Weiden et al., 1979); these data indicated that patients developing GVHD following allogeneic bone marrow transplant (BMT) from a human leukocyte antigen (HLA)-identical sibling had a decreased rate of leukemic relapse.

Eleven years passed, and in 1990 the International Bone Marrow Transplant Registry published an analysis (Horowitz et al., 1990) of 2254 patients receiving bone marrow transplantation for leukemia. Based on the data from such a large number of patients, three important conclusions regarding GVL were drawn. First, patients developing GVHD following allogeneic BMT had decreased incidence of leukemic relapse in comparison to those who did not experience GVHD. Second, among patients who did not develop any GVHD, the recipients of identical-twin donor marrow had a greater rate of leukemic relapse than the recipients of HLA-identical sibling marrow (approximately 46% versus 25%). Third, for patients who did not experience GVHD, the recipients of T cell-depleted HLA-identical sibling marrow had a greater chance of leukemic relapse than those who received non-depleted HLA-identical bone marrow (41% versus 25%). The importance of allorecognition in the antileukemic reaction became clear, and it

was also shown that T cells were at least partially responsible for these phenomena.

HLA Typing and Beyond

Human Leukocyte Antigens

The principal antigeneic barrier to transplantation—any transplantation—is a series of molecules that are products of a closely linked cluster of genes known as the major histocompatibility complex or MHC (Suthanthiran and Strom, 1994). These genes are located in a 4-Mb region of DNA on chromosome 6 (see **Figure 3-1**), and, in general, are inherited as a single unit in simple Mendelian fashion. The products of these genes, the human leukocyte histocompatibility antigens, are cell surface glycoproteins that present antigen peptide fragments to T cell receptors. They can be divided in two distinct classes, class I and class II. Class I antigens are expressed on the surfaces of virtually all nucleated cells at varying densities and present small peptide fragments to CD8+ cells. Class II molecules are more restricted to cells of the immune system, primarily B lymphocytes, monocytes, and macrophages; they present antigen peptide fragments to CD4+ cells. It is important to note the dynamic changes in the density of these molecules: Cytokines secreted by lymphocytes and monocytes during immune activation can cause dramatic increases in HLA class II antigen expression, even on cell types that normally have little or no surface expression (Halloran et al., 1986). HLA molecules provide the surface upon which the antigen receptors on T lymphocytes recognize foreign (non-self) antigens. In the last decade, due to the use of molecular biologic techniques (for example, sequencing of the human genome) an

Figure 3-1 Location and organization of the HLA complex on chromosome 6. The complex is divided into three regions: I, II, III (and IV, see text). Each region contains numerous loci (genes), only some of which are shown.

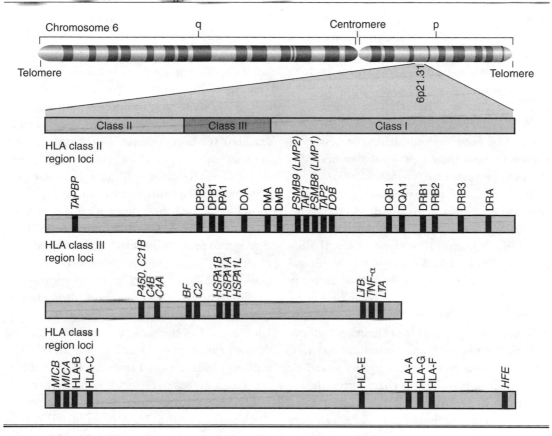

Source: Adapted from Klein et al. (2000). System—First of two parts. *N Engl J Med, 343*(10), 702–709.

ever-expanding number of immune-related genes, the class III and IV regions, lying between the class I and II genomic areas, has been found. The class III region encodes several components of the complement system, while the class IV region (located between the class III and I areas) contains a large cluster of immune-related genes, including tumor necrosis factor alpha and beta and numerous less characterized genes and gene families.

HLA Classes

As mentioned previously, the HLA region has been subdivided into class I, class II, class III, and class IV regions. Each region contains numerous gene loci and each locus may encode a large number of polymorphic alleles. Class I and class II antigens are composed of two chains, usually called the alpha and beta chains, which dimerize to form the final molecule.

Class I antigens are made up of a heavy chain containing the polymorphic regions (variations in gene sequence), which combines with the nonpolymorphic light chain, called beta-2 microglobulin, to form the final dimerized molecule. The beta-2 microglobulin is encoded on chromosome 15, not in the MHC.

The classic class I HLA antigens include HLA-A, -B, and -C antigens, which are expressed on almost all cells of the body at varying density. HLA-E, -F, and -G antigens have also been identified; these genes generally have quite restricted expression, and their functional significance is still being investigated (Geraghty, 1993).

Both the alpha (heavy) and beta (light) chains of class II antigens are encoded in MHC. The classic class II antigens are further divided into DR, DQ, and DP antigens. Class II antigens are expressed on B cells and monocytes and can be induced during inflammation on many other cell types that normally have little or no expression. The DQ and DP antigens each have polymorphic alpha and beta chains, which can dimerize in various combinations. In contrast, DR dimers all share an essentially invariant alpha chain, while the beta chain carries the extreme polymorphism characteristic of these antigens. The number of DR genes can vary among individuals.

Dozens of alleles are known to exist at each locus and more are being identified all the time (Bodmer et al., 1998; Marsh et al., 2002). However, the combination of alleles expressed in any one individual is not totally random. Instead, when a certain allele of one locus is inherited, most of the time it is closely linked to specific alleles of other loci on the same chromosome, a situation known as linkage disequilibrium. The combination of alleles on one chromosome is known as a haplotype.

HLA Typing—A Brief History and Evolution of the Nomenclature

Confusion sometimes arises from the difference in nomenclature between the genes and the proteins they encode. It is important to distinguish polymorphic variations that are defined serologically or by cellular assay from those that are defined by molecular techniques. Serologically and cellularly defined entities are referred to as antigens (or specificities), whereas the terms gene and allele refer to loci defined by nucleic acid analyses (Bodmer et al., 1998). As new loci, genes, alleles, and antigens within the MHC are recognized, the terminology used is standardized by the World Health Organization (WHO) through an HLA nomenclature committee. The reports of this committee describe the naming of new HLA genes, alleles, and serological specificities. The most recent report also contains complete lists of all the accepted genes and alleles, as well as the serologically and cellularly defined specificities (Marsh et al., 2002). The number of MHC class I and class II gene alleles are too numerous to be included here (they currently number more than 900).

Determination of HLA types, or HLA typing, has become much more accurate over the past decade. As the naming of these types reflected the methodology used and as advances were made in understanding HLA polymorphism, the nomenclature has been frequently revised. The literature is full of variations, which can be frustrating.

The earliest typing was performed by serologic methods. Women are exposed to foreign, paternally derived HLA antigens during pregnancy, and they can develop antibodies against these antigens. Sera from numerous multiparous women were screened for those reacting reproducibly to certain HLA types. The epitopes recognized by these sera were generally shared, or "public" epitopes, that are present on a family of related alleles. Thus, for example, a person would be labeled *DR4* if her cells reacted with sera characterized as seeing this epitope. The presence of a second DR antigen in some individuals was also recognized. Sera that recognized these less polymorphic antigens were characterized. For example, most individuals positive for DR4 were also positive for the second DR antigen, DRw53. Similarly, haplotypes carrying the DR3, DR5, or DR6 antigens were generally positive for DRw52, which later was split into DRw52a, DRw52b, etc., by more specific sera.

It soon became clear that human T cells are capable of distinguishing more precise splits among some of the HLA antigens recognized by these sera. As a result, mixed lymphocyte typing was developed to allow more exact typing. A mixed lymphocyte reaction involves co-culturing the stimulator cells from one individual with the responder lymphocytes from another person for several days. Stimulator cells are prevented from proliferating by irradiation or exposure to mitomycin C. The responder cells that recognize alloantigens expressed by stimulator cells are induced to proliferate. Stimulator cells are B cells and monocytes, i.e., antigen-presenting cells. Responder cells are T lymphocytes. A radioactive nucleotide (usually ^{3}H-thymidine) is added during the last 6 to 18 hours of culture to quantitate newly synthesized DNA. The amount of radioactive thymidine incorporated into the DNA of responder cells is generally proportional to the degree of HLA-D disparity between responder and stimulator cells. Cells from family members that share

both HLA-D haplotypes (e.g., HLA-identical siblings) usually do not stimulate each other. Similarly, the cells from nonrelated individuals who share both HLA-D haplotypes generally stimulate each other minimally, if at all. A panel of reference cells that were homozygous for different antigens, called homozygous typing cells, or HTCs, was generated. Homozygous typing cells were obtained from offspring of consanguineous marriages who inherited identical chromosomal HLA-D regions from each parent and were homozygous for all HLA-D region loci (DR, DQ, and DP). Cells from an individual of unknown HLA type were tested for recognition by the panel cells. HTCs do not stimulate cells from persons who have the same HLA-D haplotype, but they stimulate and respond to cells from individuals who are HLA-D heterozygous or fully disparate from them. Unfortunately, mixed lymphocyte reaction testing for patients with hematological malignancies is often not successful, as leukemic cells usually are poor stimulators with responder cells from almost any donor.

Since both the sera from multiparous women and the HTCs were continually in need of replenishment and replacement, international histocompatibility workshops, under the auspices of the WHO, were held periodically to compare and share reagents from around the world in an attempt to ensure some consistency. When consensus was reached on a new antigenic specificity, it was given a new number with the designation *w*, for workshop. After an antigen became widely reproducible and accepted, the *w* was dropped and a permanent name was given. For example, in one workshop a newly identified antigen might be given the name DRw4, and in a few years it might be revised to DR4.

Serologic and cellular recognition of HLA DP antigens was more difficult, perhaps because they are expressed at a lower density on the cell surface. A system called primed lymphocyte typing was developed to type for DP. Cells were primed by one exposure to a particular DP antigen so that a second exposure to the same antigen would generate much stronger secondary response. A panel of cells primed for different DP antigens would be available for testing an unknown individual's cells.

The development of the polymerase chain reaction has radically changed the approach to HLA typing. A number of DNA-based methods can be used in HLA typing, such as sequence-specific primer amplification (SSP), sequence-specific oligonucleotide probe hybridization (SSOP), restriction fragment length polymorphism (RFLP), single-stranded conformational polymorphism (SSCP), heteroduplex formation, and nucleotide sequencing. All involve the amplification of selected portions of HLA genes from genomic DNA with appropriate oligonucleotide primer pairs. Most frequently, exons 3 and 4 of class I genes and exon 2 of class II genes are amplified. These exons are the gene fragments encoding most of the polymorphous segments of the class I and class II molecules. As with serological typing, the HLA type of the sample is determined by the pattern with which the amplified gene fragments hybridize with the panel of different probes (SSOP) or by the pattern of products amplified in SSP.

DNA-based typing of HLA is generally performed at two levels, the first using reagents (probes or primer pairs) that detect all alleles of an HLA gene (low resolution), and the second using reagents with specificity for a selected allele (high resolution). Low-resolution typing identifies the HLA gene at the serological or antigen level; high resolution typing identifies specific alleles. If primers or probes are unavailable and it is necessary to clarify the specific allele, nucleotide sequencing of the amplified product can be done. Although nucleotide sequencing is thought by many to be the definitive method, it is costly and time consuming.

The use of molecular testing has a number of advantages over serologic typing. First, DNA-based typing does not require the isolation of viable lymphocytes but can be done using any nucleated cell source. Second, DNA-based assays have increased accuracy and specificity.

Nomenclature

The HLA-A and HLA-B antigens were defined and many antigens were named before it was recognized that the MHC is a multilocus system. Instead of changing the numbers already assigned to accepted antigens, subsequent HLA-A and HLA-B antigens and alleles continue to be numbered jointly as if they were products of a single locus (e.g., A34, B35, A36, B37). For all other HLA loci, alleles and antigens are numbered consecutively within that locus (e.g., Cw1, Cw2, etc.; DR1, DR2, etc.; DQ1, DQ2, etc.) New class I region genes are designated HLA followed by a letter in alphabetical order, omitting D (e.g., HLA-E, HLA-F, etc.). All class II genes are designated D followed by a letter that identifies the locus that is defined by the location within the class II region of the chromosome (e.g., HLA-DQ, HLA-DP, etc.). The locus letter is followed by the letters A or B for alpha or beta chain genes, and the A and B are followed by a number where there are more than one alpha or beta chain gene to a locus (e.g., DQA1, DQB1, DQA2, DQB2). Alleles are designated using the gene name (e.g., DRB1) followed by an asterisk (*), followed by a four-digit number. The first two digits of the number identify any previously characterized antigen, and the latter two identify the allele/variant. This method was chosen to maintain the relationship between alleles and serologic antigens as much as possible (please see **Figure 3-2**). For example, DRB1*1201 designates an allele of the protein formerly defined as DR12, which itself was a serologically defined variant (split) of DR5. As new alleles of a gene are sequenced and accepted, they are numbered consecutively. In some cases a five-digit number is assigned to an allele. The fifth digit indicates that alleles have different DNA nucleotide sequences, but

their amino acid sequences, and thus the proteins expressed, are the same (in other words these are silent mutations).

Alloreactions and Clinical Consequences

In laboratory circumstances, coculturing tissues that are mismatched for MHC molecules can induce a strong immune response, as reflected by the mixed lymphocyte reaction. This is manifested in vivo by allograft rejection, graft-versus-host disease (GVHD), and the graft-versus-leukemia (GVL) effect. In stem cell transplantation, the principal targets of the immune response (to the host) are the MHC molecules expressed on the surface of recipient cells (allo-MHC). The cellular and molecular basis for the recognition of alloantigens only recently became understood, as description of MHC and T cell receptor structure and function has emerged. Alloimmunity is a complex process involving donor T cells and natural killer (NK) cells interacting with certain cells of the recipient. Alloimmune reactions are responsible for three major transplant events that determine success or failure of the transplant: engraftment, GVHD, and GVL effects.

Engraftment/Rejection

Donor and recipient T cells and NK cells and donor CD34+ cells (hematopoietic stem cells) are involved in the engraftment/rejection process. To allow the graft (the donor stem cells) to stably settle and proliferate, the recipient needs to undergo substantial immunosuppression. In HLA-identical transplants, engraftment is the result of donor T cells mounting a successful alloresponse against recipient T cells, thereby

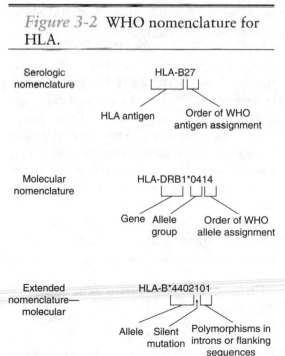

Figure 3-2 WHO nomenclature for HLA.

*This names areas of defined noncoding sequences.

eliminating the recipient's immune system. Since the introduction of more effective immunosuppressive drugs, there has been a marked improvement in allograft survival (i.e., engraftment). This immunosuppressive therapy, however, is relatively nonspecific and is associated with a number of complications, such as infections and secondary malignancies. Conditioning regimens are now designed with two specific purposes: immunoablation of the recipient and variable additional intensification to control malignancy. The introduction of peripheral blood-mobilized stem cell transplant along with sophisticated cell separation techniques provides a wide choice for the transplanting team in the dose of stem cells and lymphocytes selected for their engraftment and immunity-enhancing effects.

Graft-versus-Host Disease (GVHD)

GVHD is caused by the reaction of mature donor T cells in the stem cell transfusion against alloantigens of the host. The host is immunocompromised and therefore unable to reject the allogeneic cells in the graft. The process begins when donor T cells accompanying the stem cells encounter recipient antigens. The subsequent expansion of donor T cells leads to tissue damage either directly through T cells or indirectly through cytokine production. GVHD is the principal limitation on the use of bone marrow transplantation. GVHD (both acute and chronic) is commonly treated with intense immunosuppression. Much effort has been focused on prevention of GVHD. Cyclosporin A and the metabolic toxin methotrexate are routinely used for prophylaxis against GVHD. Accurate HLA typing and matching is also very important for preventing GVHD.

Graft-Versus-Leukemia/ Graft-Versus-Tumor Effects

The graft-versus-leukemia (GVL) effect is thought to be the main reason that allogeneic stem cell transplantation for hematological malignancies results in lower relapse rates than autologous stem cell transplantation, given identical conditioning regimens. The concept of transplants using highly immunosuppressive but low-intensity (nonmyeloablative) conditioning regimens in the treatment of hematological malignancies was largely derived from the assumption that the GVL effect has a curative potential at least as powerful as a myeloablative conditioning regimen (Battiwala and Barrett, 2002). Objective tumor regressions following allogeneic stem cell transplantation for breast, renal cell, and ovarian cancer allowed the concept of GVL effect to be extended to include a graft-versus-tumor effect (Childs and Barrett, 2004). The previously described close association between GVHD and GVL effect in both experimental and clinical transplantation suggested the possible central role of T cells in this process. At this point we know that cell populations capable of recognizing and lysing malignant targets can be divided into two broad categories based upon the mechanism of cellular recognition: cytotoxic T cells and NK cells. The separation of GVHD from GVL remains an attractive clinical goal and the target of active laboratory and clinical research.

Finding a Donor and the National Marrow Donor Program (NMDP)

In the last decade, along with the development of DNA-based HLA typing, we also learned that donor-recipient HLA compatibility has a major impact on the outcome of hematopoietic stem cell transplantation. It is now evident that complete donor-recipient matching for HLA-A, HLA-B, HLA-C, HLA-DRB1 and HLA-DQB1 genes can significantly reduce the incidence of GVHD and risk of mortality (Mickelson et al., 2002).

Inheritance of HLA Antigens

The genes of the MHC demonstrate more polymorphism than any other genetic system (i.e., multiple alleles exist for each locus). Each individual has one allele for each locus per chromosome and therefore encodes two HLA antigens per locus. The antigens at each HLA locus are expressed independently (they are codominant). The identification of each HLA antigen of an individual is called HLA-phenotype. Two unrelated persons expressing the same HLA antigens are HLA-phenotype identical.

As mentioned earlier, HLA genes are closely linked on chromosome 6, and a complete set of HLA genes is usually inherited from each parent as a unit. Recombination within the MHC is rare. The set of genes inherited from one parent are called *haplotype*. Siblings who inherit the same haplotypes from both parents are *HLA identical*. Those who inherit the same haplotype from one parent but a different haplotype from the other parent are *haploidentical*. Siblings who inherit different haplotypes from each parent are *HLA nonidentical*. As HLA genes are inherited together on a single chromosome (as haplotypes), there are four possible combinations of maternal and paternal haplotypes (provided there is no recombination within the MHC). Therefore there is a one in four (25%) chance that two siblings will be HLA identical, a two in four (50%) chance that two siblings will be HLA haploidentical, and a one in four (25%) chance that two siblings will be HLA nonidentical. All offspring are haploidentical with both of their parents, unless recombination has occurred (see **Figure 3-3**).

Figure 3-3 HLA inheritance.

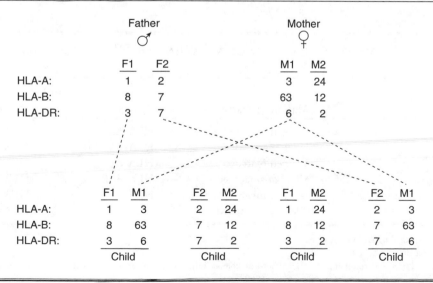

The genes of the MHC demonstrate such a high polymorphism, that the chance that two unrelated individuals would be HLA identical could be astronomical. The situation, however, is somewhat alleviated because the HLA system displays a phenomenon known as linkage disequilibrium. This means that certain HLA alleles are inherited together on the same chromosome more often than would be predicted if HLA loci were at random equilibrium. The particular alleles that are found in linkage disequilibria differ for various racial groups, but all racial groups display significant disequilibria (Beutler et al., 2001).

Unrelated Donors

Unfortunately, less than 30% of patients facing hematopoietic stem cell transplantation have an HLA-identical sibling. Thus, alternative donors, such as phenotypically matched, unrelated volunteers and partially matched family members, must be considered (please see **Table 3-1** for terminology for donor matching). In these cases, as mentioned above, the incidence of GVHD is higher, and a higher risk of transplant-related mortality can be expected, depending on the degree of HLA disparity. Again, molecular typing has improved the quality of matching unrelated donors, thus contributing to improved outcomes. Donors who are more disparate are not routinely used. Haploidentical transplants are currently under investigation, using a combination of more intense cytoreductive therapy and limited ex vivo T cell depletion followed by long-term immunosuppression (Spitzer et al., 2003).

Transplantations using stem cells from matched, unrelated donors (MUD) fostered by the National Marrow Donor Program (NMDP) and other large national donor centers such as the Anthony Nolan Center in Great Britain can be considered for patients without suitably matched, related donors. It is important to note that MUD transplants are still associated with substantial allogeneic complications, such as GVHD and prolonged and profound immunodeficiency (Casper et al., 1995).

With the current size of the pool of volunteer donors, approximately 75% of Caucasian patients can locate a suitable matched volunteer donor (Beatty et al., 1988). Patients belonging

---

Table 3-1 Terminology for donor matching of HLA class 1 alleles and antigens.

Term	Matching Status	Examples* Donor	Recipient
Matched	Antigen matched	HLA-A2	HLA-A2
	Allele matched	HLA-A*0201	HLA-A*0201
Allele mismatched†	Antigen matched	HLA-A2	HLA-A2
	Allele mismatched	HLA-A*0201	HLA-A*0205
Antigen mismatched‡	Antigen mismatched	HLA-A2	HLA-A1
	Allele mismatched	HLA-A*0201	HLA-A*0101

† Alleles are defined by DNA sequencing.

‡ Antigens are defined by serologic analysis.

Source: Adapted from Petersdorf et al. (2001). Major-histocompatibility-complex class I alleles and antigens in hematopoietic-cell transplantation. *N Engl J Med, 345*(25), 1794–1800.

to minority ethnic groups have lower rates of success in locating a fully matched donor. This is only partly due to the smaller number of donors from racial minorities, and mainly a result of their greater prevalence of uncommon HLA types. It was demonstrated, for example, that African-Americans are more polymorphic with respect to HLA, and therefore are less likely to find suitable donors at any given registry (Beatty et al., 1995). This means that a substantial increase is needed in the recruitment of minority racial groups for organ and marrow donors to alleviate the problem of access to HLA matches for patients belonging to racial minority groups.

The National Marrow Donor Program

The National Marrow Donor Program was established in 1986 to recruit and conduct HLA typing of large numbers of unrelated volunteer donors for patients in need of an allogeneic stem cell transplant but lacking an HLA-matched sibling donor. The NMDP operates the world's largest and most diverse registry of volunteer unrelated stem cell donors. By November 1, 2000, approximately 4.2 million volunteers were listed in the NMDP registry, of whom 2.4 million were typed for the HLA-A, HLA-B, and HLA-DR loci (Kollman et al., 2001). Since its founding, more than 16,000 patients worldwide have received transplants from NMDP donors (Karanes et al., 2003).

In order to initiate a search of the NMDP registry for an HLA-matched, unrelated donor, the recipient's HLA typing results with basic demographic and disease information should be submitted. When a suitable donor is identified, the NMDP coordinates the steps needed to deliver the donated stem cells to the patient. To initiate a preliminary search of the NMDP reg-

istry, contact the NMDP Office of Patient Advocacy at 1-888-999-6743 (toll free). A preliminary search request form can also be submitted through the NMDP Web site: www.marrow.org.

Issues of Stem Cell Donation

Hematpoietic stem cell donors (HSCD) provide lifesaving stem cells for more than 15,000 patients annually (Confer, 2004). Once donor selection has occurred, there are many factors to consider in the evaluation and preparation of the selected donor. Is the donor related or unrelated to the recipient? Is the donor an adult or a child? Is the donor of advanced age? Will the method of collection be bone marrow (BM) harvest or peripheral blood stem cell (PBSC) collection via apheresis? Regardless of stem cell source, numerous common denominators exist for all donors. A thorough history and physical examination must be performed at least 30 days prior to collection. The donor must be evaluated for virology history. A complete psychosocial workup is indicated to include assessment of such things as sexual history, assessment of IV drug use, and skin piercing. Additionally, donors must provide informed consent, including understanding risks and benefits of collection methods and alternatives for collection. They may also desire to know the potential outcome for the patient should the would-be donor decide to decline.

Psychosocial Elements of Donation

The psychological status of the donor must be reviewed prior to donation to anticipate and address any psychosocial issues that may be present. The motives for donation should be discussed to ensure there is no misconception of financial gain or that the donor has not been coerced. It is also worth noting that motivations for donation are intensely personal and will vary depending on whether the donor is related or unrelated (Confer, 2004). Moreover, because related donors have a direct connection to the patient, poor outcomes can have devastating effects. "Survivor's guilt" is well documented in the literature. It has been suggested that donors may experience intense feelings of guilt and self-doubt if a death is related to GVHD. Grief, however, was universally experienced by all donors on learning of the death of the patient (O'Connell, 2000).

Implications of Donor Age

The age range for eligible donors has widened considerably since the first transplants and inception of the NMDP. The literature reports successful harvest from an infant weighing 3.95 kilograms (Confer, 2004). Risks associated with donation by children include anesthesia and increased poor tolerance of blood loss. Children are more likely to require blood transfusions than adults. With respect to mobilization for peripheral harvest of blood stem cells, children are similar to adults in their tolerance of growth factors and achieve similar CD34+ cell counts (Confer, 2004). Particular attention must be paid to the psychosocial needs of the child preparing for apheresis. Involvement of a certified child life specialist is encouraged and very beneficial. In general, children tolerate stem cell donation well, with serious complications postharvest being rare (Confer, 2004).

The advent of nonmyeloablative hematopoietic stem cell transplant (NM-HSCT) has ex-panded the age continuum to include donors of advanced age who, in the infancy of transplant, would never have been selected. The donor of advanced age may present with a host of comorbid conditions ranging from hypertension to congestive heart failure and diabetes. They may also have sensory impairments and mobility issues. Although such issues may not be grounds for exclusion, they do complicate preparation and education. Much like the young donor, elder donors require tailored education and may benefit from detailed written instruction and demonstration/return demonstration as appropriate (Chouinard, 2003).

Issues Associated with Peripheral Stem Cell Harvest

Peripheral stem cell collection via apheresis has become the preferred method for autologous stem cell collection and is also widely used in allogeneic populations for both related and unrelated donors (Ng-Cashin and Shea, 2004). Risks associated with this method can be categorized as either related to mobilization therapy or related to the apheresis procedure itself. Stem cell mobilization with recombinant human growth factors such as sargramostim and filgrastim is a widely accepted practice. Potential side effects of growth factors include bone pain, headache, nausea and vomiting, myalgia, and fatigue. Pain and irritation at the injection site is another common response, though very minor. Bone pain has been experienced by as many as 86% of donors during mobilization, while injection site pain is quite rare (Confer, 2004). The long-term effects of growth factors in healthy donors is poorly understood, with documented follow-up only from 1 to 5 years postdonation. To date, no serious adverse effects have been reported (Amgen, 2004; Confer, 2004).

Minor Adverse Events Associated with Marrow Donation

The adverse events routinely experienced by marrow donors are relatively minor, though understandably noxious to the donor. The most common postdonation complication is pain. A review of 1270 patients revealed that all donors experienced pain on some level. While these experiences differ in intensity and duration, pain is universally perceived as significant (Confer, 2004). Not surprisingly, patients who received general anesthesia reported more nausea and vomiting, throat pain, and feelings of fatigue than those who received regional block anesthesia. Additional postharvest complications include bleeding at harvest sites, light-headedness, and headache (Confer, 2004; NMDP, 2004).

Serious Adverse Events Associated with Marrow Donation

RISKS OF ANESTHESIA

Bone marrow harvest under general anesthesia places the donor at significant risk, and as such, donors must be assessed according to established anesthesia guidelines. Risks include hypersensitivity/allergic reaction, infection associated with vascular access devices, and irritation of airway related to endotracheal intubation. Such events are rarely recorded; however, given that 78% of all BM donors elect general anesthesia, informed consent and patient education should include these possibilities (Confer, 2004).

RISK OF INFECTION

Infectious complications are primarily associated with aspiration sites. Vascular access device infection has also been noted in the literature. When noted, infections pose an immediate threat to the well-being of the donor; prompt intervention with organism-sensitive antibiotics is required (Confer, 2004).

RISK OF MECHANICAL INJURY

Bone marrow is typically harvested from the posterior iliac crest, though the anterior iliac crest and sternum have been used. Skin punctures are made using the proper gauge aspirate needle. Once the needle has penetrated the cortical bone, marrow is aspirated (approximately 5–10 ml). The needle is repeatedly advanced and repositioned within the original skin puncture to aspirate additional marrow. A typical harvest may involve 200–300 aspirates per side (left and right iliac crest) to obtain the volume of marrow needed to reconstitute the immune system (Confer, 2004). Given this scenario, risk of mechanical injury is obvious. Injury to the bone and nerves, particularly the sciatic nerve, has been documented. Sciatic pain lasting 18 months has been reported to the NMDP. Injury to surrounding vessels resulting in massive blood loss is another latent possibility (Confer, 2004; NMDP, 2004).

RISKS ASSOCIATED WITH TRANSFUSIONS

Blood loss during the harvest procedure places donors at risk for symptomatic anemia and hypovolemia. Risks associated with postharvest transfusion include allergic reaction, ABO incompatibility, and transference of bacterial and/or fungal organisms. To ameliorate these risks, autologous harvest and transfusion of packed red blood cells (RBCs) has all but replaced allogeneic blood transfusions. In fact, NMDP standards prohibit the transfusion of allogeneic blood to its donors. As compared with other serious risks associated with stem cell donation, blood loss is significant, with as many as 85% of all NMDP donors requiring autologous transfusions (Confer, 2004).

The use of recombinant erythropoietic growth factors plays an important role in the effort to reduce postdonation transfusions. In a study of 10 patients (including two pediatric donors), epoetin alfa administered 1 to 3 weeks preharvest resulted in stabilized postharvest hematocrits and zero transfusions (Confer, 2004).

RISK OF DEATH

Death, although rare, has been reported (NMDP, 2004). The risk of death associated with BM donation is 1:10,000 (Confer, 2004). In a review of 7857 marrow collections, only two deaths occurred, as reported to the International Bone Marrow Transplant Registry (IBMTR). Confer describes causes of deaths following marrow collection including cardiac arrest, stroke, and sickle crisis. It is not known whether stress related to impending donation contributed to the deaths. It is also difficult to determine that death in the postharvest setting was indeed related to the procedure itself. What is known is that death related to marrow or stem cell donation is very rare (Confer, 2004).

In summary, both marrow and stem cell harvest via apheresis collection methods place patients at risk for both minor and severe adverse events. However, predonation patient preparation and education can potentially affect adverse outcomes. It is also clearly documented in the literature that both collection techniques are safe (Confer, 2004). Additional research is necessary to provide long-term data for donors who receive recombinant growth factors.

Summary

A thorough understanding of HLA immunology is clearly key in the field of stem cell transplantation for a variety of reasons. Primarily, precision in HLA typing leads to improved outcomes, particularly with respect to acute and chronic graft-versus-host disease. Additionally, HLA immunology is the platform from which an understanding of nonmyeloablative stem cell transplantation and the graft-versus-tumor effect have evolved. There is an undeniable interconnectedness between graft-versus-host disease and long-term complications, immune reconstitution, relapse, and control of malignancy from this single process. Given this complexity, it is vital that continued research and study in the area of HLA immunology be supported.

Dedication

It is with thanks and gratitude that we dedicate this chapter to the many patients who have participated in the numerous clinical trials and stem cell transplant programs that have led to the improved understanding of HLA immunology. Their courage, persistence, and determination to survive despite great odds inspires us to continue and strengthens our resolve to look deeper for answers that will eventually lead to success for all.

References

Amgen, Inc. Thousand Oaks, CA. [Professional Prescribing Information]. Retrieved February 23, 2004, from http://www.neupogen.com/pi.html.

Barnes D.W., Corp, M.J., Loutit, J.F., & Neal, F.E. (1956). Treatment of murine leukemia with X rays and homologous bone marrow; preliminary communication. *British Medical Journal, 15*(32), 626–627.

Battiwala, M., & Barrett, J. (2002). Allogeneic transplantation using nonmyeloablative transplant regimens. *Best Practice & Research. Clinical Haematology, 14*, 701–722.

Beatty, P.G., Dahlberg, S., Mickelson, E.M., Nisperos, B., Opelz, G., Martin, P.J., et al. (1988). Probability of finding HLA-matched unrelated marrow donors. *Transplantation, 45*(4), 714–718.

Beatty, P.G., Mori, M., & Milford, E. (1995). Impact of racial genetic polymorphism on the probability of finding an HLA-matched donor. *Transplantation, 60*(8), 778–783.

Beutler, E., Coller, B.S., Lichtman, M.A., Kipps, T.J., & Seligsohn, U. (Eds.). (2001). *Williams Hematology* (6th ed.). New York: McGraw-Hill.

Bodmer, J.G., Marsh, S.G., Albert, E.D., Bodmer, W.F., Bontrop, R.E., Dupont, B., et al. (1998). Nomenclature for factors of the HLA system. *Tissue Antigens, 53*(4 Pt 2), 407–446.

Casper, J., Camitta, B., Truitt, R., Baxter-Lowe, L.A., Bunin, N., et al. (1995). Unrelated bone marrow donor transplants for children with leukemia or myelodysplasia. *Blood, 85*(9), 2354–2363.

Childs, R.W., & Barrett, J. (2004). Nonmyeloablative allogeneic immunotherapy for solid tumors. *Annual Review of Medicine, 55,* 459–475.

Chouinard, M.S. (2003). Nursing management of the nonmyeloablative hematopoietic stem cell transplant recipient. In Buchsel, P., & Kapustay, P.K. (Eds.), *Stem cell transplant: A clinical textbook* (pp. 20.3–20.11). Pittsburgh, PA: Oncology Nursing Society Press.

Confer, D.L. (2004). Hematopoietic stem cell donors. In Foreman, S., Blume, K., & Appelbaum, F. (Eds.), *Thomas's hematopoietic cell transplantation* (4th ed., pp. 538–548). Malden, MA: Blackwell Publishing.

Geraghty, D.E. (1993). Structure of the HLA class I region and expression of its resident genes. *Current Opinion in Immunology, 5*(1), 3–7.

Halloran, P.F., Wadgymar, A., & Autenried, P. (1986). The regulation of expression of major histocompatibility complex products. *Transplantation, 41*(4), 413–420.

Horowitz, M.M., Gale, R.P., Sondel, P.M., Goldman, J.M., Kersey, J., Kolb, H.J, et al. (1990). Graftversus-leukemia reactions after bone marrow transplantation. *Blood, 75*(3), 555–562.

Karanes C., Confer, D., Walker, T., Askren, A., & Keller, C. (2003). Unrelated donor stem cell transplantation: The role of the National Marrow Donor Program. *Oncology, 17*(8), 1036–1038, 1043–1044, 1164–1167.

Kollman, C., Howe, C.W., Anasetti, C., Antin, J.H., Davies, S.M., Filipovich, A.H., et al. (2001). Donor characteristics as risk factors in recipients after transplantation of bone marrow from unrelated donors: The effect of donor age. *Blood, 98*(7), 2043–2051.

Marsh, S.G., Albert, E.D., Bodmer, W.F., Bontrop, R.E., Dupont, B., Erlich, H.A., et al. (2002). Nomenclature for factors of the HLA system. *Tissue Antigens, 60*(5), 407.

Mickelson, E.M., Petersdorf, E.W., & Hansen, J.A. (2002). HLA matching and hematopoietic cell transplant outcome. *Clinical Transplant,* 263–271.

National Marrow Donor Program. *Sources of Stem Cells—Advanced* [Medical Information]. Retrieved February 23, 2004, from http://www.marrow.org/physician/hematopoietic_cell_sources.html

Ng-Cashin, J., & Shea, T. (2004). Mobilization of autologous peripheral blood hematopoietic cells for support of high-dose cancer therapy. In Foreman, S., Blume, K., & Appelbaum, F. (Eds.), *Thomas's hematopoietic cell transplantation* (4th ed., pp. 576–586). Malden, MA: Blackwell Publishing.

O'Connell, S. (2000). Complications of hematopoietic cell transplantation. In Yarbro, C.H., Frogge, M.H., Goodman, M., & Groenwald, S. (Eds.), *Cancer nursing: principles & practice* (5th ed., pp. 523–539). Sudbury, MA: Jones & Bartlett.

Odom, L.F., August, C.S., Githens, J.H., Humbert, J.R., Morse, H., Peakman, D. et al. (1978). Remission of relapsed leukemia during a graft-versus-host reaction: a "graft-versus-leukemia reaction" in man? *Lancet, 2*(8089), 537–540.

Petersdorf, E., Hansen, J.A., Martin, P.J., Woolfrey, A., Malkki, M. et al. (2001). Major-Histocompatibility-Complex Class I alleles and antigens in hematopoieticcell transplantation. *New England Journal of Medicine, 345*(25), 1794–1800.

Spitzer, T.R., McAfee, S.L., Dey, B.R., Colby, C., Hope, J., Grossberg, H., et al. (2003). Nonmyeloablative haploidentical stem-cell transplantation using anti-CD2 monoclonal antibody (MEDI-507)-based conditioning for refractory hematologic malignancies. *Transplantation, 75*(10), 1748–1751.

Suthanthiran, M., & Strom, T.B. (1994). Renal transplantation. *New England Journal of Medicine, 331*(6), 365–376.

Weiden, P.L., Flournoy, N., Thomas, E.D., Prentice, R., Fefer, A., Buckner, C.D., et al. (1979). Antileukemic effect of graft-versus-host disease in human recipients of allogeneic-marrow grafts. *New England Journal of Medicine, 300*(19), 1068–1073.

Blood and Marrow Transplantation: Indications, Procedure, Process

Kim Schmit-Pokorny, RN, MSN, OCN®

Blood and marrow transplantation (BMT) is being used worldwide as treatment for selected malignant and nonmalignant disorders. BMT enables patients to receive potentially lethal doses of chemotherapy or radiation therapy followed by hematopoietic rescue with marrow or blood stem cells. According to Loberiza (2003), 458 centers report to the International Bone Marrow Transplant Registry (IBMTR) and Autologous Blood and Marrow Transplant Registry (ABMTR). **Figure 4-1** shows estimates for the annual number of blood and marrow transplants worldwide from 1970–2002. During the early 1990s, there was a steep increase in the number of transplants, followed by a short decrease, and over the last few years, a plateau. The decrease in the number of autologous transplants (Figure 4-1) has been attributed to a decrease in transplants for breast cancer. The number of allogeneic transplants has also plateaued due to the decrease in the use of transplantation for chronic myelogenous leukemia. However, Loberiza (2003) indicates that there is an increase in the number of allogeneic transplants for other indications.

The treatment processes of marrow and blood stem cell transplantation vary somewhat, but the common goal for most diseases is cure. The role of transplantation in nonmalignant diseases is to replace defective marrow; in malignant diseases, the goal of stem cell infusion is to rescue the marrow after the patient has received toxic doses of myelosuppresive therapy aimed at eradicating the underlying disease (Treleaven and Barrett, 1992; Randolph, 1993). In addition, the importance of the graft-versus-tumor effect of donor stem cells has been established through the use of nonmyeloablative stem cell transplantation (NMSCT) (Slavin et al., 1998; Spitzer et al., 2000; McSweeney et al., 2001; Anagnostopoulos and Giralt, 2002).

The concept of transplanting marrow and blood cells seems simple in theory. However, life-threatening side effects and toxicities make caring for the transplant patient extremely complex. It requires sophisticated technology and procedures, a highly specialized team of healthcare workers, an adequately supportive environment, and many additional resources (Forman et al., 1994). Oncology nurses play a major role in

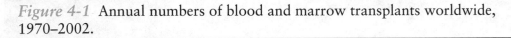

Figure 4-1 Annual numbers of blood and marrow transplants worldwide, 1970–2002.

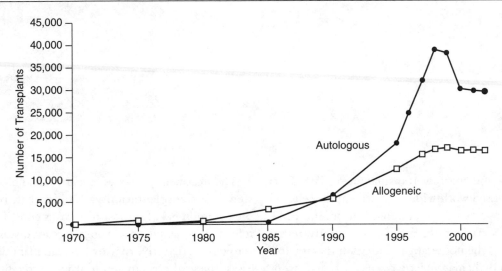

Source: Loberiza, F. (2003). Report on state of the art in blood and marrow transplantation: Part 1 of the IBMTR/ABMTR summary slides with guide. *IBMTB/ABMTR Newsletter 10*(1). Retrieved May 5, 2005, from http://www.ibmtr.org/ABOUT/NEWS/2003Nov.pdf. Used with permission of IBMTR.

the success of transplantation. Transplant scientists describe nurses' contribution this way:

> *The nursing team in particular is responsible for the day-to-day care of patients. Nurses not only provide bedside management of complex protocol studies, but also bear the burden of emotional support through the difficult hospital period. They are the most readily available source of information for patients and families day and night. Without a strong nursing team, the entire BMT program is jeopardized. (Forman et al., 1994, p. xx)*

As the field of BMT evolves, so does transplant nursing. The role of the transplant nurse is one of the most challenging oncology nursing specialties (Meyer, 1992).

Types of Transplants

Transplantation is defined as the transfer of living tissues or organs from one part of the body to another or from one individual to another. There are three major types of BMT: autologous, allogeneic, and syngeneic. Their names indicate the source of the marrow or blood cell that is transplanted, or infused, into the recipient.

Autologous

Autologous (self) BMT involves the removal, storage, and reinfusion of the patient's own healthy marrow or blood stem cells. In essence, the autologous patient is his or her own donor. The use of autologous marrow as a source of regenerating hematopoietic cells was first reported by Kurnick and colleagues (1958). They believed that increased intensity of treatment would permit the eradication of a tumor mass beyond the last viable cell. High-dose chemotherapy followed by autologous bone marrow transplantation (ABMT) appeared to offer the chance of curing malignancies in situations where myelosupression prevented the use of sufficient doses of chemotherapy without marrow rescue. The failure of early studies was due primarily to disease recurrence after inadequate doses of chemotherapy. During the late 1980s and early 1990s, interest in autologous BMT skyrocketed as a result of new technology for marrow storage, cryopreservation, and purging, as well as improvements in supportive care (Gale and Butturini, 1995). The major challenges still confronting ABMT are major organ and nonhematologic challenges, as well as dose-limiting toxicities and relapse of disease. Three theories as to the cause of relapse following autologous transplant include tumor contamination of the marrow, inadequate treatment of minimal residual disease in the patient, and the lack of a graft-versus-tumor effect (discussed later).

Allogeneic

In allogeneic transplantation, marrow or blood stem cells are removed from a donor and infused into the patient (recipient). The donor can be related (other than identical twin) or unrelated. The ideal donor is human-leukocyte-antigen identical (HLA identical) to the patient. Commonly, the stem cells are donated by a fully HLA-matched sibling. Because patients have a one in four chance of having an HLA-identical sibling, partially matched family members or matched but unrelated donors from a volunteer registry have also been donors. In **Figures** 4-2 and 4-3, Loberiza (2003) indicates the number of related and unrelated allogeneic transplants in patients. The number of unrelated transplants has grown over the last 10 years, possibly due to increased donor availability and outcomes comparable to related allogeneic transplants (Loberiza, 2003).

HLA typing involves testing leukocytes to identify genetically inherited antigens common to both donor and patient. It is important to obtain a full six-antigen match for a BMT whenever possible to prevent the donor marrow (specifically the T lymphocytes) from recognizing the recipient as foreign, leading to graft-versus-host disease (GVHD) (Freedman, 1988). GVHD is a unique complication of allogeneic transplant, and it can be a major impediment to successful transplantation (Buchsel, 1993). Alternatively, the patient's immune system can destroy the new bone marrow. This is referred to as *graft rejection*.

In the 1950s, random donors were used to attempt to rescue patients with aplastic anemia or bone marrow failure that resulted from radiation accidents. These attempts were not successful except for patients receiving marrow from an identical twin (Pegg, 1966). The most frequent causes of death from the use of random donors were graft failure and GVHD. It was not until the advent of tissue typing and compatibility testing that patients began to benefit from marrow transplant.

During the 1970s, clinical trials investigated the role of BMT in a wide variety of malignant and nonmalignant disorders. Standardized pre-transplant conditioning regimens and GVHD prevention were developed. By 1980, allogeneic BMTs using matched sibling donors were achieving disease-free survivals in hematological malignancies. During the late 1990s, allogeneic stem cell transplants using nonmyeloablative

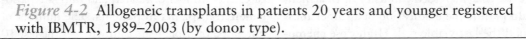

Figure 4-2 Allogeneic transplants in patients 20 years and younger registered with IBMTR, 1989–2003 (by donor type).

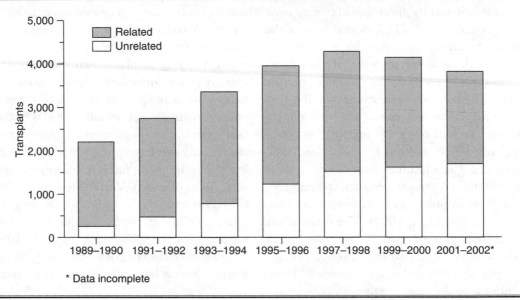

* Data incomplete

Source: Loberiza, F. (2003). Report on state of the art in blood and marrow transplantation: Part 1 of the IBMTR/ABMTR summary slides with guide. *IBMTB/ABMTR Newsletter 10*(1). Retrieved May 5, 2005, from http://www.ibmtr.org/ABOUT/NEWS/2003Nov.pdf. Used with permission of IBMTR.

conditioning regimens were explored (Slavin et al., 1998; Spitzer et al., 2000; McSweeney et al., 2001; Anagnostopoulos and Giralt, 2002). Nonmyeloablative stem cell transplantation (NMSCT) is also called mini-transplant, low intensity transplant, transplant-lite, reduced intensity transplant, or mixed chimera transplant. In NMSCT, a less intensive preparative regimen that allows prompt hematopoietic recovery even without stem cell rescue is given to the patient. Mixed chimerism should occur upon engraftment and a graft-versus-tumor effect should develop over several months. Many patients experience decreased toxicity from myelosuppression and regimen-related toxicity. NMSCT allows older patients or patients with comorbid conditions to receive the potential curative effects of a BMT. **Figure** 4-4 shows the dramatic increase in NMSCT from 1998 to 2003.

Syngeneic

Syngeneic transplantation involves harvesting stem cells from one identical twin and infusing them into the other. Identical twins have identical genetic types and are considered a perfect match. Syngeneic transplants, first attempted in the early 1960s to treat aplastic anemia, allowed investigators to learn that the hematopoietic system in humans could be replaced by that of a genetically identical donor (Whedon, 1991). This type of transplant has become relatively routine, with few complications.

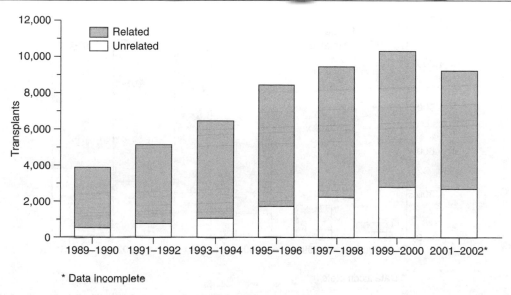

Figure 4-3 Allogeneic transplants in patients older than 20 years registered with IBMTR, 1989–2002 (by donor type).

* Data incomplete

Source: Loberiza, F. (2003). Report on state of the art in blood and marrow transplantation: Part 1 of the IBMTR/ABMTR summary slides with guide. *IBMTB/ABMTR Newsletter 10*(1). Retrieved May 5, 2005, from http://www.ibmtr.org/ABOUT/NEWS/2003Nov.pdf. Used with permission of IBMTR

Sources of Stem Cells

Peripheral blood stem cell transplantation (PBSCT) is rapidly replacing bone marrow transplantation (see **Figures 4-5** and **4-6**). PBSCT is associated with more rapid recovery of hematopoietic function than BMT and, therefore, less morbidity. Stem cells collected from the blood may have a lower risk of contamination by tumor cells (Gale et al., 1992; Sharp et al., 1992). Also, blood stem cells are collected in an outpatient setting, without general anesthesia. In allogeneic transplantation, apheresis offers donors a less invasive method than traditional marrow harvests to collect the stem cells. It is hoped that the former may serve as an incentive for the general population to serve as un-

related donors. PBSCT also offers the possibility of immunologically tailored grafts with larger numbers of T lymphocytes and natural killer cells enabling an adoptive immunotherapeutic approach (Juttner et al., 1994).

Umbilical cord blood is rich in hematopoietic stem cells, and successful allogeneic engraftment has been achieved using this source (Forman et al., 1994). Cord blood can be HLA typed and cryopreserved, and it can be a source of hematopoietic stem cells for HLA-matched, unrelated transplants. However, the relatively small amount of cord blood may render such an approach impractical except as a source of stem cells to transplant to infants and small children. This stem cell source prevents the need for marrow harvest under general anesthesia of infant donors.

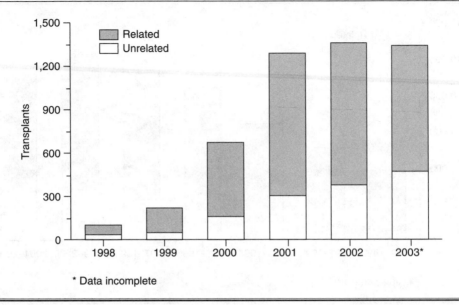

Figure 4-4 Nonmyeloablative allotransplants registered with the IBMTR, 1998–2003.

* Data incomplete

Source: Loberiza, F. (2003). Report on state of the art in blood and marrow transplantation: Part 1 of the IBMTR/ABMTR summary slides with guide. *IBMTB/ABMTR Newsletter 10*(1). Retrieved May 5, 2005, from http://www.ibmtr.org/ABOUT/NEWS/2003Nov.pdf. Used with permission of IBMTR.

Clinical Indications

Malignant Diseases

According to 2003 data from the IBMTR (Loberiza, 2003), the most common indication for an allogeneic transplant is leukemia, and the most common indication for an autologous transplant is multiple myeloma (see **Figure 4-7**). Malignant diseases that are treated with marrow or blood stem cell transplantation include:

- Acute lymphocytic leukemia
- Acute myelogenous leukemia
- Chronic myelogenous leukemia
- Chronic lymphocytic leukemia
- Myelodysplastic syndrome ("preleukemia")
- Monosomy 7 syndrome
- Non-Hodgkin's lymphoma
- Hodgkin's lymphoma
- Neuroblastoma
- Brain tumor
- Multiple myeloma
- Testicular germ cell tumors
- Breast cancer
- Lung cancer
- Ovarian cancer
- Melanoma
- Glioma
- Sarcoma
- Other solid tumors

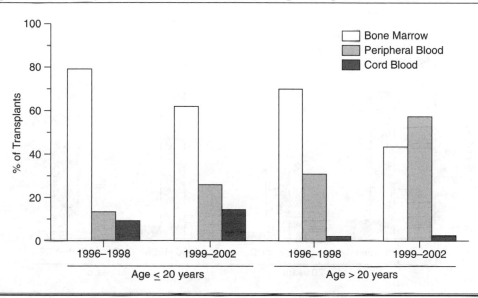

Figure 4-5 Allogeneic stem cell sources by recipient age, 1996–2002.

Source: Loberiza, F. (2003). Report on state of the art in blood and marrow transplantation: Part 1 of the IBMTR/ABMTR summary slides with guide. *IBMTB/ABMTR Newsletter 10*(1). Retrieved May 5, 2005, from http://www.ibmtr.org/ABOUT/NEWS/ 2003Nov.pdf. Used with permission of IBMTR.

Nonmalignant Diseases

Nonmalignant diseases, including congenital immunodeficiency diseases, were first treated with BMT in 1968 (Friedrich, 1994). Most of the transplants for nonmalignant diseases are done in children. Nonmalignant diseases that are treated with marrow or blood stem cell transplantation include:

- Hematologic disorders
    Severe aplastic anemia
    Diamond-Blackfan anemia
    Fanconi's anemia
    Sickle cell anemia
    Beta thalassemia major
    Chediak-Higashi syndrome
    Chronic granulomatous disease
    Congenital neutropenia
    Reticular dysgenesis

- Congenital immunodeficiencies
    Severe combined immunodeficiency
      (SCID)
    Wiskott-Aldrich syndrome
    Functional T cell deficiency
- Mucopolysaccharidoses
    Hurler's disease
    Hunter's disease
    Sanfilippo's syndrome
    Morquio's syndrome
- Lipidoses
    Adrenoleukodystrophy
    Methachromatic leukodystrophy
    Gaucher's disease
- Miscellaneous
    Osteopetrosis
    Langerhan's cell histiocytosis
    Lesch-Nyhan syndrome
    Glycogen storage diseases

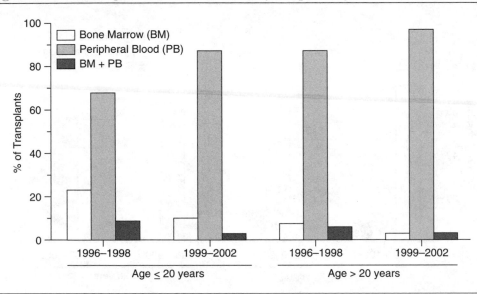

Figure 4-6 Autologous stem cell sources by recipient age, 1996–2002.

Source: Loberiza, F. (2003). Report on state of the art in blood and marrow transplantation: Part 1 of the IBMTR/ABMTR summary slides with guide. *IBMTB/ABMTR Newsletter 10*(1). Retrieved May 5, 2005, from http://www.ibmtr.org/ABOUT/NEWS/2003Nov.pdf. Used with permission of IBMTR.

Blood and Marrow Transplant Registries

The International Bone Marrow Transplant Registry receives information from more than 390 transplant centers in 48 countries and serves as a useful source of BMT statistics. Established in 1970, the database includes information for about 40% of allogeneic transplants done since 1970.

In 1991 the Autologous Blood and Marrow Transplant Registry-North and South America (ABMTR) began collecting data. More than 400 transplant centers participate in the ABMTR. This database includes about 60% of autotransplants done in North America and South America since 1989.

Patient Eligibility

Santos (1985) described several considerations for patient eligibility: 1) the malignancy is responsive to therapy; 2) the disease is in an early stage; 3) marrow toxicity is the only dose-limiting effect of the treatment; and 4) the source of stem cells is free of diseases. These considerations have been modified over time as marrow purging and newer treatment modalities have become available. Overall medical condition, psychosocial well-being, age, and compliance are also concerns when evaluating a patient's eligibility for transplant.

Disease Status

Tumor bulk and sensitivity to chemotherapy and/or radiation must be considered when select-

Figure 4-7 Indications for blood and marrow transplantation in North America, 2002.

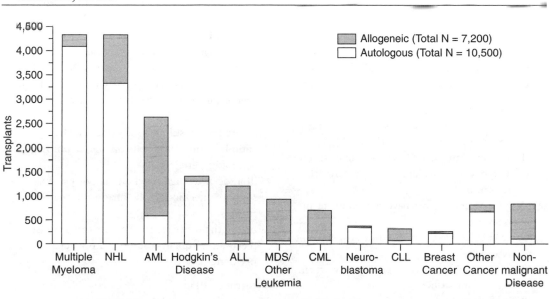

Source: Loberiza, F. (2003). Report on state of the art in blood and marrow transplantation: Part 1 of the IBMTR/ABMTR summary slides with guide. *IBMTB/ABMTR Newsletter 10*(1). Retrieved May 5, 2005, from http://www.ibmtr.org/ABOUT/NEWS/2003Nov.pdf. Used with permission of IBMTR.

ing a patient for transplant. Studies indicate that patients who have a low tumor burden and a disease responsive to chemotherapy experience an improved chance of disease-free survival following transplant (Crump et al., 1993; Jagannath et al., 1989).

The timing of a transplant in relation to disease status is integral to the overall outcome of the therapy. Outcomes of transplantation are best when the therapy is administered early in the course of the disease (Armitage and Gale, 1989).

Donor Availability

Tissue typing is usually performed on the patient's full siblings and occasionally on parents and children. If a matched, related donor is

identified, the transplant center will begin physical and psychological evaluations of the patient and potential donor. Patients without a matched related donor may be considered for an autologous transplant. If the patient's disease is not treatable with an autologous transplant, an unrelated donor search may be initiated.

Selecting a Transplant Center

The oncology nurse can play a critical role in assisting the patient and family to select a transplant center. Patients are usually overwhelmed with their diagnosis and are generally unfamiliar with treatment options. **Table 4-1** outlines

---

Table 4-1 SELECTING A TRANSPLANT CENTER.

Location

Will I need to relocate? If so, for how long?

Does the center have adequate, affordable housing?

Will the center assist me in finding housing?

What will housing cost?

Experience

How long has the center's personnel been performing BMT?

How many transplants have they done in total?

What types of transplants are they currently performing?

How many transplants have they done for my disease?

What is their success rate with transplants for my disease?

How does their success rate compare with the national statistics?

What is their mortality rate associated with transplant for patients with my disease?

How does their mortality rate compare with the national mortality rate for my disease?

What complications have they experienced with transplants for my disease?

How do these complications compare with national statistics?

Am I at high risk for developing any complication? If so, what is their experience with this complication?

BMT Team

How many physicians are working with the program?

How much experience with transplant does each physician have?

Will I have a physician caring for me?

Are there specially trained BMT nurses and staff?

How much experience does the average BMT nurse have?

How many BMT nurse coordinators are there?

Will there be one coordinator working with me during the transplant process?

Will a BMT clinical nurse specialist or nurse practitioner be working with me?

Who will be my primary medical professional in the hospital (resident, physician's assistant, nurse practitioner)? How much experience does he or she have in BMT?

Who are the consultants for various BMT complications (infectious disease, nephrology, cardiology, etc.)?

Will a social worker, psychologist, or psychiatrist support me emotionally during the transplant process?

Who are the other team members (pharmacist, dietitian, chaplain, volunteers, financial personnel, etc.)?

Treatment Plan

What is the proposed treatment plan?

Is this an investigational (research) study?

What is known to date about the treatment plan you are recommending for me?

Will my transplant be done on an outpatient basis? If so, what additional resources will I need (primary caregiver, etc.)? What percentage of outpatients are admitted for complications? Am I at any additional risk for complications?

Environment and Staffing

Do you have a designated BMT unit (or outpatient space/facility)?

How many BMT beds and outpatient rooms do you have?

Will I be in a unit with other hematology or oncology patients?

What are the infection control practices (handwashing, use of gloves, masks, gowns, air filtering system, etc.)?

Do you have dedicated BMT nurses in your unit or in your clinic?

Table 4-1 SELECTING A TRANSPLANT CENTER *continued.*

What is the nurse/patient ratio?

Will I have a primary nurse or case manager?

Are nurses with extensive experience in BMT supervising the BMT nursing staff?

If I should require critical care, will I be transferred to another unit? If so, how much training do the physicians and nurses in the critical care unit have in BMT?

How would you describe the cleanliness of the BMT unit? Can I tour the BMT unit prior to making my decision?

Can my family and friends donate blood and platelets for me if we desire? Do you have a directed donor unit at your facility? Does your center have equipment for irradiating blood products?

Are there visitor restrictions?

Patient Education and Support Groups

Does your center offer classes for patients and family members?

Do you have written information about your BMT program?

Can I talk to one or two patients with my disease who have gone through BMT at your center?

Does your center have a support group for BMT patients and their families?

Finances

How much will my transplant cost?

Is there someone at your center who will help me obtain approval for insurance coverage?

Is there someone at your center who will help me with fundraising, if needed?

Other than hospital expenses, what other expenses can I expect (parking, travel, meals, housing, child care, medications, telephone, television, etc.)?

Follow-up Care

How long can I expect to be followed at your center?

To whom will my care be transferred after I leave this center? How much training in and experience with transplantation do they have?

---

key questions the patient should ask when choosing a BMT center, although some patients may not have choices because of restrictions imposed by their insurance companies.

A successful bone marrow transplant program has a team of highly skilled health-care professionals and volunteers working to provide the best possible care for the transplant recipient and his or her family. The team is usually composed of administrators, physicians, physician's assistants, nurse practitioners, clinical nurse specialists, coordinators, staff nurses, pharmacists, social workers, psychologists or psychiatrists, dietitians, dentists, clergy, financial advisors, researchers, data management coordinators, laboratory technicians, and clerical

staff. Many consultants and ancillary staff are also involved in this enormous team effort (see **Figure 4-8**). Some centers have volunteers who are former BMT recipients. After undergoing a training program provided by the center, they give information and support to the BMT patient and family.

The nursing team "is the most important single aspect of a successful BMT unit," according to the American Society of Clinical Oncologists and the American Society of Hematologists (ASCO/ASH, 1990, p. 1209). Nurses serve in many roles on the transplant team. Advanced practice nurses (e.g., clinical nurse specialist or nurse practitioner) are integral members of the transplant team. The clinical nurse specialist

Figure 4-8 The BMT team.

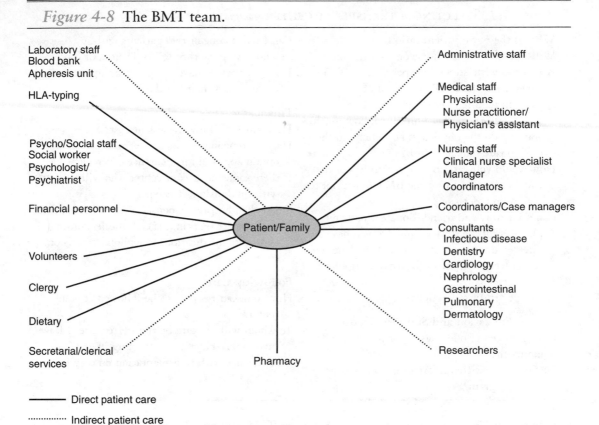

Laboratory staff
Blood bank
Apheresis unit

HLA-typing

Psycho/Social staff
Social worker
Psychologist/
Psychiatrist

Financial personnel

Volunteers

Clergy

Dietary

Secretarial/clerical
services

Pharmacy

Administrative staff

Medical staff
  Physicians
  Nurse practitioner/
  Physician's assistant

Nursing staff
  Clinical nurse specialist
  Manager
  Coordinators

Coordinators/Case managers

Consultants
  Infectious disease
  Dentistry
  Cardiology
  Nephrology
  Gastrointestinal
  Pulmonary
  Dermatology

Researchers

Patient/Family

———— Direct patient care

············ Indirect patient care

(CNS) functions as a consultant, educator, and researcher in the acute care and ambulatory care settings. The nurse practitioner (NP) works under a negotiated agreement with the institution to gather patient history and perform physical examinations and to order medications, blood products, and diagnostic studies. The NP may also perform bone marrow harvests, bone marrow biopsies and aspirations, skin biopsies, and lumbar punctures for instillation of intrathecal chemotherapy. Nurse coordinators or case managers plan and organize the pretransplant workup, harvesting of the marrow or blood cells, transplant phase, and follow-up care. Staff nurses provide direct nursing care to patients in acute care, ambulatory care, and home care settings. Nurse administrators and nurse managers facilitate the planning and development of the transplant program. It is imperative that nurses in these various roles work together closely to ensure quality and continuity of patient care (see **Table** 4-2).

Transplant Process

Patient Evaluation

Patients undergo a variety of physiological and psychological assessments to determine if they are eligible for a transplant. **Table** 4-3 lists the common tests to evaluate a patient for blood and marrow transplant. A central venous catheter is usually inserted prior to the administration of the high-dose therapy. During this work-up phase, which may last several days to one week, the patient and family are trying to learn about the transplant process. Nurses provide much of the information and education regarding the transplant and medical care.

Financial Issues

Early in the transplant process, determining financial coverage for the transplant is a necessity. Insurance benefits must be reviewed and authorization obtained. A professional, such as the transplant coordinator or case manager, who understands the patient's history, the transplant process, and insurance terminology can assist with this process (Buchsel and Kapustay, 1995).

There is a wide variation in the costs of transplantation. Estimates range from approximately $30,000 (Meisenberg et al., 1998) to $200,000 (Hillner et al., 1992) depending on the type of transplant (autologous or allogeneic), source of stem cells (bone marrow, blood, or cord blood), and whether it can be performed as an outpatient or inpatient procedure. Medicare guidelines (Department of Health and Human Services, 2003) approve allogeneic transplant for patients with leukemia, aplastic anemia, severe combined immunodeficiency disease (SCID), and Wiskott-Aldrich syndrome. Allogeneic transplant for multiple myeloma is specifically noted not to be covered. Autologous transplant coverage includes acute leukemia, resistant non-Hodgkin's lymphomas or those presenting with poor prognostic features following an initial response, recurrent or refractory neuroblastoma, advanced Hodgkin's disease, newly diagnosed or responsive multiple myeloma (tandem transplant for multiple myeloma is not covered), and primary amyloidosis. Diseases specifically listed as not covered are acute leukemia not in remission, chronic granulocytic leukemia, and solid tumors (other than neuroblastoma). The Medicare guidelines should be consulted for detailed descriptions of coverage or noncoverage. Coverage for other types of transplants is left to the individual intermediary's discretion.

Efficacy of transplantation for patients with solid tumors is highly debated (Wodinsky et al., 1994). Autologous transplant for breast cancer probably is the most widely discussed and controversial therapy. Welch and Mogielnicki (2002) summarize the early reports and media hype that led women to sue their insurance companies to obtain coverage. They further describe the political pressure and lawsuits that caused insurance companies to cover transplant for breast cancer. Finally, it was discovered upon review (McGreal, 2000; Weiss, et al. 2000) that potential problems and inconsistencies existed in a report by South African oncologists (Bezwoda et al., 1995). Welch and Mogielnicki (2002) report that the findings of "no benefit" for transplant for patients with breast cancer (Lippman, 2000) caused insurance companies to no longer cover the procedure. They conclude that effectiveness of transplant must be proven before raising arguments about money.

Obtaining insurance coverage or raising funds may delay the transplant procedure. During this delay, the patient's cancer may progress, making him or her physically ineligible for the transplant. Patients and their families may experience frustration over the delay in treatment.

Patient Education

Complete discussion of the entire transplant process can be conducted by the BMT coordinator, physician, nurse practitioner, and staff

Table 4-2 Adult BMT Patient Care Delivery Process.

Consultation	Salvage Chemotherapy?	Evaluation	Harvest Stem Cells	High-Dose Therapy and Transplant	Recovery	Long-Term Follow-Up
Referral Received —Transplant coordinator/case manager (TC) obtains patient information, including radiology scans, pathology, and patient medical records. —TC schedules appointments for consultation visit. —Insurance authorization obtained for consultation visit. **Consultation Visit** —Patient attends transplant educational session (Presentation: Blood and Marrow Stem Cell Transplantation). —Physician/NP/PA and TC review all medical information, perform history and physical, provide patient education, outline treatment options, provide protocol consents, outline plan of care, and dictate letter to referring physician.	**Salvage Chemotherapy if Indicated** —Additional chemotherapy may be necessary to assure that the patient has the least amount of disease prior to transplant. —This may take place at transplant center or through the patient's local oncologist.	**Pretransplant Testing** —TC arranges pretransplant tests and communicates to the physician. —Continued patient education includes 1:1, classroom instruction, and written material. —Social work interview. —Meeting with financial counselor. —Insurance authorization obtained prior to proceeding with transplant. —Consents for transplant signed.	**Blood Stem Cell Collection** —Meeting with stem cell collection physician/case manager. —Evaluation of clinical status, education provided. —Mobilization of stem cells with growth factors and/or chemotherapy initiated. —Daily apheresis procedures to obtain stem cells. **Bone Marrow Harvest** —History and physical by harvesting physician/NP/PA. —Evaluation of clinical status,	**Transplant** —Transplant team determines if transplant will occur in the inpatient or outpatient setting. —TC coordinates schedule of high-dose therapy. —High-dose therapy begins ("minus" days). —Daily physical assessments. —Day 0, or transplant day, the stem cells are infused.	**Inpatient and/or Outpatient Recovery** —Daily assessments until absolute neutrophil count > 500. —Continued patient education includes discussion of medications, treatments, precautions during recovery. —Physician or TC communicates with referring physician. —Follow-up tests and procedures as needed. —TC schedules physician visits.	**100-Day and Annual Evaluation** —TC schedules +100-day and yearly follow-up. —Allogeneic patients may return home and may be scheduled to be seen on a frequent basis (e.g., every 3–6 months) —Re-immunizations scheduled for 1 year posttransplant.

—Central
venous
catheter
inserted.

education
provided, and
consents
signed.
—Harvest
performed.

—Autologous
patients
return home
about day
+25–30.
—Allogeneic
patients
return home
after day
+100.
—Primary
physician
continues
physical
assessments.

Source: The University of Nebraska Medical Center, Blood and Marrow Stem Cell Transplantation Program, Omaha, Nebraska.

Table 4-3 Evaluation of a patient
for BMT.

Laboratory Tests
  Complete blood count
  Serum tests for major organ function (renal,
    hepatic, endocrine)
  Infectious disease tests (hepatitis B surface
    antigen, hepatitis B core antigen, hepatitis
    C antibody, human immunodeficiency
    virus [HIV-1] antibody, HIV-2 antibody,
    HIV antigen, human T cell lymphotropic
    virus [HTLV], and syphilis)
  CMV
  Herpes simplex virus
  PT/PTT
  ABO/Rh blood group typing
Pulmonary function tests
Chest x-ray
MUGA/echocardiogram
Electrocardiogram
Nutritional evaluation
Psychological evaluation
Social work evaluation
Dental exam
Pregnancy test

Staging Tests
  Bone marrow aspirate and biopsy
  Radiological tests (computerized tomogra-
    phy, magnetic resonance imaging, bone
    scans, x-rays, gallium scans)
  Tumor markers

**Additional Tests for Allogeneic Transplant
  Candidates**
ABO and Rh
  Histocompatible tissue typing
HLA typing (A, B, DR)

---

nurse during the initial evaluation or BMT interview. The patient usually receives a variety of
educational materials (pamphlets, notebooks,
videos, computer programs) that describe the
transplant process. The initial interview may be
quite overwhelming for the patient and family.
During the evaluation and eligibility workup,
reinforcement and frequent encouragement to
ask questions are essential. The transplant coordinator is a primary, consistent contact during
this phase. Outpatient nurses also provide much
of the information regarding transplant. In addition to individual contact, patients and families may benefit from small group presentations
and discussions. Prior to the start of the high-
dose therapy, the main objective is clarifying
and describing the transplant process.

Although informed consent for children is
obtained from the parent, information should be
given to the child in an age-appropriate manner
(Schmit-Pokorny and Nuss, 2000).

Donor Search

Patients have approximately a one in four (25%)
chance of having an HLA-identical sibling. For
patients who do not have a sibling match, a
matched, unrelated donor (MUD) search may be
performed through the National Marrow Donor
Program (NMDP). In 2004, there were more
than 5.5 million potential marrow and blood
stem cell donors and more than 40,000 cord
blood units listed on the NMDP registry
(NMDP, 2005). The NMDP preliminary search
automatically includes a search of the Bone
Marrow Donor Worldwide (BMDW) database.
The BMDW database lists volunteers from 48
registries in 37 countries. Currently, 40% of the
transplants facilitated by the NMDP involve either a foreign donor or a foreign recipient. In
2004, more than 170 stem cell transplants were
coordinated each month by the NMDP.

Tissue Typing

A critical component of allogeneic blood or
marrow transplantation is to determine the

compatibility of the donor and the recipient. The degree of compatibility is determined by comparing their HLA typing. The HLA histocompatibility system includes at least six antigen groups that are located on the sixth chromosome: HLA-A, -B, -C, -DR, -DQ, and -DP (Welte, 1994). This HLA code, or fingerprint, allows the body's immune system to differentiate self and nonself cells and to mount an immune reaction against nonself cells (Weinberg, 1991). Individuals inherit two sets of antigens, a maternal haplotype and a paternal haplotype. Antigens are in two classes. Class I antigens are found on the surface of most nucleated body cells and are readily detected on leukocytes. They include antigens, or loci, A, B, and C. They are identified or typed serologically or molecularly by a small blood sample (see Chapter 3). Class II antigens are typed using DNA technology, which is very accurate. Methods currently used are sequence-specific primer amplification (SSP), sequence-specific oligonucleotide probe hybridization (SSOP), and single-stranded conformational polymorphism (SSCP). DNA typing is performed at low resolution (it detects all alleles of an HLA gene) at the antigen level and at high resolution to detect selected alleles.

The search for a compatible marrow donor involves comparing the most significant antigens, HLA-A, -B, and -DR, that are most involved in developing a response to graft-versus-host disease. The ideal donor is identical to the recipient at all three loci, resulting in a six-antigen match. The NMDP has provided guidelines for donor selection for unrelated transplants (Hurley et al., 2003). It suggests that it is advantageous to the patient's survival to match at the allele level for HLA-A, -B, -C, and -DRB1. See Chapter 3 for a complete discussion.

Donor Preparation

Once HLA typing has been reviewed to determine the most appropriate donor, education and medical evaluation of the transplant donor is conducted by the donor center. The standard physical evaluation of a donor includes:

- Medical history
- Physical exam, including vaccination, travel, and recent blood transfusion history
- Psychosocial evaluation
- Laboratory evaluation
    CBC with differential
    Serum tests for major organ function (renal, hepatic)
    Infectious disease tests (hepatitis B surface antigen, hepatitis B core antigen, hepatitis C antibody, human immunodeficiency virus [HIV-1] antibody, HIV-2 antibody, HIV antigen, human T cell lymphotropic virus [HTLV], and syphilis)
    Cytomegalovirus
    Herpes simplex virus
    ABO and Rh
    HLA typing
- Prothrombin time (PT) Partial thromboplastin time (PTT) Internormal Ratio (INR)
- Pregnancy test
- Electrocardiograph (bone marrow donor only)
- Chest x-ray (bone marrow donor only)

Storage of autologous blood, which may be reinfused at the time of the bone marrow harvest, is done prior to the harvest. The blood will replace the blood lost during the bone marrow harvest, and may also decrease the donor's anxiety regarding exposure to viruses in the blood donation from the community (Dannie, 1991). A thorough description of the collection or harvesting procedure and the general transplant process is discussed. Assessment of the potential impact that stem cell collection or harvest may have on the donor's lifestyle and the relationship with the recipient should also be discussed. A social worker may also evaluate or follow up with the patient or family to help them to deal with stress related to the donation or concerns for the recipient.

Unrelated donors also receive counseling prior to the donation of stem cells. The healthcare provider must remember that the donor is a volunteer and should not be pressured into donating marrow or blood stem cells. The identity of an unrelated donor remains unknown to both the patient and the transplanting center.

Stem Cell Collection

Stem cells may be harvested from circulating blood or bone marrow. The method depends on the patient's type of disease and the protocol.

Peripheral Blood Stem Cell Transplant

The use of peripheral blood stem cells is replacing marrow stem cells for both autologous and allogeneic transplant (see Figures 4-5 and 4-6). Because there are fewer stem cells in the blood stream than in bone marrow, mobilizing or enhancing the number of stem cells in the blood by using chemotherapy and/or growth factors is a common practice.

Chemotherapy causes an increase in the number of circulating progenitor cells in the peripheral blood above the baseline level. During this increase, the stem cells are collected. Mobilizing stem cells with chemotherapy results in earlier engraftment (To et al., 1990). A single agent that has been used to mobilize stem cells is cyclophosphamide (Juttner et al., 1994). Using chemotherapy for mobilization has several disadvantages. Myelosuppressive chemotherapy may result in neutropenia and infection requiring antibiotic therapy (To et al., 1990). Also, stem cell mobilization does not occur until approximately 2 weeks following the myelosuppressive chemotherapy. If not enough stem cells are collected, the patient must undergo this chemotherapy again and continue the collections (Kessinger, 1993).

Hematopoietic growth factors are also used to mobilize stem cells (Socinski et al., 1988). Common growth factors used for mobilization are granulocyte-macrophage colony-stimulating factor (GM-CSF, sargramostim) and granulocyte colony-stimulating factor (G-CSF, filgrastim). Other growth factors that have been reported to mobilize stem cells are IL-3, (Vose et al., 1992), PIXY321 (Bishop et al., 1996), recombinant human stem cell factor (Glaspy et al., 1997), FLT3 ligand (Lebsack et al., 1997), and erythropoietin (Kessinger and Sharp, 1996). Kessinger and Sharp (2003) summarized the results from these studies and concluded that they are not as useful as sargramostim or filgrastim. Additional studies are currently being conducted for recombinant pegfilgrastim (Steidl et al., 2003) and Mpl ligands.

An apheresis machine collects the stem cells from the peripheral blood. Usually, the white blood count (WBC) is monitored to determine when to initiate the collection of stem cells. When growth factors are used for mobilization, collections may be started when the WBC reaches 10^9/liter, approximately day 4–5 following the start of growth factor. If chemotherapy is used for mobilization, the collections may begin when the WBC reaches 1.0^9/liter, approximately 10–14 days following chemotherapy. If both hematopoietic growth factors and chemotherapy are used for mobilization, apheresis begins when the WBCs start to recover, approximately when the WBC reaches 1.0^9/liter. The antecubital vein may be used; however, if it is inadequate, the patient usually has a central venous catheter placed, most commonly in the subclavian vein. The apheresis machine centrifuges blood drawn from the patient, drawing the stem cell layer into a collection bag and returning the rest to the patient. Depending on the type of apheresis machine, the machine may process 12 to 15 liters of blood in 2 to 4 hours. Large-volume apheresis procedures in which up to 40 liters of blood are processed have been reported (Kapustay and Buchsel, 2000). The collection procedures are repeated daily until the target cell yield is obtained.

An adequate number of stem cells may be collected in one apheresis procedure. The average number of collections is four; however, some patients may need many collections in order to achieve an adequate amount (Schmit-Pokorny, 2004).

A variety of methods have been used to determine an adequate collection of stem cells for transplant. Evaluating the number of mononuclear cells (MNC) present in the collection was the initial method used. The assay to detect committed progenitors, colony-forming units granulocyte-macrophage (CFU-GM), became the most common method to determine an adequate collection. Currently, the use of flow cytometric analysis to measure the number of cells expressing the CD34 antigen in the product is the most common method for determining an adequate number of stem cells.

Side effects during the collection procedure are minimal and usually well tolerated by the patient (see **Table 4-4**). Small children may re-

quire blood products to prime the apheresis tubing to prevent removal of too much blood. Also, the overall collection time will be longer and a lesser amount of blood should be processed. Age-appropriate activities should also be available during the lengthy apheresis procedure.

Collecting stem cells from peripheral blood offers the donor a less invasive procedure than bone marrow harvesting (Juttner et al., 1994). Also, stem cells collected from a donor's blood may result in more rapid engraftment. Another potential advantage of collecting donor stem cells is that the product may contain natural killer cells, promoting an adoptive immunotherapeutic approach (Juttner et al., 1994).

The first allogeneic peripheral blood stem cell transplant was reported by Kessinger and colleagues (1989). Ten apheresis collections were obtained from the donor. The T lymphocytes were depleted to decrease graft-versus-host disease. Although the patient died from an infectious complication at approximately 1 month following the transplant, hematopoietic recovery was established. Currently, most centers are collecting peripheral blood stem cells from related donors. Usually the donor is mobilized with a growth factor, G-CSF, and 10–15 liter apheresis procedures are conducted. Related donors often donate in one to two collections (Kessinger and Sharp, 2003).

To and colleagues (1992) noted patients who received autologous PBSCT recovered neutrophils and platelet counts faster and required less supportive care than patients who received an allogeneic or autologous bone marrow transplant. This decrease in supportive care and inpatient length of stay translates into decreased cost of transplantation for patients who receive a PBSCT. Henon and colleagues (1992) noted more rapid granulocyte and platelet recovery

Table 4-4 Some side effects of blood stem cell collection.

Potential Side Effects	Etiology	Assessment	Intervention
Citrate toxicity	Hypocalcemia caused by citrate's binding of ionized calcium	Baseline serum calcium Patient age Paresthesias of the extremities or circumoral area during the procedure	Notify physician if low. Do not exceed 1.5 ml/kg/minute flow in pediatric patients. Slow flow rate and offer oral calcium. Increase calcium-containing foods. Give calcium supplements.
Hypovolemia	Extracorporeal volume greater than patient's tolerance	Baseline pulse and blood pressure, Hgb/Hct, and health history Brief physical assessment and vital signs every 5 minutes initially, gradually decreasing frequency as patient's tolerance is established Assess for: 　Hypotension 　Tachycardia 　Light-headedness 　Diaphoresis 　Dysrhythmias	Notify physician of abnormal or unexpected findings before proceeding. Interrupt the procedure until the patient is stable, then resume at a slower flow rate and minimal extracorporeal volume. Monitor physical status and vital signs closely. Notify physician if symptoms persist or progress. Administer blood products. Administer fluid.
Thrombocytopenia	Collection of platelets into product	Baseline platelet count Ascertain whether platelet-rich plasma will be returned at the procedure's completion	Notify physician if less than 50,000/mm^3. Monitor for signs of postprocedure bleeding. Administer platelet products.

Table 4-4 SOME SIDE EFFECTS OF BLOOD STEM CELL COLLECTION *continued.*

Potential Side Effects	Etiology	Assessment	Intervention
Miscellaneous Chilling	Cooling of blood while circulating in apheresis machine	Note any unusual response	Provide warmth (e.g., blankets, heating pad).
Severe headache	Intracranial metastases unique to patient with cancer	CT or MRI of brain in patients prone to intracranial metastasis prior to apheresis (e.g., breast cancer)	Treat the problem (e.g., analgesics for; headache, transfusion support).
Prolonged cytopenia	Pediatric patients with less developed hematopoietic progenitor pool	Observe CBC, PH, Diff daily	Watch for patterns of emergencies in subsequent patients and report findings to the professional community. • Provide transfusion support.

Source: Data from Hooper, P. and Santas, E. 1993. Peripheral blood stem cell transplantation. *Oncol Nurs Forum* 20(8): 1215–1221; Kessinger, A. and Schmit-Pokorny, K. 1990. Toxicities associated with cryopreserved autologous peripheral stem cell infusions: influence of purification methods. *J Clin Apheresis* 5:156. Used with permission.

following PBSCT. They also noted a decrease in the documented infections, transfusions, and length of hospitalization. Cost was reduced by 45% (Henon et al., 1992).

Bone Marrow Transplant

Bone marrow, which contains more stem cells than peripheral blood (McCarthy and Goldman, 1984), can be harvested as an inpatient or outpatient procedure, under general or spinal anesthesia. The patient is placed in a prone position and multiple needle aspirations from both posterior iliac crests are obtained. Marrow may also be aspirated from the anterior iliac crests and the sternum if the cell yield is not adequate from the posterior iliac crests. The amount of bone marrow or

the number of nucleated cells necessary for transplant is not established; however, most institutions attempt to harvest a minimum of 1 to 2.5 $\times$ 10^8 nucleated cells per kilogram (Keating, 1995). The total fluid volume obtained is usually between 500 ml and 1000 ml. The entire harvest procedure usually takes 1 to 2 hours and the patient can be discharged following recovery. The bone marrow is filtered to remove fat and bone particles and processed similarly to blood stem cells. Marrow obtained from a donor will be depleted of red cells or plasma if there is a major ABO incompatibility of donor and recipient.

Following the harvest and recovery, the donor may experience pain at the collection sites. Mild analgesics can be prescribed. The donor's body will replace the bone marrow cells that were removed in a few weeks. The risks involved with a bone marrow harvest are minimal.

Human Cord Blood

The use of umbilical cord blood (UCB) transplants in children has risen in the last few years, but it still accounts for less than 20% of allogeneic transplants (Loberiza, 2003). The most common method used to harvest cord blood is puncturing the umbilical vein with a 16-gauge needle once the placenta has been delivered. The blood is drained by gravity or withdrawn into a syringe. Wagner and colleagues (1995) reported that the median volume of cord blood harvested was 100 ml (range 42.1 to 282 ml). The New York Blood Center, established in 1992, is the largest UCB bank in the United States. The NMDP also began to facilitate UCB transplants in 1999.

Cryopreservation

Two methods of cryopreservation are commonly used to store stem cells from blood or bone marrow. The first method uses 10% by volume of dimethylsulfoxide (DMSO), followed by controlled-rate freezing and storage in a liquid nitrogen freezer. The second method uses 5% DMSO and 6% hydroxyethyl starch (HES). The cells are then stored between $-80°C$ and $-196°C$ in a freezer (Kessinger, 1993).

Stem Cell Manipulation

If there is a concern that the autologous stem cell product contains malignant cells, removal of tumor cell contamination may be attempted by purging. Two main methods of purging are negative cell selection and positive cell selection. Negative cell selection involves attempts to remove tumor cells from the product. A variety of methods including physical separation, chemotherapy, monoclonal antibodies, toxins, magnetic beads, and radionuclides are described by Blume and Thomas (2000). They conclude that even though some studies showed promising results, delayed engraftment was noted in some studies. Further randomized trials are needed to determine if purged products are preferable.

Positive cell selection involves removing the stem cells necessary for transplant from the product. Blume and Thomas (2000) describe the use of sorting devices that target specific cell antigens (e.g., CD34 antigens). The targeted cells are removed and have been used for transplant. This method is very labor intensive and has a high cost. Further studies must be conducted before this method becomes standard.

Ex Vivo Expansion of Stem Cells

Another approach to obtaining an adequate amount of stem cells for transplant is ex vivo expansion, or growth of the cells in the laboratory following harvest or collection. Several growth factors are added to the stem cell cultures; this is followed by incubation to increase the number of cells (Brugger et al., 1995).

Preconditioning Chemotherapy

Patients with bulky disease or high tumor burden may benefit from standard-dose chemotherapy prior to the high-dose chemotherapy to decrease tumor burden. It may also be given to test chemosensitivity. This chemotherapy (i.e., cyclophosphamide) may be combined with the process of peripheral blood stem cell collection and serve as a mobilizer for blood stem cells.

Preparative Regimens

Following the physical and psychological evaluations and harvesting of the blood or marrow cells, the patient receives the high-dose chemotherapy and/or radiation. The ideal preparative regimen is capable of eradicating malignancy, has tolerable morbidity without mortality, and has sufficient immunosuppressive effect in allogeneic marrow recipients to avoid graft rejection (Forman et al., 1994). Preparative regimens vary according to the disease and medical condition of the patient and the institution's protocol. The preparative regimen consists of high-dose chemotherapy with or without radiation therapy and is capable of eradicating the disease. No ideal preparative regimen has been determined; it is selected based on the chemosensitivity of the tumor. Determining appropriate antineoplastic transplant therapy has been the major focus of marrow transplant researchers for more than 30 years. Disease recurrence, treatment-related mortality, and graft failure all remain important causes of treatment failure. High-dose chemotherapy is usually given over a course of 2 to 6 days. For more detailed preparative regimen information, see Chapter 5.

Total body irradiation (TBI), total lymphoid irradiation (TLI), or total abdominal irradiation (TAI) can be used for immunosuppression of patients or to eradicate disease. In addition, localized irradiation ("boost" treatment) may be used for areas of presumed higher concentrations of malignant cells (Shank, 1994). If TBI is part of the preparative regimen, it may be given in one dose or in multiple doses over the course of several days (fractionated radiation therapy). Fractionated dosing schedules appear to minimize the risk of side effects and are generally preferred over single doses. Considerations relevant to the effective therapy delivered include the nature of the radioactive source, source distance, patient positioning, total dose, and dose rate.

The preparative regimens may take place as an inpatient or outpatient. The patient may be admitted to a room in a unit designated for transplant patients. Isolation techniques during transplantation include reverse isolation, or reverse isolation with special air handling systems, high efficiency particulate air (HEPA) filters, or laminar air flow (LAF) (Zerbe et al., 1994). Zerbe and colleagues (1994) reported that admitting patients to LAF caused more anxiety than simple reverse isolation. However, they concluded that these findings need to be replicated due to lack of research-based evidence to demonstrate efficacy of many reverse isolation techniques.

The efficacy of different isolation techniques was studied by Passweg et al. (1998). They reviewed IBMTR records for 5065 patients who received an allogeneic BMT between 1988 and 1992. HEPA and/or LAF isolation was compared to single patient room isolation with any combination of hand-washing, gloves, masks, or gowns. Their conclusion was that transplant-related mortality during the first 100 days post-transplant was significantly lower in patients who were transplanted in HEPA/LAF isolation. This decrease in mortality resulted in a significantly higher 1-year survival rate for patients treated in HEPA/LAF isolation.

Cohen, Ley, and Tarzian (2001) reported a phenomenological study in which they explored the perceptions of 20 patients following autologous BMT. Patients reported that physical isolation, regardless of the type of isolation, was experienced by all patients. Cohen, Ley, and Tarzian found that physical isolation often led to emotional isolation. They suggest the need for support groups, increased education for the family, and professional emotional support.

Some institutions administer high-dose chemotherapy on an outpatient basis, admitting the patient to the hospital only if physical conditions necessitate (Jagannath et al., 1997; Meisenberg et al., 1997). Other centers administer the high-dose chemotherapy on an inpatient basis, discharging the patient prior to the transplant or shortly after (Meisinger et al., 1996).

An innovative approach to delivering care to transplant patients is the use of the Cooperative Care Model (Schmit-Pokorny et al., 2003). In this model, a family member or friend serves as the primary caregiver for the patient during the acute phase of the transplant. The patient and care partner learn skills necessary to care for the patient that will later be used at home. The patients are admitted to an inpatient home-like setting, with hotel-style service and amenities. The patient's suite consists of a sitting area, kitchenette, bedroom, and bathroom. Patients receive chemotherapy, blood products, monitoring, infusion of stem cells, and many other treatments and procedures in the treatment center, open 24 hours a day, 7 days a week.

Schmit-Pokorny (2005) reviewed the various models of outpatient transplantation, including advantages and disadvantages. Schmit-Pokorny states that there are several critical components to maintaining a patient in the outpatient setting, including having a dedicated care partner, a strong education program, and a diverse multidisciplinary team with excellent transplant nurses.

Regardless of where the chemotherapy or radiation therapy is given, patient education, including mouth care, incentive spirometry, skin care, hand-washing, diet, neutropenic precautions, and activity, is crucial.

Stem Cell Infusion

The day of the transplant or infusion of the stem cells is generally referred to as day 0. The patient is usually premedicated to lessen the side effects associated with cell infusion (transplant). Premedications may include lorazepam, diphenhydramine hydrochloride, meperidine hydrochloride, hydrocortisone, acetaminophen, furosemide, or methylprednisolone. The patient is usually hydrated prior, during, and following the infusion. The stem cells are thawed in a water bath at approximately 37°C until the product is liquid. The stem cells are then quickly infused via a central venous catheter, using a syringe or infusion pump (Kessinger, 1993). During the infusion and for several hours following, the patient may experience side effects associated with the dimethylsulfoxide preservative, volume of infusate, or amount of red blood cells infused (see **Table 4-5**).

Kessinger and Schmit-Pokory (1990) noted that patients who received larger volumes containing a greater number of red cells had a larger number and greater severity of side effects. Children tend to tolerate complications associated with transplant better than adults (Shannon et al., 1987).

The transplant patient may experience a variety of complications or side effects during the preparative regimen and continuing throughout recovery (see **Table 4-6**). These complications are covered in detail in the rest of this publication.

Engraftment and Recovery

It takes approximately 7 to 15 days following the transplant for the cells to find their home (*homing*) and begin to produce normal blood cells.

Table 4-5 SOME SIDE EFFECTS OF MARROW AND BLOOD CELL REINFUSION (TRANSPLANT).

Potential Side Effect	Etiology	Assessment	Intervention
Nausea Vomiting	DMSO	Evaluate amount and frequency	Give antiemetics Lorazepam Diphenhydramine hydrochloride Ondansetron Prochlorperazine
Hemoglobinuria Elevated serum creatinine Elevated serum bilirubin	Lysis of RBCs DMSO	Baseline creatinine and bilirubin Hematest urine	Hydration
Chest tightness Cough Dyspnea Increased weight Hypertension Tachycardia Tachypnea	Volume of infusate	Vital signs every 15–30 minutes I/O hourly	Decrease rate of infusion Administer furosemide or mannitol Give oxygen
Chills, fever	Coldness of product	Temperature every 15–30 minutes	Provide warmth Give meperidine hydrochloride Give acetaminophen PRN
Garlic taste or smell	DMSO	Ask patient if taste noticed	Provide mints or gum
Anaphylactic reaction	DMSO	Notify physician for c/o itching, wheezing, skin rash, or erythema	Stop infusion Administer epinephrine
Miscellaneous Diarrhea Headache Flushing Abdominal cramping Malaise	DMSO	Evaluate frequency and duration	Treat symptoms Decrease rate of infusion

Table 4-6 COMPLICATIONS OF HIGH-
DOSE THERAPY AND TRANSPLANTATION.

Infection
— Bacterial
— Viral
— Fungal
Anemia
Bleeding
Fatigue
Hair loss
Gastrointestinal complications
— Mucositis
— Stomatitis
— Nausea
— Vomiting
— Diarrhea
— Anorexia
— Taste changes
— Loss of appetite
Renal toxicity
— Acute renal failure
Hepatic toxicity
— Veno-occlusive disease
— Hepatic injury
Bladder toxicity
— Hemorrhagic cystitis
Pulmonary toxicity
— Pneumonia
— Edema
— Diffuse alveolar hemorrhage
— Infections
Neurologic complications
Cardiac toxicity
Skin toxicity
Vision changes
Failed or delayed engraftment
Psychosocial
Graft-versus-host disease
— Acute
— Chronic

Hematopoietic and immunological recovery of the transplant patient occur at variable speeds and are influenced by a number of factors, including the nature and status of the primary disease, previously administered chemotherapy and radiation, the type of preparative regimen, the type of GVHD prophylaxis, viral complications (particularly CMV), and the use of antiviral agents (Messner and McCulloch, 1994).

The average length of hospital stay varies according to the patient's condition, type of transplant, and protocol. The use of peripheral blood stem cell transplants and use of growth factors has dramatically reduced the length of hospital stay. Discharge planning should begin early in the course of the hospitalization. Transplant centers vary in their criteria for discharge from the acute-care setting. Common criteria for discharge following transplant include:

- Patient's absolute neutrophil count (ANC) is greater than $500/mm^3$ for 2 consecutive days.
- Patient is afebrile and has been off antibiotics for 48 hours.
- Patient's oral intake is greater than 1000 Kcal per day.
- Nausea and vomiting is controlled.
- Diarrhea is less than 500 ml per day.
- Patient tolerance of oral medications has lasted at least 48 hours.
- Caregivers are able and willing to provide 24-hour care for as long as needed.
- The patient or caregiver is able to care for central venous catheter.

Discharge from the transplant center is often a time of both excitement and anxiety for patients and their families. Patients look forward to recuperating in their own homes, sleeping in their own beds, eating home-cooked foods, and resuming their previous lifestyles. At the same time, they are hesitant to "cut the cord" with the health-care team that has provided vigilant care in the hospital. Families may feel inadequate in providing the necessary care for the patients. It may also put an additional burden on families if someone must take time off from work or change daily living patterns. It is important for the nurse to discuss these common feelings with patients and families when planning discharge. Patients need to be reassured that their discharge depends on competent caregivers and adequate supports and resources in the home. Additionally, the BMT team is available 24 hours a day, 7 days a week.

It is critical that the BMT nurse provides verbal and written discharge instructions to patients and their families prior to discharge. These instructions should include signs and symptoms to report to the transplant center, bleeding precautions, infection control practices, central line care, dietary restrictions, medication instructions, dates of outpatient appointments and blood counts, and what to do in an emergency. **Figure** 4-9 illustrates common written discharge instructions given to marrow and blood stem cell transplant patients. It is not all-inclusive of written instructions given to the patients regarding follow-up care.

Follow-up Care

Follow-up care of the blood or marrow cell recipient for the first 100 days after transplant can be provided in an outpatient, ambulatory, or home-care setting. The focus of the healthcare team is to prevent and treat complications and to assess engraftment and disease status in the post-BMT recipient. Major complications that may occur 30 to 100 days postallogeneic transplant include acute GVHD, interstitial pneumonia (CMV and idiopathic), and disseminated fungal infection. Other complications that may occur during this phase are varicella-zoster virus, bacteremia, herpes simplex virus, and restrictive lung disease. Routine care includes thorough physical assessments; blood

work; blood product transfusions; administration of TPN, antibiotics, immunoglobulin, and IV fluids; symptom management; skin biopsies; bone marrow biopsies and aspirations; spinal taps with the instillation of intrathecal chemotherapy; close monitoring of medication administration and drug levels; and care of the central venous catheter. Additionally, psychosocial support and physical therapy are continued during this posttransplant phase.

It is crucial that nurses working in the outpatient and home-care setting provide consistent care and communicate regularly. It is extremely beneficial for the home-care nurse to meet the patient and family prior to discharge. This will alleviate anxiety the patient and family may feel about the patient's going home.

Posttransplant Evaluation

Most centers evaluate disease status and major organ toxicity 100 days following transplant. Patients may undergo the following tests: CBC, PLt, Diff, pulmonary function test, and liver and kidney function tests. Additional testing of tumor response is done individually for the particular disease and may include bone marrow biopsy and aspirate, tumor markers, CT scans, MRI, bone scans, and skeletal scans. Annual evaluations are recommended to examine the patient for transplant-related problems.

Delayed Complications after Transplant

The number of BMT recipients is increasing rapidly. Most patients are able to live a relatively normal productive life. Some, however, develop delayed or long-term complications that compromise quality of life. Common delayed complications following transplant include:

- Chronic graft-versus-host disease
- Pulmonary disease

- Neurologic complications
- Disease relapse
- Secondary malignancies
- Cataracts
- Infertility
- Growth and development disorders in children
- Psychosocial dysfunction
- Avascular necrosis
- Late infectious complications
- Dental problems
- Genitourinary dysfunction

- Chronic fatigue
- Depression
- Thyroid dysfunction

Some delayed complications are transplant related (e.g., GVHD, immunodeficiency); others are due to the intensity of the preparative regimen (e.g., infertility, cataracts). Some of the delayed complications are related to the underlying disease (e.g., recurrence of disease) and many are multifactorial in etiology (e.g., secondary malignancies, chronic pulmonary disease) (Deeg, 1994). Chapter 12 discusses other

---

Figure 4-9 Blood and marrow transplant discharge instructions.

Now you are entering the phase of transplant where a great deal of your successful recovery depends on you and your caregiver. This short list of instructions is designed to help you with this process.

Post page 1 in a prominent place for easy reference.

EMERGENCIES AND WHEN TO CALL:

A blood and marrow transplant (BMT) physician and a physician's assistant are available to you 24 hours a day, 7 days a week.

WHOM TO CALL:

Between 8 AM and 5 PM, Monday through Friday, call or page your case manager, or call the operator at 555-555-5555 and ask to have your case manager paged.

Your case manager is: _____

Telephone number: _____

Digital pager number: _____

Before 8 AM and **after** 5 PM, Monday through Friday and weekends, Call 555-555-5555 and ask the operator to speak to the **BMT physician assistant (PA) on call**.

CALL IMMEDIATELY IF:

- Your temperature reaches or exceeds 101.5 F. Take your temperature twice daily and record. <u>Do not</u> take Tylenol or acetaminophen to bring your temperature down.
- You notice any rashes on your skin.
- You have serious stomach cramping.
- You get the "chills."
- You have excessive bleeding from the nose, mouth, or catheter, or if you notice blood in your stool.
- You experience severe headache or dizziness.

1

- You see any new drainage from your central line, or if the site is red or tender.
- You have diarrhea with more than five stools a day, or your stool pattern changes in color or consistency.
- You develop a new cough, or become short of breath.

MEDICATIONS: Your medications are very important to treat and prevent complications and other problems

- List all your medications, their dosages, and when you take them. Keep this information in a notebook or folder. This will help you to track changes in your medications. If you are unsure of a medication name, dose, or its use, please ask your physician or nurse.
- Keep your notebook with you at all times; bring it with you to each clinic visit.
- Do *NOT* use aspirin, Excedrin, or ibuprofen products, such as Advil, Motrin, or Nuprin if your platelet count is below normal. These medications can affect your platelets. Always ask your physician before taking any over-the-counter medication.

REST:

Many patients have difficulty sleeping at night the first few nights after dismissal from the transplant unit. Rest during the day as needed, but remember that napping too often may interfere with your sleep at night. Please inform your physician or case manager if you experience extreme fatigue.

EXERCISE:

Exercise is important in gaining strength and maintaining or increasing lung function.

- Increase your activity as tolerated.
- Try to do a little more each day without becoming exhausted.
- You may walk outside if the weather is good.
- Avoid construction areas or any areas where there is likely to be a lot of dust.
- Avoid crowds. Use common sense. Go to the mall or a movie at nonpeak times.

ENVIRONMENT:

You should make sure that your external environment is such that it promotes healing.

- Always wear a mask outside your room or apartment while around the hospital.
- Screen guests for coughs, colds, flu, or recent exposure to illness.
- Due to the bacteria and fungi content, you may not have fresh flowers, plants, or artificial flowers or plants until you are off all immunosuppressive therapy.

SEXUAL ACTIVITY:

Sexual activity can still be enjoyed while you are here. There are some precautions to take, however, to minimize potential problems.

- Kissing is encouraged!
- Men must wear a condom during intercourse while on steroids or immunosuppressive therapy.
- Female partners should also have their partner wear a condom and use a water-soluble, nonirritating lubricant (i.e., Replens) to help relieve vaginal dryness.

QUESTIONS:

Please speak with your case manager or physician if you have questions.

long-term effects. The causes of death after transplants done from 1996 to 2000 and reported to the IBMTR/ABMTR are shown in **Figure 4-10**.

Blood and marrow stem cell transplantation offers patients a potential cure from their malignant or nonmalignant disease. Transplant nurses, who play a major role in the suc-

cess of the transplant, must have a thorough understanding of the entire process.

Acknowledgment

I would like to acknowledge and thank Susan O'Connell for her contributions as co-author for the second edition of this chapter.

Figure 4-10 Causes of death after transplants done in 1996–2000.

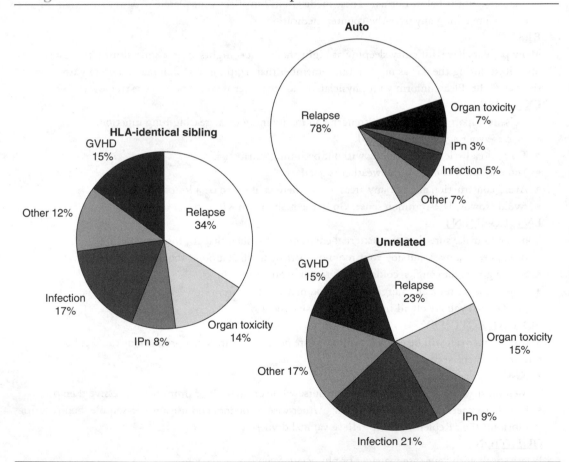

Source: Loberiza, F. (2003). Report on state of the art in blood and marrow transplantation: Part 1 of the IBMTR/ABMTR summary slides with guide. *IBMTB/ABMTR Newsletter 10*(1). Retrieved May 5, 2005, from http://www.ibmtr.org/ABOUT/NEWS/2003Nov.pdf. Used with permission of IBMTR.

References

Anagnostopoulos, A., Giralt, S. (2002). Critical review on non-myeloablative stem cell transplantation (NST). *Crit Rev Oncol Hemat*, 44:175–190.

Armitage, J., Gale, R. (1989). Bone marrow autotransplantation. *Am J Med* 86:203–206.

ASCO/ASH. (1990). Recommended criteria for the performance of bone marrow transplantation. *Blood* 75(5):1209.

Bezwoda, W., Seymour, I., Dansey, R. (1995). High-dose chemotherapy with hematopoietic rescue as a primary treatment for metastatic breast cancer: a randomized trial. *J Clin Oncol* 13:2483–2489.

Bishop, M.R., Jackson, J.D., O'Kane-Murphy, B., Schmit-Pokorny, K., Vose, J., Bierman, P.J., et al. (1996). Phase I trial of recombinant fusion protein PIXY321 for mobilization of peripheral-blood cells. *J Clin Oncol* 14:2521–2526.

Blume, K.G., Thomas, E.D. (2000). A review of autologous hematopoietic cell transplantation. *Biol Blood Marrow Transplant* 6:1–12.

Brugger, W., Heimfeld, S., Berenson, R., Mertelsmann, R., Kanz, L. (1995). Reconstitution of hematopoiesis after high-dose chemotherapy by autologous progenitor cells generated ex vivo. *N Engl J Med* 333:5, 283–287.

Buchsel, P. (1993). Bone marrow transplantation. In Groenwald, S., Frogge, M., Goodman M., et al. (eds.), *Cancer Nursing: Principles and Practice*, 3rd ed. Boston: Jones and Bartlett, 393–434.

Buchsel, P., Kapustay, P. (1995). Peripheral stem cell transplantation. *Oncol Nurs* 2(2):1–14.

Cohen, M., Ley, C., Tarzian, A. (2001). Isolation in blood and marrow transplantation. *West J Nurs Res* 23(6): 592–609.

Crump, M., Smith, A., Brandwein, J., et al. (1993). High-dose etoposide, melphalan and autologous bone marrow transplantation for patients with advanced Hodgkin's disease: importance of disease status at transplant. *Clin Oncol* 1(4):704–711.

Dannie, E. (1991). Assessment of bone marrow donors. *Nurs Stand* 5(32):28–31.

Deeg, J.H. (1994). Delayed complications after bone marrow transplantation. In: Forman, S.J., Blume, K.G., Thomas, E.D. (eds.), *Bone Marrow Transplantation*. Boston: Blackwell Scientific.

Department of Health and Human Services. Centers for Medicare and Medicaid Services. (2003, April 25). Medicare Intermediary Manual. Retrieved from www.cms.hhs.gov/manuals/pm_trans/r1880A3.pdf.

Forman, S.J., Blume K.G., Thomas, E.D. (eds.) 1994. *Bone Marrow Transplantation*. Boston: Blackwell Science.

Freedman, S.E. (1988). An overview of bone marrow transplantation. *Semin Oncol Nurs* 4:3–8.

Friedrich, W. (1994). Marrow transplantation for primary immunodeficiency diseases. *Marrow Transplant Rev* 4(2):17–22.

Gale, R., Butturini, A. (1995). What is the best strategy for bone marrow and blood cell autotransplants in cancer? In: Armitage, A., Antman, K. (eds.), *High-Dose Cancer Therapy: Pharmacology, Hematopoietins, Stem Cells*. Baltimore: Williams & Wilkins, 117–119.

Gale, R.P., Henon, P., Juttner, C. (1992). Blood stem cell transplants come of age. *Bone Marrow Transplantation* 9:151–155.

Glaspy, J.A., Shpall, E.J., LeMaistre, C.F., Briddell, R.A., Menchaca, D.M., Turner, S.A., et al. (1997). Peripheral blood progenitor cell mobilization using stem cell factor in combination with filgrastim in breast cancer patients. *Blood* 90:2939–2951.

Henon, P., Liang, H., Beck-Wirth, G., et al. (1992). Comparison of hematopoietic and immune recovery after autologous bone marrow or blood stem cell transplants. *Bone Marrow Transplantation* 9:285–291.

Hillner, B., Smith, T., Desch, C. (1992). Efficacy and cost-effectiveness of autologous bone marrow transplantation in metastatic breast cancer. *JAMA* 267(15): 2055–2061.

Hooper, P., Santas, E. (1993). Peripheral blood stem cell transplantation. *Oncol Nurs Forum* 20(8):1215–1221.

Hurley, C.K., Lowe, L.A., Logan, B., Karanes, C., Anasetti, C., Weisdorf, D., et al. (2003). National marrow donor program HLA-matching guidelines for unrelated marrow transplants. *Biol Blood Marrow Transplant* 9:610–615.

Jagannath, S., Armitage, J., Dicke, K., et al. (1989). Prognostic factors for response and survival after high-dose cyclophosphamide, carmustine, and etoposide with autologous bone marrow transplantation for relapsed Hodgkin's disease. *J Clin Oncol* 7(2):179–185.

Jagannath, S., Vesole, D., Zhang, M., Desikan, K., Copeland, N., Jagannath, M., et al. (1997). Feasibility and cost-effectiveness of outpatient autotransplants in multiple myeloma. *Bone Marrow Transplantation* 20:445–450.

Juttner, C., Fibbe, W., Nemunaitis, J., et al. (1994). Blood cell transplantation: report from an international consensus meeting. *Bone Marrow Transplantation* 14: 689–693.

Kapustay, P.M., Buchsel, P.C. (2000). Process, complications, and management of peripheral stem cell transplantation. In: Buchsel, P.C., Kapustay, P.M. (eds.), *Stem Cell Transplantation: A Clinical Textbook.* Pittsburgh, PA: Oncology Nursing Press, Inc., 5.1–5.28.

Keating, A. (1995). Autologous bone marrow transplantation. In: Armitage, A., Antman, K. (eds.), *High-Dose Therapy: Pharmacology, Hematopoietins, Stem Cells.* Baltimore: Williams & Wilkins, 172–195.

Kessinger, A. (1993). Utilization of peripheral blood stem cells in autotransplantation. *Hematol Oncol Clin North Am* 7(3):535–545.

Kessinger, A., Schmit-Pokorny, K. (1990). Toxicities associated with cryopreserved autologous peripheral stem cell infusions: influence of purification methods. *J Clin Apheresis* 5:156.

Kessinger, A., Sharp, G. (1996). Mobilization of hematopoietic progenitor cells with epoetin alfa. *Seminars in Hematology* 33(suppl 1):10–15.

Kessinger, A., Sharp, G. (2003). The whys and hows of hematopoietic progenitor and stem cell mobilization. *Bone Marrow Transplantation* 31:319–329.

Kessinger, A., Smith, D., Strandjord, S., et al. (1989). Allogeneic transplantation of blood derived, T cell-depleted hemopoietic stem cells after myeloablative treatment in a patient with acute lymphoblastic leukemia. *Bone Marrow Transplantation* 4:643–646.

Kurnick, N.B., Montano, A., Gerdes, J.C., et al. (1958). Preliminary observations on the treatment of post irradiation hemapoietic depression in man by the infusion of stored autologous bone marrow. *Ann Intern Med* 49:973.

Lebsack, M.E., McKenna, H.J., Hoek, J.A., et al. (1997). Safety of FLT3 ligand in healthy volunteers. *Blood* 90(suppl 1):17a (Abstr. 751).

Lippman, M. (2000). High-dose chemotherapy plus autologous bone marrow transplantation for metastatic breast cancer. *N Engl J Med* 342:1119–1120.

Loberiza, F. (2003). Report on state of the art in blood and marrow transplantation—Part 1 of the IBMTR/ABMTR summary slides with guide. *IBMTR/ABMTR Newsletter* 10:1, 7–10.

McCarthy, D., Goldman, J. (1984). Transfusion of circulating stem cells. *CRC Crit Rev Clin Lab Sci* 20(1):1–24.

McGreal, C. (2000). Top researcher falsified breast cancer results. *Guardian* 19(February):18.

McSweeney, P.A., Niederwieser, D., Shizuru, J.A., Sandmaier, B.M., Molina, A.J., Maloney, D.G., et al. (2001). Hematopoietic cell transplantation in older patients with hematologic malignancies: replacing high-dose cytotoxic therapy with graft-versus-tumor effects. *Blood* 97(11):3390–3400.

Meisenberg, B.R., Ferran, K., Hollenbach, K., Brehm, T., Jollon, J., Piro, L.D. (1998). Reduced charges and costs associated with outpatient autologous stem cell transplantation. *Bone Marrow Transplantation* 21: 927–932.

Meisenberg, B., Miller, W., McMillan, R., Callaghan, M., Sloan, C., Brehm, T., et al. (1997). Outpatient high-dose chemotherapy with autologous stem-cell rescue for hematologic and nonhematologic malignancies. *J Clin Oncol* 15(1):11–17.

Meisinger, D., Sasse, S., Schmit-Pokorny, K. (1996). "Early discharge" autologous bone marrow or peripheral stem cell transplant patients: outcomes. *Oncol Nurs Forum* 23(2):328 (abstr).

Messner, H.A., McCulloch, E.A. (1994). Mechanisms of human hematopoiesis. In Forman, S.J., Blume, K.G., Thomas, E.D. (eds.), *Bone Marrow Transplantation.* Boston: Blackwell Science, 41–71.

Meyer, C. (1992). The richness of oncology nursing. *Am J Nurs* 92(5):71–78.

National Marrow Donor Program. Addition of public cord units grow cord blood registry by 20 percent: National Marrow Donor Program increases cord blood units available for life-saving transplants. NMDP Web site. Retrieved May 5, 2005, from www.marrow.org.

Passweg, J., Rowlings, P., Atkinson, K., Barrett, A., Gale, R., Gratwohl, A., et al. (1998). Influence of protective isolation on outcome of allogeneic bone marrow transplantation for leukemia. *Bone Marrow Transplantation* 21:1231–1238.

Pegg, D.E. (1966). Syngeneic bone marrow transplantation in man. In Pegg, D.E. (ed.), *Bone Marrow Transplantation.* London: Lloyd-Luke, 102.

Randolph, S. (1993). Home care of the bone marrow transplant recipient. *Home Health Nurse* 11(1):24–28.

Santos, G. (1985). Overview of autologous bone marrow transplantation. *Int J Cell Cloning* 3:215–216.

Schmit-Pokorny, K. (2004). Stem cell collection. In Ezzone, S. (ed.), *Hematopoietic Stem Cell Transplantation: A Manual for Nursing Practice.* Pittsburgh, PA: Oncology Nursing Press, Inc., 23–42.

Schmit-Pokorny, K. (2005). Hematopoietic stem cell transplant outpatient models. In Buchsel, P.C., Yarbro, C.H. (eds.), *Oncology Nursing in the Ambulatory Setting*. Sudbury, MA: Jones and Bartlett Publishers, 211–230.

Schmit-Pokorny, K., Franco, T., Frappier, B., Vyhlidal, R. (2003). The Cooperative Care Model: an innovative approach to deliver blood and marrow stem cell transplant care. *Clin J Oncol Nurs* 7(5):509–514, 556.

Schmit-Pokorny, K., Nuss, S. (2000). Pediatric peripheral stem cell transplantation. In Buchsel, P.C., Kapustay, P.M. (eds.), *Stem Cell Transplantation: A Clinical Textbook*. Pittsburgh, PA: Oncology Nursing Press, Inc., 16.1–16.24.

Shank, B. (1994). Radiotherapeutic principles of bone marrow transplantation. In Forman, S.J., Blume, K.G., Thomas, E.D. (eds.), *Bone Marrow Transplantation*. Boston: Blackwell Science, 96–113.

Shannon, K, Cowan, M., Matthay, K. (1987). Pediatric bone marrow transplantation: intensive care management. *J Intensive Care Med* 2:328–344.

Sharp, J.G., Kessinger, A., Vaughan, W.P., Mann, S., Crouse, D.A., Dicke, K., et al. (1992). Detection and clinical significance of minimal tumor cell contamination of peripheral stem cell harvests. *Int J Cell Clon* 10(suppl 1):92–94.

Slavin, S., Nagler, A., Naparstek, E., Kapelushnik, Y., Aker, M., Cividallli, G., et al. (1998). Nonmyeloablative stem cell transplantation and cell therapy as an alternative to conventional bone marrow transplantation with lethal cytoreduction for the treatment of malignant and nonmalignant hematologic diseases. *Blood* 91(3):756–763.

Socinski, M., Cannistra, S., Elias, A., et al. (1988). Granulocyte-macrophage colony stimulating factor expands the circulating haemapoietic progenitor cell compartment in man. *Lancet* 1:1194.

Spitzer, T.R., McAfee, S., Sackstein, R., Colby, C., Toh, H.C., Multani, P., et al. (2000). Intentional induction of mixed chimerism and achievement of antitumor responses after nonmyeloablative conditioning therapy and HLA-matched donor bone marrow transplantation for refractory hematologic malignancies. *Biol Blood Marrow Transplantation* 6:309–320.

Steidl, U., Fenk, R., Kondakci, M., Henze, L., Hoyer, B., Graef, T., et al. (2003). Transplantation of peripheral blood stem cells mobilized by single dose application of pegylated G-CSF in patients with multiple myeloma. *Blood* 102(11), abstract no. 3554.

To, L., Roberts, M., Haylock, D., et al. (1992). Comparison of haematological recovery times and supportive care requirements of autologous recovery phase peripheral blood stem cell transplant, autologous bone marrow transplants and allogeneic bone marrow transplants. *Bone Marrow Transplantation* 9(4): 277–284.

To, L., Shepperd, K., Haylock, D., et al. (1990). Single dose of cyclophosphamide enables the collection of high numbers of hemapoietic stem cells from the peripheral blood. *Exp Hematol,* 190(18):442–447.

Treleaven, J., Barrett, J. (1992). *Bone Marrow Transplantation in Practice*. New York: Churchill Livingstone.

Vose, J.M., Kessinger, A., Bierman, P.J., Sharp, G., Garrison, L., Armitage, J.O. (1992). The use of rhIL-3 for mobilization of peripheral blood stem cells in previously treated patients with lymphoid malignancies. *Int J Cell Clon* 10(suppl 1):62–65.

Wagner, J., Kernan, N., Steinbuch, M., et al. (1995). Allogeneic sibling umbilical-cord-blood transplantation in children with malignant and non-malignant disease. *Lancet* 346:214–219.

Weinberg P.A. (1991). The human leukocyte antigen (HLA) system, the search for a matching donor, National Marrow Donor Program development, and marrow donor issues. In Whedon, M. (ed.), *Bone Marrow Transplantation: Principles, Practice, and Nursing Insights*. Boston: Jones and Bartlett Publishers, 105–131.

Weiss, R., Rifkin, R., Stewart, F., Theriault, R., Williams, I., Herman, A., et al. (2000). High-dose chemotherapy for high-risk primary breast cancer: an on-site review of the Bezwoda study. *Lancet* 355:999–1003.

Welch, H.G., Mogielnicki, J. (2002). Presumed benefit: lessons from the American experience with marrow transplantation for breast cancer. *BMJ* 324: 1088–1092.

Welte, K. (1994). Matched unrelated transplants. *Semin Oncol Nurs* 10(1):20–27.

Whedon, M.B. (1991). *Bone Marrow Transplantation: Principles, Practice, and Nursing Insights*. Boston: Jones and Bartlett Publishers.

Wodinsky, H., Dillman, R., MacDonald, S. (1994). Assessing peripheral stem cell transplant technology. *J Oncol Manage* 3(4):22–27.

Zerbe, M., Parkerson, S., Spitzer, T. (1994). Laminar air flow versus reverse isolation: nurses' assessments of moods, behaviors, and activity levels in patients receiving bone marrow transplants. *Oncol Nurs Forum* 21(3):565–568.

Chapter 5

Conditioning Regimens in Hematopoietic Stem Cell Transplantation

Cathleen M. Poliquin, MS, APRN-BC, AOCN®

Introduction

The first step in the stem cell transplant process is the conditioning regimen, also referred to as the preparative regimen. After the patient has been thoroughly evaluated and deemed medically and psychologically ready to undergo the hematopoietic stem cell transplant (HSCT), the conditioning phase of the HSCT process begins. The conditioning regimen is the phase of HSCT whereby the patient is physiologically prepared for the HSCT. Conditioning involves administering chemotherapy, radiation therapy, and immunosuppressive therapy singly, but more often in combination, during the days immediately preceding the HSCT. This chapter describes the rationale and types of conditioning regimens, chemotherapy/radiation therapy/immunotherapy used, the acute toxicities, and the nursing management of the acute toxicities.

Types of HSCT

There are several types of HSCT. In autologous HSCT, hematopoietic stem cells (HSC) from the bone marrow or the peripheral circulation are harvested or collected from the patient (recipient) and cryopreserved to be used at a later date. The patient serves as both the donor and recipient of the HSC. The purpose of the conditioning regimen in the autologous setting is eradication of malignant disease, and the components of the conditioning regimen consist of high-dose (myeloablative) chemoradiotherapy. Autologous HSCT is the treatment modality for hematologic malignancies and solid tumors.

In allogeneic HSCT, the source of stem cells is another individual (donor). The donor may be related or unrelated to the recipient. The HSCT may be fully HLA-matched or HLA-mismatched with the recipient. The purpose of the conditioning regimen in allogeneic HSCT is disease eradication, as in autologous HSCT, and additionally suppression of the host immune system and creation of space for the donor cells in the recipient marrow. The conditioning regimen can be myeloablative or nonmyeloablative. Allogeneic HSCT is the treatment modality for hematologic malignancies and many nonmalignant diseases, such as severe aplastic anemia, immunodeficiency diseases, and genetic diseases.

Conditioning Regimen

The days of conditioning are designated by negative or minus numbers. The day of the infusion of stem cells is referred to as day 0. All days following the stem cell infusion are designated by positive, or plus, numbers. For example, for a conditioning regimen that includes 4 days of total body irradiation (TBI) followed by 2 days of cyclophosphamide, the days of TBI would be called days -7, -6, -5, and -4, while the days of cyclophosphamide would be days -3 and -2. In this example, day -1 is considered a recovery day whereby no chemoradiotherapy is administered. The length of conditioning regimens varies depending on the specific protocol. Most conditioning regimens are completed in 2 to 8 days.

There is no standard conditioning regimen. Conditioning regimens vary in terms of chemotherapeutic drugs, other immunosuppressants and radiation administered, dosages, and scheduling. Consequently, many different conditioning regimens are used in HSCT. Conditioning regimens may be broadly classified as myeloablative or nonmyeloablative. Conditioning regimens may include high-dose/dose-intensive (myeloablative) chemotherapy alone or in combination with TBI, or reduced intensity (nonmyeloablative) chemotherapy alone or in combination with other immunomodulator drugs. Whatever the combination of chemotherapy, radiotherapy, or immunotherapy, conditioning regimens share similar goals.

The goals of the conditioning phase of the HSCT include the following:

1. Cytoreduction of malignant cells in patients undergoing HSCT for malignancy

2. Creation of "space" for the donor cells in the recipient marrow

3. Suppression of the host immune system

Although not a specific goal of the conditioning, the ideal conditioning regimen should limit severe nonhematological toxicity.

Although conditioning regimens share the same goals, choosing the appropriate regimen depends on many factors. In the early days of transplant, few conditioning regimens were available, so selecting the appropriate one was a fairly straightforward decision. However, now with a growing list of diseases treatable with HSCT, new chemotherapeutic agents, new combinations of chemoradiotherapy used in conditioning regimens, the availability of more sources of stem cells, and an increased patient population now eligible for HSCT, selecting the appropriate conditioning regimen is a complex decision for the transplant physician.

Mangan (2000) described several factors that must be considered when choosing an appropriate conditioning regimen. Please see **Table 5-1**.

Ablative Potency

Myeloablative conditioning regimens are very aggressive treatment modalities whereby dose-intensive chemotherapy, with or without total body irradiation, is administered. The goal is to eradicate malignant disease and, in the situation of allogeneic HSCT, to suppress the immune system to prevent graft rejection. Myeloablative regimens can cause profound, irreversible damage to the microenvironment of the bone marrow with subsequent severe life-threatening aplasia. Without the infusion of hematopoietic stem cells following these myeloablative conditioning regimens, bone marrow recovery would be unlikely or so severely prolonged that mortality due to complications of profound and pro-

Table 5-1 FACTORS TO CONSIDER WHEN CHOOSING A CONDITIONING REGIMEN.

1. Ablative potency of the chemoradiotherapy
2. Immunosuppressive therapy
3. Disease-related factors
   Malignancy versus nonmalignancy
   Treatment of bulky versus minimal residual disease
   Anticipation of graft-versus-leukemia or graft-versus-tumor effect
   Degree of tumor resistance at time of transplant
   Presence of medullary versus extramedullary disease
   Presence of sanctuary sites
   Need for posttransplant therapy or second (tandem) transplant
4. Patient-related factors
   Preexisting cardiac disease (use caution with cyclophosphamide)
   Preexisting pulmonary disease (use caution with BCNU, busulfan, total body irradiation)
   Preexisting renal disease (use caution with carboplatin, cisplatin)
   Preexisting liver disease (use caution with busulfan, methotrexate)
5. Influence of stem cells
   Source of stem cells (bone marrow, peripheral, cord blood)
   Purged
   Enriched
6. Pharmacologic and radiobiologic factors
7. Setting (in-patient versus out-patient/ambulatory setting)

tracted aplasia, such as infection and bleeding, is almost certain.

Nonmyeloablative conditioning regimens employ reduced doses of chemotherapy with less toxicity to the bone marrow. In fact, when nonmyeloablative conditioning regimens are used, hematopoietic recovery is likely even without the infusion of stem cells. The goal of a nonmyeloablative conditioning regimen is to eradicate disease while preserving immune function through a graft-versus-tumor mechanism.

Immunosuppression

Conditioning regimens vary in their effects on the immune system. In the allogeneic setting, suppression of the host immune system is an essential requirement to prevent graft rejection and promote successful engraftment. However, in autologous HSCT, there is no need to suppress the host immune response to prevent graft rejection, and rapid hematopoiesis is desirable. High-dose etoposide, carboplatin, cisplatin, carmustine (BCNU), and busulfan are chemotherapeutic agents often used in the autologous setting because they are less immunosuppressive, yet demonstrate effective cytoreductive activity.

Disease-Related Considerations

For patients with malignant disease, the tumor must be sensitive to the conditioning agents. However, in patients undergoing allogeneic HSCT for nonmalignant diseases such as severe aplastic anemia (SAA) and severe combined immunodeficiency syndrome (SCIDS) or congenital diseases such as sickle cell anemia, the goal of conditioning is to eradicate abnormal nonmalignant clones, not malignant cells.

A goal of conditioning chemoradiotherapy is to eliminate minimal residual disease. Conditioning chemoradiotherapy was never intended to eradicate diffuse or bulky disease. Current conditioning regimens generally cannot cure patients with bulky disease (tumor mass > 5 cm) or patients in chemoresistant relapse. Therefore, these patients require chemoradiotherapy prior to starting the transplant process to decrease the tumor burden, or they must receive consolidative chemotherapy/immunotherapy following transplant.

Graft-versus-Leukemia/ Tumor/Malignancy (GVL/GVT/GVM) Effect

In some hematological malignancies, especially chronic myelogenous leukemia (CML), a potent antileukemic effect, called graft-versus-leukemia (GVL) or graft-versus-tumor (GVT), can eliminate minimal residual disease following allogeneic stem cell transplant. Therefore, by relying on that GVL response following HSCT, in some allogeneic settings total elimination of the malignant cell population is not required. Subsequently, lower doses of conditioning chemotherapy with less toxicity and less morbidity and mortality may be administered. Although the GVL effect is clearly established in some hematologic malignancies, its effectiveness against solid tumors, such as breast cancer, is largely unknown and warrants continued research.

Medullary versus Extramedullary Disease

For hematologic malignancies, where the disease may arise in a malignant bone marrow stem cell, conditioning regimens that include total body irradiation (TBI), busulfan, and BCNU are often used for their well-known toxicity to these hematopoietic stem cells. However, such agents may not be as useful in patients with solid tumors that arise outside the bone marrow.

Sanctuary Sites

Well-known sanctuary sites for malignant cells are the central nervous system (CNS), testes,

and ovaries. Conditioning regimens that contain TBI and CNS-penetrating chemotherapeutic agents such as nitrosoureas, cytarabine, and high-dose methotrexate may be used in patients with hematological malignancies with CNS involvement or to prevent future CNS disease. However, conditioning therapy alone is not expected to be efficacious in eliminating disease from these known sanctuary sites. Therefore, patients with disease in these sites require additional treatment to these areas before or following HSCT.

Posttransplant Therapy and Second Transplants

Patients with a large tumor burden will likely require additional consolidation chemoradiotherapy after HSCT or, possibly, a planned second (consolidative) autologous HSCT. When a second HSCT is planned, it is referred to as a tandem, or sequential, transplant. The need for treatment following the HSCT will, therefore, influence the chemoradiotherapy components of the conditioning regimen. For example, if it is known that radiation therapy is planned following HSCT, TBI dosing may be altered or entirely omitted from the conditioning regimen. In the autologous setting, in which less toxic conditioning chemotherapy may be given, relapse following HSCT may be a significant possibility. In this situation, allogeneic HSCT may be the anticipated treatment of choice following such relapse. Therefore, the choice of conditioning regimen for the prior autologous HSCT may be influenced by the possibility of needing an allogeneic HSCT in the future.

Patient-Related Factors

Virtually all conditioning regimens have potentially life-threatening toxicities. Therefore, all patients undergo a thorough pretransplant medical evaluation to identify any preexisting comorbidities and to assess their ability to undergo the treatment. Cyclophosphamide, which can be cardiotoxic, must be used with caution in patients with cardiac disease. Pulmonary toxicity such as interstitial pneumonitis is a well-known potential long-term effect of BCNU, busulfan, and TBI; therefore, these treatment modalities must be used cautiously in patients with pulmonary dysfunction. Carboplatin and cisplatin, both potentially renal toxic, must be used carefully in patients with known renal disease. Optimal liver function is crucial because veno-occlusive disease (VOD) is often associated with dose-intensive chemotherapy. Patients who have been heavily pretreated with chemotherapy often have resultant damage to the microenvironment of the bone marrow and may not be eligible to undergo myeloablative conditioning due to the increased risk of failed, delayed, or unsustainable engraftment. However, these patients may be eligible for therapy that is less toxic to the hematopoietic stem cell, such as a nonmyeloablative conditioning regimen followed by allogeneic stem cell transplant. These are some examples of patient-related factors that may influence the type of conditioning regimen chosen for the patient.

Influence of Stem Cells

The source and quality of stem cells may influence the choice of conditioning regimens. Hematopoietic stem cells may come from the bone marrow, peripheral circulation, or umbilical cord blood. Peripheral stem cells usually engraft in 8 to 12 days, whereas bone marrow–derived hematopoietic stem cells take a longer time to engraft, generally 14 to 24 days. Stem cells may be enriched with CD34+ cells

or "purged" by removing T lymphocytes or contaminating malignant cells. Bone marrow and T cell–depleted stem cells may take more time to engraft. Consequently, acute toxicities such as bone marrow depression, febrile neutropenia, or bleeding may be more prominent in patients who have received these types of transplants.

Myeloablative Conditioning Regimens

Total Body Irradiation (TBI)

The first conditioning regimens used TBI as the primary treatment component for patients undergoing HSCT for hematologic malignancies. The advantages of TBI include the following (Bensinger & Buckner, 1999; Shank, 1999; Copelan & Penza, 2000):

1. Excellent immunosuppressive properties
2. Activity against a wide variety of malignancies, especially hematologic
3. Activity against chemotherapy-resistant malignancies
4. Penetration of sanctuary sites (CNS/testes)
5. Homogeneous effect regardless of blood supply
6. Lack of cross-resistance with chemotherapeutic agents
7. No detoxification or excretions requirements
8. Ability to shield vital organs

However, TBI is toxic to normal cells and can cause significant acute and long-term/delayed effects. The cells of the gastrointestinal (GI) tract and bone marrow are acutely sensitive to the effects of TBI, while the lungs and lenses are at risk for delayed effects of TBI (see **Table 5-2**).

Table 5-2 ACUTE AND DELAYED TOXICITIES OF TBI.

Acute Toxicities of TBI	Delayed Toxicities of TBI
Bone marrow depression	Pulmonary complications
GI toxicities: Anorexia	Cataracts
Nausea and vomiting	Alterations in growth and development
Diarrhea	Development of a secondary malignancy
Xerostomia	Gonadal dysfunction
Esophagitis	Increased sensitivity to sunlight
Oral mucositis (onset 4–5 days)	Endocrine dysfunction
Cutaneous manifestations: Alopecia	
Erythema	
Hyperpigmentation	
Parotitis	
Fever	
Fatigue	
Hepatotoxicity	

TBI DOSING

Evaluation of the dose of TBI given has been studied. The goal of this research is to determine whether the dose of TBI affects the occurrence and severity of toxicities or long-term survival.

Two studies, both by Clift and associates (1990, 1991), compared the dose of TBI given (12 cGy versus 15.75 cGy). One study involved patients with acute myelogenous leukemia (AML) in first remission and the other involved patients with CML in chronic phase. In both studies, patients who received the higher dose of TBI (15.75 cGy) had a decreased incidence of relapse. Unfortunately, however, the patients who received the higher dose of TBI (15.75 cGy) had increased treatment-related complications. Therefore, overall survival was not improved due to fatal conditioning regimen–related pulmonary and hepatic toxicities. Results of these studies demonstrate that lower dose TBI is more favorable than higher dose TBI because disease relapse is a more tolerable and potentially treatable situation than is early death due to regimen-related complications.

FRACTIONATION OF TBI

In the early days of transplant, TBI was given in a single dose. Patients who received single-dose TBI quickly developed acute and severe side effects such as nausea, vomiting, diarrhea, and mucositis. In addition, single-dose TBI often resulted in some form of interstitial pneumonitis, which can be severely disabling and can cause or exacerbate pneumonia. Of those affected by this pulmonary syndrome, two thirds died (Shank, 1999).

Fractionated or hyperfractionated TBI means that the TBI treatments are given 2 to 3 times each day over 3 to 4 days. Giving TBI in fractionated doses has a number of advantages: (1) it decreases toxicity to normal cells, thus making TBI more tolerable to the patient; (2) it allows time between treatments for normal tissue recovery; (3) it decreases damage to lung tissue;

and (4) it allows for achievement of higher dose of TBI, which increases tumor cell kill (Shank, 1999).

SHIELDING

An advantage of TBI is that specific organs can be shielded, or protected, to minimize the toxic effect of TBI. Because the lungs are particularly sensitive to the effects of TBI, most institutions use some form of lung shielding. The lungs can be shielded during some or all of the fractions (Shank, 1999).

Shielding of the liver has been done to decrease the incidence of veno-occlusive disease (VOD). However, VOD is more often associated with advanced age, graft-versus-host disease (GVHD), prior hepatitis, and certain chemotherapeutic agents than it is with TBI. A potential disadvantage of shielding of the liver is that it may contribute to leukemic relapse. Some transplant centers use eye shielding. However, it is not generally recommended for patients with leukemia due to the potential for recurrence in the eye or orbit (Shank, 1999). Partial shielding of the kidneys has also been used.

BOOSTING

Boosting is a process whereby additional radiation is given to areas that have been shielded from TBI but that do require some radiation or to areas that may have a higher concentration of malignant cells. Areas that may be boosted include the chest wall (if lung shields were used), the testes (in patients with leukemia), the spleen (in patients with CML), or other sites of gross/bulky disease.

ADMINISTRATION OF TBI

There is no standard delivery technique for the administration of TBI. Each transplant program has a specific method of giving TBI designed to accommodate the treatment room size, distance from the source of radiation, type of shielding desired, concerns over reproducibility, attempts to achieve homogeneity, and patient comfort (Shank, 1999).

Although TBI can be administered in a variety of patient positions, it is crucial that the patient assume the same position for each treatment to assure dose and accurate reproducibility. Generally, TBI can be delivered with the patient standing, sitting, or lying flat. Some transplant centers can administer TBI with the patient lying on a standard treatment delivery table, while some centers have developed a treatment stand/apparatus specifically for patients requiring TBI (see **Figure 5-1**). This treatment stand/apparatus requires the patient to stand, but features an adjustable bicycle seat and adjustable handles on the side to assure accurate reproducibility and to promote patient comfort and safety while standing during the TBI treatment. Customized lung shields are mounted on the surface of an acrylic plastic plate. After the patient has been properly positioned in the treatment stand, with attention to correct placement of the handles, height of the bicycle seat, and position of the feet, the acrylic plastic plate is attached to the treatment stand to protect the lungs. The radiation therapy personnel leave the room and the TBI treatment begins. Actual treatment time varies, but generally occurs over a few minutes.

During the actual treatment, the patient is alone in the lead-shielded room and must remain very still. For optimal patient safety, the patient is observed on a closed-circuit monitor. Audio monitoring is usually available so the patient can communicate with the radiation staff should a need arise. The patient may bring a

Figure 5-1 TBI treatment stand.

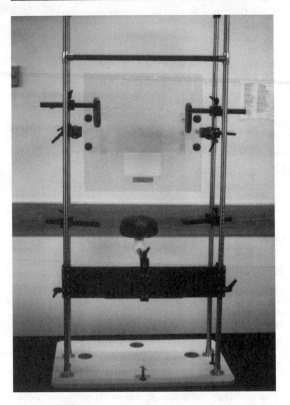

photograph to focus on as a means of distraction during the treatment session. Some patients may choose to bring a meaningful item as a source of comfort or to provide a sense of normalcy during this stressful time. A cassette or CD player is usually available so the patient can listen to music during positioning and the treatment session.

The patient is transported via wheelchair or stretcher directly from the transplant unit to the radiation therapy department. Patient transport differs among transplant centers. Some require the patient to be completely covered by wearing a head covering, face mask, gown, gloves, and shoe protectors, while others require only a face mask and hand-washing. Some radiation therapy departments require that their staff wear protective garb as well. Some transplant centers require that the patient be accompanied to each TBI treatment by a nurse, and some even require the assistance of hospital security to clear hallways to decrease patient exposure to hospital personnel and visitors who may be in the hospital corridors. Some centers provide staff who transport patients to radiation therapy with a security key to the elevators so they can summon an elevator car to expedite travel between the transplant unit and radiation therapy.

Because the patient has gone outside the protected environment of the hospital room, some centers require that the patient bathe after each TBI treatment to remove any microorganisms that may have accumulated on the skin or hair during the TBI process.

NURSING IMPLICATIONS FOR THE PATIENT UNDERGOING TBI

Nursing care during TBI is focused on patient and family education and support and symptom management. Ongoing patient and family education includes reinforcement of the rationale for TBI, the treatment schedule, the components of the conditioning regimen, the potential acute side effects, and the management of the side effects.

TBI can cause many acute toxicities with the potential to cause significant symptom distress for the patient. The role of the HSCT nurse is to know the potential acute toxicities of TBI, to prevent or minimize the acute side effects, and to accurately identify and manage side effects when they occur.

TBI is highly emetogenic treatment. Therefore, patients should be premedicated with antiemetics to prevent nausea and vomiting. Antiemetics should be given regularly throughout the TBI course. Antianxiety agents are given as needed. Standing in the treatment stand, even for short times, during a TBI treatment can be difficult for the patient who may have nausea, vomiting, diarrhea, or drowsiness due to medication effect or postural hypotension. To avoid the risk of light-headedness, hypotension, and possibly fainting during a TBI treatment, especially if the patient is standing during the treatment, it is advisable that the patient eat a light snack before going to the radiation department. If TBI is administered using two separate fields (anterior and posterior) per session, the patient usually comes out of the treatment stand between treatment of each field for a brief rest period. Intravenous (IV) hydration can usually be interrupted before leaving the transplant unit to facilitate transport to the radiation therapy department, patient positioning for treatment, and delivery of TBI.

There are other aspects of TBI that may be stressful for the HSCT patient. TBI treatment sessions require careful coordination between the radiation department and the transplant unit. Several factors, including radiation department scheduling, accurate TBI dosing, and administration of premedications, necessitate that the patient arrives for each TBI session in a timely fashion. The patient may feel pressure simply getting to the radiation department, arriving on schedule, and completing the preparations that must be accomplished before leaving the transplant unit, such as donning protective garb, if required, and receiving all premedications. All of these may seem a daunt-

ing undertaking for the patient who may be feeling some acute side effects of TBI such as fatigue, nausea, vomiting, or parotitis.

TBI is not only a difficult challenge physically for the patient due to significant acute side effects and other peripheral aspects, but it is psychologically difficult as well. During the TBI treatment session, the patient is alone in the room. This may increase a sense of isolation and loneliness or a sense of being untouchable or radioactive. During the quiet, solitary time of the treatment session, thoughts, fears, and uncertainties may surface. It is a time during which the patient may forecast or anticipate the ability to withstand the physical demands of TBI or wonder which side effects will develop, the severity of the side effects, and the effectiveness of interventions to treat the side effects. The patient may also contemplate the effectiveness of TBI in eradicating the disease or in suppressing the immune system so that the HSCT will be a success. Some patients have referred to TBI as the "point of no return" because TBI causes irreversible aplasia, and the patient knows that without the infusion of stem cells, a fatal outcome is almost certain.

Clearly, the nurse has a significant role in caring for the patient undergoing TBI. Although the patient cannot feel, hear, see, smell, or taste the radiation, it does not lessen the toxicity. Preventing treatment-related toxicities and effective symptom management are essential. The nurse can be a source of information, comfort, reassurance, and safety for the patient. Through keen insight into the significant physical and emotional impact of TBI, the nurse can enable the patient to express any concerns or vulnerabilities regarding TBI. The nurse has the privilege of being present for the patient during this phase of transplant when a patient may be fraught with thoughts on the irreversibility of treatment or the threat of distressing symptoms.

Total Lymphoid Irradiation (TLI)

TLI was first used to treat patients with Hodgkin's disease (Whedon, 1991). In these patients, TLI showed extensive immunosuppression (Shank, 1999). TLI has also been used as a means of immunosuppression to decrease the incidence of graft failure in patients with CML receiving T cell–depleted marrow from matched or partially matched marrow.

In the early days of marrow transplantation, TLI was used alone only when immunosuppression was needed, such as in aplastic anemia. TLI has been given as a single dose and in fractionated doses (Shank, 1999). In the HSCT experience, TLI has been added to TBI to increase engraftment when T cell–depleted marrow is given. TLI has also been successfully used in combination with etoposide and cyclophospharride in patients with relapsed or refractory Hodgkin's disease treated with autologous bone marrow transplantation (Yahalom et al., 1989). An advantage of TLI for immunosuppression is decreased organ toxicity because organs outside the treatment field—brain, eyes, lungs, kidneys and much of the small bowel—are spared.

Thoracoabdominal Irradiation (TAI)

Though not commonly used, TAI has been used in combination with cyclophosphamide for transplantation for Fanconi anemia and severe aplastic anemia. As with TLI, organ toxicity is limited only to the radiation field involved.

Chemotherapeutic Agents Used in Myeloablative Conditioning Regimens

Many chemotherapeutic agents are used singly, but most often in combination with others, for conditioning regimens. Following is a brief description of the more common chemotherapeutic agents used, including acute side effects that the nurse should know about when caring for a patient undergoing conditioning chemotherapy prior to HSCT. This section does not provide comprehensive information such as dosing, potential interactions, scheduling, or administration for each drug. Please refer to appropriate drug information textbooks, specific protocols, and institutional policies and procedures for that important, detailed information.

Cyclophosphamide (Cytoxan)

Cyclophosphamide is an alkylating agent that is cell cycle nonspecific. It causes cross-linkage of DNA strands and thereby prevents DNA synthesis and cell division. Cyclophosphamide is commonly used to treat Hodgkin's disease, non-Hodgkin's lymphoma, acute and chronic leukemia, multiple myeloma, and solid tumors such as neuroblastoma, retinoblastoma, rhabdomyosarcoma, and cancer of the breast, ovary, testes, and lungs. Cyclophosphamide is also given to treat nonmalignant diseases such as severe rheumatoid disorders, multiple sclerosis, lupus, lupus nephritis, and others. It is a component of many conditioning regimens in HSCT.

Acute side effects of cyclophosphamide include bone marrow depression, hemorrhagic cystitis, gastrointestinal (GI) symptoms (anorexia, nausea, vomiting, diarrhea, stomatitis), hepatotoxicity, cardiomyopathy, and syndrome of inappropriate antidiuretic hormone (SIADH). Other side effects include alopecia, nail changes (hyperpigmentation and transverse ridging), and, rarely, pulmonary toxicity. It is mutagenic and teratogenic (Wilkes, Ingwersen, & Barton-Burke, 2003).

CYCLOPHOSPHAMIDE AND TBI

Cyclophosphamide, a potent immunosuppressive alkylating agent, was added to TBI as a component of the conditioning regimen for its antileukemic and additional immunosuppressive effects. (See **Table 5-3** for a list of TBI-based regimens.) In one study (Thomas et al., 1977), 100 patients with acute leukemia were given TBI and cyclophosphamide for conditioning regimen followed by an HLA-identical sibling allogeneic bone marrow transplant. Thirteen percent became long-term leukemia-free survivors. Subsequently, TBI and cyclophosphamide were used increasingly for conditioning regimens. This combination continues to be a frequently used and efficacious treatment modality for hematological malignancies. It has withstood the test of time and

---

Table 5-3 **TBI-BASED REGIMENS.**

TBI + CY
TBI + VP-16 + CY
TBI + VP-16 + BU
TBI + Melphalan
TBI + Ara-C
TBI + Ara-C + CY

Ara-C, cytarabine; CY, cyclophosphamide; TBI, total body irradiation; VP-16, etoposide.

---

has served as a standard to which other regimens are compared.

Busulfan (Myleran/Busulfex)

Busulfan is an alkylating agent that causes cross-linkage of DNA strands and prevents DNA replication and RNA transcription. Because busulfan damages hematopoietic cell lines, myelosuppression may be prolonged. Acute side effects include bone marrow depression, GI effects (anorexia, nausea, vomiting, diarrhea, stomatitis), neurological effects (dizziness, headache, insomnia, anxiety, and generalized tonic-clonic seizures, especially at high doses), and hepatotoxicity, including VOD. Later effects include alopecia, rash, hyperpigmentation, and interstitial pulmonary fibrosis.

CYCLOPHOSPHAMIDE AND BUSULFAN

It has been well documented that the combination of TBI and cyclophosphamide is an effective conditioning regimen. However, over time, it has become clear that a non-TBI-containing regimen was needed for several reasons. First, many patients with hematological malignancies have been previously treated with dose-limiting radiotherapy and would be unable to receive TBI. Many received radiation therapy to the mediastinum. If TBI was given to these patients, they would likely develop fatal interstitial pneumonitis. Second, many institutions lack the facilities and equipment to administer TBI. TBI puts an additional strain on personnel, equipment, and time of already-busy radiation resources. A third consideration for the development of a non-TBI-containing regimen is to lessen the potential delayed effects of TBI, including cataracts, sterility, impaired growth and development in children, and the development of secondary malignancies (Bensinger & Buckner, 1999). Consequently, busulfan was substituted for TBI in TBI + cyclophosphamide regimens. (See **Table 5-4** for a list of busulfan-based regimens.)

Busulfan is an alkylating agent with three properties that make it beneficial in treating patients with AML: It is a potent antineoplastic, immunosuppressive, and myeloablative agent. Busulfan is active against many malignancies, including acute leukemia, lymphoma, multiple myeloma, testicular carcinoma, Ewing's sarcoma, and breast cancer (Bensinger & Buckner, 1999).

Early dose-finding studies in patients with AML demonstrated that busulfan (20 mg/kg) frequently caused severe, often dose-limiting, mucositis and VOD. Subsequent studies showed that decreasing the dose of busulfan (16 mg/kg) given over 4 days combined with cyclophosphamide (200 mg/kg) given over 4 days was very effective in treating patients with AML undergoing transplant because of busulfan's antileukemic, immunosuppressive, and myeloablative effects. This combination was referred to as "big BU/CY," or BuCy 4. However, busulfan + cyclophosphamide given at these doses resulted in severe and dose-limiting mucositis and liver toxicities (VOD). Of these patients, 20–30% developed

VOD, and of these, 50% were fatal (Jones et al., 1987).

Because of the high level of these treatment-related toxicities, this regimen was modified by decreasing the dose of cyclophosphamide to 120 mg/kg over 2 days (Tutschka et al., 1987). This regimen became known as "little Bu/Cy," or BuCy 2. This change resulted in a decreased incidence of VOD to approximately 10–15% and decreased fatal VOD to 5% (Copelan et al., 1991). There was no increase in disease relapse.

Because BuCy 2 may not be as immunosuppressive as previous busulfan + cyclophosphamide regimens, failure to engraft using BuCy 2 was a concern. There was an increased incidence of graft failure in T cell–depleted marrow using BuCy 2 (Copelan & Deeg, 1992). When non-T-cell–depleted marrow was used, failure to engraft was rare, though probably more frequent than with TBI-containing regimens (Sahebi et al., 1996).

Cisplatin (Platinol)

Cisplatin is a heavy metal that acts like an alkylating agent and is cell cycle nonspecific. Acute toxicities include bone marrow depression (at high doses), GI toxicities (anorexia, dysgeusia, severe nausea, and vomiting), anaphylaxis, neurotoxicities (numbness, tingling, sensory loss in the arms and legs, areflexia, loss of proprioception and vibratory sense), and ototoxicity. Cardiotoxicity (angina, myocardial infarction, thrombotic microangiopathy) can occur when used in combination with other chemotherapeutic agents (Wilkes et al., 2003).

Cytosine Arabinoside (Cytarabine/Ara-C)

Cytarabine is an antimetabolite that is most effective when cells are undergoing rapid DNA synthesis, and therefore is often given to pa-

---

Table 5-4 BUSULFAN-BASED REGIMENS.

BU + CY
BU + Melphalan
BU + Melphalan + Thiotepa
BU + CY + Melphalan
BU + CY + Thiotepa
BU + VP-16
BU + CY + VP-16

BU, busulfan; CY, cyclophosphamide; VP-16, etoposide.

tients with leukemia and may be included in conditioning regimens for leukemia. Side effects include bone marrow depression, anorexia, nausea, vomiting, diarrhea, and mucositis. It can also cause erythema and skin sloughing of the palmar and plantar surfaces, especially at higher doses. Corticosteroids and/or skin moisturizers are helpful in preventing or treating this syndrome. Neurological toxicities include cerebellar toxicities (nystagmus, dysarthrias, ataxia, slurred speech, disdiadochokinesia, and difficulty with fine motor movements). Ocular manifestations include conjunctival injection, decreased visual acuity, blurred vision, photophobia, increased lacrimation, and conjunctivitis. Corticosteroid eyedrops are usually given in concert with cytarabine to prevent conjunctivitis. If the patient has significant tumor burden, as is often the case with acute leukemia and lymphoma, tumor lysis syndrome may develop in patients receiving cytarabine (Wilkes et al., 2003).

Etoposide (VP-16)

Etoposide is a plant alkaloid that inhibits DNA synthesis in the S and G2 phases of the cell cycle so that cells do not enter mitosis and multiply. Etoposide has significant antineoplastic properties and is included in many conditioning regimens for treatment of hematological malignancies. Etoposide is a poor immunosuppressive agent. Acute side effects include bone marrow depression, hypotension if the drug is infused too quickly, anorexia, nausea, vomiting, and mucositis, especially at high doses. Cutaneous manifestations include radiation recall and alopecia. Etoposide is mutagenic and teratogenic.

Etoposide (60 mg/kg) has been added to the BuCy 2 regimen by multiple investigators. (See **Table 5-5** for a list of etoposide-based

Table 5-5 VP-16–BASED REGIMENS.
VP-16 + Carbo + Ifos (ICE)
VP-16 + CY + Cisplatin
VP-16 + Carbo + Dox
VP-16 + Carbo + CY
VP-16 + CY

Carbo, carboplatin; CY, cyclophosphamide; Dox, doxorubicin; Ifos, ifosfamide; VP-16, etoposide.

regimens.) It is given as a component of conditioning for patients with advanced hematologic malignancies followed by allogeneic bone marrow transplant. Major toxicities observed after using etoposide include VOD, mucositis, and skin rash. Overall, disease-free survival rate has been encouraging when etoposide is used as a component of conditioning.

Etoposide has also been combined with fractionated TBI and cyclophosphamide (etoposide 60 mg/kg and cyclophosphamide 100 mg/kg) and has been used in the treatment of non-Hodgkin's lymphoma and Hodgkin's disease (Cagnoni, Nieto, & Jones, 2000). Two- to 3-year disease-free survival rates following autologous HSCT with this regimen have been reported at 55–59%, with a fatal treatment-related mortality rate of less than 10%.

Carmustine (BCNU)

BCNU is a nitrosourea commonly used as a myeloablative agent because it is active against a variety of malignancies. BCNU and cyclophosphamide are often combined and may have synergistic activity (Bensinger & Buckner, 1999). See **Table 5-6** for a list of nitrosourea-based regimens.

BCNU has been combined with cyclophosphamide and etoposide (CBV) and has been frequently used in patients with lymphoma, followed by autologous transplants. BCNU-based

Table 5-6 NITROSOUREA-BASED REGIMENS.

Carm + CY + VP-16 (CBV)

Carm + VP-16 + Ara-C + Melp (BEAM)

Carm + VP-16 + Ara-C + CY (BEAC)

Carm + CY + Cisplatin

Carm + Amsacrine + Ara-C + VP-16 (BAVC)

Carm + Melp + VP-16

Carm + VP-16 + Cisplatin

Ara-C, cytarabine; Carm, carmustine; CY, cyclophosphamide; Melp, melphalan; VP-16, etoposide.

regimens are often used as a substitute for TBI-based regimens in patients with lymphoma because many of these patients have previously received thoracic radiation therapy as part of their initial treatment and therefore cannot receive TBI.

Acute toxicities include bone marrow depression (delayed); GI toxicity such as anorexia, nausea, and vomiting; nephrotoxicity (hemorrhagic cystitis); and hepatotoxicity (Wilkes et al, 2003). It is well known that BCNU can cause pulmonary toxicity. At doses of greater than 450 mg/m^2 there is significant pulmonary toxicity, including pulmonary fibrosis. Patients who receive BCNU must be carefully monitored for signs and symptoms of pulmonary dysfunction, such as cough, dyspnea, exercise intolerance, fatigue, and worsening pulmonary function tests. Generally, steroid treatment is promptly initiated at the first signs and symptoms of respiratory compromise.

Other BCNU-based conditioning regimens are BEAM (BCNU + etoposide + cytarabine + melphalan) and BEAC (BCNU + etoposide + cytarabine + cyclophosphamide).

BEAM is used as conditioning in patients with Hodgkin's disease and non-Hodgkin's lymphoma undergoing autologous and allogeneic HSCT. The use of melphalan rather than cyclophosphamide avoids hemorrhagic cystitis and the need for administering the uroprotectant mesna and/or instilling bladder irrigation. Complete remission rates of 50% have been reported in refractory Hodgkin's disease. Regimen-related toxicities include mucositis and pulmonary toxicities (Chopra et al., 1993)

BEAC is similar to CBV. It has been widely evaluated and usually is used as a preparative therapy for malignant lymphoma. Toxicities include liver dysfunction, interstitial pneumonitis, renal dysfunction, and mucositis.

Carboplatin (Paraplatin)

Carboplatin is a cell cycle nonspecific alkylating agent with similar, though less severe, nephrotoxicity as cisplatin. Acute side effects include bone marrow depression, GI disturbances (anorexia, nausea, vomiting, stomatitis), metabolic abnormalities, hepatic toxicity, ototoxicity, and renal toxicity. Neurotoxicities are infrequent. It is mutagenic and teratogenic (Wilkes et al., 2003). Carboplatin has a broad scope of antitumor activity and is often used in combination with other antineoplastics as conditioning for patients with cancer of the breast or ovary, germ cell neoplasms, neuroblastoma, and sarcomas. Dose-limiting toxicities include renal dysfunction, hepatotoxicity, and ototoxicity.

Ifosfamide (IFEX)

Ifosfamide is an alkylating agent that is cell cycle nonspecific. Acute side effects include bone marrow depression, GI toxicities (anorexia, nausea, vomiting), and hemorrhagic cystitis. Neurotoxicity (dizziness, somnolence, lethargy, confusion, hallucinations, seizures) may occur with higher doses. Ifosfamide is mutagenic and teratogenic. It is effective in patients with Hodgkin's disease, non-Hodgkin's lymphoma, and acute and chronic leukemias, and in some patients with solid tumors such as of the lung, breast, and ovary. It has been shown to be effective in tumors previously resistant to cyclophosphamide (Wilkes et al., 2003). Ifosfamide is used in combination with other antineoplastics in conditioning regimens.

Melphalan

Melphalan, an alkylating agent, is a derivative of nitrogen mustard. Although myelosuppression is the most common side effect, anorexia, nausea, vomiting, stomatitis, hemorrhagic cystitis, and transaminitis may occur acutely.

Melphalan (150 to 240 mg/m^2) is used as a single conditioning agent in patients with multiple myeloma and breast cancer followed by autologous stem cell infusion and, in patients with hematological malignancies, allogeneic transplant. It has been widely used in dose-intensive regimens for patients with breast or ovarian cancer, multiple myeloma, and lymphoma. Melphalan is a part of other conditioning regimens (see **Table 5-7**), including those using TBI, busulfan, BCNU, etoposide, cisplatin, cytarabine, and cyclophosphamide (Chan, 2000). Whereas melphalan is generally well tolerated at conventional doses, at the high doses used in conditioning regimens, melphalan can cause severe myelosuppression, GI toxicities, and hepatic toxicity (Bensigner & Buckner, 2000; Chan, 2000).

Thiotepa

Thiotepa is an alkylating agent that is cell cycle nonspecific. It inhibits malignant cell reproduction by interfering with DNA replication

Table 5-7 MELPHALAN-BASED REGIMENS.

Melphalan alone
Melphalan + Ara-C
Melphalan + Mito
Melphalan + Mito + Carbo
Melphalan + CY + Cisplatin
Melphalan + Mito + Tax
Melphalan + TBI

Ara-C, cytarabine; Carbo, carboplatin; CY, cyclophosphamide; Mito, mitoxantrone; Tax, Taxol; TBI, total body irradiation.

and RNA transcription. High doses of thiotepa can cause severe myelosuppression, mucositis, esophagitis, neurotoxicities (somnolence, confusion, dizziness, headache, blurred vision), hepatic dysfunction, and cutaneous manifestations (Chan, 2000). Hypotension can occur if thiotepa is infused rapidly. Gastrointestinal toxicities are minimal even at high doses. It is mutagenic and teratogenic. Thiotepa is used in combination with several chemotherapy agents (see **Table 5-8**), including busulfan, carboplatin, cyclophosphamide, etoposide, or mitoxantrone for conditioning in autologous and allogeneic HSCT for breast cancer, lymphoma, melanoma, and other solid tumors.

Nonmyeloablative Conditioning Regimens

Since the 1960s, allogeneic HSCT has been the treatment of choice for a variety of hematological malignancies. Autologous and allogeneic HSCT are aggressive and potentially curative treatment modalities. The success of these transplants relies on myeloablative conditioning regimens to create space for the donor marrow, to

Table 5-8 Thiotepa-based regimens.

Thio + CY
Thio + CY + Cisplatin
Thio + Mito
Thio + Mito + CY
Thio + CY + Carbo

Carbo, carboplatin; CY, cyclophosphamide; Mito, mitoxantrone; Thio, thiotepa.

Table 5-9 Nonmyeloablative (reduced-intensity) regimens.

FLU + CY
FLU + BU
FLU + TBI
FLU + MEL
CY + ATG + TI
FLU + Ida + Ara-C
FLU + BU + ATG
2′-deoxycoformycin + Photopheresis + TBI
TBI
VP-16

Ara-C, cytarabine; ATG, antithymocyte globulin; BU, busulfan; CY, cyclophosphamide; Flu, fludarabine; Ida, idarubicin; Mel, melphalan; TBI, total body irradiation; TI, thymic irradiation; VP-16, etoposide.

severely suppress the host immune system to promote engraftment, and to eradicate malignant disease. However, these toxic myeloablative conditioning regimens do not come without a high cost to the patient in terms of morbidity and mortality. Conventional myeloablative conditioning regimens produce considerable organ toxicity with resultant morbidity and mortality. As a result, these regimen-related toxicities have limited this treatment option to patients who are generally younger (< 55 years old) and to patients with few, if any, comorbidities. Heavily pretreated patients are often excluded due to poor performance status, organ toxicity due to previous chemoradiotherapy, and concern regarding the potential for delayed hematopoietic engraftment following transplant due to poor bone marrow microenvironment from previous antineoplastic therapy. The need for conditioning regimens with fewer and less severe toxicity has become obvious.

Nonmyeloablative or reduced-intensity conditioning regimens have recently been developed and show promising results (see **Table 5-9**). Nonmyeloablative conditioning regimens administer lower doses of chemotherapy so as to avoid completely eradicating host hematopoiesis and immunity. The goals of these nonmyeloablative regimens are to reduce regimen-related

toxicities, which would then make this treatment option available to older patients, patients with other comorbidities, and patients who have received a significant amount of prior chemotherapy and/or radiation therapy, and to capture or enhance the curative potential of the graft-versus-tumor effect.

Because these conditioning regimens are generally nonmyeloablative, there is residual host hematopoiesis and immune function so that upon engraftment of donor cells a state of mixed chimerism exists. Mixed chimerism is a condition in which both donor and host hematopoietic stem cells are present in the recipient. This state of mixed chimerism allows for recovery from conditioning regimen–induced toxicities, a more gradual engraftment, and less cytokine release, which may be protective against acute GVHD. This induced state of mixed chimerism may then serve as an immunological platform for adoptive cellular immunotherapy (Spitzer et al., 2003). An optimal GVL effect hopefully occurs with conversion of mixed chimerism to full donor hematopoiesis, either spontaneously or after the administration of donor lymphocyte infusion(s) (DLI).

The graft-versus-tumor (GVT)/graft-versus-leukemia (GVL) effect is an immunological response in the recipient mediated by immuno-competent donor T lymphocytes and relies on differences in histocompatibility antigens between the donor and recipient. The donor T lymphocytes recognize malignant cells in the host as foreign, mount an attack against them, and, hopefully, induce a remission. However, it is a delicate balancing act for the transplant physician to achieve the desired GVT effect in an attempt to cure a malignancy and, at the same time, minimize GVHD (Kim, 2002).

GVL has been particularly successful in curing many patients with recurrent CML following bone marrow transplantation (Kolb et al., 1990). This phenomenon may also be useful in patients with chronic lymphocytic leukemia (CLL), follicular non-Hodgkin's lymphoma (NHL), and multiple myeloma. The GVT effect may be present, though less potent, in the setting of CML in blast crisis, AML, acute lymphocytic leukemia (ALL), and aggressive large cell lymphomas (Mangan, 2000). GVT may play a role in patients with breast cancer, renal cell carcinoma, malignant melanoma, and other tumors that may respond to the immunological effects of donor T cells or natural killer cells (Mangan, 2000).

Many terms are used to describe nonmyeloablative HSCT, including mini-transplant, transplant-lite, drive-through transplant, and reduced-intensity transplant. However, some of these terms may be misleading, causing the patient, family, and possibly some health-care professionals to think that these transplants are easy. Though patients receive less intense doses of chemoradiotherapy, they are still at risk for developing serious side effects such as bone marrow depression, fevers, bleeding, hepatic and renal toxicities, and GVHD. Thus, despite the decreased conditioning regimen–related toxicities, a nonmyeloablative HSCT can be a difficult and challenging treatment modality.

Chemotherapeutic Agents Used in Nonmyeloablative Conditioning Regimens

The chemotherapeutic drugs described in the myeloablative conditioning regimens may also be used in the nonmyeloablative conditioning regimens. However, other chemotherapeutic agents are often used in the nonmyeloablative setting. Following is a brief description of the more common chemotherapeutic agents used, including acute side effects that the nurse should know about when caring for a patient undergoing a nonmyeloablative conditioning regimen. This section does not provide comprehensive information such as dosing, potential interactions, scheduling, or administration for each drug. Please refer to the appropriate drug information textbooks, specific protocols, and institutional policies and procedures for that important, detailed information.

Fludarabine (Fludara)

Fludarabine is an antimetabolite used primarily in patients with B cell chronic lymphocytic leukemia (Bashey, 2002; Wilkes et al., 2003). It has also been used, though on an investigational basis, for the treatment of other B cell and T cell malignancies. The major route of excretion is the kidneys. When fludarabine is used as part of a conditioning regimen, the dose is 25 to 30 mg/m^2 over 5 to 6 days. A lower dose of 25 mg/m^2 given for 3 days has also been used (Bashey, 2002).

Myelosuppression and neurotoxicity are the most common adverse reactions, and the severity of the reactions are dose related. Neurotoxicities observed in up to 20% of patients treated with standard doses include weakness, blurred vision, and hearing disturbances (Bashey, 2002).

Fludarobine-containing conditioning regimens include fludarabine + busulfan + cyclophosphamide + antithymocyte globulin (Slavin et al., 1998), fludarabine + cyclophosphamide, and fludarabine + melphan.

Cladribine (2-CdA)

Cladribine is a highly immunosuppressive antimetabolite that interferes with DNA synthesis and prevents repair of DNA strand breaks (Wilkes et al., 2003). It is usually given to patients with hairy cell leukemia and has limited use in nonmyeloablative conditioning regimens. Acute side effects include bone marrow depression (particularly neutropenia and lymphopenia), fever, headache, and rash. Gastrotintestinal toxicities such as nausea, vomiting, diarrhea, or constipation are rare and are generally mild. Although cladribine is generally well tolerated, it can cause severe neurotoxicity and renal toxicity when given in higher doses in combination with other antineoplastics in preparation for ablative or nonmyeloablative HSCT (Bashey, 2002).

Pentostatin (Nipent, 2'-deoxycoformycin)

Pentostatin is also an immunosuppressive antimetabolite and an antibiotic-derived antineoplastic agent. It is a highly immunosuppressive drug that causes a marked decrease in circulating B cells. It is used in the treatment of hairy cell leukemia, chronic lymphocytic leukemia, non-Hodgkin's lymphoma, and T cell lymphoma. In addition, it may be effective in patients with steroid-resistant GVHD. Adverse effects include bone marrow depression (particularly leukopenia and thrombocytopenia), nausea and vomiting, dose-dependent neurotoxicity (headache, lethargy, paresthesia, seizures), and reversible nephrotoxicity.

Other Agents Used in Nonmyeloablative Conditioning Regimens

In nonmyeloablative HSCT, additional agents, such as immunosuppressants or monoclonal antibiodies, are combined with the chemotherapy component of the conditioning regimen.

Alemtuzumab (CamPath)

Alemtuzumab is a humanized monoclonal antibody that targets the CD52 antigen, which is expressed on the surface of most normal human lymphocytes, as well as on malignant T cell and B cell malignant lymphoma. Acute toxicities include bone marrow depression (especially neutropenia and lymphopenia), skeletal pain, asthenia, peripheral edema, headache, malaise, hypotension, hypertension, and tachycardia (Wilkes et al., 2003). Alemtuzumab is used in patients with B cell CLL who have received alkylating agents or have failed fludarabine. Other uses for alemtuzumab include low grade lymphoma, GVHD, and autoimmune diseases. Its use in HSCT as part of the preparatory regimen is limited at this time (Bashey, 2002).

Antithymocyte Globulin (Equine) (Atgam)

Atgam is a highly selective lymphocyte immunosuppressant agent used in some conditioning regimens. It is also used to treat GVHD and aplastic anemia. The dose is 10 to 40 mg/kg/day over several days.

Due to the profound immunosuppressive effects of Atgam, opportunistic infections are common when Atgam is used. When it is a component of a nonmyeloablative conditioning regimen, there is an increased risk of reactivation of cytomegalovirus (CMV) (Bashey, 2002).

Fever and chills are common side effects and occur in approximately 50% of patients who receive Atgam (Bashey, 2002). Other side effects include rash, pruritus, hypotension, hypertension, chest pain, dyspnea, respiratory distress, anxiety, leukopenia, thrombocytopenia, and phlebitis at the IV site. Anaphylaxis is a possible side effect, occurring in 1–10% of those who receive Atgam. Serum sickness may occur 7 to 18 days after the initiation of Atgam. It is characterized by fever, sore throat, arthralgias, myalgias, fatigue, nausea, and skin rash.

It is recommended that an intradermal skin test be done prior to the administration of the initial dose of Atgam. The dose is 0.1 ml of a 1:1000 dilution of Atgam in normal saline. The site should be clearly circumscribed and checked 30 to 60 minutes after placement. Pruritus, erythema, and swelling may indicate a possible sensitivity to Atgam. A positive skin reaction consists of wheal > 10 mm in diameter. If a positive skin test occurs, the first infusion should be administered very cautiously with emergency equipment readily available. The absence of a reaction does not preclude the possibility of a systemic reaction during the Atgam infusion.

Patients are premedicated with antipyretics, antihistamines, corticosteroids, and histamine H2 antagonists, which may eliminate or decrease the intensity of the side effects. Meperidine may be indicated for rigors associated with fevers. Antiemetics may be given as needed.

During the infusion of Atgam, the patient must be carefully monitored for adverse reactions, especially anaphylaxis.

Antithymocyte Globulin (Rabbit) (Thymoglobulin)

Thymoglobulin is another lymphocyte-selective immunosuppressant. When compared to Atgam, studies have shown that there are fewer adverse reactions when thymoglobulin is used, but leukopenia is more severe and more persistent (lasting as long as a year after therapy). Serious infections were no different with thymoglobulin than with Atgam. The incidence of CMV infections was decreased.

Examples of Nonmyeloablative Conditioning Regimens

Slavin et al. (1998) treated 26 patients with acute and chronic myelogenous leukemia (22 patients) and other genetic disorders (4 patients). The conditioning regimen was busulfan 4 mg/kg for 2 consecutive days, fludarabine 30 mg/m^2/day for 6 days (total 180 mg/m^2), and Atgam 10 mg/kg over 4 days, followed by HLA-matched allogeneic HSCT. Cyclosporine was given for GVHD prophylaxis. Sustained, predominantly full donor chimerism was achieved in all 26 patients. Acute GVHD occurred in 12 of 26 patients. Six patients developed grade 3 and grade 4 GVHD, and limited chronic GVHD occurred in 9 of 25 evaluable patients. Three patients who relapsed received DLI, which successfully induced remission.

Spitzer et al. (2003) treated 57 patients with advanced hematological malignancies with bone marrow transplantation. The age range was 16 to 62 years with a median age of 43 years. Thirty-six patients received HLA-matched stem cells and 21 patients received HLA-mismatched HSCT. The preparative regimen consisted of cyclophosphamide 150–2000 mg/m^2, Atgam 15–30 mg/kg/day for 3 to 4 days, and one dose of thymic irradiation 700 cGy on day -1. The first 14 mismatched patients were treated with Atgam, the subsequent 7 were treated with a T cell–depleting monoclonal antibody (MEDI-507). Cyclosporine was begun on day -1 for GVHD prophylaxis. The cyclosporine was tapered and discontinued as soon as day $+35$ for patients with no evidence of GVHD. Treatment-related toxicities included cyclophosphamide-induced cardiomyopathy, ATG infusion-related toxicity, pulmonary hemorrhage, unexplained CNS toxicity, and posttransplant lymphoproliferative disease (PTLD). Late posttransplant-related deaths (day 108, 180, 405, 559) were due to opportunistic infections. Potent, sustained responses in some patients with chemorefractory hematologic malignancies were observed.

McSweeney et al. (2001) treated 44 patients with hematologic malignancies who were ineligible for conventional myeloablative conditioning due to advanced age, prior treatment, organ dysfunction, or poor performance status. The conditioning regimen consisted of only low-dose irradiation, 200 cGy. Cyclosporine and mycophenolate mofetil (MMF) were given for GVHD prophylaxis. The regimen was tolerated well, with only minimal myeloablation and no GI toxicities, mucositis, or alopecia.

Graft rejection occurred in 20% of the patients within 4 months. Of the nine patients with graft rejection, eight had persistent disease. Seventy percent realized disease response, and of 36 patients who maintained engraftment, 19 achieved a complete response.

Kottaridis et al. (2001) treated 24 patients with Hodgkin's disease (6 patients were in complete remission, 13 in partial remission, and 6 had refractory disease). The conditioning regimen consisted of alemtuzumab 20 mg/day, fludarabine 30 mg/m^2, and melphalan 140 mg/m^2. Sixteen recipients received unmanipulated granulocyte colony stimulating factor (G-CSF) mobilized HLA-identical sibling peripheral blood stem cells and six patients received unmanipulated marrow from matched, unrelated donors. GVHD prophylaxis was with cyclosporine alone, although one patient also received methotrexate. All 24 patients sustained donor engraftment, and chimerism studies using microsatellite polymerase chain reaction (PCR) showed 70% of patients to be full donor chimeras in both myeloid and lymphoid lineages. The incidence of GVHD was very low, and only 5 patients (20%) developed grade 1 or grade 2 GVHD. Two patients died of treatment-related toxicities; 3 patients with refractory disease at the time of transplant died within 3 months of transplant; and 5 patients relapsed. Of the 5 who relapsed, 3 received salvage chemotherapy and DLI, and 2 received DLI only. Four of these 5 patients achieved and maintained remission, but 1 died of grade 4 GVHD. These results show that this regimen is associated with a high incidence of durable engraftment and low incidence of GVHD. Initial response to DLI suggests that this regimen can facilitate adoptive immunotherapy. Longer follow-up will be needed to assess the impact of this protocol on disease control and ultimate cure.

Nonmyeloablative conditioning regimens are increasingly used in an older patient population. Flowers et al. (2001) described 22 patients with CLL who failed prior therapy with alkylating agents and/or fludarabine, who were not eligible for or failed prior autologous transplant, and who underwent HLA-matched related donor HSCT. The age range was 46 to 67 years with a mean age of 54 years. The median number of treatment regimens prior to HSCT was 4 (range 1 to 10). The conditioning regimen consisted of 2 Gy TBI with (12 patients) or without (10 patients) fludarabine 90 mg/m^2. GVHD prophylaxis consisted of cyclosporine and mycophenolate mofetil (MMF). Twenty-one patients engrafted. Four developed grade 3 and grade 4 GVHD, and 6 developed grade 2 GVHD. Four had disease progression or relapse, 3 had stable disease, 2 achieved a partial response, and 10 achieved a complete response. Ten died of progressive disease, GVHD, sepsis, and metastatic small cell lung cancer (present before treatment). This demonstrated that a nonmyeloablative conditioning regimen can be performed in older, heavily pretreated patients with advanced CLL and can produce marked disease responses. It offers a treatment with curative potential to older patients who failed conventional chemotherapy.

In a study by Shapira et al. (2004), 17 "older" patients with hematological malignancies (median age 62.5 years) were conditioned with fludarabine and busulfan (14 patients), fludarabine and low-dose TBI (3 patients), or busulfan alone (1 patient), followed by G-CSF mobilized allogeneic stem cells from fully matched siblings (12 patients), fully matched unrelated donors (3 patients), and partially mismatched siblings (2 patients). Cyclosporine was used for GVHD prophylaxis. Cyclosporine was tapered during the second or third month after the transplant, depending on chimeric status and presence of GVHD. All patients displayed evidence of trilineage engraftment and none exhibited immune-mediated rejection. Treatment-related toxicities included fever, acute GVHD, acute renal failure, VOD, and nonischemic paroxysmal atrial fibrillation. Transplant-related mortality was 33%. Twelve of the 17 patients were discharged home. Five of 17 (29%) survived follow-up (8 to 53 months). Whereas overall survival was 29%, these were elderly, high-risk patients who would otherwise not be considered for this potentially curative treatment.

Maris et al. (2003) described 89 patients with various hematological malignancies, including myelodysplastic syndrome (MDS), AML, ALL, CML, non-Hodgkin's lymphoma, chronic lymphocytic leukemia, Hodgkin's disease, and multiple myeloma. They were classified as low risk, 22% (AML or ALL in first complete remission, MDS refractory anemia or CML chronic phase), or high risk, 78% (advanced-stage AML, ALL, MDS, or CML in accelerated or blast phase and B cell malignancy). Median age was 53 years (range 5 to 69 years). The conditioning regimen, based on the high graft loss rate with low-dose TBI alone, added fludarabine 30 mg/m^2 for 3 days to 2 Gy TBI on day 0. Following conditioning, the patients received HLA-matched and mismatched, unrelated bone marrow or G-CSF stimulated HSC. GVHD prophylaxis consisted of cyclosporine and MMF. In patients without GVHD, MMF was tapered at day 40 and cyclosporine at day 100. Treatment-related toxicities included grade 3 and grade 4 cardiac toxicities (27%), pulmonary (20%), hepatic (18%), neurological (10%), GI (8%), renal (5%), and hematologic (5%) toxicities. Grade 2 to grade 4 GVHD developed in 52% of the patients. New onset alopecia, mucositis, and VOD were not observed in any patient. Median time to neutrophil recovery was 15 days (range 0 to 55 days), and 27% of patients did not develop neutropenia (absolute neutrophil count < 500). Median time to platelet recovery was 4 days (range 0 to 53 days), and 55% did not develop thrombocytopenia (platelet count < 20,000). Donor engraftment (> 5% donor chimerism) at day 28 was observed in 77 of 89 (87%) patients and was sustained in 70 of 89 (79%). Nonrelapse mortality at day 100 was 11% and at 1 year was 16%. Causes of death included GVHD, infection, bleeding, congestive heart failure, pulmonary failure, hepatic toxicity, and suicide. One-year overall survival and disease-free survival were 52% and 38%, respectively.

Toxicity of Conditioning Regimens

Patients undergoing conditioning chemotherapy with or without TBI followed by HSCT are at substantial risk for developing multiple-organ toxicities and complications associated with this aggressive treatment modality. Etiologies for these toxicities and complications include the conditioning regimen, underlying disease, prior treatment, GVHD, and GVHD prophylaxis with immunosuppressive therapy.

With so many conditioning regimens used and most involving two or more chemotherapeutic agents, some including TBI and some using immunosuppressive agents, it is understandable that every organ can be affected by the conditioning regimen. Some toxicities may be short term and reversible, such as mucositis, gastroenteritis, vomiting, and diarrhea. Others may be long term and potentially life-threatening,

such as VOD or interstitial pneumonitis (Spitzer & McAfee, 1999).

Bearman et al. (1988) developed a toxicity grading system designed to measure organ toxicity caused only by the conditioning regimen. The goal was to determine whether toxicities were due to the preparatory regimen or influenced by other transplant-related factors. One hundred ninety-five patients were selected. Most of the 195 patients selected for the study were in remission (128 patients); others were in relapse (67 patients). The transplants were autologous and matched and mismatched allogeneic. The TBI dose was 12 Gy (74 patients) versus 15.75 Gy (12 patients). GVHD prophylaxis included no prophylaxis, methotrexate (MTX), cyclosporine (CSA), and CSA + MTX. The results show that toxicity was most common in the liver, mouth, and GI tract, and most of the toxicities were rated mild to moderate (grade 1 and grade 2) in severity. Severe regimen-related toxicity was most common in the liver, kidneys, and lungs.

Of 30 patients who developed grade 3 and grade 4 toxicities, 20 patients had one organ involved (liver, 10 patients; lungs, 4 patients; mucosa, 3 patients; heart, 1 patient; CNS, 1 patient; kidney, 1 patient). Seven patients had two organs involved, and 3 patients had three or more organs involved. Seventeen of 19 patients with grade 3 toxicity died within the first 100 days.

In this study, patients who developed the most regimen-related toxicities were the following: those with advanced disease, those who received a higher dose of TBI, those who received allografts, and those who received MTX and CSA for GVHD prophylaxis.

Nevill and colleagues (1991) from Vancouver, Canada, used this grading system to evaluate regimen-related toxicities of busulfan (16 mg/kg)

+ cyclophosphamide (120 mg/kg) in patients with hematological malignancies undergoing allogeneic transplant. Stomatitis and hepatic toxicity were the most frequently observed toxicities. Grade 2 or higher mucositis was reported in 63% of the patients, and grade 2 or higher hepatic toxicity occurred in 44% of the patients. Hepatic toxicity of grade 2 or higher was more common in those patients who received MTX for GVHD prophylaxis. Grade 2 or greater toxicity was rare (< 10%) in other organ systems. Amphotericin B and prolonged antibiotic use were associated with grade 2 to grade 4 hepatic toxicities. Hemorrhagic cystitis occurred in 21% of the patients. Pulmonary and cardiac toxicity were rare. Overall, 17% of the patients in the study developed grade 3 or grade 4 regimen-related toxicities.

Nursing Implications During the Conditioning Regimen

Nursing care during the conditioning regimen is focused on prevention of acute side effects and prompt and accurate identification of the acute toxicities and their management. (See **Table 5-10.**) It is incumbent on the nurse to know all the aspects of the conditioning regimens, including the rationale for use, the agents used, doses, schedule, and duration of therapy. The HSCT nurse must know the potential acute toxicities of the conditioning chemoradiotherapy, the clinical manifestations of the toxicities, and appropriate preventative and treatment strategies.

Many supportive medications such as antiemetics, antianxiety agents, analgesics, antidiarrheals, and multiple antibiotics are given as clinically indicated during this phase of HSCT. Prophylactic medications such as phenytoin (Dilantin®) to decrease the risk of busulfan-induced seizure activity, and mercaptoethane sodium sulfonate (mesna) to decrease the risk of cyclophosphamide/ifosfamide-induced hemorrhagic cystitis are usually given during conditioning chemoradiotherapy. Ursodiol (Actigall) may be given to decrease the risk of dose-intensive chemotherapy-induced VOD. The HSCT nurse must know the rationale for these supportive medications and their potential side effects.

A complete baseline nursing assessment is done prior to the initiation of the conditioning regimen. This includes obtaining height, weight, and vital signs, and thorough assessment of the cardiopulmonary system, the GI system, the hepatic and renal function, the neurological system, and the skin and mucous membranes. Because prompt identification of conditioning-induced acute toxicity is crucial in decreasing the morbidity and mortality associated with HSCT, it is incumbent on the nurse to carefully monitor vital signs, daily weights, intake and output, laboratory results (complete blood counts and serum chemistries, and therapeutic drug levels), and to do a thorough nursing assessment on a regular basis during the conditioning phase of HSC transplantation.

The nurse should assess for any risk factors the patient may have that may trigger or exacerbate toxicities (such as smoking and alcohol history, previous treatment with anthracyclines, pre-existing comorbidities). The nurse should ascertain the patient's previous chemoradiotherapy history, including the side effects experienced and strategies that were effective, or ineffective, in treating the symptoms or cause of distress.

Infection

Infection is the most significant cause of morbidity and mortality due to immunosuppression

Table 5-10 SIDE EFFECTS OF PREPARATIVE REGIMENS BY AGENT AND SYSTEM.

System	Cyclophosphamide	Busulfan	Carboplatin	Thiotepa	Melphalan	Carmustine	Cytarabine	Etoposide	Fludarabine	Mitoxantrone	ATG	TBI
Hematopoietic												
Anemia	X	X	X	X	X	X	X	X	X	X	X	X
Leukopenia	X	X	X	X	X	X	X	X	X	X	X	X
Thrombocytopenia	X	X	X	X	X	X	X	X	X	X		X
Gastrointestinal												
Nausea/vomiting	X	X	X	X	X	X	X	X	X	X	X	X
Anorexia	X			X	X		X	X		X	X	X
Mucositis/stomatitis	X	X	X	X	X		X	X	X	X		X
Diarrhea	X		X	X	X		X	X				X
Constipation												
Hepatotoxicity	X					X	X					X
Genitourinary												
Hemorrhagic cystitis	X	X		X				X			X	
Nephrotoxicity	X	X	X			X			X		X	X
Electrolyte imbalances	X	X	X						X			
Cardiovascular												
Cardiotoxicity	X									X		
Hypo- or hypertension								X				X
Pulmonary												
Fibrosis	X				X	X						X
Pneumonitis	X											X
Reproductive												
Infertility	X		X	X	X	X		X				X
Gynecomastia		X										
Integumentary												
Dermatitis			X	X	X		X	X			X	X

Hyperpigmentation

Alopecia

Erythema

Immunologic

Fever/chills

Hypersensitivity/
allergic reaction/
anaphylaxis

Neurologic

Ototoxicity

Peripheral
neuropathy

Seizures

Headache/altered
mental status

Miscellaneous

Secondary
malignancy

Cataracts

Nasal congestion

Conjunctivitis

Parotitis

Source: From McAdams and Burgunder (2004).

and myelosuppression with subsequent neutropenia following conditioning chemoradiotherapy. The neutropenia can be severe and prolonged depending on the class of antineoplastics used and the number, dosages, and scheduling of the chemotherapeutic and immunosuppressive agents or radiation that may be a part of the conditioning regimen.

Other risk factors for infection that may be present during the conditioning phase of HSCT include older patient age, preexisting comorbidities, hematological disease, preexisting infection, relapse at time of transplant, impaired skin and mucous membranes, less-than-optimal nutritional status, and presence of indwelling venous catheter, or urinary catheter for bladder irrigation to decrease risk of hemorrhagic cystitis. It is not uncommon that an HSCT patient has one, and likely more, of these risk factors at the initiation of the conditioning regimen.

Infection prevention, therefore, is an important aspect of the medical and nursing management of the patient undergoing HSCT. The administration of polyantimicrobial therapy for infection prophylaxis is a common practice in the care of HSCT patients. Often, the patient is unable to mount an inflammatory response because the leukocyte count is extremely low. Consequently, the usual signs and symptoms of infection may be minimal or even absent, which hinders early and accurate diagnosis of an infectious process. When caring for the neutropenic HSCT patient, it is essential that the nurse maintains a reduced microbial environment, adheres to the established neutropenic guidelines, and continually and thoroughly assesses the patient for signs and symptoms of infection. The nurse must monitor the leukocyte count, paying particular attention to the absolute neutrophil count, and must monitor the results of all cultures of bodily fluids and secretions. Any infection in the HSCT patient during this period of moderate to severe neutropenia can quickly become life-threatening. Therefore, at the first indication of infection, prompt treatment is indicated.

Bleeding

As a result of the conditioning regimen, the patient becomes thrombocytopenic and at risk for bleeding. Bleeding can be mild, such as petechiae, or potentially life-threatening, such as hemorrhagic cystitis or diffuse alveolar hemorrhage. It is important to keep in mind that even mild bleeding can progress quickly. Other risk factors for bleeding that may be present during the conditioning phase of HSCT include mucositis or any mucosal injury, hemorrhagic cystitis, prolonged nausea, vomiting, and diarrhea.

Providing a safe environment to decrease the risk of patient injury, frequent and thorough nursing assessments, and timely management of bleeding are essential components in preventing hemorrhage in the thrombocytopenic HSCT patient. Platelet count is monitored every day.

Generally, for patients undergoing HSCT, platelet transfusions are given when the platelet count is 10,000/ml to 20,000/ml or lower, with the appearance of petechiae, increased bruising, or in the setting of any active bleeding. All platelet transfusions are irradiated to inactivate T lymphocytes, thereby decreasing the risk of transfusion-acquired GVHD. All transfusions should be leukocyte filtered to decrease the risk of allosensitization, febrile transfusion reactions, and the transmission of cytomegalovirus (CMV). Many HSCT transplant patients can receive CMV-safe platelets. However, allogeneic HSCT patients who are CMV seronegative and whose donors are CMV seronegative should receive

CMV-negative transfusions. Single-donor and HLA-matched platelets may be indicated if the patient becomes platelet refractory or develops anti-HLA antibodies.

Gastrointestinal Toxicities

Nausea and vomiting are common during conditioning chemoradiotherapy. Nausea and vomiting can occur within hours of starting chemotherapy and persist until after its completion. The severity of the nausea and vomiting depends on the chemotherapeutic agents given, the combination of agents given, dose, route of administration, rate of the IV infusion, schedule, and the emetogenic potential of each agent. TBI, often a component of the conditioning regimen, is highly emetogenic. In addition, nausea and vomiting are potential side effects of many supportive medications given during this time.

Antiemetics are given prior to and at regular intervals during and after the conditioning chemoradiotherapy. A spectrum of antiemetics may be given to prevent or manage the nausea and vomiting associated with the conditioning phase of HSCT. Often, a combination of different types of antiemetics is effective due to the different mechanisms of action. Antiemetics commonly used are serotonin antagonists (dolasetron mesylate [Anzemet], ondansetron hydrochloride [Zofran], granisetron hydrochloride [Kytril]), antihistamines (diphenhydramine hydrochloride [Benadryl], promethazine hydrochloride [Phenergan]), phenothiazines (prochlorperazine [Compazine], perphenazine [Trilafon]), corticosteroids (dexamethasone [Decadron]), benzodiazepimes (lorazepam [Ativan]), and butyrophenones (haloperidol [Haldol]). For some patients, the cannabinoid Marinol is an effective antiemetic.

Scopolamine may be added to the antiemetic regimen if position changes and movement trigger or exacerbate the nausea and vomiting.

Nursing interventions for nausea and vomiting during the conditioning regimen include the administration of antiemetics, providing frequent mouth care (especially after each episode of vomiting), and reducing unpleasant or noxious noise, sights, and smells in the room. Dietary interventions include frequent, small meals and bland/dry/cool/nonspicy foods. Clear liquids may be an effective option. It may be beneficial for the patient to stop eating and drinking altogether during the conditioning regimen if nausea and vomiting persist. Once the conditioning is completed, the GI distress may lessen.

Nonpharmacological measures that may be used during conditioning that may assuage nausea and vomiting include relaxation techniques, guided imagery, music, meditation, prayer, and gentle yoga stretches.

Diarrhea occurs as a result of the direct toxicity of the conditioning chemoradiotherapy on the gastrointestinal mucosa. Antineoplastics that can cause diarrhea include busulfan, melphalan, cytarabine, etoposide, methotrexate, and thiotepa. Diarrhea is a common acute side effect of TBI. Some supportive medications such as antacids, metoclopramide, magnesium, and antibiotics can cause or exacerbate diarrhea (Rust, 1997). Diarrhea may be accompanied by abdominal cramps, bloating, and rectal pain or bleeding.

Antidiarrheals may be administered and dietary interventions, such as bland, low-residue diet and avoidance of dairy products, may be implemented. A BRAT (banana, rice, applesauce, toast) diet may be helpful in decreasing diarrhea.

Mucositis

Mucositis is a significant side effect of the conditioning regimen. It is caused by the direct and indirect toxicity of chemoradiotherapy on the epithelium of the mucosa. The development and severity of mucositis are dependent on the types and dosages of chemotherapy given. Conditioning regimens that contain etoposide, cytarabine, busulfan, high-dose cyclophosphamide, thiotepa, cisplatin, BCNU, methotrexate, or TBI frequently cause mucositis. It has been demonstrated that 69–75% of patients undergoing either allogeneic or syngeneic bone marrow transplantation with regimens that include cyclophosphamide, with or without TBI, experience some degree of mucositis (Vargus & Silverman, 2000). It usually develops during and/or after the administration of conditioning chemoradiotherapy.

Early signs and symptoms of mucositis are xerostomia, mild mucosal edema and erythema, soreness, and pseudomembrane formation. As mucositis progresses, there is worsening mucosal edema and erythema, ulceration, tissue sloughing, ulceration, and pain (often requiring continuous narcotic analgesia). The potential sequelae of mucositis include pain, bleeding, anorexia, inability to eat and drink, dehydration, fluid and electrolyte imbalance, weight loss, infection, and drowsiness, nausea, vomiting, and other side effects due to narcotics given to relieve the pain.

Mucositis begins to resolve 2 to 3 weeks after the completion of the conditioning regimen once engraftment begins and there is neutrophil recovery.

Hemorrhagic Cystitis

Conditioning regimens that contain cyclophosphamide, ifosfamide, or busulfan can cause hemorrhagic cystitis. Hemorrhagic cystitis is an inflammation of the epithelial lining of the urinary bladder. It occurs when acrolein, a metabolite of Cytoxan and ifosfamide, binds to the urothelium and causes mucosal hyperemia, ulceration, and bleeding. Hemorrhagic cystitis usually occurs during or days after the completion of the conditioning regimen, but it can also occur weeks to months after the completion of the conditioning. Late hemorrhagic cystitis is often caused by a viral infection such as adenovirus or polyoma virus. Thrombocytopenia increases the risk for hemorrhagic cystitis. The incidence of hemorrhagic cystitis in patients undergoing HSCT is 10–40% (Chan, 2000). Hemorrhagic cystitis can range from mild (microscopic hematuria) to severe (exsanguinating, life-threatening hematuria). Hemorrhagic cystitis can cause significant pain and bleeding. Signs and symptoms of hemorrhagic cystitis include hematuria (microscopic or gross with clots), dysuria, burning on urination, urinary frequency or urgency, painful bladder spasms, and flank pain.

Several strategies are used to prevent or minimize the risks of developing hemorrhagic cystitis. The uroprotectant drug mesna is given intravenously before and 4 and 8 hours after the completion of each dose of cyclophosphamide. Mesna binds to the acrolein, rendering it an inactive compound. Forced diuresis with vigorous IV hydration (often two to three times the maintenance dose) and the administration of diuretics are done to prevent or decrease the contact of acrolein with the urothelium, thereby decreasing bladder irritation and the risk of bleeding. This aggressive IV hydration, combined with diuretics, is started several hours before the initiation of the conditioning regimen and continues for 24 to 48 hours after the completion of chemotherapy or until there is no evidence of hematuria. A three-way urinary catheter may be placed to keep the bladder empty, with or without a continuous bladder instillation, to flush the bladder and remove the acrolein. Some transplant centers require that the patient voids every 2 hours to flush the bladder and remove the acrolein.

Urine should be dipsticked frequently for microhematuria. Intake and output and daily weight and serum chemistries should be frequently and carefully monitored in this setting of aggressive hydration and diuretic administration. Analgesics, antispasmodics, and platelet transfusions are also used to manage this urotoxicity following conditioning chemotherapy. If the bleeding persists, cystoscopy and cauterization of the ulcerated and bleeding areas may be required (Rust, 1997).

Hemorrhagic cystitis usually responds with supportive treatment and resolves soon after the completion of conditioning chemotherapy. Long-term effects on the bladder are infrequent, but can occur.

Veno-Occlusive Disease (VOD)

VOD is a frequent cause of nonrelapse mortality among patients receiving high-dose cytoreductive conditioning regimens (Bearman, 1995). For some preparative regimens used in HSCT, VOD is the dose-limiting toxicity (McDonald et al., 1993). VOD is believed to result from chemoradiotherapy-induced injury to hepatocytes and vascular endothelium in zone 3 of the liver acinus, from local hypercoagulability, and from microvenular/sinusoid hepatic vascular obstruction secondary to thrombosis and fibrosis (Spitzer & McAfee, 1999). Renal insufficiency is often associated with VOD.

Clinical manifestations of VOD are hyperbilirubinemia, weight gain, fluid retention, abdominal discomfort, painful hepatomegaly, ascites, peripheral edema, thrombocytopenia, hepatic encephalopathy, and multiorgan failure.

There are many risk factors for VOD. Please refer to **Table 5-11**. Patients undergoing HSCT can easily have several of these risk factors that significantly increase the possibility of developing VOD.

Table 5-11 RISK FACTORS FOR VOD.

Pretransplant Risk Factors	Transplant-Related Risk Factors
History of hepatitis or other liver disease	TBI used in the conditioning regimen
Liver metastases	Intensity and type of conditioning regimens
Elevated liver function tests prior to HSCT	Hepatotoxic medications
Intensity of conventional chemotherapy prior to HSCT	Receiving antimicrobial treatment for bacterial/ fungal infection before starting conditioning
Prior radiation to the liver or in a field that included the liver	GVHD prophylaxis with MTX
Diagnosis of CML	Mismatched or unrelated transplant
CMV-positive serology	
Older patient age	
Recipient of a second transplant	

Source: Bearman (1995) and McDonald et al. (1993).

The reported incidence of VOD is variable with ranges from 5% (Carreras et al., 1998) to 54% (Bearman, 1995) to 70% (Essell et al., 1992). Generally, VOD occurs in 20–50% of patients undergoing HSCT.

In a study by Jones et al. (1987), of 235 patients undergoing autologous or allogeneic HSCT for severe aplastic anemia, ALL, AML, and CML, VOD occurred in 23% of patients prepared with cyclophosphamide (200 mg/kg) + TBI (1200 cGy) and 24% of patients prepared with busulfan (16 mg/kg) + cyclophosphamide (200 mg/kg). McDonald et al. (1993) compared the incidence of VOD in patients who received cyclophosphamide (120 mg/kg) + TBI (1200 cGy) with three other more intensive conditioning regimens. They included cyclophosphamide (120 mg/kg) + TBI (> 1200 cGy); busulfan (16 mg/kg) + cyclophosphamide (120 to 200 mg/kg); and cyclophosphamide + etoposide + BCNU. The incidence of severe VOD was 8% in patients who received cyclophosphamide + TBI and 23–33% in patients who received the more intense conditioning regimens. In this study, multiorgan failure was more common in patients who developed VOD. One half of the patients with severe VOD developed renal, cardiac, and pulmonary failure. VOD can be fatal in up to 40% of patients who develop this conditioning-induced hepatic toxicity (Vinayek, Demetris, & Rakela, 2000).

GVHD prophylaxis is a risk factor for VOD. In one study (Essell et al., 1992), the incidence of VOD was 18% in 67 patients who received cyclosporine (CSA) + methylprednisolone (MP) for GVHD prophylaxis versus 70% of 20 patients who received CSA + methotrexate (MTX) for GVHD prophylaxis. VOD was fatal in 4.5% of the patients treated with CSA + MP versus 25% treated with CSA + MTX.

Although the conditioning regimen is the antecedent for the development of VOD, the onset of signs and symptoms generally does not occur during the conditioning regimen. VOD usually occurs 1 to 3 weeks after the completion of the conditioning chemoradiotherapy. During the conditioning regimen, the nurse should carefully monitor intake and output and daily weights and assess for signs and symptoms suggestive of early VOD, such as sudden weight gain, fluid retention, and increased serum bilirubin, aspartate aminotransferase (SGOT), alanine aminotransferase (SGPT), and alkaline phosphatase. Ursodiol may be given for VOD prophylaxis. Its mechanism of action in preventing hepatic toxicity is unclear.

Cardiac Toxicity

Cardiac complications account for approximately 5% of early transplant-related fatalities (Oblon, 2000). The major cause of cardiac toxicity in HSCT is the conditioning regimen, particularly dose-intensive cyclophosphamide. Other potentially cardiotoxic chemotherapeutic agents often used in preparatory regimens include BCNU, cytarabine, etoposide, ifosfamide, cisplatin, and busulfan (Keller, 2004). There are many risk factors for cardiac toxicities. Please see **Table 5-12.**

Cyclophosphamide can cause hemorrhagic necrosis, thickening of the left ventricular wall, transmural hemorrhage, coronary artery vasculitis, pericardial effusion, fibrinous pericarditis, arrythmias, and cardiomyopathy (Wikle, 1991; Wilkes et al., 2003). Approximately 1–5% of patients who receive more than 120 mg/m^2 of cyclophosphamide develop acute cardiac injury.

Cardiac toxicity may be manifested by palpitations, EKG changes (low voltage), arrhythmias,

Table 5-12 RISK FACTORS FOR CARDIAC TOXICITIES.

Patient Related	Cancer Treatment Related
Extremes of age (pediatric/elderly)	History of anthracyclines
Renal or hepatic impairment	Cumulative chemotherapy and radiation therapy doses
History of cardiac disease	History of radiation therapy to the chest
History of mitral valve disease	Total dose of cyclophosphamide >150 mg/kg
History of ischemic heart disease	Cyclophosphamide and TBI used in the conditioning
Cardiac ejection fraction < 50%	regimen

Sources: Wikle (1991) and Camp-Sorrell (1999).

chest pain, dyspnea on exertion, orthopnea, syncopy, fatigue, anxiety, weight gain, hypotension, hypertension, and pericardial friction rub.

Ongoing assessment of the patient's cardiac status to detect any signs and symptoms of conditioning regimen–induced cardiac toxicity is essential. A baseline EKG and echocardiogram, including the ejection fraction, are usually obtained as part of the patient evaluation done prior to the HSCT. A 12-lead EKG is done before each dose of cyclophosphamide and 24 to 48 hours after the final dose. Each EKG should be reviewed with the physician to detect any changes that may have occurred subsequent to cyclophosphamide administration. Some transplant centers require cardiac monitoring during cyclophosphamide administration and for 24 to 48 hours after the completion. Vital signs must be carefully monitored, paying particular attention to heart and lung sounds and the rate, rhythm, and quality of the heart rate. Fluid and electrolyte balance must be monitored. Weighing the patient twice each day on the days of cyclophosphamide administration is a common practice.

Pulmonary Toxicity

Many conditioning regimens cause mucosal injury in the nose, mouth, and pharynx. The mucosal lining may become edematous and ulcerated, causing dysphagia and bleeding, which can cause airway obstruction or aspiration of blood, saliva, or sloughed tissue (Kreit, 2000). Pulmonary edema can occur during the conditioning regimen. Although not directly related to the conditioning chemoradiotherapy, pulmonary edema can be triggered by aggressive hydration given to prevent hemorrhagic cystitis.

Acute respiratory toxicity, such as diffuse alveolar hemorrhage, interstitial pneumonitis, and infection, generally do not occur during the conditioning phase of HSCT. These are potential sequelae of the conditioning regimen and usually occur weeks to months after the conditioning is completed.

Patient risk factors that may increase the possibility of the development of pulmonary toxicity during conditioning include tobacco use, prior lung damage, preexisting lung disease, previous radiation to the chest, previous treatment with bleomycin, conditioning with TBI, and conditioning with cyclophosphamide or BCNU.

Prevention of respiratory complications is a nursing priority. A key component of prevention is educating the patient and family regarding the importance of activity in decreasing the risks of developing respiratory complications.

The patient should be encouraged to be as active as possible. Activity such as getting out of bed, sitting in a chair, ambulating, using the treadmill or stationary bike, and doing the exercises recommended by the physical therapist are helpful in decreasing the risk of developing pulmonary complications during the conditioning regimen. Additional preventive measures include frequent coughing and deep breathing and incentive spirometry. However, these activities can be difficult for patients experiencing nausea, vomiting, diarrhea, or drowsiness due to medications that are given to manage symptom distress caused by the conditioning chemoradiotherapy. Therefore, the HSCT nurse must diligently, yet at the same time gently, encourage and support the patient in these important preventive activities.

Nursing care also encompasses early recognition of signs and symptoms of respiratory complications through ongoing assessment of respiratory function, including respiratory rate and rhythm and quality of breath sounds. Oxygen saturation should be checked with vital signs. The nurse should assess for cyanosis, pallor, cough, sputum production, dyspnea, and hemoptysis. The nurse should know the recent results of laboratory tests, sputum cultures, and diagnostic tests such as chest x-rays and lung scans.

It is important for the nurse to keep in mind that sometimes seemingly small changes in the patient's respiratory status, such as mild dyspnea after performing activities of daily living such as showering or a seemingly benign nonproductive cough, can escalate and the patient's condition can quickly deteriorate and require transfer to an intensive care setting.

Neurological Toxicity

During the conditioning phase of HSCT, neurological complications are primarily due to the neurotoxicity of the chemotherapy agents administered. Neurotoxic drugs often included in conditioning regimens include cytarabine, busulfan, ifosfamide, BCNU, cisplatin, and cyclophosphamide.

Cytarabine is an antimetabolite used in the conventional treatment of leukemia, as well as a component of many conditioning regimens. Because cytarabine crosses the blood–brain barrier and has a long half-life in the cerebral spinal fluid (Walker & Brochstein, 1988), it has a high propensity to induce neurotoxicity. Cerebellar toxicity is a neurological side effect particularly characteristic of cytarabine. Signs and symptoms of cerebellar toxicity are ataxia, nystagmus, dysarthria, intention tremors, muscle weakness, slurred speech, and disdiadochokinesia.

Other cytarabine-induced neurotoxicities include headache, somnolence, confusion, seizures, personality changes, memory loss, intellectual impairment, and peripheral neuropathies. Ocular toxicities associated with cytarabine include conjunctival injection, corneal opacities, decreased visual acuity, increased lacrimation, blurred vision, photophobia, and eye pain (Wilkes et al., 2003).

Busulfan is an alkylating agent that also crosses the blood–brain barrier. Busulfan is known to cause seizure activity. Therefore, phenytoin is often given as a prophylaxis for busulfan-induced seizures. It is usually given during the days of busulfan administration and for 24 to 48 hours after the completion of busulfan. Other neurotoxicities of busulfan include insomnia, anxiety, headache, dizziness, depression, confusion, lethargy, and hallucinations (Wilkes et al., 2003).

Ifosfamide is an alkylating agent that can cause neurological toxicity when given at high doses. Neurotoxicities include somnolence, amnesia, mental status changes, seizures, ataxia, confusion, depressive psychosis, hallucinations, dizziness, disorientation, and cranial nerve dysfunction (Wilkes et al., 2003). The etiology of ifosfamide-induced neurotoxicty is unclear.

During the conditioning phase of HSCT, patients receive many supportive medications (such as analgesics for pain, antiemetics, corticosteroids and antianxiety agents for nausea and vomiting). Each of these medications has neurological side effects or may potentiate the neurotoxicity of the conditioning agents. Supportive medications must be given with caution and the patient must be regularly and carefully assessed.

Metabolic abnormalities can cause neurological signs and symptoms. The etiologies of metabolic abnormalities that may occur during the conditioning regimen include vigorous IV hydration, diuretics, vomiting, diarrhea, bleeding, tumor lysis syndrome, and some antineoplastics (cyclophosphamide, cisplatin, cytarabine). Conditioning-induced metabolic abnormalities include hypercalcemia, hypocalcemia, hypokalemia, hypomagnesemia, hypernatremia, hyponatremia, hyperammonemia, and metabolic acidosis. Neurological manifestations of these metabolic abnormalities are varied and may present as headache, lethargy, drowsiness, irritability, muscle twitching or weakness, confusion, seizures, obtundation, and coma (Preston & Cunningham, 1998). It is important to monitor intake and output, electrolytes, creatinine, blood urea nitrogen (BUN), liver function tests, phosphorus, calcium, magnesium, and ammonia.

Nursing implications during conditioning chemotherapy containing neurotoxic agents include ongoing assessment of the patient's neurological status during conditioning, paying particular attention to any subtle neurological changes. Such changes may be a harbinger of more serious neurotoxicities. Patients who receive busulfan as part of the conditioning phase are at risk of busulfan-induced seizure activity. Additionally, patients with a history of seizures, epilepsy, brain tumor, or head injury present an increased risk of seizure activity. All patients receiving conditioning busulfan must be carefully monitored for any signs or symptoms of seizure activity. An airway and suction equipment should be placed near the bedside and the side rails padded to provide patient safety.

With changes in the patient's mental status comes an increased risk of injury; therefore, providing a safe environment is essential. Some strategies to decrease the risk of injury include maintaining the bed in the low position, raising and padding the side rails, placing the nurse call light in easy reach, and minimizing equipment and clutter in the room to decrease the chance of a fall. Providing a calm environment and reassurance to the patient and family may assuage fears and anxiety and contribute to patient safety and comfort (Simpson, 2000).

Generally, neurotoxicities that occur during the conditioning regimen are dose-related and reversible. However, long-term sequelae of these neurotoxic agents are possible. Long-term follow-up of these patients is crucial to aid in the understanding of the occurrence and severity of delayed effects associated with high-dose chemotherapy.

Tumor Lysis Syndrome (TLS)

Most patients who undergo conditioning chemotherapy followed by HSCT are in remission or have minimal residual disease. However, if the patient has significant tumor burden, as may be the situation with acute leukemia and lymphoma, TLS may develop in patients receiving a conditioning regimen. Nursing interventions when caring for a patient at risk for TLS include vigorous IV hydration, alkalinization of the urine, strict measurement of intake and output, allopurinal to prevent excess serum and urinary uric acid formation, cardiac monitoring, and frequent monitoring of electrolytes, BUN, creatinine, phosphorus, uric acid, and calcium.

Outpatient/Ambulatory Conditioning Regimens

Most conditioning regimens are administered in the inpatient setting because the recipient requires careful, comprehensive medical and nursing monitoring. However, some conditioning regimens may be safely administered in an outpatient setting on each day of the regimen. For example, high-dose melphalan can be administered as a single dose over a short period, making it an outpatient option. In some situations, oral busulfan and TBI may be safely administered on an outpatient basis (Mangan, 2000). Maris et al. (2003) safely administered fludarabine and 2 Gy TBI as conditioning to 89 patients in the ambulatory setting. However, most (91%) had to be admitted to the hospital (median time was day +8.5) for management of treatment-related toxicities.

For a recipient to receive conditioning on an outpatient basis, many things must be considered, including the toxicity of the agents used, the ability of the recipient to come to the outpatient setting, transportation issues, availability and cost of parking, distance from the transplant center, and competency/ability of the recipient to take all medications (chemotherapy and supportive) exactly as directed. The med-

ications may be administered orally, subcutaneously, or intravenously, and the patient and caregiver must be competent with these various modes of medication delivery.

Patient and caregiver education is ongoing throughout the HSCT process. During the conditioning phase of HSCT, topics discussed should include rationale for conditioning chemoradiotherapy, name of the chemotherapeutic medications, dosages, schedule, potential acute side effects of the chemotherapy/TBI, and management of the side effects. Potential long-term effects of the conditioning chemotherapy/TBI should be addressed.

There must also be a competent caregiver readily available. The caregiver must be given instructions to safely and effectively monitor the patient at home. The caregiver must be able to do the following:

- Assist/monitor the administration of medications
- Administer IV hydration if needed
- Take the patient's temperature
- Read the thermometer
- Recognize signs and symptoms that must be reported to the transplant team
- Promptly notify the transplant team if worrisome signs or symptoms appear
- Transport the patient to the transplant center as clinically indicated
- Attend to the patient's physical needs, such as fever, vomiting, diarrhea, and mucositis
- Provide encouragement to the patient in terms of eating, drinking, activity, and rest periods

Education during the conditioning phase of HSCT is complex with many medical terms unfamiliar to the patient and caregiver. As with all patient and family education, this information must be explained in terms the patient and caregiver understand and it must be reinforced regularly. Many transplant centers provide written material that includes specific interventions for managing acute conditioning regimen–induced toxicities, as well as caregiver classes addressing these issues.

In addition to caring for the patient, caregivers may have other ongoing responsibilities such as work and child care or elder care issues that must be addressed during this already stressful time. Summers and associates (2000) reported that the greatest impact on caregivers was related to alterations in their routines. Caregivers who were employed were particularly burdened. If an outpatient conditioning regimen is undertaken, this caregiver burden should be acknowledged. Health-care professionals may need to advocate on behalf of the patient and family for understanding from employers regarding this challenging, but hopefully temporary, situation.

Conclusion

A myriad of conditioning regimens that incorporate various combinations of chemotherapy, radiation therapy, and immunotherapy are used in HSCT. Many disease-related factors such as malignant versus nonmalignant condition, bulky disease versus minimal resistant disease, as well as patient-related factors such as age, preexisting morbidities, and number and type of previous treatments must be considered so that the transplant physician can choose an appropriate, effective, and safe conditioning regimen.

Myeloablative conditioning regimens use dose-intensive chemotherapy with or without TBI in an attempt to eradicate disease, create space for the new stem cells to establish hematopoiesis, and suppress the host immune system. These conditioning regimens are aggressive and often result in significant treatment-related toxicity. Some of the toxicities may be fatal. Because myeloablative conditioning regimens are so aggressive, they are appropriate for a limited patient population that includes those who are younger ($<$ age 60 years), those with minimal previous antineoplastic treatment, and those with few, if any, preexisting comorbidities.

Recently, however, nonmyeloablative conditioning regimens have been developed for allogeneic HSCT. These regimens use lower doses of chemotherapy and radiation therapy and often include immunosuppressive therapy. These regimens result in fewer treatment-related toxicities and rely on the GVT effect to promote remission. Because nonmyeloablative conditioning regimens are less toxic, they are viable treatment modalities for those patients who are older, have a less than optimal performance status, or have other comorbidities. Until the advent of nonmyeloablative conditioning regimens, such patients were generally ineligible for consideration for the potentially curable HSCT.

Whether the conditioning regimen is myeloablative or nonmyeloablative, and regardless of whether it is done in the inpatient or ambulatory setting, it is a difficult, stressful, and challenging time for the patient and the patient's family. The nurse must be knowledgeable about the types and rationale of the various regimens as well as the potential side effects and complications to competently care for these patients. The nurse plays a vital role within the transplant team in providing potentially complex, comprehensive physical care and psychosocial and spiritual support to the patient and the patient's family.

References

Bashey, A. (2002). Immunosuppression with limited toxicity: the characteristics of nucleoside analogs and anti-lymphocyte antibodies used in non-myeloablative hematopoietic cell transplantation. In A. Bashey and E.D. Ball (eds.), *Non-myeloablative allogeneic transplantation* (pp. 39–49). Norwell, MA: Kluwer Academic Publishers.

Bearman, S.I. (1995). The syndrome of hepatic veno-occlusive disease after marrow transplantation. *Blood,* 85, 3005–3020.

Bearman, S.I., Appelbaum, F.R., Back, A., Petersen, F.B., et al. (1989). Regimen-related toxicity and early posttransplant survival in patients undergoing marrow transplantation for lymphoma. *J Clin Oncol,* 7, 1288–1294.

Bearman, S.I., Appelbaum, F.R., Buckner, C.D., Petersen, F.B., Fisher, L.D., Clift, R.A., & Thomas, E.D. (1988). Regimen-related toxicity in patients undergoing bone marrow transplantation. *J Clin Oncol,* 6, 1562–1568.

Bensinger, W.I., & Buckner, C.D. (1999). Preparative regimens. In E.D. Thomas, K.G. Blume, & S.J. Foreman (eds.), *Hematopoietic cell transplantation* (pp. 123–134). Malden, MA: Blackwell Science.

Bensinger, W.I., Buckner, C.D., Clift, R.A., et al. (1992). Phase I study of busulfan and cyclophosphamide in preparation for allogeneic bone marrow transplantation for patients with multiple myeloma. *J Clin Oncol,* 10, 1492–1497.

Cagnoni, P.J., Nieto, Y., and Jones, R.B. (2000). High dose chemotherapy conditioning regimens for autologous or allogeneic hematopoietic stem cell transplantation. In E.D. Ball, J.Lister, & P. Law (eds.), *Hematopoietic stem cell therapy* (pp. 382–402). Philadelphia, PA: Churchill Livingstone.

Camp-Sorrell, D. (1999). Surviving the cancer, surviving the treatment: acute cardiac and pulmonary toxicity. *Oncol Nurs Forum,* 26, 983–990.

Carreras, E., Bertz, H., Arcese, W., Vernant, J.P., Tomas, J.F., & Hagglund, H. (1998). Incidence and outcome of hepatic veno-occlusive disease after blood or marrow transplantation: a prospective cohort study of the European group for blood and marrow transplantation. *Blood,* 92, 3599–3604.

Chan, B. (2000). The pharmacology of peripheral stem cell transplantation. In P.C. Buchsel & P.M. Kapustay (eds.), *Stem cell transplantation: a clinical textbook* (pp. 8.1–8.23). Pittsburgh, PA: Oncology Nursing Press.

Chopra, R., McMillan, A.K., Linch, D.C., et al. (1993). The place of high dose BEAM therapy and autologous bone marrow transplantation in poor risk Hodgkin's disease: a single center 8 year study of 155 patients. *Blood,* 81, 1137–1145.

Clift, R.A., Buckner, C.D., Appelbaum, F.R., et al. (1990). Allogeneic marrow transplantation in patients with acute myeloid leukemia in 1st remission: a randomized trial of two irradiation regimens. *Blood,* 76, 1867–1871.

Clift, R.A, Buckner, C.D., Appelbaum, F.R., et al. (1991). Allogeneic marrow transplantation in patients with chronic myeloid leukemia in the chronic phase: a randomized trial of two irradiation regimens. *Blood,* 77, 1660–1665.

Copelan, E.A. (2000). Are busulfan-based preparative regimens equivalent, worse or better than total body irradiation regimens? In B.J. Bolwell (ed.), *Current controversies in bone marrow transplantation* (pp. 53–67). Totowa, NJ: Humana Press.

Copelan, E.A., Biggs, J.C., Thompson, J.M., et al. (1991). Treatment of acute myelocytic leukemia with allogeneic bone marrow tranplantation following preparation with Bu/Cy2. *Blood,* 78, 838–843.

Copelan, E., & Deeg, H. (1992). Conditioning for allogeneic marrow transplantation in patients with lymphohematopoietic malignancies without the use of total body irradiation. *Blood,* 80, 1648–1658.

Copelan, E.A., & Penza, S.L. (2000). Preparative regimens for stem cell transplantation. In R. Hoffman, E.J. Benz, S.J. Shattil, B. Furie, H.J. Cohen, L.E. Silberstein, & P. McGlave (eds.), *Hematology basic principles and practice* (3rd ed., pp. 1628–1642). New York: Churchill Livingstone.

Essell, J.H., Thompson, J.M., Harman, G.S., Halvorson, R.D., Snyder, M.J., Johnson, R.A., et al. (1992). Marked increase in veno-occlusive disease of the liver associated with methotrexate use for graft-versus-host disease prophylaxis in patients receiving busulfan/cyclophosphamide. *Blood,* 79, 2784–2788.

Flowers, C.R., Maloney, D.G., Sandmaier, J.A., Shizuru, J.A., McSweeney, P.A., Chauncey, T.R., et al. (2001). Allogeneic hematopoietic stem cell transplantation with nonmyeloablative conditioning for patients with chronic lymphocytic leukemia [Abstract No. 1755]. *Blood,* 98, 418a.

Forman, S.J., & O'Donnell, M.R. (2003). Hematopoietic stem cell transplantation. In B. Furie, P.A. Cassileth, M.B. Atkins, & R.J. Mayer (eds.), *Clinical hematology and oncology. Presentation, diagnosis and treatment* (pp. 391–418). Philadelphia, PA: Churchill Livingstone.

Jones, R.J., Lee, K.S.K., Beschorner, W.E., Vogel, V.G., Grochow, L.B., Braine, H.G., et al. (1987). Veno-occlusive disease of the liver following bone marrow transplantation. *Transplantation,* 44, 778–783.

Keller, C.A. (2004). Cardiopulmonary effects. In S. Ezzone (ed.), *Hematopoietic stem cell transplantation: a manual for nursing practice* (pp. 177–199). Pittsburgh, PA: Oncology Nursing Society.

Kim, H. (2002). Mini-allogeneic stem cell transplantation. Past, present and future. *Cancer Practice,* 10, 170–172.

Kolb, J.H., Mittermuller, J., Clkemin, C., et al. (1990). Donor leukocyte transfusions for treatment of recurrent chronic myelogenous leukemia in marrow transplant patients. *Blood,* 76, 2462–2465.

Kottaridis, P.D., Milligan, D.W., Chopra, R., Craddock, C., Kyriacou, C., Peggs, K., et al. (2001). Nonmyeloablative transplantation for patients with Hodgkin's disease: limited transplant related mortality and possible evidence of a graft-versus Hodgkin's effect [Abstract No. 747]. *Blood,* 98, 416a.

Kreit, J.W. (2000). Respiratory complications. In E.D. Ball, J. Lister, & P. Law (eds.), *Hematopoietic stem cell therapy* (pp. 567–577). Philadelphia, PA: Churchill Livingstone.

Mangan, K.F. (2000). Choice of conditioning regimens. In E.D. Ball, J. Lister, & P. Law (eds.), *Hematopoietic stem cell therapy* (pp. 403–413). Philadelphia, PA: Churchill Livingstone.

Maris, M.B., Niederwieser, D., Sandmaier, B.M., Storer, B., Stuart, M., Maloney, D., et al. (2003). HLA-matched unrelated donor hematopoietic cell transplantation after non-myeloablative conditioning for patients with hematologic malignancies. *Blood,* 102, 2021–2030.

McAdams, F.W., & Burgunder, M.R. (2004). Transplant course. In S. Ezzone (ed.), *Hematopoietic stem cell transplantation: a manual for nursing practice* (pp. 43–59). Pittsburgh, PA: Oncology Nursing Society.

McDonald, G.B., Hinds, M.S., Fisher, L.D., Schoch, H.G., Wolford, J.L., Banaji, M., et al. (1993). Veno-occlusive disease of the liver and multiorgan failure after bone marrow transplantation: a cohort study of 355 patients. *Ann Intern Med,* 118, 255–267.

McSweeney, P.A., Niederwieser, D., Shizuru, J.A., et al. (2001). Hematopoietic cell transplantation in older patients with hematologic malignances: replacing high dose cytotoxic therapy with graft-vs-tumor effects. *Blood,* 97, 3390–3400.

Nevill, T., Barnett, M., Klingemann, H., et al. (1991). Regimen-related toxicity of a busulfan-cyclophosphamide conditioning regimen in 70 patients undergoing allogeneic bone marrow transplantation. *J Clin Oncol,* 9, 1224.

Oblon, D.J. (2000). Evaluation of the patient before hematopoietic stem cell transplantation. In E.D. Ball, J. Lister, & P. Law (eds.), *Hematopoietic stem cell therapy* (pp. 225–232). Philadelphia, PA: Churchill Livingstone.

Preston, F.A., & Cunningham, R.S. (eds.). (1998). *Clinical guidelines for symptom management in oncology. A handbook for advanced practice nurses.* New York: Clinical Insights Press.

Rust, D.M. (1997). Conditioning regimens and management of common toxicities. In T.W. Shapiro, D.B. Davison, & D.M. Rust (eds.), *A clinical guide to stem cell and bone marrow transplantation* (pp. 39–80). Sudbury, MA: Jones and Bartlett Publishers.

Sahebi, R., Copelan, E., Cilly, P., et al. (1996). Unrelated allogeneic bone marrow transplantation using high dose busulfan and cyclophosphamide (BU-CY) for preparative regimen. *Bone Marrow Transplant,* 17, 685–693.

Shank, B. (1999). Radiotherapeutic principles of hematopoietic cell transplantation. In E.D. Thomas, K.G. Blume, & S.J. Foreman (eds.), *Hematopoietic cell transplantation* (pp. 151–167). Malden, MA: Blackwell Science.

Shapira, M.Y., Resnick, I.B., Bitan, M., Ackerstein, A., Samuel, S., Elad, S., et al. (2004). Low transplant-related mortality with allogeneic stem cell transplantation in elderly patients. *Bone Marrow Transplant,* 34, 155–159.

Simpson, J.K. (2000). Specialized nursing. In E.D. Ball, J. Lister, & P. Law (eds.), *Hematopoietic stem cell therapy* (pp. 683–687). Philadelphia, PA: Churchill Livingstone.

Slavin, S., Naglet, A., Naparstek, E., Kapelushink, Y., Aka, M., Cividelli, G., et al. (1998). Nonmyeloablative stem cell transplantation and cell therapy as an alternative to conventional bone marrow transplantation with lethal cytoreduction for the treatment of malignant and non-malignant hematological diseases. *Blood, 91,* 756–763.

Spitzer, T.R., Deeg, H.J., Torrisi, J., et al. (1990). Total body irradiation (TBI) induced emesis is universal after small dose fractions (120 Gy) and is not cumulative dose related [abstract]. *Proc Am Soc Clin Oncol,* 9(14).

Spitzer, T.R., & McAfee, S.L. (1999). Bone marrow transplantation. In L.C. Ginns & A.B. Cosimi (eds.), *Transplantation* (pp. 560–587). Cambridge, MA: Blackwell Science.

Spitzer, T.R., McAfee, S.L., Dey, B.R., Colby, C., Hope, J., Grossberg, H., et al. (2003). Nonmyeloablative haploidentical stem-cell transplantation using anti-CD2 monoclonal antibody (MEDI-507)-based conditioning for refractory hematologic malignancies. *Transplantation, 75,* 1748–2003.

Summers, N., Dawe, U., & Stewart, D.A. (2000). A comparison of inpatient and outpatient ASCT. *Bone Marrow Transplant, 26,* 389–395.

Thomas, E.D., Buckner C., Banaji, M., et al. (1977). 100 patients with acute leukemia treated by chemotherapy, total body irradiation and allogeneic marrow transplantation. *Blood, 49,* 511–533.

Tutschka, P.J., Copelan, E.A., & Klein, J.P. (1987). Bone marrow transplantation for leukemia following a new busulfan and cyclophosphamide regimen. *Blood, 70,* 1382–1388.

Vargus, E.H., & Silverman, W.B. (2000). Mucositis and other gastrointestinal complications. In E.D. Ball, J. Lister, & P. Law (eds.), *Hematopoietic stem cell therapy* (pp. 557–561). Philadelphia, PA: Churchill Livingstone.

Vaugh, W.P., Dennison, J.D., Reed, E.C., et al. (1991). Improved results of allogeneic bone marrow transplantation for advanced hematological malignancy using busulfan, cyclophosphamide and etoposide as cytoreductive and immunosuppressive therapy. *Bone Marrow Transplant, 8,* 489–495.

Vinayek, R., Demetris, J., & Rakela, J. (2000). Liver disease in hematopoietic stem cell transplant recipients. In E.D. Ball, J. Lister, & P. Law (eds.), *Hematopoietic stem cell therapy* (pp. 541–556). Philadelphia, PA: Churchill Livingstone.

Walker, R.W., & Brochstein, J.A. (1988). Neurological complications of immunosuppressive agents. *Neuro Clinics,* 6(2), 261–278.

Warnick, E. (2004). Neurologic complications. In S. Ezzone (ed.), *Hematopoietic stem cell transplantation: a manual for nursing practice* (pp. 191–199). Pittsburgh, PA: Oncology Nursing Society.

Whedon, M.B. (1991). Allogeneic bone marrow transplantation: clinical indications, treatment, process and outcomes. In M.B. Whedon (ed.), *Bone marrow transplantation: principles, practice and nursing insights* (pp. 20–48). Boston: Jones and Bartlett Publishers.

Wikle, T.J. (1991). Pulmonary and cardiac complications of bone marrow transplantation. In M.B. Whedon (ed.), *Bone marrow transplantation: principles, practice and nursing insights* (pp. 182–205). Boston: Jones and Bartlett Publishers.

Wilkes, G.M., Ingwersen, K., & Barton-Burke, M. (2003). *Oncology nursing drug handbook.* Sudbury, MA: Jones and Bartlett Publishers.

Wujcik, D., Ballard, B., & Camp-Sorrell, D. (1994). Selected complications of allogeneic bone marrow transplantation. *Semin Oncol Nurs, 10,* 28–41.

Yahalom, J., Gulati, S., Shank, B., Clarkson, B., & Fuks, Z. (1989). Total lymphoid irradiation, high-dose chemotherapy and autologous bone marrow transplantation for chemotherapy-resistant Hodgkin's disease. *Int J Radiat Oncol Biol Phys, 17,* 915–922.

Chapter 6

Graft-Versus-Host Disease: Complex Sequelae of Stem Cell Transplantation

Viki Anders, RN, MSN, CRNP

Margaret Barton-Burke, PhD, RN, AOCN®

Introduction

The scientific knowledge and therapeutic use of hematopoietic stem cell transplantation (HSCT) has increased dramatically since 1957, when the first attempted human bone marrow transplantation occurred (Mathe, 1959). There was a greater understanding of the immune system and more precise laboratory tests in the 1960s, which led to effective prophylaxis of the life-threatening complication called graft-versus-host disease (GVHD) in the 1970s (Deeg et al., 1984). Interest grew from the use of stem cells collected directly from the bone marrow to the use of stem cells mobilized and collected from the peripheral blood for transplantation. An understanding of graft-versus-tumor effect and reduced-intensity transplants (RIT) has broadened the use of HSCT as a treatment option for many diseases. Despite all the scientific gains in HSCT the complication of GVHD remains a complex posttransplant problem.

GVHD is an immunologically mediated disease that contributes substantially to transplant-related morbidity and mortality. This chapter presents an overview of GVHD, including pathophysiology, incidence and risk factors, clini-

cal manifestations, methods of diagnosis, staging and grading, and medical management and a standard of nursing care for the patient with this potentially life-threatening complication of HSCT.

GVHD in animals was reported in the mid-1950s (Barnes and Loutit, 1995; Barnes et al., 1956) when a fatal syndrome was observed in irradiated mice receiving transplanted spleen cells collected from an allogeneic donor mouse. The syndrome was marked by skin abnormalities, diarrhea, and wasting. These first animal experiments compared mice receiving syngeneic stem cell grafts to those receiving stem cells from different strains of mice. Mice receiving stem cells with major histocompatibility complex (MHC) mismatches recovered from their primary disease (the radiation toxicity) but developed "secondary disease" that we now know as GVHD. In this secondary disease, the animals developed erythema, diarrhea, liver disease, and severe wasting, and ultimately died (Billingham, 1966; Ezzone, 2004; Sullivan, 1999). These same symptoms were seen in humans receiving allogeneic bone marrow transplants.

This response occurs when immunologically competent T cells from the donor graft attack the host. At a cellular level, GVHD is a complex response where preparative regimen damage causes the release of inflammatory cytokines and increases the expression of MHC antigens within the recipient.

Acute GVHD (aGVHD) is the clinical manifestation of this immune reaction. The pathophysiology of chronic GVHD (cGVHD) is not really known at this point. The clinical results are varying degrees of damage to three target organs—the skin, gastrointestinal (GI) tract, and liver—in aGVHD, and to additional organ systems in cGVHD. The three criteria specified for the development of GVHD are 1) that the graft must contain immunologically competent cells; 2) that the host must appear foreign to the graft and be capable of stimulating the donor cells; and 3) that the host immune system must be incapable of mounting an effective immunologic reaction against the graft long enough for the graft to become sensitized and mount an immunologic assault on the host. These antigenic differences stimulate the donor lymphocytes to attack epithelial cells and mucous membranes in the skin, intestinal tract, and biliary ducts (Billingham, 1966; Dean and Bishop, 2003; Mitchell, 2004).

Pathophysiology

An understanding of the major histocompatibility complex (MHC) is helpful when discussing the current approach to HSCT and the consequent GVHD. This is described well by Erlich et al. (2001). The MHC is involved in many of the steps leading to T cell activation and contains the genes that encode tissue antigens used for tissue typing. The genes first identified in rodents as transplantation antigens responsible for rejection of tissue grafts between unmatched animals are from the MHC. In humans, these genes lie on the short arm of chromosome 6 and are called the human leukocyte antigen (HLA). Not all of the genes in the HLA region are involved in immune activation. There are two classes of antigens, class I and class II, each composed of two chains. Class I antigens are made up of a heavy chain and are involved in the presentation of peptides to CD8+ T cells. They contain polymorphic regions and the nonpolymorphic light chain, beta-2 microglobulin, from chromosome 15. The antigens of class I include HLA-A, -B, and -C. Other class I HLA antigens have a more restricted expression, and their significance is not clear. Class II antigens have two chains, which are encoded in the MHC. These class II antigens also further divide into DR, DQ, and DP antigens. Class II antigens are expressed on monocytes and B cells, and following injury or inflammation can be seen on many other cell types. Since HLA types are now identified at a molecular level, accuracy has been increased. Polymerase chain reaction (PCR) technology, based on the exact nucleotide sequences of individual alleles, is a rapid method now used for HLA typing. One would think finding an HLA-identical unrelated donor would be impossible because of the millions of potential haplotypes. Through evolution and inheritance, however, certain haplotypes are far more commonly identified than would be expected by chance alone. Homogenous populations such as that in Japan have less GVHD because of the lower degree of genetic diversity. Patients who have a background of mixing of racial groups find it much more difficult to find a matched, unrelated donor (Mori et al., 1997). Even when HLA typing appears matched, patients still develop GVHD. This is thought to be secondary to minor histocompatibility antigen differences, which are expressd on the cell surface as degraded peptides bound to specific HLA molecules. Petersdorf et al. (2001) feel that matching C antigens decreases the incidence of GVHD in unrelated donor HSCT.

GVHD is the result of an immunologic response occurring in the recipient, whereby immunologically competent T cells from the donor attack the seemingly foreign recipient, resulting in varying degrees of damage to the three target organs. Allogeneic reactivity between transplant-recipient antigens is a prerequisite for GVHD. The recipient must be immunoincompetent and unable to reject the donor cells. The current model of GVHD presents GVHD induction as a multistep process. The conditioning regimen results in tissue damage with release of cytokines. In the first phase, the transplant conditioning regimen intentionally causes recipient tissue injury and ablates the recipient immune response in order that the HSCT will engraft. The high-dose conditioning regimens used are toxic to many organ systems including the skin, liver, and GI tract. Preparative regimens, using chemotherapy such as cyclophosphamide and radiation therapy, directly damage recipient tissue, and this damage begins an inflammatory cytokine cascade. The production and release of inflammatory cytokines, such as tumor necrosis factor-α (TNF-α), interleukin-1 (IL-1), and interleukin-12 (IL-12) enhance antigen presentation and adhesion molecule expression. The antigen presentation is caused by the upregulation of the MHC and minor histocompatible antigens (mHA). The adhesion molecule expression causes white blood cells (WBCs) to be attracted and retained in the damaged area, and donor T lymphocytes attack recipient tissues (Deeg, 2001; Mitchell, 2004).

These cytokines then support and drive the proliferation of donor T cells responding to the host antigens. The greater the immunologic disparity between the donor and recipient, the greater the T cell response. The inflammatory cytokine cascade continues with subsets of T lymphocytes, T helper-1 (or Th-1) lymphocytes, also producing proinflammatory cytokines, including IL-12, interleukin-2 (IL-2), and interferon-γ (INF-γ). Additionally, cytotoxic T lymphocytes (CTL) and natural killer (NK) cells respond and stimulate monocytes to produce IL-1 and TNF-α (Mitchell, 2004) resulting in direct tissue damage of the skin and gut. T cells also directly attack host tissue. The ongoing tissue damage results in further cytokine production, thus perpetuating the cascade. The resulting cytokine production is often referred to as a cytokine storm.

Chronic GVHD (cGVHD) is one of the most common problems affecting survivors of allogeneic HSCT. It is considered a syndrome of immune dysfunction that results in immunodeficiency and autoimmunity (Martin, 1999; Williams, 2004). The pathophysiology of cGVHD remains largely unknown, but there are two basic theories. Chronic GVHD may be simply end-stage alloreactivity from T cells that have evolved to approach a Th-2 phenotype (Kataoka et al., 2001). The second theory is that cGVHD is caused by poor or dysfunctional immunologic recovery (Vogelsang et al., 2003). Other investigators, noting the similarity between chronic GVHD and auto immune disorders, have suggested that cGVHD is the result of autoreactive clones, which are normally deleted in the thymus, escaping into the periphery. If the thymus becomes damaged, as with chemotherapy or radiation therapy, it cannot function properly and may not be able to eliminate these cells. This damage to the thymus results in the formation of autoantibodies similar to those seen in autoimmune disease (Biedermann et al., 2002; Lister et al., 1987; Sullivan, 1999). Thymic damage may help to explain the GVHD that develops in autologous and syngeneic transplant.

Graft-Versus-Tumor Effect

Graft versus leukemia (GVL), or graft versus tumor (GVT), is the attack of residual tumor cells by the new donor cells. The GVL/GVT effect is the main reason that allogeneic HSCT results in a lower relapse rate than syngeneic HSCT given an identical conditioning regimen. Retrospective data analysis has repeatedly shown that relapse occurred less frequently in patients who developed GVHD after allogeneic transplant compared to patients who did not develop GVHD (Goldman et al., 1988; Martin, 1999; Williams, 2004). Another example of this effect is reported in a study by Perez-Simon and colleagues (2003) that suggests a graft-versus-myeloma effect is the main weapon for disease control after nonmyeloablative transplant in multiple myeloma. In addition, a GVL/GVT effect may be obtained in patients receiving donor lymphocyte infusions (DLI) after relapse from HSCT (Giralt et al., 1997; Margolis et al., 2000; McSweeney et al., 2001; Michallet et al., 2001; Nash et al., 1992).

The current and increasingly common practice of reduced-intensity transplant (RIT) makes use of the GVL/GVT effect. RIT SCT was first explored in patients with suboptimal performance, older patients, and those who had relapsed after an autologous SCT (Giralt, 2002). Achievement

of stable donor cell engraftment with nonmyeloablative stem cell transplantations provides a framework for adoptive immune cell treatments and is promising for extended indications of SCT in the future.

Alloimmunity Concepts

There is a fine balance that is being attempted when a patient is being treated with HSCT. The desired balance is an attempt to cure a malignancy while minimizing GVHD, and this is often difficult when dealing with the donor's and recipient's immune systems, engraftment or rejection, GVHD, and the GVL/GVT effect.

A delicate balance occurs among the factors GVHD, GVL/GVT effect, and graft rejection. On the donor side of the balance, there is the potential for GVHD as mature donor T cells react against the alloantigens of the recipient. On the recipient side of the balance there is a complex interplay between the pretransplantation conditioning regimen, the posttransplantation immunosuppressive regimen, and the effects of donor T cells in the graft to govern the ability of the recipient-derived hematopoietic and lymphoid cells to survive after HSCT while risking GVHD, rejection, and recurrent malignancy.

Chimerism

Chimerism is the term used to describe the relative balance of donor and host lymphohematopoietic cells. The word is derived from the mythological creature, the chimera, which had a lion's head, a goat's body, and a serpent's tail. Stem cell transplant recipients are described as having full chimerism when all hematopoietic cells and lymphoid cells are derived from the allogeneic donor. Partial chimerism and mixed chimerism (Spitzer et al., 1999; Spitzer et al., 2003) are used when the recipient's hematopoietic and lymphoid lineage persist together with the donor's cells after HSCT. Finally, the term *split chimerism* is sometimes used when donor cells are present within some hematopoietic or lymphoid lineage but not in others.

Incidence, Risk Factors, and Prognosis

The overall incidence of GVHD remains between 30% and 60% and carries approximately a 50% mortality rate (Antin, 2002; Ringden and Deeg, 1997). Acute GVHD occurs in 30–50% of all allogeneic transplant recipients, while the incidence of cGVHD is even higher (Deeg and Storb, 1984; Gilman et al., 2000; Goerner et al., 2002). Collins et al. (1997) reported the incidence of GVHD in 140 patients after DLI for relapsed malignancy after allogeneic BMT. Acute GVHD was seen in 60% and cGVHD in 60.7% of these patients. Chronic GVHD occurs in at least 30–50% of recipients of transplants from HLA-matched siblings, and at least 60–70% of recipients from unrelated donors (Lee et al., 2003). A recent analysis of 4174 HLA-identical sibling transplants for CML showed at 3 years, survival was 74%, 74%, 64%, 37%, and 10% for patients with aGVHD Grades 0, I, II, III, and IV, respectively (Bacigalupo and Palandri, 2004).

There are risk factors that predispose the recipient to developing both acute and chronic GVHD. Donor-recipient histoincompatibilities and human leukocyte antigen (HLA) disparities are the primary cause of GVHD for reasons discussed previously in this chapter. There is an increased incidence of GVHD seen with cumulative blood transfusions, once again suggesting a histological incompatibility and a donor allosensitization. Risk is lowest in fully matched sibling transplants and increases with mismatched and unrelated transplants (Dean and Bishop, 2003). Risk increases for donor-recipient pairs with age and stem cell source and dose; cytokine mobilized peripheral stem cells (PSC) contain more lymphocytes and may increase the risk of GVHD. Przepiorka et al. (2001) reported an increased risk for cGVHD in patients who had prior acute GVHD Grades 2–4, the use of corticosteroids on day 100, prophylaxis other than tacrolimus and methotrexate, and a correlation between total nucleated cell dose of stem cells and development of cGVHD. Socie et al. (2003) list increased donor and recipient age, prior acute GVHD, use of alloimmune female donors, type of GVHD prophylaxis, and history of recipient herpes virus infection as factors that increase the development of cGVHD. Wingard et al. (1989) analyzed 85 patients with cGVHD and in a multivariate proportion hazards analysis discovered three baseline factors that predicted for death: progressive presentation of cGVHD, lichenoid changes on skin histology, and elevated serum bilirubin level. An expanded analysis of 151 patients (Wingard et al., 1989) found that skin involvement (< 50%), platelet count < 100,000, and progressive onset were predictors of poor survival at diagnosis. When cGVHD progresses, diffuse skin involvement, progressive onset, poor performance status, and hyperbilirubinemia level predicted poor outcome. In a similar analysis by Sullivan et al. (1988), progressive onset, advanced stage of malignancy, and thrombocytopenia were independent risk factors for death in 143 patients treated with alternate-day cyclosporine and prednisone. Patients with extensive, rather than limited, disease also had higher death rates.

There is conflicting data to both support and refute the use of peripheral blood stem cells over bone marrow as a means of decreasing GVHD (Cutler et al., 2001; Dean and Bishop, 2003; Mitchell, 2004; Ustun et al., 1999). Cutler et al (2001) reported an increase in both acute and chronic GVHD when patients received PSC. Further analysis of this data by Flowers et al. (2002) found the incidence the same with PSC and marrow, with the cGVHD being more protracted and less responsive to treatment when patients received PSC. Finally, conditions such as higher doses of radiation, advanced disease, and viral infections in either the donor or the recipient may predispose a patient to a higher risk for GVHD (Anagnostopoulos and Giralt, 2002; Dean and Bishop, 2003; Kim, 2002; Mitchell, 2004; Sullivan, 1999).

RIT are becoming more common. Since RIT patients have comparable rates of aGVHD when compared to those who receive full myeloablative conditioning, it suggests rates of cGVHD may be similar (Giralt et al., 2001; Kouri et al., 1998; McSweeney et al., 2001). Couriel et al. (2004) evaluated 137 patients who received nonmyeloablative and ablative conditioning regimens. They found a reduced incidence of Grade II–IV aGVHD and cGVHD in the nonmyeloablative group. Both groups received the same GVHD prophylaxis. Nonrelapse and GVHD-related mortality were low in both groups.

Presentation

Most authors use day 100 as the demarcation between acute and chronic GVHD, with aGVHD occurring before day 100 and cGVHD occurring after day 100 posttransplant (Antin, 2002; Dean and Bishop, 2003; Mitchell, 2004; Sullivan, 1999). The separating of acute and chronic

GVHD by date is no longer used due to the changes within transplantation protocols being used and studied. For example, after relapse from an HSCT, a RIT may be used, followed by the use of donor lymphocyte infusions (DLI) until a GVHD reaction occurs. This new way of manufacturing GVHD may not fit into the pre-100- and post-100-day parameters used for diagnosing acute or chronic GVHD. Currently, the diagnosis of acute and chronic GVHD is determined by assessing clinical manifestations, histology of the target organs, and the number of days away from the actual HSCT. This suggests that GVHD diagnosis criteria may have to be redefined at some point in the future (Dean and Bishop, 2003; Kim, 2002).

Acute GVHD after a myeloablative transplant usually occurs with engraftment of white cells. The time to aGVHD after RIT depends on the preparative regimen and donor type, and can range from 2 weeks to years after transplant. The median time after HLA-identical sibling transplant to diagnosis of cGVHD is day 201; day 159 after mismatched, related transplant; and day 133 after unrelated donor transplant (Sullivan et al., 1991). Bhushan and Collins (2003) report cGVHD occurring 4 to 7 months after transplant but as early as 2 months or as late as 2 or more years, with an earlier presentation in patients from mismatched or unrelated donors.

Although aGVHD usually begins in the skin, Martin et al. (1990) found that 81% had skin involvement, 54% had GI involvement, and 50% had liver involvement at the initiation of therapy. Chronic GVHD can involve almost any organ, and many symptoms resemble those of spontaneously occurring autoimmune disorders. The skin, liver, and mouth are the most frequent targets (Vogelsang et al., 2003).

Immune function is the main effect of cGVHD, with infections accounting for the majority of deaths in these patients (Parkman, 1993; Weinberg et al., 1995; Weinberg et al., 2001). This problem is multifactorial, including disruption of mucosal barriers, thymic injury, functional asplenia, hypogammaglobulinemia, as well as qualitative T cell and B cell abnormalities. Infections are the cause of death in most cases, including invasive fungal infections and *Pneumocystis jiroveci* pneumonia. Functional asplenia increases the risk of infections caused by encapsulated organisms. Other systems that may be involved include gastrointestinal, ocular, dermal appendages, neuromuscular, respiratory, hematologic, and reproductive. Patients who develop aGVHD or cGVHD months to years after transplant or are refractory to treatment may develop depression. Those with cGVHD have been associated with a decreased quality of life (QOL) (Sutherland et al., 1997).

The diagnosis of aGVHD and cGVHD should be confirmed with biopsy. A review of 123 patients referred to Johns Hopkins for the management of refractory chronic GVHD revealed that nine patients had no evidence of ever having chronic GVHD and that 26 additional patients had no evidence of ongoing active disease (Jacobsohn et al., 2001).

Clinical and Histologic Manifestations

Skin Manifestations

Initial symptoms of aGVHD may include a maculopapular rash starting on the ears, face, palms (**Figure 6-1**), and soles and spreading to the trunk, arms, and legs, generally sparing the

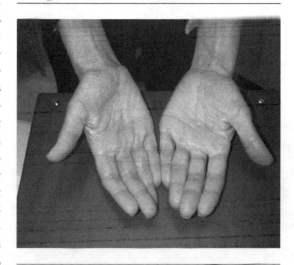

Figure 6-1 Acute GVHD skin.

scalp. In severe cases bullae, ulcerations, and epidermal necrosis may occur and may progress to generalized desquamation of skin. A follicular pattern may also be present with destruction of hair follicles (Ferrara and Deeg, 1991). Patients receiving DLI may develop acute manifestations that can progress rapidly to a chronic skin GVHD. Histologic confirmation is necessary to rule out other possible causes such as drug reactions and viral infections. Although there is no definitive pathologic finding that differentiates aGVHD from other skin eruptions, apoptosis at the base of dermal crypts is the characteristic finding. Other features include basal vacuolization, dermal lymphocytic infiltrate, exocytosis, and dyskeratosis (Horn, 1994). Dermal–epidermal separation is seen in patients with blistering disease.

The skin is the most frequently affected system in cGVHD. Patients initially develop a macular eruption, with an erythematous, papular rash and no typical distribution pattern;

however the rash is usually symmetrical, occuring on both sides of the body in affected areas.

Skin that has been previously damaged from herpetic infection, aGVHD, sun, or drug rashes may be more susceptible to the development of cGVHD. A later form of chronic skin GVHD clinically resembles systemic sclerosis and may involve the dermis and/or the muscular fascia. Histologic changes in early cGVHD include a band-like infiltrate of lymphocytes into the epidermis and dermis that has been described as a lichenoid eruption (**Figure 6-2**) (Shulman et al., 1980). Thickening of the dermis with dropout of hair follicles and sweat glands is seen in later scleroderma-like cGVHD (**Figure 6-3**).

The skin is thickened and tight sometimes with either hypo- or hyperpigmentation. There is poor wound-healing capacity and there are often problems with poor lymphatic drainage or ulcerations from minor trauma. Hair loss and lack of sweating is caused by destruction of the dermal layer of skin. A commonly missed form

Figure 6-3 Chronic GVHD skin, sclerodermoid changes.

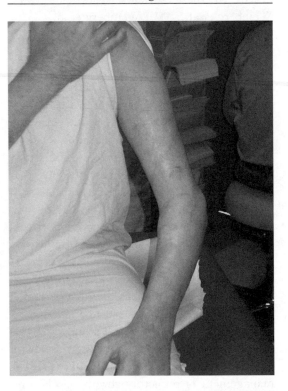

Figure 6-2 Chronic GVHD skin, lichenoid eruption.

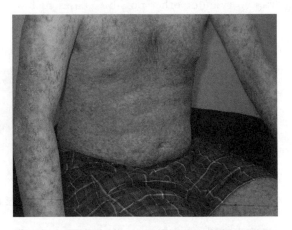

of cGVHD is isolated fascial scleroderma, which presents with normal-appearing skin but tightness and decreased mobility. The skin may appear fixed to the fascia, making pinching of the skin difficult, or the fascia may become fixed to the muscle, decreasing the range of motion of affected joints. Fasciitis has been thought to be rare and atypical, starting with sudden and painful skin swelling, and leading to disabling skin tightness, joint stiffness, contractures, and sores (Janin et al., 1994). It is possible that this type of cGVHD is underreported, since the skin may look normal with patients only reporting symptoms when range of motion is significantly altered and functional ability decreased.

Gastrointestinal Manifestations

Gastrointestinal (GI) aGVHD usually, but not always, occurs simultaneously with acute skin and liver GVHD, and it is a panintestinal process. There can be varying degrees of severity in the upper and lower GI tract. The patient may present with complaints of nausea, vomiting, anorexia, diarrhea, and/or abdominal cramping. The vomiting may not always be preceded by nausea and its pathogenesis is unclear. Upper tract GVHD can be extremely devastating. There can be massive protein and fluid loss with desquamation of the small bowel, increased susceptibility to infection due to loss of the mucosal barrier, ileus, and possibly perforation. Diffuse thickening of the small bowel wall, seen as a ribbon sign, is seen on abdominal-computed tomography. Abdominal flat plates or small bowel series may show luminal dilatation with thickening of the wall of the small bowel and air/fluid levels suggest an ileus (Vogelsang et al., 2003). Gastroparesis is seen after HSCT but it is not usually associated with the gastric involvement of GVHD (Eagle et al., 2001). The diarrhea in the lower GI tract may have a stringy appearance, which is a clue to the provider that there is sloughing of intestinal mucosa, especially in more severe cases, and it is secretory (the small and large bowel secrete more electrolytes and water than they absorb). Tumor necrosis factor alpha (TNF-α) may mediate the diarrhea by inducing chloride and potassium secretion in the distal colon, driven by prostaglandin E2 (Schmitz et al., 1996). Significant bleeding from mucosal ulceration is associated with a poor prognosis (Nevo et al., 1999). Large quantities of diarrhea (> 2 liters/day) caused by water and protein exudation across a severely injured mucosa, as well as diffuse, severe abdominal pain and distention, is seen in advanced disease.

Biopsies of the intestinal mucosa are necessary for a diagnosis, since there is little relationship between extent of disease and endoscopic appearance. Since aGVHD occurs throughout the entire GI tract, biopsies can be obtained from the upper or lower GI tract, but rectal biopsies do not seem to be as diagnostic as gastric biopsies. Gastric biopsies may have a higher diagnostic yield (Snover et al., 1985). The gastric, intestinal, or colonic mucosa may appear deceptively normal. In severe disease, mucosal sloughing of the esophagus, duodenum, and colon has been described (Ponec et al., 1999). The histology of GI GVHD is characterized by the presence of apoptotic bodies in the base of crypt cells, sometimes accompanied by an acute or chronic inflammatory infiltrate (Igbal et al., 2000). Other common features include crypt cells abscess, flattening of the surface of the epithelium, and loss of crypt cells, but these findings may also be present secondary to mucosal damage due to the preparative regimen and infection.

Although many patients with cGVHD have GI complaints, they may be attributable to other disease states, including infection, dysmotility, lactose intolerance, pancreatic insufficiency, and drug-related side effects (Akpeck, Valladares, et al., 2001). There is a wasting syndrome that is seen in patients with cGVHD, and this syndrome occurs despite an adequate intake of calories (Vogelsang, 2001).

Liver Manifestations

In most cases, patients with acute liver GVHD have no presenting symptoms. Jaundice occurs as the serum bilirubin levels rise in the bloodstream. Some patients with elevated bilirubin levels complain of generalized pruritis without a skin rash. Abnormalities in serum liver function tests are common after transplant, but since many patients with liver involvement are not biopsied, the incidence of hepatic GVHD is not known. The incidence is thought to be approximately 50% in those developing aGVHD (Arai, Lee, et al., 2002). These abnormalities may have various etiologies, including iron overload, venoocclusive disease (VOD), drug toxicity, viral infection, sepsis, and extrahepatic biliary obstruction. Medications such as antifungals (fluconazole, voriconazole) and GVHD prophylactic agents (tacrolimus, cyclosporine, methotrexate) may cause liver toxicity, which, without a liver biopsy, may be confused with GVHD. In acute liver GVHD, injury occurs to the biliary tract epithelium, causing an increase in both the bilirubin and alkaline phosphatase blood levels.

More recently, a variant of acute hepatic GVHD has been described in the literature (Fugii et al., 2001). In this hepatitis variant of GVHD, there is an increase in the serum transaminase levels similar to those seen in patients with viral hepatitis. Akpek et al. (2002) reported this hepatic variant after donor lymphocyte infusion. After viral hepatitis and recent drug exposures were excluded, 50% of those diagnosed with liver GVHD were given a diagnosis of a hepatic variant of GVHD. This was based on histologic evidence of lobular hepatitis with an elevation of maximum serum alanine aminotransferase (ALT) or aspartate aminotransferase (AST) level more than 10 times the upper normal limit. There was a significant difference in the maximum ALT and AST. Since this occurs after DLI, it is difficult to describe this as either acute or chronic hepatic GVHD.

Cholestasis is the most common presentation of hepatic disease in cGVHD. Evaluation reveals elevated alkaline phosphatase and elevated serum bilirubin (Vogelsang et al., 2003).

Mouth Manifestations

Although oral lesions can occur with aGVHD, it is usually at the time patients also have mucositis from their preparative regimen, making definitive diagnosis difficult. Xerostomia and food sensitivities are the most common symptoms of oral cGVHD. A lichenoid reaction (**Figure 6-4**) of the oral mucosa may cause a spider web appearance, and patients describe burning with toothpaste, spicy foods, citrus fruits, and carbonation.

There is a destruction of salivary glands causing this xerostomia, subsequently resulting in an increase in dental caries. Odynophagia

Figure 6-4 Chronic GVHD mouth, lichenoid changes.

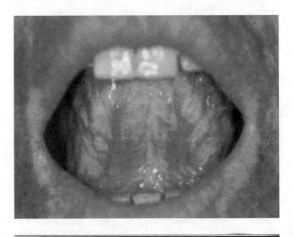

(painful swallowing) occurs and may be due to lichenoid eruption, ulcerations, and infection. Esophageal strictures are rare but may occur and may require further treatment with esophageal dilation. It is important to culture the affected areas to rule out infection. Yeast infections occur frequently, especially when steroids are used to treat oral GVHD. Infection should always be considered when there is an increase in symptoms with little change on physical exam. Salivary gland and mucosal involvement can be demonstrated by biopsy with the histopathological features of lichenoid oral lesions similar to those seen in the lichenoid form of cutaneous chronic GVHD. Minor salivary glands may show fibrosing sialoadenitis as seen in Sjögren's syndrome, with symptoms of severe dry mouth. A study of 66 specimens from 59 patients with oral cGVHD, taken an average of 136 days after allogeneic BMT, showed no significant associations between any oral change and the overall binary survival outcome, and did not correlate with the occurrence of lichenoid or sclerodermoid chronic skin disease. These observations led to the conclusion that histologic changes in the oral cavity do not correlate with overall BMT outcome, chronic cutaneous disease, or earlier acute GVHD (Horn et al., 1995).

Eye Manifestations

Patients with severe aGVHD, especially of the skin, may develop a pseudomembrane of the conjunctiva, which holds a poor prognosis for survival (Jabs et al., 1989). Patients with dry mouth syndrome from cGVHD frequently develop dry, gritty eyes with reduced tear flow, and in severe disease, corneal epithelial defects and corneal ulceration (Johnson and Jabs, 1997). Keratoconjunctivitis sicca syndrome reaches

nearly 40% in patients with cGVHD, compared with less than 10% in those without GVHD (Socie et al., 2003).

Dermal Appendages Manifestations

Erythema around the nail beds is commonly seen with the development of aGVHD of the skin. Patients with cGVHD may develop vertical ridges and cracking of fingernails, and periungual infection around the nails is common. Nail problems and hair loss may continue even after the skin changes have resolved, although new hair growth is often a sign of recovery. Brittle hair, scalp dryness, and flaking may occur before alopecia, and premature graying is often seen with cGVHD, affecting scalp hair and eyebrows, even in children. Sweat glands can be destroyed in patients with sclerotic skin disease, leading to the inability to sweat and a high risk of serious hyperthermia.

Neuromuscular Manifestations

The neuromuscular system is affected by cGVHD in a number of ways. The range of joint motion is commonly affected with sclerodermatous and fascial cGVHD. Muscle cramping is a common complaint; however, the pathophysiology is not understood. Myositis with tender muscles and elevated muscle enzymes is rare and does not explain the symptoms. The cramping may be secondary to impingement of muscles or nerves with sclerodermatous GVHD, and sometimes worsens as skin softens with successful treatment. Electrolyte imbalances, especially low magnesium, may contribute to muscle cramping. Decreased sensation of skin with numbness and tingling is commonly described in sclerotic disease, increasing the risk of injury and infection. Case reports of myasthenia gravis have also been reported with the tapering of steroids after treatment for cGVHD. This may be confused with the steroid myopathy frequently seen with long-term steroid use. Bolanos-Meade et al. (2005) report severe vacuolar myopathy in a patient receiving hydroxychloroquine for cGVHD.

Respiratory Manifestations

Bronchiolitis obliterans (BO) is a late and serious manifestation of cGVHD, with patients complaining of cough and dyspnea on exertion. It occurs in 2–14% of those receiving allogeneic HSCT with a 50% mortality rate (Chan et al., 1987; Holland et al., 1988; Ralph et al., 1984; Sharples et al., 1996). The symptoms usually develop slowly over time and can be confused with infection, reactive airway disease, fluid overload, cardiac disease, and other etiologies. Bronchiolitis obliterans is often confused with bronchiolitis obliterans organizing pneumonia (BOOP). Radiographic changes with BO may show hyperinflation of the lungs from air trapping but usually do not show the infiltrates that are seen in BOOP. Pulmonary function tests (PFTs) in a patient with BO reveal an obstructive pattern, which is not responsive to bronchodilators, and there is a marked decrease in the functional end volume (FEV1), with an increase in the residual volume caused by air trapping. Pulmonary function tests in the patient with BOOP have more of a restrictive pattern, and both the functional vital capacity (FVC) and FEV1 are uniformly decreased. The only way to definitively diagnosis BO is with an open lung biopsy, especially if bronchoscopy does not provide adequate tissue to visualize the small airways. The histologic changes seen with BO

include scarring of small airways, while with BOOP there are inflammatory changes. Afessa et al. (2001) compared BO to BOOP, with one of the significant differences being the responsiveness to steroids in BOOP. Symptoms of shortness of breath and dyspnea on exertion may be present in patients with external restriction from sclerosis or fasciitis in the chest wall. Complete pulmonary function tests, including spirometry before and after bronchodilators, lung volumes, and diffusing capacity, as well as radiographic imaging are important to help localize the problem. Sinusitis is also seen frequently with cGVHD, and CT scans with coronal cuts may show air fluid levels despite minimal symptoms (Thompson et al., 2002).

Hematopoietic Manifestations

Cytopenias can be seen in aGVHD. Chronic GVHD affects the hematologic system by damaging the stroma. Autoimmune neutropenia, anemia, and/or thrombocytopenia may occur as well. Thrombocytopenia at the time of cGVHD diagnosis is associated with a poor prognosis (Akpek, Zahurak, et al., 2001; Anasetti et al., 1989; Jacobsohn et al., 2001; Sullivan et al., 1988). Eosinophilia may also occur and may be used as a tool to track disease activity (Jacobsohn, et al., 2004).

Reproductive Manifestations

The reproductive system in both women and men is affected by cGVHD. Women with severe cGVHD may have inflammation, mucosal dryness, adhesions, and stenosis of the vagina (Corson et al., 1982). Topical application of steroids and estrogen may be helpful, but surgery may be required in extreme cases. Hormone replacement therapy is controversial but should be considered, especially in patients under the age of 40 to 50.

Men frequently complain of impotence and erectile dysfunction, which may be secondary to chronic disease or low testosterone level.

Psychosocial Manifestations

Many patients with GVHD, especially those with cGVHD that is refractory to treatment, develop signs of depression and may even become suicidal. Unless asked, they may not admit that they are having coping problems. Lee, Cook, and colleagues (2002) used a cohort of 107 patients with active cGVHD to develop and validate a scale to measure symptoms of cGVHD. They found that the cGVHD symptom scale is a short, simple, valid measurement of cGVHD manifestations, and when combined with the Functional Assessment of Chronic Illness Therapy with Bone Marrow Transplant subscale (FACIT-BMT), quality of life can be determined (see **Table 6-1**).

Staging and Grading

Acute GVHD is staged by assessing the three major organ systems involved, the skin, the GI tract, and the liver. There are many systems now in use including the Glucksberg, the Keystone, and the IBMTR systems. All of these systems use a numerical staging scale ranging from 0 to 4 except for the IBMTR system, which uses an alphabetical staging of A, B, C, and D. An example of a useful staging system can be found in **Table 6-2**. The Glucksberg Scale (Glucksberg et al., 1974) uses a system where an overall clinical stage ranges from 0 (none) to IV (severe), and is determined by grading individual organ systems. The skin is staged by assessing the percentage of body involved plus the presence or absence of blisters. The gastrointestinal system is staged by the quantity and quality of the pa-

tient's diarrhea. The liver is measured by the level of the patient's serum bilirubin. An overall grade is determined by the highest stage among the four body organ systems. See **Table 6-3** for the criteria used by the International Bone Marrow Transplant Registry (IBMTR) for grading aGVHD.

There is no one clear method of staging and grading cGVHD. In 1980, a system of limited and extensive cGVHD was devised after looking at the outcome of 20 patients. It was thought that limited disease, defined as localized skin involvement with or without hepatic dysfunction, did not require treatment. Extensive disease requiring treatment included those patients with generalized skin involvement, or limited skin involvement with eye and/or oral disease, hepatic dysfunction, or involvement of any other target organ (Shulman et al., 1980). Although this method is highly reproducible, little information is provided about prognosis and it provides little clinical utility (Lee, Vogelsang, et al., 2002).

Atkinson and colleagues expanded on this method by using previous history of aGVHD as a predetermining factor for risk of cGVHD. They described the presentation and severity of cGVHD. The presentation of cGVHD is described in three ways: progressive, quiescent, and de novo. Progressive presentation is a direct extension from aGVHD, whereas quiescent occurs after the resolution of aGVHD, and de novo is diagnosed when there is no history of aGVHD. The severity is described as either limited or extensive. In limited cGVHD, there is mild involvement of ≤ 2 organ systems, while extensive severity involves ≥ 2 organ systems (Atkinson et al., 1989). Also, patients' symptoms may be described by the type of skin manifestations that are present, either lichenoid (lichen planus) or

Table 6-1 CLINICAL MANIFESTATIONS OF GVHD.

	Acute	Chronic
Skin	Erythema	Dry skin
	Maculopapular rash	Pruritis
	Follicular rash	Lichenoid rash (plaquelike)
	Bullae formation	Sclerodermoid changes
	Pruritis	(thick and tight)
	Burning pain	Fascial changes
		(tight with normal skin)
		Hypo-/hyperpigmentation
		Ulcerations
		Hair loss
		Gray hair
		Fragile skin
Gastrointestinal	Diarrhea	Weight loss
	Abdominal cramping	Dysphagia
	Nausea/vomiting	
	Anorexia	
	Electrolyte imbalance	
	Thickening small bowel CT	
	Air/fluid levels consistent with ileus flat plate	
	GI bleeding	
Liver	Liver function tests elevation (TB, enzymes, alkaline phosphatase)	Liver function tests elevation (TB, enzymes, possibly isolated increase in alkaline phosphatase)
	Generalized pruritis and/or jaundice with elevated bilirubin	Cholestasis
		Jaundice
Oral	Erythema	Lichenoid changes (white, spiderweb appearance)
	Ulcerations	Sensitivity to spicy food, toothpaste, citrus fruit
	Superinfections (thrush, herpes simplex virus)	Erythema and ulcerations
	Pain	Dry mouth
		Sclerotic changes less often
		Superinfections (thrush, herpes simplex virus)
		Pain
Eyes	Erythema	Erythema
	Pain	Dry and gritty
	Conjunctival pseudomembrane formation	Scarring

Table 6-1 CLINICAL MANFESTATIONS OF GVHD *continued.*

	Acute	Chronic
Dermal appendages	Periungual erythema	Vertical ridging nails
		Hair loss
		Loss of sweating
Neuromuscular	Weakness/steroid myopathy	Decreased range of motion
		Muscle cramping (more with sclerodermoid and fascial)
		Decreased sensation
		Neuropathic pain
		Weakness/steroid myopathy
		Myasthenia gravis
Respiratory	Infections	Infections
		Sinusitis
		External restriction with tight skin
		Bronchiolitis obliterans (dyspnea on exertion, cough, air trapping on chest radiograph/computerized tomography)
Hematopoietic	Cytopenias	Cytopenias
	Eosinophilia	Thrombocytopenia predicts for poor outcome
		Eosinophilia
Reproductive		Functional asplenia
		Vaginal inflammation, dryness, adhesions, stenosis
Psychosocial	Anxiety	Anxiety
		Depression
		Suicidal ideations

sclerodermatous. The lichenoid changes usually occur early and may progress to sclerodermatous GVHD. Akpek, Lee, and colleagues (2001) described a grading system that classifies patients by risk factors according to the clinical characteristics that are present at diagnosis. Multivariate analysis of data from 151 patients with cGVHD found that three variables were risk factors for a shortened survival. These variables are extensive skin GVHD involving > 50% of a patient's total body surface area (BSA), a platelet count of < 100,000, and the progressive onset of cGVHD (Akpek, Lee, et al., 2001). This model was validated using data from the IBMTR ($n = 711$), Fred Hutchinson Cancer Center ($n = 188$), University of Nebraska ($n = 60$), and University of Minnesota ($n = 149$) (Akpek et al., 2003). This grading system may help improve clinical management, trial designs, and communication among transplant centers, as it is highly predictive of outcome. There is a National Institutes of Health–sponsored effort under way now to define a staging system and response criteria.

Table 6-2 Consensus conference criteria for staging and grading of acute graft-versus-host disease.

| Stage | Extent of Organ Involvement | | |
	Skin	Liver	Gastrointestinal Tract
1	Maculopapular rash < 25% of body surface*	Total bilirubin 2–3 mg/dl[†]	Diarrhea 500–1000 ml/day[‡] or persistent nausea[§]
2	Maculopapular rash 25–50% of body surface	Total bilirubin 3–6 mg/dl	Diarrhea 1000–1500 ml/day
3	Maculopapular rash > 50% of body surface	Total bilirubin 6–15 mg/dl	Diarrhea 1500 ml/day
4	Generalized erythroderma with bullous formation	Total bilirubin > 15 mg/dl	Severe abdominal pain ± ileus
Grade Criteria for grading given as the minimum degree of organ involvement required to confer grade.			
I	Stage 1–2	None	None
II	Stage 3, or	Stage 1, or	Stage 1
III	_____	Stage 2–3, or	Stage 2–4
IV[§§]	Stage 4, or	Stage 4	_____

*Use "Rule of Nines" or burn chart to determine extent of rash.
[†]Downgrade one stage if an additional cause of hyperbilirubinemia is documented.
[‡]Volume of diarrhea applies to adults.
[§]Persistent nausea with histologic evidence of GVHD in the stomach or duodenum.
[§§]Grade IV may also include lesser organ involvement, with extreme decrease in performance status.
Source: Adapted from Przepiorka, D., et al. (1995). 1994 consensus conference on acute GVHD grading. *Bone Marrow Transplant,* *15,* 825–828. Dean, R.M., & Bishop, M.R. (2003). Graft versus host disease: Emerging concepts in prevention and therapy. *Current Hematology Reports, 2*(4), 287–294.

Prophylaxis

The two basic strategies used to prevent aGVHD are lymphocyte depletions of the donor graft and pharmacologic therapy. A comprehensive review of lymphocyte depletion to re-move mature lymphocytes that are responsible for the initiation of aGVHD was provided by Ho and colleagues (2001). The major techniques involve lymphocyte depletion resulting in the loss of stem cells, which may increase the risk of failed engraftment and cause an increased

Table 6-3 CRITERIA FOR INTERNATIONAL BONE MARROW TRANSPLANT REGISTRY SEVERITY INDEX FOR ACUTE GRAFT-VERSUS-HOST DISEASE.

Index*	Skin Involvement		Liver Involvement		Gut Involvement	
Stage, maximum	Extent of rash, %		Stage, maximum	Total bilirubin, Mol/L	Stage, maximum	Volume of diarrhea
A	1	<25	or	1	<34	0	<500 cc
B	2	25–50	or	2	34–102	1–2	550–1500 cc
C	3	>50	or	3	103–255	3	>1500 cc
D	4	Bullae		4	>255	4	Severe pain and ileus

*Assign index based on maximum involvement in an individual organ system.

Source: Adapted from Atkinson, K., Horowitz, M.M., Gale, R.P., et al. (1989). Consensus among bone marrow transplanters for diagnosis, grading and treatment of chronic graft versus host disease: Committee of the International Bone Marrow Transplant Registry. *Bone Marrow Transplant, 4*(3), 247–254.
Dean, R.M., & Bishop, M.R. (2003). Graft versus host disease: Emerging concepts in prevention and therapy. *Current Hematology Reports, 2,* 287–294.

relapse rate and higher rates of infection (Vogelsang et al., 2003). T cell depletion ex vivo has declined over the past decade. T cell depletion in vivo using 15 mg/kg of rabbit ATG significantly reduced the risk of Grade III–IV aGVHD, but overall survival is unchanged compared to more standard approaches due to a higher risk of lethal infections (Bacigalupo et al., 2001).

The most commonly used pharmacologic approach for prophylaxis of aGVHD is cyclosporine A (CSA) or tacrolimus (FK506) in combination with methotrexate (MTX). Several large, prospective randomized clinical trials demonstrated the superiority of CSA and MTX versus CSA alone (Locatelli et al., 2000;Ruutu et al., 2000; Storb, 1986). The regimens range from CSA alone, to CSA and MTX, to CSA and MTX with the addition of steroids (Locatelli et al., 2000; Ruutu et al., 2000; Storb, 1986). A large randomized trial showed no advantage to the addition of steroids (Chao et al., 2000). The combination of tacrolimus and MTX appears to offer results similar to CSA and MTX; however, controversy remains over the use of tacrolimus in matched-sibling HSCT (Nash et al., 2000). More recently, sirolimus (rapamycin) was added to tacrolimus and low-dose methotrexate with a low rate of aGVHD compared to historical data (Antin et al., 2003).

Retrospective analysis suggests therapeutic CSA blood levels ≥ 200 ng/mL and tacrolimus levels of 5–15 ng/mL decrease the risk of developing GVHD. Bacigalupo and Palandri (2004) reviewed the following prophylactic strategies: infusion of mesenchymal stem cells, which is being tested in a prospective randomized trial; inactivation of antigen-presenting cells, which is in preclinical studies, and which suggests that depleting the host antigen presenting cell

(APC) before the conditioning regimen should eliminate GVHD; and the use of anti-IL-2 and anti-TNF antibodies, which have been tested in the clinical setting with inconsistent results. Visilizumab, a humanized anti-CD3 monoclonal antibody that induces apoptosis in activated T cells, has been shown in a phase I trial to be well tolerated and that it has activity in advanced GVHD (Carpenter et al., 2002).

Treatment

Glucocorticoid steroids are the treatment of choice as initial therapy for aGVHD. Steroids act as lympholytic agents and inhibit the release of inflammatory cytokines. Methylprednisolone is available in an intravenous form, making it the most commonly used steroid for aGVHD. No clear advantage has been described by using different dosing schedules. Although high doses of steroids (10–20 mg/kg or 500 mg/m^2) have higher initial response rates, flares are seen on tapering, opportunistic infections are common, and a randomized clinical trial of 10 mg/kg showed no clinical advantage (Van Lint et al., 1998).

The hematopoietic stem cell transplant programs at Seattle, Washington, and Minneapolis, Minnesota reviewed their experiences with initial therapy for Stages II–IV of aGVHD. Although many of these patients were treated before CSA was available, possibly skewing results, what these programs found was as effective as, or more effective than, other therapies or combination of therapies. Durable long-term responses were seen in 20–40% of patients. Long-term salvage rates were ≤ 20% in patients who failed to respond to steroids, with most dying of infection and acute and/or chronic GVHD. Patients who flared on low doses of steroids or after a steroid taper appeared to respond to a second course of steroids and did relatively well (Martin et al., 1990; Martin et al., 1991; Weisdorf et al., 1990); however, as stated previously, patients who continued steroids past day 100 have an increased risk of developing cGVHD.

Antithymocyte globulin (ATG) is the most commonly used secondary treatment, especially among pediatric transplant centers, with a response in 19–56% of patients but a 1-year mortality that approaches 90% (Antin et al., 2004). Arai, Margolis and colleagues (2002) reported a 5% long-term survival rate in 69 patients treated with ATG. The use of ATG is complicated by the use of at least 14 different formulations of horse- and rabbit-derived products currently available worldwide, and because a standard dose and schedule has not been established. Psoralen and ultraviolet A irradiation (PUVA) has been shown to be an effective therapy for steroid-resistant acute GVHD of the skin (Furlong et al., 2002). Sirolimus (rapamycin) is an immunophilin binding agent that inhibits T lymphocyte activation and proliferation. Although it appears to have activity in steroid-refractory patients, it has been associated with frequent complications including myelosuppression and hemolytic uremic syndrome (Benito et al., 2001). Monoclonal antibodies are being studied in high risk and steroid refractory patients with aGVHD. Daclizumab, which is an anti-interleukin-2 receptor monoclonal antibody, has been used in patients with gut or steroid-refractory aGVHD, with a 37% complete response but a 60% mortality rate at 6 months (Przepiorka et al., 2000). However, several randomized trials using daclizumab were stopped due to excess mortality in the daclizumab group (Lee et al., 2004). Infliximab,

an immunoglobulin G1 murine/human chimeric monoclonal antibody composed of human constant and murine variable regions that binds both the soluble subunit and the membrane-bound precursor of TNF-α, has been used for gastrointestinal GVHD but reports suggest frequent infectious deaths (Kobbe et al., 2001). Pentostatin is a nucleoside analog that is a potent, irreversible inhibitor of adenosine deaminase. Encouraging results have been reported using a 3-day course of the drug, with most patients achieving a CR with no evidence of aGVHD within 4 weeks of treatment. However, a minority of the patients experienced disease flares and required a second course of therapy, and mortality remained high (Bolanos-Meade et al., 2005; Margolis and Grever, 2000; Margolis and Vogelsang, 2000). Mycophenolate mofetil (MMF) is a morpholinoethyl ester of mycophenolic acid that has antibacterial, antifungal, antiviral, antitumor, and immunosuppressive properties. It has a good therapeutic index and is a relatively selective inhibitor of T cell metabolism. It seems to have significant activity in phase II studies of primary and secondary therapy of aGVHD (Vogelsang and Arai, 2001). A comparison of 93 patients receiving CSA and methotrexate versus CSA and MMF was reviewed retrospectively and showed no differences in overall survival rate. Relapse rate, treatment related mortality, and acute or chronic GVHD and time to myeloid recovery were shorter in those receiving CSA and MMF (Neumann et al., 2005). The use of MMF as prophylaxis for patients receiving nonmyeloablative conditioning for stem cell transplantation is currently being studied. Denileukin difitox is a recombinant fusion protein with selective cytotoxicity against activated T lymphocytes based on its preferential binding to high-affinity IL-2R.

It seems to have significant clinical activity in steroid-refractory aGVHD; however, overall survival rates were disappointing, and infections remained a common cause of late mortality (Ho et al., 2003). In a phase II trial of 22 patients with steroid refractory GVHD, 9 patients showed a complete response by study day 3; 6 patients had a complete response and 2 showed a partial response by day 100 (Shaughnessy et al., 2005). Greinin et al. (1998) reported the successful use of extracorporeal photo chemotherapy in the treatment of severe acute and chronic GVHD.

The standard treatment for cGVHD is cyclosporine (CSA) and prednisone. Initial studies showed prednisone alone in standard risk cGVHD is superior to prednisone and azathioprine; however, in high-risk patients, based on platelet counts < 100,000, there was only a 26% survival rate with prednisone alone. When a similar group of high-risk patients was treated with alternating prednisone and CSA, the 5-year survival rate increased to > 50% (Sullivan et al., 1988). This led most centers to adopt the regimen of treating patients initially with 1 mg/kg/day of prednisone and 10 mg/kg/day of CSA (CSA in two divided doses). After two weeks if the patient is stable to improved, a taper of steroids is initiated to either 1 mg/kg every other day or 0.5 mg/kg daily. Due to pharmacokinetic considerations, the current recommendation is to treat cGVHD with twice daily CSA or tacrolimus (Flowers et al., 2003).

Patients are treated for 3 months after there are signs of active disease, then tapered off of one medication at a time, usually every 2 weeks. Patients who have an incomplete response are evaluated every 3 months, and if they are not responding or have progressive disease, salvage therapies are considered. Although this regimen of daily dosing of CSA and every other day prednisone has been widely used in extensive, high-risk (< 100,000 platelets) cGVHD, there was no data on how effective the treatment is in standard-risk patients. The Seattle group reported results on a group of 307 patients with extensive cGVHD without thrombocytopenia. A total of 287 patients were evaluated, and the incidence of transplant-related mortality was similar in both arms of the study. However, survival without recurrent malignancy was lower in the two-drug arm of the study, and there was an increased risk of avascular necrosis in the prednisone-only arm of the study. What is not clear is whether the addition of CSA to prednisone reduces transplant-related mortality in patients with cGVHD (Koc et al., 2002).

Hydroxychloroquine is an anti-malarial drug used in the treatment of autoimmune diseases, which interferes with antigen presentation and cytokine production, and is synergistic with CSA and tacrolimus in vitro. In a study of 32 patients with cGVHD, more than half showed improvement (Gilman et al., 1996), which has led to a Children's Oncology Group (COG) trial comparing CSA and prednisone with or without hydroxychloroquine. Further study of 40 patients with steroid-resistant or steroid-dependent GVHD showed a 53% response rate (Gilman et al., 2000). Clofazimine, an antimycobacterial drug used to treat leprosy and *Mycobacterium avium* complex, is also used to treat chronic autoimmune skin disorders. A study of 22 patients showed greater than a 50% response rate with a decrease in sclerodermatous skin disease, flexion contractures, and oral manifestations (Lee et al., 1997). Mycophenolate mofetil (MMF) is an ester prodrug of the active immunosuppressant mycophenolic acid, which inhibits DNA and RNA synthesis, and thus is effective in preventing and reversing rejection of allogeneic donor organs (Fulton and Markham, 1996). The City of Hope National Medical Center reported that MMF is well tolerated and may have a beneficial effect on survival in patients with GVHD (Lopez et al., 2005). A multicenter clinical trial planned by the Fred Hutchinson Cancer Research Center is looking at the addition of MMF to CSA or tacrolimus plus prednisone in patients with extensive cGVHD. Many patients are switched from CSA to tacrolimus when there is liver disease, since tacrolimus is better concentrated in the liver. The combination of tacrolimus and MMF has been studied in steroid refractory patients with 46% responding to this therapy (Mookerjee et al., 1999). Breukman et al. (2004) published a thorough research review on the use of PUVA (psoralen and UVA light treatment) in sclerodermoid and lichenoid cGVHD. Although it is difficult to manage PUVA in patients with severe sclerodermoid skin cGVHD because of the risk of burning, lichenoid eruptions tend to respond well to this treatment (Vogelsang, 2001). Extracorporeal photopheresis (ECP) concentrates leukocytes, which are incubated with 8-methoxypsoralen (MOP), then passed through a sterile cassette surrounded by an ultraviolet A (UVA) bulb, then returned to the patient. Antigen-presenting cells and T lymphocytes are susceptible to photoinactivation. This treatment takes about 4 hours and requires that the patient have a 16-gauge peripheral line or temporary central access. Seaton et al. (2003) reported on 28 patients with advanced cGVHD, all of whom had failed conventional immunosuppressive therapy for at least 2 years. Their results showed an improvement in median skin scores by 53% in patients with both sclerodermoid and lichenoid skin eruptions. Seaton et al. (2003) also reported pos-

itive results treating both lichenoid and sclerodermoid GVHD with ECP. Thalidomide has also been reported to be active against cGVHD, but the drug is difficult to obtain and is associated with significant sedation (Vogelsang et al., 1992). A more recent randomized trial did not show a benefit to adding thalidomide to CSA and prednisone for initial treatment (Arora et al., 2001). Pentostatin is currently being studied in patients with refractory disease, with about a 50% response rate in patients who are heavily pretreated with multiple agents (Margolis et al., 2000). Acetretin, a synthetic retinoid, was studied in a group of 27 patients with sclerotic and/or fascial cGVHD based on its use in systemic scleroderma. Twenty of 27 patients showed improvement in skin lesions and/or range of motion (Marcellus et al., 1999). Etretinate is no longer commercially available because it accumulates in the fat with blood levels present in patients even years after stopping the drug. It has been replaced with acetretin, which, after 2 years, is no longer detectable in the patient's blood. Since this drug is cleared through the liver, it should not be used in patients with abnormal liver function. It also can cause redness of the skin and open sores, making it undesirable for patients with open wounds or breakdown of the skin. Clofazimine has activity in a number of chronic autoimmune skin disorders. Based on the response in that patient population, it was studied in 22 patients with cGVHD where half of patients had sclerodermatous skin involvement and demonstrated improvement in skin manifestations, range of motion, and oral involvement (Lee et al., 1997). Hydroxychloroquine has been used in the treatment of autoimmune diseases and is synergistic with CSA and tacrolimus in vitro (Gilman et al., 2000). Although not formally studied, it appears to soften skin and improve range of motion when added to immunosuppressive therapy in patients who are showing a response to treatment. Sirolimus (rapamycin) is also being explored in sclerodermatous cGVHD because of its anti-fibrotic properties (Vogelsang and Morris, 1993; Benito et al., 2001; Johnston et al., 2005).

Table 6-4 lists medications used in the prophylaxis and treatment of GVHD.

A retrospective analysis of 751 patients with cGVHD was completed to evaluate outcomes. The median duration of treatment for cGVHD was 23 months in the 274 patients who had resolution of GVHD and were able to discontinue immunosuppressive therapy. The remaining 477 patients either relapsed or died (Stewart et al., 2004).

Nursing and Supportive Care

The management of patients with GVHD is challenging. The first step in caring for patients with this treatment sequelae is to assess the early clinical manifestations and distinguish GVHD from other possible etiologies. Once the diagnosis of GVHD is confirmed, frequent assessment is necessary to determine the patient's response to therapy and to assist with the patient's comfort and healing. Patient and caregiver education also is essential . This is especially true when the patient is discharged from the transplant center back to his or her referring physician. At some HSCT centers, patients and caregivers attend a GVHD class prior to discharge and may be given a card with reportable signs and symptoms and contact phone numbers. Acute and chronic GVHD should be discussed with patients before discharge, and they should be urged to call the GVHD team or the HSCT physician if symptoms occur. Patients should be monitored for their GVHD in a standardized fashion, by consistent individuals. Patients may be followed at a GVHD clinic by a specific HSCT team member who utilizes a formal set of GVHD documentation tools within the medical record. It is important that patients be monitored consistently for early and effective intervention of this major complication of HSCT.

Nurses are in a unique role when caring for patients with GVHD. The remainder of the chapter focuses on the nursing care involved when caring for a patient with GVHD.

Infection Care

The primary cause of death in patients with cGVHD is infections. There must be a high index of suspicion for infection in patients with GVHD, with aggressive investigation of potential infections. All patients should receive antimicrobial prophylaxis. Patients with aGVHD should receive prophylaxis for *Pneumocystis Jiroveci* pneumonia with agents such as a trimethoprim sulfamethoxazole, dapsone, atovaquone, or pentamadine. Patients with cGVHD should also receive prophylaxis, such as penicillin, against encapsulated organisms including *Pneumococcus*. Poor splenic function may persist even after immunosuppressive therapy has been decreased or stopped, and *Pneumocystis* prophylaxis should be maintained for 6 months after stopping immunosuppressive therapy. Patients are maintained for a lifetime on antimicrobials for prophylaxis against *Pneumococcus*.

Additionally, all patients should receive antibiotic prophylaxis for dental and all other

Table 6-4 MEDICATIONS USED IN PROPHYLAXIS AND TREATMENT OF GVHD.

Medication	Action	Adverse Effects
Corticosteroids	Direct lymphocyte toxicity; suppress proinflammatory cytokines (TNF-α).	Hyperglycemia; acute psychosis; severe myopathy; cataract development; avascular necrosis.
Methotrexate (MTX)	Antimetabolite; aids in inducing tolerance after BMT; may downregulate T lymphocytes by inhibiting proliferation.	Significant renal, hepatic, and gastrointestinal toxicities.
Cyclosporine A (CSA)	IL-2 suppressor; blocks calcium-dependent signal transduction distal to engagement of T cell receptor.	Renal and hepatic insufficiency; hypertension; hyperglycemia; headache; nausea and vomiting; hirsutism; gum hypertrophy; seizure with severe toxicity.
Tacrolimus (FK506)	Similar to CSA.	Similar to CSA.
Mycophenolate mofetil (MMF)	Inhibits de novo purine synthesis; lymphocytes are highly dependent on de novo synthesis.	Body aches; abdominal pain; nausea and vomiting; diarrhea; neutropenia.
Antithymocyte globulin	Polyclonal immunoglobulin capable of destroying human T cells.	Anaphylaxis; serum sickness.
Sirolimus	Inhibits T lymphocyte activation and proliferation that occurs in response to antigenic and cytokine stimulation.	Muscle aches; hypertension; cytopenias, especially thrombocytopenia; renal insufficiency; peripheral edema.
Pentostatin	Potent transition state inhibitor of the enzyme adenosine deaminase (ADA) found in lymphoid cells, especially T cells.	Nausea/vomiting; fever; leucopenia; myalgias; hepatic dysfunction; adjust for renal insufficiency.
Hydroxychloroquine	Antimalarial; beneneficial in autoimmune disorders; exact mechanism of action not known.	Irreversible retinal damage; headache; mild GI symptoms.
Acetretin	Retinoid used to treat psoriasis.	Must not be used in women who plan on getting pregnant; erythema and breakdown of skin; elevation in LFTs and lipids; dry eyes; dry skin.
Daclizumab	IL-2 receptor antagonist; in circulation impairs response of immune system to antigenic challenges.	Increased mortality when used with steroids.

invasive procedures according to the endo-carditis prophylaxis recommendations of the American Heart Association. Topical antifungal prophylaxis with clotrimazole troches or nystatin swish and swallow should be used in all patients receiving topical steroids for oral GVHD. The use of the newer antifungals, such as caspofungin and voriconazole, against aspergillosis have not been studied for prophylactic use but may be useful in patients with a history of fungal disease.

Reactivation of virus is a problem in patients with acute and chronic GVHD (Lin et al., 2002). All patients should be monitored for cytomegalovirus (CMV) and be treated with antivirals, such as ganciclovir and valganciclovir, if there is evidence of the CMV antigen with polymerase chain reaction (PCR) or antigenemia testing. Immunoglobulin infusions should be given if there is documented disease, especially in the lungs. Patients with frequent infection should be monitored for quantitative immunoglobulins monthly.

Many patients have outbreaks of oral and genital herpes and should receive prophylaxis if they are on high doses of immunosuppression. It is unclear if patients with cGVHD benefit from prophylaxis with antivirals unless they are having frequent outbreaks.

Since most patients with cGVHD are unlikely to respond to vaccinations, it is best to delay these immunizations until one year after treatment has been completed and ensure there is no evidence of active disease. Antibody titers can be checked to assess response to inactivated vaccines such as polio, diphtheria, and tetanus toxoid. The Centers for Disease Control has specific recommendations for immunizations in an immune-compromised host. These include delaying measles vaccines until the pa-tient has been off immunosuppression for 2 years. Polyvalent influenza and pneumococcal vaccinations may be given at any time, but the patient may not elicit a response, although it is highly recommended that family members and friends receive flu shots yearly.

Skin Care

Lubrication of skin is essential. An oil- or petroleum-based agent without perfumes or additives is helpful and should be applied to the skin at least twice a day, preferably after a luke-warm shower. Many patients complain about the messiness of petroleum jelly and find it more tolerable to use it in the evening before bedtime and cover the skin with old night-clothes. Patients report that the use of baby oil after a shower is helpful, but they should be reminded to apply it *after* stepping out of the shower or tub to prevent falls.

Most lotions have a high percentage of water and do not lubricate adequately; therefore, it should be stressed that a solid product, such as petroleum jelly, may be better than a watery cream. Patients should test any new skin product by applying it to a small area of skin two nights in a row. If there are signs of redness or rash this product should be avoided. When using topical steroids it is best to use a petroleum-based product, since creams may contribute to dry skin.

If aGVHD progresses to bullae, the blisters should be kept intact, when possible. Once the skin is desquamated, it is important to prevent infection. If small areas of skin are involved, an antibacterial ointment may be useful; however, with diffuse desquamation, bathing and removing ointments can be quite painful. The area can be cleaned with saline, and a 0.5–1% silver nitrate solution (1:4 dilution with normal saline) can be applied to the open areas. Generalized debridement is not advisable unless there are necrotic areas. Carefully trimming dead skin to within about 1/8 inch of the intact skin can promote healing.

Patients with ongoing ulcerations associated with aGVHD or sclerodermatous cGVHD may benefit from a wound care consult. There are many products available to treat ulcerations, but specific recommendations depend on the moistness of the wound, the signs of infection, and the fragility of the skin surrounding the ulcerations. Patients should be careful to avoid trauma, especially of the lower legs, since that skin may be fragile and susceptible to abrasions, which can lead to ulcerations. Patients should use sunblock with a sun protection factor (SPF) of 15 or higher and avoid sunburns. The sunblock should be tested on the skin for a sensitivity or allergic reaction before use.

Patients with sclerotic or fascial disease may not sweat normally and should take precautions so that they avoid getting overheated, since heat prostration and heat stroke can occur in patients who do not take precautions in hot and/or humid weather.

Eye Care

All patients with severe aGVHD or with the onset of cGVHD should be assessed by an ophthalmologist. Patients with severe aGVHD should be evaluated for evidence of pseudomembrane formation. A Schirmer's test, the use of topical anesthetic drops applied to the conjunctiva, followed by the measurement of millimeters of wetting over 5 minutes, should be performed in patients who complain of dry eyes and when patients are first diagnosed with cGVHD. Infections should be ruled out, especially CMV. Patients with sicca syndrome should use preservative-free artificial tears at least every 4 hours during the day and preservative-free ointment at night to prevent corneal abrasions. Scleral lenses, which are placed in the eye and continuously lubricate, are now available. They were FDA approved in 1994. The Boston Foundation for Sight was the first to develop this lens; however, it is now available at other facilities.

Mouth Care

Agents available to treat symptoms of dry mouth have not been found to be very effective with this patient population. Patients report that sugar-free, non-sorbitol-containing candies help to stimulate saliva production. A sorbitol-free product prevents diarrhea. The use of topical agents prior to eating can help decrease mouth pain; however, topical lidocaine should be avoided before meals as it increases the risk of trauma to the oral mucosa, as well as risk of aspiration.

Patients with sicca syndrome are at high risk for dental caries and should be seen by a dentist at least every 6 months. Many patients with cGVHD complain of burning when using toothpaste and mouthwash. This is most likely from the mint added for flavoring. Pediatric toothpastes with fruit or bubble gum flavoring may be more easily tolerated.

A swallowing study may be helpful in identifying strictures when patients complain of difficulty swallowing. Endoscopy may be necessary to rule out infections like esophageal candida and to dilate the esophagus. Repeat esophageal dilation may become necessary.

Gastrointestinal Care

Careful monitoring of diarrhea is important with aGVHD, and with the onset of diarrhea, cultures should be sent to rule out infection. A GI consult is helpful if nausea, vomiting, and/or diarrhea become persistent symptoms. Endoscopies with biopsy are helpful in confirming the diagnosis of GVHD.

Patients' nutritional status should be monitored carefully. Patients with severe aGVHD of the upper or lower GI tract benefit from resting their gut by taking nothing by mouth. These patients require parenteral or enteral feedings. Patients with the wasting syndrome associated with cGVHD may need to have enteral feedings through surgically placed tubes. Many patients, especially those with cGVHD, develop symptoms of reflux. This symptom should be assessed and monitored by a gastroenterologist, with appropriate medications given for treatment.

Liver Care

Liver function tests should be monitored closely along with hepatitis screens. Patients should be advised to avoid supplemental vitamins unless recommended by their physician because many, especially vitamin A, may be liver toxic. Many over-the-counter medications, such as acetaminophen, may be toxic to the liver. Alcohol also may affect the liver.

Some patients complain of itching when liver disease is present; this pruritis is frustrating and not easily managed. Ursodiol may be helpful in decreasing the bilirubin, and many of the skin lubricants recommended earlier in this section may help eliminate the pruritis. Unfortunately, the best way to manage this symptom is to treat the underlying GVHD.

Respiratory Care

Computerized axial tomography (CAT) scans of the sinuses and lungs should be considered at the initiation of high-dose therapy for aGVHD and cGVHD and at least quarterly while the patient is on immunosuppression. Many patients complaining of shortness of breath and dyspnea of exertion (DOE) have clear scans of the lungs but positive findings with air fluid levels in their sinuses. Lung CAT scans should utilize high resolution when ruling out infection, and sinus CAT scans should be coronal to better visualize the sinuses.

Patients with new onset of shortness of breath or dyspnea on exertion should have pulmonary function tests (PFTs) before and after the administration of bronchodilators to assist with the diagnosis. Chien and colleagues (2005) suggest that comparing PFTs posttransplant may be important to identify patients at high risk for developing pulmonary complications and/or mortality. Some patients have no response to bronchodilators with PFTs but have some symptomatic relief if they are used regularly. Patients with respiratory symptoms should be followed by an ear, nose, and throat specialist or pulmonologist if symptoms persist or recur.

Neuromuscular Care

Muscle cramping is a frequent complaint with an unknown etiology. Electrolyte disorders, including calcium, magnesium, and potassium, contribute to these symptoms but may decrease or even resolve with adequate supplementation. Oral agents such as quinine, dantrolene, and baclofen have also been effective for persistent and disabling cramping.

Patients should be monitored carefully if oral agents are used since these agents have specific side effects. The side effects may include muscle weakness, drowsiness (for which quinine should be given at bedtime), diarrhea, abnormal liver function tests, and sun sensitivity. Dantrolene should not be used for patients who are being treated with PUVA or extracorporeal photopheresis (ECP).

Patients should be monitored by physical therapists for signs of myopathy, a common complication of steroid use, and for decreased range of motion that is common with sclerodermatous and fascial cGVHD. It is best for a patient to develop a relationship with one therapist who can assess for changes and give a personalized prescription for activities and exercises. Occupational therapy can also be helpful in assessing functional capabilities in activities of daily living, employment opportunities, and sexual satisfaction. These therapists are helpful when upper extremities are affected by either the GVHD or the side effects of treatment. Consultation with a physiatrist specializing in rehabilitation medicine may be helpful when the use of splints or adaptive devices are necessary.

Genitourinary Care

Symptoms of vaginal dryness and painful intercourse may occur with GVHD. Lubricants may be helpful, but with severe GVHD there is a possibility of narrowing or even obstruction of the vaginal canal, leading to pelvic inflammatory disease. Women should be advised to see a gynecologist for routine care and assessment. Hormone replacement therapy is controversial. Replacement therapy for women under 40 years old, especially if they are having severe menopausal symptoms, may be considered.

Men with GVHD often complain of erectile dysfunction and decreased libido. Testosterone levels should be checked and testosterone patches or injections could be used if there are no liver abnormalities.

Psychosocial Care

Graft-versus-host disease, regardless of the type, is a difficult and oftentimes frustrating complication of HSCT. Imagine having your disease cured or in remission, only to be confronted with aGVHD or cGVHD, the sequelae of HSCT. All patients should be assessed by a social worker or behavioral medicine professional and be referred for a psychiatric consult if there appears to be history of depression or suicidal ideation. Antianxiety or sleep medications may need to be ordered. Patient education that includes relaxation techniques such as music, movies, television, guided imagery, or biofeedback may offer the patient some personal control over the psychosocial aspects of GVHD.

Table 6-5 outlines many nursing issues for patients with GVHD.

Conclusions

Great strides have been made in HSCT over the past 50 years, and within the past decade the scientific knowledge has grown exponentially. However, one of the major treatment complications, GVHD, continues to be the clinical condition that not only affects the transplant recipient's quality of life, but also is life threatening. Although our understanding of the pathophysiology, risk factors, and their relationship to treatment regimens continues to grow, there is more to be learned about GVHD. Clinical trials are needed to advance the knowledge of GVHD, including determining the most appropriate combination and duration of drugs for prophylaxis and whether conditioning

Table 6-5 NURSING MANAGEMENT.

Problem	Nursing Action
Infection	Educate patients about increased risk of infection, even if not treating with immunosuppression; monitor prophylactic antibiotics, antifungals, antivirals; CMV PCR if CMV positive; monitor for herpes simplex virus (HSV) and varicella zoster virus (VZV) reactivation; flu and *Pneumococcal* vaccines OK, no live vaccines until off immunosuppression for 2 years.
Skin	Lubricate with petroleum-based ointments; test all new products on small area of skin to rule out hypersensitivity; keep bullae intact; use antibacterial ointment on small desquamated areas; use silver nitrate solution (1:4 silver nitrate to normal saline) on large desquamated areas; debride only necrotic or contaminated wounds; wound care consult for severe ulcerations.
Eyes	Preservative-free tears and ointments; arrange for ophthalmology consult to rule out infection and evaluate for dry eyes.
Mouth	Sugar-free candies for dry mouth (avoid sorbitol); mint-free toothpastes (pediatric bubble gum or fruit flavored); topical agents for pain but cautious use of viscous lidocaine, especially with dysphagia; culture for fungus and virus if symptoms increase.
GI	Monitor nutritional status; food diary if losing weight; swallowing study and possible endoscopy for dysphagia; prophylaxis with H2 blocker if on steroids, MMF, pentostatin.
Liver	Hepatitis screen if LFTs increase; monitor patient OTC medications.
Respiratory	CT chest and sinus monthly or if symptoms present, monitor PFTs yearly or more often if new DOE, otolaryngology consult for chronic sinusitis.
Neuromuscular	Physical therapy/occupational therapy for all patients with sclerosis, fasciitis, or on steroids; magnesium supplements for muscle cramping.
Reproductive	Monitor for vaginal dryness; possible hormone replacement, especially for younger females; monitor male testosterone levels
Psychosocial	Social work evaluation at diagnosis of cGVHD; monitor for depression and suicidal ideations; pain team consult for refractory pain.

regimens for particular diseases have any bearing on clinical outcomes.

The clinical area of HSCT nursing not only is challenging, but also is fertile with the need and the possibilities for evidence-based research and practice related to patient complications including GVHD. It is the authors' hopes that nurses working in the field of HSCT will be encouraged to help further the knowledge base of GVHD and other HSCT patient-related topics.

References

Afessa, B., Litzow, M.R., Tefferi, A. (2001). Bronchiolitis obliterans and other late onset non-infectious pulmonary complications in hematopoietic stem cell transplantation. *Bone Marrow Transplant, 28*(5), 425–434.

Akpek, G., Ambinder, R.F., Piantadosi, S., Abrams, R.A., Brodsky, R.A., Vogelsang, G.B., et al. (2001). Long-term results of blood and marrow transplantation for Hodgkin's lymphoma. *J Clinical Oncol, 19*(23), 4314–4321.

Akpek, G., Boitnott, J.K., Lee, L.A., Hallick, J.P., Torbenson, M., Jacobsohn, D.A., et al. (2002). Hepatitic variant of graft-versus-host disease after donor lymphocyte infusion. *Blood, 100*(12), 3903–3907.

Akpek, G., Lee, S.M., Anders, V., Vogelsang, G.B. (2001). A high-dose pulse steroid regimen for controlling active chronic graft-versus-host disease. *Biol Blood Marrow Transplant, 7*(9), 495–502.

Akpek, G., Lee, S., Flowers, M.E., Pavetic, S., Arora, M., Lee, S., et al. (2003). Performance of a new clinical grading system for chronic graft-versus-host disease: A multicenter study. *Blood, 102*(3), 802–809.

Akpek, G., Valladares, J.L., Lee, L., Margolis, J., Vogelsang, G.B. (2001). Pancreatic insufficiency in patients with chronic graft-versus-host disease. *Bone Marrow Transplant, 27*, 163–166.

Akpek, G., Zahurak, M.L., Piantadosi, S., Margolis, J., Doherty, J., Davidson, R., et al. (2001). Development of a prognostic model for grading chronic graft-versus-host disease. *Blood, 97*, 1219–1226.

Alcindor, T., Gorgun, G., Miller, K.B., Roberts, T.F., Sprague, K., Schenkein, D.P., et al. (2001). Immunomodulatory effects of extracorporeal photochemotherapy in patients with extensive chronic graft versus host disease. *Blood, 98*(5), 1622–1625.

Anagnostopoulos, A., Giralt, S. (2002). Critical review on non-myeloablative stem cell transplantation. *Crit Rev Oncol Hemat, 44*(2), 175–190.

Anasetti, C., Rybka, W., Sullivan, K.M., Banaji, M., Slichter, S.J. (1989). Graft-v-host disease is associated with autoimmune-like thrombocytopenia. *Blood, 73*(4), 1054–1058.

Antin, J. (2002). Long-term care after hematopoietic-cell transplantation in adults. *N Engl J Med, 347*, 36–42.

Antin, J.H., Chen, A.R., Couriel, D.R., Ho, V.T., Nash, R.A., Weisdorf, D. (2004). Novel approaches to the therapy of steroid-resistant acute graft-versus-host disease. *Biol Blood Marrow Transplant, 10*(10), 655–668.

Antin, J.H., Kim, H.T., Cutler, C., Ho, V.T., Lee, S.T., Miklos, D.B., et al. (2003). Sirolimus, tacrolimus, and low-dose methotrexate for graft-versus-host disease prophylaxis in mismatched related donor or unrelated donor transplantation. *Blood, 102*(5), 1601–1605.

Arai, S., Lee, L.A., Vogelsang, G.B. (2002). A systematic approach to hepatic complications in hematopoietic stem cell transplantation. *J Hematother Stem Cell Res, 11*(1), 215–230.

Arai, S., Margolis, J., Zahurak, M., Anders, V., Vogelsang, G. (2002). Poor outcome in steroid refractory graft-versus-host disease with antithymocyte globulin treatment. *Biol Blood Marrow Transplant, 8*, 155–160.

Arora, M., Wagner, J.R., Davies, S.M., Blazer, B.R., Defor, T., Enright, H., et al. (2001). Randomized clinical trials of thalidomide, cyclosporine, and prednisone versus cyclosporine and prednisone as initial therapy for chronic graft-versus-host disease. *Biol Blood Marrow Transplant, 7*(5), 265–273.

Atkinson, K., Horowitz, M.M., Gale, R.P., Lee, M.B., Rim, A.A., Burtin, M.M. (1989). Consensus among bone marrow transplantation for diagnosis, grading and treatment of chronic graft-versus-host disease: Committee of International Bone Marrow Transplant Registry. *Bone Marrow Transplant, 4*, 247–254.

Bacigalupo, A., Oneto, R., Lamparelli, T., Gualandi, F., Bregante, S., Rajola, A.M., et al. (2001). Pre-emptive therapy of acute graft-versus-host disease: A pilot study with antithymocyte globulin (ATG). *Bone Marrow Transplant, 28*(12), 1093–1096.

Bacigalupo, A., Palandri, F. (2004). Management of acute graft versus host disease (GvHD). *Hematol J, 5*, 189–196.

Barnes, D.W., Corp, M.J., Loutit, J.F., Heal, F.E. (1956). Treatment of murine leukemia with X rays and homologous bone marrow: Preliminary communication. *Br Med J, 15*(4993), 626–627.

Barnes, D.W., Loutit, J.F. (1995). Spleen protection: The cellular hypothesis. In Bacq, Z.M. (Ed.). *Radiobiology Symposium* (pp. 135–136). London: Butterworth.

Beiderman, T., Schwarzler, C., Lametschwandtner, G., Thoma, G., Carballido Perrig, N., Kund, J. (2002). Targeting CLA/E-selectin interactions prevents

CCR4-mediated recruitment of human Th2 memory cells to human skin in vivo. *Eur J Immunol, 32*(11), 3178–3180.

Benito, A.L., Furlong, T., Martin, P.J., Anasetti, C., Allelbaum, F.R., Doney, K., et al. (2001). Sirolimus (rapamycin) for the treatment of steroid-refractory acute graft-versus-host disease. *Transplantation, 72*(12), 1924–1929.

Bhushan, V., Collins, R.H. (2003). Chronic graft-vs-host disease. *JAMA, 290,* 2599–2603.

Billingham, R.E. (1966). The biology of graft-versus-host reactions. *Harvey Lectures, 62*(61), 21–28.

Bishop, M.R. (2003). Graft versus host disease: Emerging concepts in prevention and therapy. *Curr Hematol Rep, 2,* 287–294.

Bolanos-Meade, J., Jacobsohn, D.A., Margolis, J., Ogden, A., Wientjes, M.G., Byrd, J.C. (2005). Pentostatin in steroid refractory acute graft-versus-host-disease. *J Clin Oncol, 23*(12), 2661–2668.

Bolanos-Meade, J., Zhou, L., Hoke, A., Corse, A., Vogelsang, G., Wagner, K.R. (2005). Hydroxychloroquine causes severe vacuolar myopathy in a patient with chronic graft-versus-host disease. *Am J Hematol, 78*(4), 306–309.

Breukman, F., Gambickler, T., Altmeyer, P., Kreuter, A. (2004). UVA/UVA1 phototherapy and PUVA photochemotherapy in connective tissue disease and related disorders: A research based review. *BMC Dermatol, 4*(11), 1471–1594.

Carpenter, P.A., Appelbaum, F.R., Corey, L.H., Deeg, J., Doney, K., Gooley, T., et al. (2002). A humanized non-FcR-binding anti-CD3 antibody, visiluzumab, for treatment of steroid-refractory acute graft-versus-host disease. *Blood, 99*(8), 2712–2719.

Chan, C.K., Hyland, R.H., Hutcheon, M.A., Minden, M.D., Alexander, M.A., Kossakowska, A.E., et al. (1987). Small-airways disease in recipients of allogeneic bone marrow transplants: An analysis of 11 cases and a review of the literature. *Medicine* (Baltimore), 66, 327–340.

Chao, N.J., Snyder, D.S., Jain, M., Wong, R.M., Niland, J.C., Negrin, R.S., et al. (2000). Equivalence of 2 effective graft-versus-host disease prophylaxis regimens: Results of a prospective double-blind randomized trial. *Biol Blood Marrow Transplant, 6,* 254–261.

Chien, J.W., Madtes, D.K., Clark, J.G. (2005). Pulmonary function testing prior to hematopoietic stem cell transplantation. *Bone Marrow Transplant, 35*(5), 429–435.

Collins, R.H., Shpilberg, O., Drobyski, W.R., Porter, D.L., Giralt, S., Champlin, R., et al. (1997). Donor leukocyte infusions in 140 patients with relapsed malignancy after allogeneic bone marrow transplantation. *J Clin Oncol, 15,* 433–444.

Corson, S.L., Sullivan, K., Batzer, F., August, C., Storb, R., Thomas, E.D. (1982). Gynecologic manifestations of chronic graft-versus-host disease. *Obstet Gynecol, 60*(4), 488–492.

Couriel, D.R., Saliba, R.M., Giralt, S., Khouri, I., Andersson, B., de Lima, M., et al. (2004). Acute and chronic graft-versus-host disease after ablative and nonmyeloablative conditioning for allogeneic hematopoietic transplantation. *Biol Blood Marrow Transplant, 10,* 178–185.

Cutler, C., Giri, S., Jeyapalan, S., Paniagua, D., Viswanathan, A., Antin, J. (2001). Acute and chronic graft-versus-host disease after allogeneic peripheral blood stem-cell and bone marrow transplantation: A meta-analysis. *J Clin Oncol, 19*(16), 3685–3691.

Dean, D.M., Bishop, M.R. (2003). Graft versus host disease: Emerging concepts in prevention and therapy. *Curr Hematol Rep, 2*(4), 287–294.

Deeg, H.J. (2001). Cytokines in graft-versus-host disease and the graft-versus-leukemia reaction. *Int J Hematol, 74*(1), 26–32.

Deeg, H.J., Storb, R. (1984). Graft-versus-host disease: Pathophysiological and clinical aspects. *Annu Rev Med, 35,* 11–24.

Deeg, H.J., Storb, R., Thomas, E.D. (1984). Bone marrow transplantation: A review of delayed complications. *Brit J Hematol, 57*(2), 185–208.

Eagle, D.A., Gian, V., Lauwers, G.Y., Manivel, J.C., Moreb, J.S., Mastin, S., et al. (2001). Gastroparesis following bone marrow transplantation. *Bone Marrow Transplant, 28*(1), 59–62.

Erlich, H.A., Oelz, G., Hansen, J. (2001). HLA DNA typing and transplantation. *Immunity, 14,* 347–356.

Ezzone, S. (2004). *Hematopoietic Stem Cell Transplantation: A Manual for Nursing Practice.* Pittsburgh, PA: Oncology Nursing Society.

Ferrara, J.L., Deeg, H.J. (1991). Graft-versus-host disease. *N Engl J Med, 324,* 667–674.

Flowers, M.E., Lee, S., Vogelsang, G. (2003). An update on how to treat chronic GVHD. *Blood, 102*(6), 2312.

Flowers, M.E., Parker, P.M., Johnston, L.J., Matos, A.V.B., Storer, B., Bensinger, W.I., et al. (2002). Comparison of chronic graft-versus-host disease after transplantation of peripheral blood stem cells versus bone marrow in allogeneic recipients: Long-term follow-up of a randomized trial. *Blood, 100*(2), 415–419.

Fujii, N., Takenaka, K., Shinagawa, K., Ikeda, K., Maeda, Y., Sunami, K., et al. (2001). Hepatic graft-versus-host disease presenting as an acute hepatitis after allogeneic peripheral blood stem cell transplantation. *Bone Marrow Transplant, 27*, 1007–1010.

Fulton, B., Markham, A. (1996). Mycophenolate mofetil: A review of its pharmacodynamic and pharmacokinetic properties and clinical efficacy in renal transplantation. *Drugs, 51*, 278–298.

Furlong, T., Leisenring, W., Storb, R., Anasetti, C., Appelbaum, F.R., Carpenter, P.A., et al. (2002). Psoralen and ultraviolet A irradiation (PUVA) as therapy for steroid-resistant cutaneous acute graft-versus-host disease. *Biol Blood Marrow Transplant, 8*, 206–212.

Gilman, A.L., Beams, F., Tufft, M., Mazumder, A. (1996). The effect of hydroxychloroquine on alloreactivity and its potential use for graft-versus-host disease. *Bone Marrow Transplant, 17*, 1069–1075.

Gilman, A.L., Chan, K.W., Mogul, A., Morris, C., Goldman, F.D., Boyer, M., et al. (2000). Hydroxychloroquine for the treatment of chronic graft-versus-host disease. *Biol Blood Marrow Transplant, 6*(3A), 327–334.

Giralt, S. (2002). Update on non-myeloablative stem cell transplantation for hematologic malignancies. *Int J Hematol, 76*(Suppl 1), 368–375.

Giralt, S., Estey, E., Albitar, M., van Besien, K., Rondon, G., Anderlini, P., et al. (1997). Engraftment of allogeneic hematopoietic progenitor cells with purine analog-containing chemotherapy: Harnessing graft-versus-leukemia without myeloablative therapy. *Blood, 89*, 4531–4536.

Giralt, S., Thall, P.F., Khouri, I., Wang, X., Braunschweig, I., Ippolitti, C., et al. (2001). Melphalan and purine analog-containing preparative regimens: Reduced-intensity conditioning for patients with hematologic malignancies undergoing allogeneic progenitor cell transplantation. *Blood, 97*, 631–637.

Glucksberg, H., Storb, R., Fefer, A., Buckner, C.D., Neiman, P.E., Clift, R.A., et al. (1974). Clinical manifestations of graft-versus-host disease in human recipients of marrow from HL-A-matched sibling donors. *Transplantation, 18*, 295–304.

Goerner, M., Gooley, T., Flowers, M., Sullivan, K.M., Kiem, H.P., Sanders, J.E. (2002). Morbidity and mortality of GVHD after stem cell transplant. *Biol Blood Marrow Transplant, 8*, 47–56.

Goldman, J.M., Gale, R.P., Horowitz, M.M., Biggs, J.C., Champlin, R.E., Gluckman, E. (1988). Bone marrow transplant for chronic myelogenous leukemia in chronic phase: Increased risk for relapse associated with T-cell depletion. *Ann Intern Med, 108*(6), 806–814.

Gratwohl, A., Moutsopoulos, H.M., Chused, T.M., et al. (1977). Sjogren-type syndrome after allogeneic bone-marrow transplantation. *Ann Intern Med, 87*, 703–706.

Greinin, H., Volc-Platzer, B., Rabitsch, W., Gmeinhart, B., Guevara-Pineda, C., Kalhs, P. (1998). Successful use of extracorporeal photochemotherapy in the treatment of severe acute and chronic graft-versus-host disease. *Blood, 92*(9), 3098–3104.

Ho, V.T., Soiffer, R.J. (2001). The history and future of T-cell depletion as graft-versus-host disease prophylaxis for allogeneic hematopoietic stem cell transplantation. *Blood, 98*(12), 3192–3204.

Ho, V.T., Zahrieh, D., Hochberg, E., Micale, E., Levin, J., Reynalds, C., et al. (2003). Safety and efficacy of denileukin difitox in patients with steroid refractory graft-versus-host disease (GVHD) after allogeneic hematopoietic stem cell transplantation (HSCT). [Abstract 850]. *Blood, 102*(11).

Holland, H.K., Wingard, J.R., Beschorner, W.E., Santos, G.W. (1988). Bronchiolitis obliterans in bone marrow transplantation and its relationship to chronic graft-vs-host disease and low serum IgG. *Blood, 72*, 621–627.

Horn, T.D. (1994). Acute cutaneous eruptions after marrow ablation: Roses by other names? *J Cutan Path, 21*, 385–392.

Horn, T.D., Rest, E.B., Mirenski, Y., Corio, R.L., Zahurak, M.L., Vogelsang, G.B., et al. (1995). The significance of oral mucosal and salivary gland pathology after allogenic bone marrow transplantation. *Arch Dermatol, 131*, 964–965.

Igbal, N., Salzman, D., Lazenby, A.J., Wilcox, C.M. (2000). Diagnosis of gastrointestinal graft-versus-host disease. *Am J Gastroenterol, 95*, 3034–3038.

Jabs, D.A., Wingard, J., Green, W.R., Farmer, E.R., Vogelsang, G., Saral, R., et al. (1989). The eye in bone marrow transplantation. *Arch Ophthalmol, 107*, 1343–1348.

Jacobsohn, D.A., Margolis, J., Doherty, J., Anders, V., Vogelsang, G.B. (2002). Weight loss and malnutrition in patients with chronic graft-versus-host disease. *Bone Marrow Transplant, 29*, 231–236.

Jacobsohn, D.A., Montross, S., Anders, V., Vogelsang, G.B. (2001). Clinical importance of confirming or excluding the diagnosis of chronic graft-versus-host disease. *Bone Marrow Transplant, 28*, 1047–1051.

Jacobsohn, D.A., Schechter, T., Seshadri, R., Thormann, K., Duerst, R., Kletzel, M. (2004). Eosinophilia correlates with the presence of development of chronic graft-versus-host disease in children. *Transplantation,* 77(7), 1096–1100.

Janin, A., Socie, G., Devergie, A., Aractingi, S., Esperou, H., Verola, O., Gluckman, E. (1994). Fasciitis in chronic graft-versus-host disease. A clinicopathologic study of 14 cases. *Ann Intern Med, 120*(12), 993–998.

Johnson, D.A., Jabs, D.A. (1997). The ocular manifestations of graft-versus-host disease. *Int Ophthalmol Clin,* 37, 119–133.

Johnston, L.J., Brown, J., Shirzuro, J.A., Stockerl-Goldstein, K.E., Stuart, M.J., Blume, K.G. (2005). Rapamycin (sirolimus) for treatment of chronic graft-versus-host disease. *Biol Blood Marrow Transplant,* 11(1), 47–55.

Kataoka, Y., Iwasaki, T., Kuroiwa, T., Seto, Y., Iwata, N., Kaneda, Y., et al (2001). The role of donor T cells for target organ injuries in acute and chronic graft-versus-host diseas. *Immunology, 103*, 310–318.

Khouri, I.F., Keating, M., Korbling, M., Przepiorka, D., Anderlini, P., O'Brien, S., et al. (1998). Transplant-lite: Induction of graft-versus-malignancy using fludarabine-based non-ablative chemotherapy and allogeneic blood progenitor-cell transplantation as treatment for lymphoid malignancies. *J Clin Oncol, 16*, 2817–2824.

Kim, H. (2002). Mini-allogeneic stem cell transplantation. *Cancer Pract, 10*(3), 170–172.

Kobbe, G., Schneider, P., Rohr, U., Fenk, R., Neumann, F., Aivado, M., et al. (2001). Treatment of severe steroid refractory acute graft-versus-host disease with infliximab, a chimeric human/mouse anti-TNF alpha antibody. *Bone Marrow Transplant, 28*, 47–49.

Koc, S., Leisening, W., Flowers, M.E., Anasetti, C., Deeg, H.J., Nash, R.A., et al, (2002). Therapy for chronic graft-versus-host disease: A randomized trial comparing cyclosporine plus prednisone versus prednisone alone. *Blood, 100*(1), 48–51.

Lee, S.J., Cook, E.F., Soiffer, R., Antin, J.H. (2002). Development and validation of a scale to measure symptoms of chronic graft-versus-host disease. *Biol Blood Marrow Transplant, 8*, 444–452.

Lee, S.J., Kelin, J.P., Barrett, A.J., Ringden, O., Antin, J.H., Cuhn, J., et al. (2002). Severity of chronic graft-versus-host disease: Association with treatment-related mortality and relapse. *Blood, 100*, 406–414.

Lee, S.J., Vogelsang, G., Flowers, M.E. (2003). Chronic graft-versus-host disease. *Biol Blood Marrow Transplant, 9*, 215–233.

Lee, S.J., Vogelsang, G., Gilman, A., Weisdorf, D.J., Pavletic, S., Antin, J.H., et al. (2002). A survey of diagnosis, management, and grading of chronic GVHD. *Biol Blood Marrow Transplant, 8*, 32–39.

Lee, S.J., Wegner, S.A., McGarigle, C.J., Bierer, B.E., Antin, J.H. (1997). Treatment of chronic graft-versus-host disease with clofazimine. *Blood, 89*, 2298–2302.

Lee, S.J., Zahrieh, D., Agura, E., MacMillan, M.L., Maziarz, R.T., McCarthy, P.L., et al. (2004). Effect of up-front daclizumab when combined with steroids for the treatment of acute graft-versus-host disease: Results of a randomized trial. *Blood, 104*(5), 1559–1564.

Lin, T.S., Zahrieh, D., Weller, E., Alyea, E.P., Antin, J.H., Soiffer, R.J. (2002). Risk factors for cytomegalovirus reactivation after CD6+ T-cell depleted allogeneic bone marrow transplantation. *Transplantation, 74*, 49–54.

Lister, J., Messner, H., Keystone, E., Miller, R., Fritzler, M.J. (1987). Autoantibody analysis of patients with graft-versus-host disease. *J Clin Lab Immun, 24*(1), 19–23.

Locatelli, F., Zecca, M., Rondelli, R., Bonetti, F., Dini, G., Prete, A., et al. (2000). Graft versus host disease prophylaxis with low-dose cyclosporine-A reduces the risk of relapse in children with acute leukemia given HLA-identical sibling bone marrow transplantation: Results of a randomized trial. *Blood, 95*, 1572–1579.

Lopez, F., Parker, P., Nademanee, A., Rodriguez, R., Al-Kadhimi, Z., Bhatia, R. (2005). Efficacy of mycophenolate mofetil in the treatment of chronic graft-versus-host disease. *Biol Blood Marrow Transplant, 11*(4), 307–313.

Marcellus, D.C., Altomonte, V., Farmer, E.R., Horn, T.D., Freener, G.S., Grant, J., et al. (1999). Etretinate therapy for refractory sclerodermatous chronic graft-versus-host disease. *Blood, 93*, 66–70.

Margolis, J., Borrello, I., Flinn, I.W. (2000). New approaches to treating malignances with stem cell transplantation. *Semin Oncol, 27*(5), 524–530.

Margolis, J., Grever, M.R. (2000). Pentostatin (Nipent): A review of potential toxicity and its management. *Semin Oncol, 27*(2 Suppl 5), 9–14.

Margolis, J., Vogelsang, G. (2000). An old drug for a new disease: Pentostatin (Nipent) in acute graft-versus-host disease. *Semin Oncol, 27*(2 Suppl 5), 72–77.

Martin, P.J. (1999). Overview of marrow transplantation immunology. In Thomas, E.D., Blume, K.G., Forman, S.J. (Eds.). *Hematopoietic Cell Transplantation* (2nd ed., pp. 19–27), Malden, MA: Blackwell Science, Inc.

Martin, P.J., Schoch, G., Fisher, L., Byers, V., Anasetti, C., Appelbaum, F.R., et al. (1990). A retrospective analysis of therapy for acute graft-versus-host disease: Initial treatment. *Blood, 76*, 1464–1472.

Martin, P.J., Schoch, G., Fisher, L., Byers, V., Appelbaum, F.R., McDonald, G.B., et al. (1991). A retrospective analysis of therapy for acute graft-versus-host disease: Secondary treatment. *Blood, 77*, 1821–1828.

Mathe, G. (1959). Transfusions et greffes de moelle osseuse homologue chez les humains irradies a hautes dose accidentellement. *Rev Fr Etudes Clin Bio, 4*, 675–704.

McSweeney, P.A., Niederwieser, D., Shizuru, J.A. (2001). Hematopoietic stem cell transplantation in older patients with hematologic malignancies: Replacing high-dose cytotoxic therapy with graft-versus-tumor effects. *Blood, 97*, 3390–3400.

Michallet, M., Bliger, K., Garban, F. (2001). Allogeneic hematopoietic stem cell transplantation after non-myeloablative preparative regimens: Impact of pretransplantation and posttransplantation factors on outcome. *J Clin Oncol, 19*, 3340–3349.

Mitchell, S.A. (2004). Graft versus host disease. In S. Ezzone (Ed.). *Hematopoietic Stem Cell Transplantation: A Manual for Nursing Practice* (pp. 85–131). Pittsburgh, PA: Oncology Nursing Society.

Mookerjee, B., Altomonte, V., Vogelsang, G. (1999). Salvage therapy for refractory chronic graft-versus-host disease with mycophenolate mofetil and tacrolimus. *Bone Marrow Transplant, 24*(5), 517–520.

Mori, M., Beatty, P.G., Graves, M., Boucher, K.M., Milford, E.L. (1997). HLA gene and haplotype frequencies in the North American population: The National Marrow Donor Program Donor Registry. *Transplantation, 64*, 1017–1027.

Nash, R., Pepe, M.S., Storb, R. (1992). Acute graft versus host disease: Analysis of risk factors after allogeneic marrow transplantation and prophylaxis with cyclosporine and methotrexate. *Blood, 8*, 1838–1845.

Nash, R.A., Antin, J.H., Karanes, C., Fay, J.W., Avalos, B.R., Yeager, A.M., et al. (2000). Phase 3 study comparing methotrexate and tacrolimus with methotrexate and cyclosporine for prophylaxis of acute graft-versus-host disease after marrow transplantation from unrelated donors. *Blood, 96*(6), 2062–2068.

Neumann, F., Graef, T., Tapprich, C., Vaupel, M., Steidl, U., Germing, U. (2005). Cyclosporine A and mycophenolate mofetil vs cyclosporine A and methotrexate for graft-versus-host disease prophylaxis after stem cell transplantation from HLA-identical siblings. *Bone Marrow Transplant, 35*(11), 1089–1093.

Nevo, S., Enger, C., Swan, V., Wojno, R.J., Fuller, A.K., Altomonte, V., et al. (1999). Acute bleeding after allogeneic bone marrow transplantation: Association with graft versus host disease and effect on survival. *Transplantation, 67*, 681–689.

Parkman, R. (1993). Is chronic graft-versus-host disease an autoimmune disease? *Curr Opin Immunol, 5*(5), 800–803.

Perez-Simon, J.A., Martino, R., Alegre, A., Tomas, J.F., De Leon, A., Caballero, D., et al. (2003). Chronic but not acute graft-versus-host disease improves outcome in multiple myeloma patients after non-myeloablative allogeneic transplantation. *Brit J Haematol, 121*(1), 104–108.

Petersdorf, E.W., Hansen, J.A., Martin, P.J., Woolfrey, A., Malkki, M., Gooley, T, et al. (2001). Major-histocompatibility-complex class I alleles and antigens in hematopoietic-cell transplantation. *N Eng J Med, 345*, 1794–1800.

Ponec, R.J., Hackman, R.C., McDonald, G.B. (1999). Endoscopic and histologic diagnosis of intestinal graft-versus-host disease after marrow transplantation. *Gastrointest Endosc, 49*, 612–621.

Przepiorka, D., Anderlini, P., Saliba, R., Cleary, K., Mehra, R., Khouri, I., et al. (2001). Chronic graft-versus-host disease after allogeneic blood stem cell transplantation. *Blood, 98*(6), 1695–1700.

Przepiorka, D., Kernan, N.A., Ippoliti, C., Papadopoulos, E.B., Giralt, S., Khouri, I., et al. (2000). Daclizumab, a humanized anti-interleukin-2 receptor alpha chain antibody, for treatment of acute graft-versus-host disease. *Blood, 95*, 83–89.

Przepiorka, D., Weisdorf, D., Martin, P., Klingmann, H., Beatty, P., Hows, J., et al. (1995). 1994 consensus conference on acute GVHD grading. *Bone Marrow Tranplant, 15*, 825–828.

Ralph, D.D., Springmeyer, S.C., Sullivan, K.M., Hackman, R.C., Sturb, R., Thomas, E.P. (1984). Rapidly progressive air-flow obstruction in marrow transplant recipients: Possible association between obliterative bronchiolitis and chronic graft-versus-host disease. *Am Rev Respir Dis, 129*, 641–644.

Ringden, O., Deeg, H.G. (1997). Clinical spectrum of graft-versus-host disease. In Ferrara, J.L.M., Deeg,

H.J., Burakoff, S.J. (Eds). *Graft versus Host Disease* (pp. 525–550). New York: Dekker.

Ruutu, T., Volin, L., Parkkali, T., Juvonen, E., Elonen, E. (2000). Cyclosporine, methotrexate, and methylprednisolone compared with cyclosporine and methotrexate for the prevention of graft-versus-host disease in bone marrow transplantation from HLA-identical sibling donor: A prospective randomized study. *Blood, 96*, 2391–2398.

Schmitz, H., Fromm, M., Bode, H., Scholz, P., Riecken, E.O., Schulzke, J.D. (1996). Tumor necrosis factor-alpha induces Cl and K secretion in human distal colon driven by prostaglandin E2. *Am J Physiol Gastrointest Liver Physiol, 271*, G669–G674.

Seaton, E.D., Szydlo, R.M., Kanfer, E., Apperley, J.F., Russell-Jones, R. (2003). Influence of extracorporeal photopheresis on clinical and laboratory parameters in chronic graft-versus-host disease and analysis of predictors of response. *Blood, 102*(4), 1217–1223.

Sharples, L.D., Tamm, M., McNeil, K., Higenbottam, T.W., Stewart, S., Wallwork, J. (1996). Development of bronchiolitis obliterans syndrome in recipients of heart-lung transplantation: Early risk factors. *Transplantation, 61*, 560–566.

Shaughnessy, P.J., Bachier, C., Grimley, M., Freytes, C.O., Callander, N.S., Essell, J.H., et al. (2005). Denileukin difitox for the treatment of steroid-resistant acute graft-versus-host disease. *Biol Blood Marrow Transplant, 11*(3), 188–193.

Shulman, H.M., Sullivan, K.M., Weiden, P.L., McDonald, G.B., Striker, G.E., Sale, G.E., et al. (1980). Chronic graft-versus-host disease in man. *Am J Pathol, 92*, 545–570.

Snover, D.C., Weisdorf, S.A., Vercellotti, G.M., Rank, B., Hutton, S., McGlave, P. (1985). A histopathologic study of gastric and small intestinal graft-versus-host disease following allogeneic bone marrow transplantation. *Hum Pathol, 16*(4), 387–392.

Socie, G., Salooja, N., Cohen, A., Rovelli, A., Carreras, E., Locasciulli, A., et al. (2003). Nonmalignant late effects after allogeneic stem cell transplantation. *Blood, 101*(9), 3373–3385.

Spitzer, T.R., Delmonico, F., Tolkoff-Rubin, N., McAfee, S., Sacksein, R., Saidman, S., et al. (1999). Combined histocompatibility leukocyte antigen-matched donor bone marrow and renal transplantation for multiple myeloma with end stage renal disease: The induction of allograft tolerance through mixed lymphohematopoietic chimerism. *Transplantation, 68*(4), 480–484.

Spitzer, T.R., McAfee, S., Sacksein, R., Colby, C., Toh, H.C., Multani, P., et al. (2003). Intentional induction of mixed chimerism and achievement of antitumor responses after nonmyeloablative conditioning therapy and HLA-matched donor bone marrow transplantation for refractory hematologic malignancies. *Biol Blood Marrow Transplant, 6*(Suppl 3), 309–320.

Stewart, B.L., Storer, B., Storek, J., Deeg, H.J., Storb, R., Hansen, J.A., et al. (2004). Duration of immunosuppressive treatment for chronic graft-versus-host disease. *Blood, 104*(12), 3501–3506.

Storb, R. (1986). Graft-versus-host disease after marrow transplantation. In *Transplantation: Approaches in Graft Rejection* (p. 139). New York: Alan R. Liss.

Sullivan, K.M. (1999). Graft-versus-host-disease. In Thomas, E.D., Blume, K.G., Forman, S.J. (Eds.). *Hematopoietic Cell Transplantation* (2nd ed., pp. 515–536). Malden, MA: Blackwell Science, Inc.

Sullivan, K.M., Agura, E., Anasetti, C., Appelbaum, F., Badger, C., Bearman, S., et al. (1991). Chronic graft-versus-host disease in other late complications of bone marrow transplantation. *Semin Hematol, 28*(3), 250–259.

Sullivan, K.M., Witherspoon, R., Storb, A., Deeg, H.J., Dahlberg, S., Sanders, J.E., et al. (1988). Prednisone and azathioprine compared with prednisone and placebo for treatment of chronic graft-versus-host disease: Prognostic influence of prolonged thrombocytopenia after allogeneic marrow transplantation. *Blood, 72*, 546–554.

Sutherland, H.J., Fyles, G.M., Adams, G., Hao, Y., Lipton, J.H., Minden, M.D., et al. (1997). Quality of life following bone marrow transplantation: A comparison of patient reports with population norms. *Bone Marrow Transplant, 19*, 1129–1136.

Thompson, A.M., Couch, M., Zahurak, M.L., Johnson, C., Vogelsang, G.B. (2002). Risk factors for post stem cell transplant sinusitis. *Bone Marrow Transplant, 29*, 257–261.

Ustun, C., Arslan, O., Beksac, M., Koc, H., Gurman, G., et al. (1999). A retrospective comparison of allogeneic peripheral blood stem cell and bone marrow transplant results from a single center: A focus on the incidence of graft-vs-host disease and relapse. *Biol Blood Marrow Transplant, 5*(1), 28–35.

Van Lint, M.T., Uderzo, C., Locasciulli, A., et al. (1998). Early treatment of acute graft-versus-host disease with high- or low-dose 6-methylprednisolone: A multicenter randomized trial from the Italian Group for Bone Marrow Transplantation. *Blood, 92*, 2288–2293.

Vogelsang, G.B. (2001). How I treat chronic graft-versus-host disease. *Blood, 97*(5), 1196–1201.

Vogelsang, G.B., Arai, S. (2001). Mycophenolate mofetil for the prevention and treatment of graft-versus-host disease following stem cell transplantation: Preliminary findings. *Bone Marrow Transplant, 27*, 1255–1262.

Vogelsang, G.B., Farmer, E.R., Hess, A.D., Altomonte, V., Beschorner, W.E., Jabs, D.A., et al. (1992). Thalidomide for the treatment of chronic graft-versus-host disease. *N Engl J Med, 326*(16), 1055–1058.

Vogelsang, G.B., Lee, L., Bensen-Kennedy, D.B. (2003). Pathogenesis and treatment of graft versus host disease after bone marrow transplant. *Ann Rev Med, 52*, 29–52.

Vogelsang, G.B., Morris, L.E. (1993). Prevention and management of graft-versus-host disease. Practical recommendations. *Drugs, 45*(5), 668–676.

Weinberg, K., Annett, G., Kashyap, A., Lenarsky, C., Forman, S.J., Parkman, R. (1995). The effect of thymic function on immunocompetence following bone marrow transplantation. *Biol Blood Marrow Transplant, 1*(1), 18–23.

Weinberg, K., Blazar, B.R., Wagner, J.E., Agura, E., Hill, B.J., Smogorzewska, M., et al. (2001). Factors affecting thymic function after allogeneic hematopoietic stem cell transplantation. *Blood, 97*, 1458–1466.

Weisdorf, D., Haake, R., Blazar, B., Miller, W., McGlave, P., Ramsay, N., et al. (1990). Treatment of moderate/severe acute graft-versus-host disease after allogeneic bone marrow transplantation: An analysis of clinical risk features and outcome. *Blood, 75*(4), 1024–1030.

Williams, L. (2004). Comprehensive review of hematopoiesis and immunology: Implications for hematopoietic stem cell recipients. In Ezzone, S. (Ed.). *Hematopoietic Stem Cell Transplantation: A Manual for Nursing Practice* (pp. 1–12). Pittsburgh, PA: Oncology Nursing Society.

Wingard, J., Piantadosi, S., Vogelsang, G., Farmer, E.R., Jabs, D.A., Levin, L.S., et al. (1989). Predictors of death from chronic graft versus host disease after bone marrow transplantation. *Blood, 74*, 1428–1435.

Chapter 7

Hematologic Effects of Transplantation

Shelley Burcat, RN, MSN

Francis McAdams, RN, MSN, AOCN®

Hematopoietic dysfunction remains a major complication of hematopoietic stem cell transplantation (HSCT). Patients undergoing HSCT receive chemotherapy and/or radiotherapy as part of the conditioning regimen. These treatments eradicate hematopoietic function, resulting in profound pancytopenia and immune dysfunction (Schuening et al., 1994; Storb, 2003; Devine et al., 2003; Centers for Disease Control and Prevention et al., 2000).

During the time of pancytopenia, patients are at risk for complications such as infection and bleeding. The greater the degree and the longer the duration of pancytopenia, the greater the associated morbidity and mortality. The use of colony stimulating factors and newer transplant regimens have lessened the duration of neutropenia but not eliminated it. The delayed immune reconstitution and donor lymphoid chimerism seen with nonmyeloablative HSCT may be associated with changes in the pattern of infections seen in these patients (Yeager, 2004; Junghanss et al., 2002).

Nurses must be knowledgeable about hematologic side effects of transplantation. Assessments should be done for anticipated as well as unexpected reactions (Ford and Eisenberg, 1990). Appropriate nursing interventions can minimize or eliminate complications. This chapter provides an overview of common hematologic complications associated with HSCT.

Hematologic Effects

Leukopenia and Neutropenia

In patients who receive transplants, treatment-related factors may produce profound leukopenia, or a decrease in the number of circulating white blood cells to fewer than 100 cells per microliter (Lin et al., 1993). High-dose chemotherapy causes both neutropenia and lymphopenia, a decrease in the number of lymphocytes in the blood. Stem cells and immature neutrophils and lymphocytes in the process of differentiation are the most sensitive to the effects of chemotherapy.

Total body irradiation (TBI) may be used to ablate marrow function in HSCT patients. Radiation causes marrow suppression due to the inclusion in the active radiation field sites of bone marrow (skull, sternum, ribs, vertebrae, pelvis, and long bones). Radiation therapy destroys stem cells; therefore, the duration of neutropenia is prolonged. The patterns of neutropenia seen with chemotherapy may be exaggerated or prolonged when radiation therapy is administered prior to or during chemotherapy. In addition, certain marrow-purging techniques interfere with hematopoietic function, resulting in prolongation of the neutropenic recovery period (Shafer, 1993).

Other factors may also complicate neutropenia in some transplant patients. Protein-calorie malnutrition is associated with the gastrointestinal side effects of chemotherapy and radiation therapy; the effects include anorexia, taste alterations, stomatitis, esophagitis, nausea, vomiting, and diarrhea. Disruption of the integrity of the skin or mucous membranes, as well as failure to provide an adequate protective environment, may also complicate the neutropenic period by predisposing the patient to infection (Caudell and Whedon, 1991). The immunosuppressive effects of steroids can also predispose the patient to complications during the neutropenic period by inhibiting the inflammatory response and by causing impaired cell-mediated immunity and protein-calorie malnutrition through increased catabolism (Shafer, 1993).

Infection remains a leading cause of death among allogeneic transplants and is a major cause of morbidity among autologous HSCT recipients (Centers for Disease Control and Prevention et al., 2000; Devine et al., 2003). Infection occurs when the body or a specific anatomical site is invaded by pathogenic microbes (bacteria, viruses, protozoa, fungi, or yeast) that have the ability to multiply under favorable conditions and cause cellular injury or destruction (Shafer, 1993). Increased susceptibility to infection is a characteristic complication of HSCT. Immediately after transplant, risks are loss of barrier integrity and agranulocytosis. After neutrophil recovery, defects in both cell-mediated and humoral immunity predominate. It can take 2 years or longer for immunologic reconstitution to be complete (Antin, 2002). The risk of infection in transplant patients is divided into three phases: 1) the pre-engraftment phase; 2) the early postengraftment phase; and 3) the late postengraftment phase. Each phase is characterized by a susceptibility to infection correlating with the state of immune recovery that occurs during that post-HSCT time frame (Spitzer, 2003). The predominant host problem during the pre-engraftment phase (within 30 days after transplantation) is neutropenia (Wujcik et al., 1994; Nash, 2003). The infections most commonly seen at this time are bacterial and fungal, similar to those seen in neutropenic patients with leukemia (Shaffer and Wilson, 1993).

Bacterial Infections

Bacterial infections may complicate HSCT at any time but pose a particular risk when the patient is neutropenic. The main sources of infection include central venous catheters, oral flora, and gut flora via bacterial translocation (Sullivan et al., 2001; Spitzer and Anderlini, 2002; Devine et al., 2003). Prophylactic use of antibiotics has shifted the spectrum of gastrointestinal flora to potentially pathogenic organisms like clostridium difficile. Agents of bacteremia include coagulase-negative staphylococci, viridans streptococci, and less common, though more virulent, gram-negative bacilli (Van Burik and Weisdorf, 1999). Gram-positive organisms are responsible for one half of the bacteremias that occur after HSCT. Gram-negative organisms are the second most common cause of bloodstream infection (Van Burik and Weisdorf, 1999).

There are no specific recommendations about the use of prophylactic antibiotics in the HSCT patient. If a physician chooses to use prophylactic antibiotics among asymptomatic, afebrile, neutropenic recipients, he or she should weigh the potential immediate benefit against the longer-term consequence (Sullivan et al., 2001). He or she should also routinely review hospital and HSCT center antibiotic susceptibility profiles, particularly when using a single antibiotic for antibacterial prophylaxis (Centers for Disease Control and Prevention et al., 2000). Because of the potential severity of antibiotic-resistant infections, particularly among HSCT recipients, every effort should be made to use preventive antibacterials with restraint (Sullivan et al., 2001).

The progression of infection in neutropenic patients can be rapid, and such patients with early bacterial infections cannot be reliably distinguished from noninfected patients at presentation. Empirical antibiotic therapy should be administered promptly to all neutropenic patients at the onset of fever (Hughes et al., 2002). Afebrile patients who have signs or symptoms compatible with an infection should also have empirical antibiotic therapy begun in the same manner as do febrile patients (Hughes et al., 2002). In the setting of changing flora and susceptibility patterns to antibiotics, guidelines as to best therapy for infection in the neutropenic patient must be evaluated on the basis of local patterns of infection and local and regional resistance patterns (Donowitz et al., 2001). Several standard regimen choices for antibiotic therapy listed in **Table 7-1** are associated with response rates of 65–85%, without modification of the initial regimen (Donowitz et al., 2001).

Table 7-1 STANDARD ANTIBIOTIC REGIMENS FOR TREATMENT OF BACTERIAL INFECTIONS.

Aminoglycoside + antipseudomonal penicillin
Aminoglycoside + extended spectrum
   cephalosporin
Aminoglycoside + quinolone
Vancomycin + anti-pseudomonal penicillin
Vancomycin + quinolone
Double β-lactam combination
Carbapenem or extended spectrum
   cephalosporins

Fungal Infections

Fungal infections in the HSCT patient population are difficult to diagnose and treat and are associated with high mortality rates. Fungal infections can be divided into three general categories: invasive infection due to *Candida* and *Aspergillus* species, which account for > 90% of fungal infections occurring in the HSCT population; infection due to geographically restricted systemic mycoses (e.g., *Blastomyces dermatitides, Coccidioides immitis*, and *Histoplasma capsulatum*); and invasive infection due to newly emerging fungi (e.g., *Fusarium, Paecilomyces,* the *Zygomycetes,* and such dematiaceous fungi as *Scedosporium, Scopulariopsis*, and *Dactylaria* (Sullivan et al., 2001). The mortality rate of established invasive fungal infections in recipients of allografts remains unacceptably high despite administration of newer antifungal drugs (Brown, 2004).

Risk factors in the development of invasive fungal infections include disruption of anatomical barriers, including placement of central venous catheter (CVC) and mucositis. Another risk factor is the state of immunosuppression of the patient, which includes duration of neutropenia, GVHD and its treatment, administration of corticosteroids, broad-spectrum antibiotic use, and immunomodulating viral infections, as well as protein-calorie malnutrition, uremia, and possibly hyperglycemia (Sullivan et al., 2001; Donowitz et al., 2001). It is important to be aware of sources of nosocomial transmission, which can be found in areas of construction, as well as the need for good hand washing (Sullivan et al., 2001; Marr, 2001). *Aspergillus* infections are associated with long duration of neutropenia, use of corticosteroids and other immunosuppressants, and chronic GVHD (Donowitz et al., 2001). The pattern of risk for *Aspergillus* infection has been described as bimodal but may be trimodal, as patients are developing *Aspergillus* very late post-HSCT (> 180 days) (Marr, 2001).

General recommendations for the prevention of exposure to fungal pathogens include instructing HSCT patients to avoid certain areas and substances, including foods that might increase risk for fungal exposure. This includes avoiding areas of high dust, construction, occupations involving soil, and foods that contain molds (e.g., blue cheese) (Centers for Disease Control and Prevention et al., 2000). Because *Aspergillus* species are ubiquitous and found in the air, avoidance is unlikely. It is important to be aware of sources of nosocomial transmission (areas of construction) and be aware of extended risk in allogeneic HSCT patients with GVHD (Marr, 2001).

There are three modes in which antifungal drugs can be administered to prevent invasive fungal infection: prophylactic mode, empiric mode, and preemptive mode (Sullivan et al., 2001). Administration of topical (nonabsorbable) antifungal agents to the skin has been shown to decrease the colonizing fungal burden, particularly with yeasts, when applied to specific skin sites or the gastrointestinal tract. Mucosal manifestations of superficial yeast infection are probably decreased by topical therapy. However, such topical therapy does not reduce the incidence of either invasive candidiasis or invasive mold infection (Sullivan et al., 2001).

Prophylactic administration of fluconazole 400 mg/day orally or intravenously beginning at the time of HSCT and continuing until at least the time of engraftment provides clinically important protection against invasive yeast infection. If breakthrough candidal infection occurs despite such a regimen, it should be assumed that the isolate is fluconazole resistant. The increasing incidence of *C. krusei, C. glabrata*, and other non-albicans strains is in large part related to the widespread use of fluconazole prophylaxis (Sullivan et al., 2001).

Itraconazole is another antifungal currently available for use for prophylaxis of fungal yeast infections. It has activity against *C. albicans* and non-albicans spp., *A. flavus, A. fumigatus, B. dermatitidis*, and *H. capsulatum* and is available in well-absorbed oral and IV formulations. Satisfactory and predictable levels were obtained in most patients in one pharmacokinetic study using itraconazole capsules at a dose of 600 mg/day (Prentice and Donnelly, 2001). Absorption of the capsule form of intraconazole is improved when the drug is taken with food. Absorption of the capsule formulation is reduced when taken with H2 antagonists and in patients with severe mucositis or GVHD (Prentice and Donnelly, 2001). Currently there is a lack of data regarding toxicities and drug interactions. Amphotericin B is only available intravenously, and its primary disadvantage as a prophylactic agent is its toxicities. Lipid formulations of amphotericin B have less toxicity but are expensive for prophylactic administration (Marr, 2001). No regimen has been shown to be clearly effective in the prevention of invasive mold infection, which makes environmental protection strategies important for the HSCT patient (Sullivan et al., 2001).

Early initiation of empiric fungal therapy for the febrile neutropenic HSCT patient has become the standard of care. Empiric therapy is defined as the initiation of systemic antifungal therapy to neutropenic patients who remain febrile after 4 days of empiric broad-spectrum antibacterial therapy and whose clinical laboratory evaluation remains negative (Sullivan et al., 2001). Amphotericin B has been established as the therapy of choice for empiric treatment of invasive fungal infections. Recently, liposomal amphotericin B has been shown to have equal efficacy to conventional amphotericin B, with significantly less infusion-related toxicity and dose-related nephrotoxicity, but at greater cost (Sullivan et al., 2001). In a recent study, liposomal amphotericin at 3 mg/kg/day was compared to voriconazole at a dose of 3 mg/kg twice a day intravenously (or 200 mg orally) following two loading doses of 6 mg/kg every 12. Voriconazole, a new broad-spectrum triazole agent available in oral and intravenous formulations, was equal or superior to liposomal amphotericin (Sullivan et al., 2001). Empiric therapy of the febrile, neutropenic HSCT patient has been accepted as standard care. Amphotericin B, liposomal amphotericin B, and voriconazole have comparable efficacy (Sullivan et al., 2001). Caspofungin has also been shown to be as effective and better tolerated than liposomal amphotericin B when given as empirical antifungal therapy in patients with persistent fever and neutropenia (Walsh et al., 2004).

Caspofungin is the first echinocandin available for clinical use. A small, unpublished experience with caspofungin for salvage therapy of invasive aspergillosis was the background for FDA approval. In spite of having demonstrated that these drugs work by inhibiting growth of hyphal cells, there is concern over the utility of caspofungin as a single agent for primary therapy. Caspofungin has demonstrated equal efficacy to amphotericin B for the treatment of invasive *Candida* infections (Marr, 2003).

Preemptive therapy is defined as the administration of an antimicrobial regimen to a patient population felt to be at high risk of life-threatening infection before the onset of a clinically recognizable event (Sullivan et al., 2001). Three opportunities for preemptive fungal therapy have been described. First, colonization of the respiratory tract with *Aspergillus* species as demonstrated by positive cultures of respiratory secretions. The problem with this approach is absence of early colonization in a significant percentage of patients and lack of clear-cut information as to which is the best regimen for accomplishing preemptive therapy (Sullivan et al., 2001). Second, high-resolution computerized tomographic scans of the lungs at regular intervals in HSCT patients during periods of high risk for invasive aspergillosis can result in earlier diagnosis of disease and the opportunity for preemptive therapy (Sullivan et al., 2001). Finally, detection of fungal antigens or fungal metabolites could give early evidence of invasive infection at a time when therapy would be most effective. PCR-based assays that will detect both yeast and mold are of particular interest (Sullivan et al., 2001). Screening studies on the detection of circulating galactomannan with aspergillus galactomannan antigenassay showed galactomannan detection had a sensitivity and specificity > 90% for the diagnosis of aspergillosis, and antigenemia preceded antifungal therapy in most patients (Marr, 2003). Because of these studies, the U.S. Food and Drug Administration has approved the galactomannan enzyme immunoassay using the Platelia *Aspergillus* test as an aid to diagnose aspergillosis. Continued research is needed to evaluate this assay for different patient populations (Marr, 2003). A number of groups are also developing PCR assays to diagnose multiple fungal infections (Marr, 2003).

Viral Infections

If viral infection occurs, reactivation of a latent virus is the most common cause. Herpes viruses include herpes simplex virus (HSV) types I and II, cytomegalovirus (CMV), and varicella-zoster (VZ). Reactivation of herpes simplex virus can be reduced from 80% to less than 5% among HSV-seropositive recipients by initiating acy-

clovir treatment at the time of conditioning and continuing until mucositis has diminished (Van Burik and Weisdorf, 1999). Valacyclovir may be used instead of oral acyclovir (Sullivan et al., 2001).

In the preengraftment period, infections of HSV type I are manifested by oral ulcerative mucositis, and type II reactivation appears as genital or extragenital vesicles. Because oral ulceration is a common side effect of chemotherapy and irradiation, a viral culture is necessary to distinguish viral etiology. Although acyclovir is highly effective when given as prophylaxis and treatment, there is evidence of an increasing frequency of acyclovir-resistant herpes viruses (McLaren et al., 1985; Englund et al., 1990; Van Burik and Weisdorf, 1999). In cases of acyclovir-resistant herpes virus, foscarnet may be indicated (Van Burik and Weisdorf, 1999).

At 30 to 100 days posttransplant (the early postengraftment phase), patients are at risk for infection from viruses, principally cytomegalovirus and herpes simplex, and intracellular

---

Table 7-2 CDC RECOMMENDATIONS FOR PREVENTION OF EXPOSURE TO CMV INFECTIONS IN THE HSCT RECIPIENT.

1. HSCT candidates should be tested for the presence of serum anti-CMV IgG antibodies before transplantation to determine risk for primary CMV infection and reactivation after HSCT.
2. HSCT recipients should avoid sharing drinking glasses and eating utensils with others.
3. Sexually active patients should wear a latex condom during sexual contact.
4. HSCT recipients should practice regular hand-washing, especially after handling or changing a diaper or wiping oral or nasal secretions.
5. CMV seronegative recipients of allogeneic transplant should receive leukocyte-reduced or seronegative blood products.

Source: Centers for Disease Control and Prevention et al. (2000). Guidelines for preventing opportunistic infections among hematopoietic stem cell transplant recipients. *Biol Blood Morrow Transplant,* 6(6a), 659–713; and Sullivan, K.M., et al. (2001). Preventing opportunistic infections after hematopoietic stem cell transplantation: The Centers for Disease Control and Prevention, Infectious Diseases Society of America and American Society for Blood and Marrow Transplantation practice guidelines and beyond. *Hematology,* 392–421.

Table 7-3 CDC RECOMMENDATIONS FOR PREVENTION OF CMV DISEASE AND/OR RECURRENCE.

1. CMV disease prevention program for all HSCT recipients who are CMV-positive or have a CMV-positive donor, from the time of engraftment until day 100.
2. Physicians should use either prophylaxis or preemptive treatment with ganciclovir for allogeneic recipients.
3. CMV surveillance and preemptive therapy if CMV viremia or antigenemia is detected or if the recipient has two consecutively positive CMV-DNA PCR tests.
4. IVIG or CMV-IVIG for prevention of CMV infection and disease.
5. High-dose acyclovir for prevention of CMV infection and disease in HSCT recipients with positive CMV antigenemia.

Sources: Centers for Disease Control and Prevention et al. (2000). Guidelines for preventing opportunistic infections among hematopoietic stem cell transplant recipients. *Biol Blood Morrow Transplant,* 6(6a), 659–713; 715; 717–727; and Sullivan, K.M., et al. (2001). Preventing opportunistic infections after hematopoietic stem cell transplantation: The Centers for Disease Control and Prevention, Infectious Diseases Society of America and American Society for Blood and Marrow Transplantation practice guidelines and beyond. *Hematology,* 392–421.

organisms such as mycobacteria, fungi, and protozoa (Wingard, 1990; Winston and Gale, 1991; Van Burik and Weisdorf, 1999). Illnesses may be the result of a new infection in seronegative patients or represent reactivation in a seropositive patient. These infections are related to deficient cell-mediated immunity. Neutrophil recovery has usually occurred by this time. Immunologic recovery is related to delayed recovery of the immune system, immunosuppressive therapy, and/or acute graft-versus-host-disease (GVHD) in allogeneic patients (Atkinson, 1990; Wingard, 1990).

CMV infections have been reduced from 40% to less than 3% in the CMV-seronegative HSCT recipient with the use of seronegative or leukocyte-filtered blood products for transfusions (Van Burik and Weisdorf, 1999; Tabbara et al., 2002). Strategies to prevent new CMV infections or disease reactivation include ganciclovir administered prophylactically from time of engraftment until day 100 (Sullivan et al.,

Table 7-4 CDC GUIDELINES FOR PREVENTION OF EXPOSURE TO HSV DISEASE.

1. HSCT candidates should be tested for serum anti-HSV IgG prior to transplant.
2. HSCT candidates should be educated about methods of prevention for HSV infections.
3. HSCT recipients should be counseled in the use of latex condoms with sexual activity.
4. Contact isolation should be enacted for patients with disseminated primary or severe mucocutaneous HSV disease.

Sources: Centers for Disease Control and Prevention et al. (2000). Guidelines for preventing opportunistic infections among hematopoietic stem cell transplant recipients. *Biol Blood Morrow Transplant,* 6(6a), 659–713; 715; 717–727; and Sullivan, K.M., et al. (2001). Preventing opportunistic infections after hematopoietic stem cell transplantation: The Centers for Disease Control and Prevention, Infectious Diseases Society of America and American Society for Blood and Marrow Transplantation practice guidelines and beyond. *Hematology,* 392–421.

Table 7-5 CDC GUIDELINES FOR PREVENTION OF PRIMARY HSV DISEASE OR RECURRENCE OF HSV.

1. Acyclovir prophylaxis for all allogeneic HSCT recipients who are HSV-seropositive.
2. HSV prophylaxis with acyclovir at the start of conditioning therapy and continuing until engraftment or mucositis resolves, whichever is longer.

Sources: Centers for Disease Control and Prevention et al. (2000). Guidelines for preventing opportunistic infections among hematopoietic stem cell transplant recipients. *Biol Blood Morrow Transplant,* 6(6a), 659–713; 715; 717–727; and Sullivan, K.M., et al. (2001). Preventing opportunistic infections after hematopoietic stem cell transplantation: The Centers for Disease Control and Prevention, Infectious Diseases Society of America and American Society for Blood and Marrow Transplantation practice guidelines and beyond. *Hematology,* 392–421.

2001; Van Burik and Weisdorf, 1999). Preemptive dosing of ganciclovir is 5 mg/kg twice a day for 7 to 14 days followed by maintenance with 5 mg/kg/day until day 100 (Van Burik and Weisdorf, 1999). The strategy involves virologic surveillance using antigenemia or PCR-guided detection methods and starting ganciclovir for early evidence of subclinical CMV infection (Sullivan et al., 2001; Van Burik and Weisdorf, 1999). Late CMV disease is an emerging problem in HSCT recipients given ganciclovir prophylaxis or preemptive therapy. Risk factors for late CMV disease include chronic GVHD, low CD4 counts ($< 50/mm^3$), and CMV infection before day 100 (Sullivan et al., 2001). End-organ manifestations of CMV disease, including pneumonia, enteritis, and retinitis, are treated with an extended course of ganciclovir induction therapy (14 to 21 days) followed by a maintenance dosage. For CMV pneumonia, ganciclovir treatment is combined with intravenous immune globulin (IVIG), 500 mg/kg every other day for 14 to 21 days (Van Burik and Weisdorf, 1999).

Prevention of viral infections in the HSCT recipient includes risk assessment based on viral

Table 7-6 CDC GUIDELINES FOR PREVENTION OF VARICELLA-ZOSTER VIRUS (VZV) EXPOSURE.

1. HSCT candidates should be tested for the presence of serum anti-VZV IgG antibodies.
2. Educate all HSCT candidates about the seriousness of VZV infections and how to prevent exposure.
3. HSCT candidates and recipients who are VZV-seronegative or VZV-seropositive and immunocompromised should avoid exposure to persons with active VZV infections.
4. Family members, household contacts, and health-care workers who come in contact with HSCT recipients and who have no history of varicella infection and are VZV-negative should be immunized.
5. HSCT recipients who develop VZV should be placed on airborne and contact precautions.

Sources: Centers for Disease Control and Prevention et al. (2000). Guidelines for preventing opportunistic infections among hematopoietic stem cell transplant recipients. *Biol Blood Morrow Transplant,* 6(6a), 659–713; 715; 717–727; and Sullivan, K.M., et al. (2001). Preventing opportunistic infections after hematopoietic stem cell transplantation: The Centers for Disease Control and Prevention, Infectious Diseases Society of America and American Society for Blood and Marrow Transplantation practice guidelines and beyond. *Hematology,* 392–421.

Table 7-7 CDC GUIDELINES FOR PREVENTION OF PRIMARY VZV OR VZV
RECURRENCE.

1. VZV-seronegative HSCT recipients should be treated with varicella-zoster immune globulin
   (VZIG) within 96 hours of close contact or household contact of a person with either chickenpox or
   shingles.
2. All HSCT recipients or candidates undergoing conditioning therapy who experience a VZV-like
   rash should receive preemptive intravenous acyclovir until all lesions have crusted.

Sources: Centers for Disease Control and Prevention et al. (2000). Guidelines for preventing opportunistic infections among
hematopoietic stem cell transplant recipients. *Biol Blood Morrow Transplant,* 6(6a), 659–713; 715; 717–727; and Sullivan, K.M.,
et al. (2001). Preventing opportunistic infections after hematopoietic stem cell transplantation: The Centers for Disease Control
and Prevention, Infectious Diseases Society of America and American Society for Blood and Marrow Transplantation practice
guidelines and beyond. *Hematology,* 392–421.

and host factors as well as the time patterns of infections after transplant (Sullivan et al., 2001). (See **Tables 7-2, 7-3, 7-4, 7-5, 7-6, 7-7,** and **7-8.**)

Parasitic Infections

The incidence rate of *Pneumocystis carinii* pneumonia (PCP) was 7% in 1978, prior to the advent of trimethoprim-sulfamethoxazole (TMP-SMX). Prophylaxis with TMP-SMX has decreased the incidence of PCP to 0.2% (Boeckh, 2003). When infection with PCP occurs, it is usually because of an error in adherence to the prophylaxis schedule (Van Burik and Weisdorf, 1999). Current practice for prophylaxis of PCP in allogeneic recipients is to treat throughout all periods of immunocompromise after engraftment (CDC et al., 2000). Prophylaxis should be administered from engraftment until 6 months after HSCT. At 6 months, the patient's risk is assessed and patients who remain immunosuppressed or have

---

Table 7-8 CDC RECOMMENDATIONS FOR PREVENTION OF COMMUNITY
RESPIRATORY VIRUS INFECTION.

1. Infection-control guidelines should be instituted to minimize risk of community-acquired
   respiratory virus.
2. Clinical surveillance for community-acquired respiratory infections should be conducted on all
   hospitalized HSCT recipients and patients undergoing conditioning therapy.
3. Contact isolation should be enacted for all HSCT recipients with upper respiratory infection (URI)
   or lower respiratory infection (LRI) symptoms.
4. Family members, close household contacts, and health-care workers involved with HSCT recipients
   should receive influenza vaccinations.

Sources: Centers for Disease Control and Prevention et al. (2000). Guidelines for preventing opportunistic infections among
hematopoietic stem cell transplant recipients. *Biol Blood Morrow Transplant,* 6(6a), 659–713; 715; 717–727; and Sullivan, K.M.,
et al. (2001). Preventing opportunistic infections after hematopoietic stem cell transplantation: The Centers for Disease Control
and Prevention, Infectious Diseases Society of America and American Society for Blood and Marrow Transplantation practice
guidelines and beyond. *Hematology,* 392–421.

GVHD or delayed engraftment should continue on TMP-SMX (Boeckh, 2003; Spitzer, 2003).

TMP-SMX is associated with drug intolerance, neutropenia, gastrointestinal side effects, and rash. (Boeckh, 2003; Spitzer, 2003). These issues may be significant with up to 38% of patient's requiring alternative agents for PCP prophylaxis (Boeckh, 2003). For patients who are intolerant of TMP-SMX, desensitization with TMP-SMX can be attempted prior to using dapsone, inhaled pentamidine, or atovaquone (Van Burik and Weisdorf, 1999; Boeckh, 2003).

Dapsone is sometimes administered once daily as a 100 mg dose. Because high-peak serum levels may correlate with hematologic toxicity of dapsone, it is preferentially administered at a dosage of 50 mg twice daily (Boeckh, 2003). Dapsone is not recommended for patients with glucose-6-phosphate dehydrogenase deficiency. Other side effects include gastrointestinal adverse events, methemoglobinemia, and myelosuppression. Hemolytic anemia remains the most important side effect, but its clinical relevance cannot be evaluated because of a paucity of data on transfusional requirements after its onset (Boeckh, 2003).

Pentamidine may be administered either aerosolized or intravenously. Aerosolized pentamidine is administered at 300 mg once every 3 to 4 weeks via nebulizer. Nebulized pentamidine has a high prophylaxis failure rate. There are virtually no reports on the efficacy of intravenous pentamidine in the prophylaxis of PCP. Dosage of IV pentamidine is 4 mg/kg every other week (Boeckh, 2003).

Atovaquone is a new agent for prophylaxis of PCP in individuals who are unable to tolerate TMP-SMX. It has convenient once-daily dosing and published studies report fairly low incidence of side effects. The main disadvantage of atovaquone is its lack of antibacterial coverage. Because of its poor bioavailability as a capsule, it is currently available in a suspension formulation that is distasteful. Currently a number of studies are looking at the efficacy of atovaquone in the HSCT population (Spitzer, 2003)

Anemia

The intense antineoplastic regimens used in BMT create a deficiency in circulating red blood cells (anemia). Chemotherapy creates a hypoproliferative anemia because of its effects on the bone marrow. In addition, radiation therapy results in a decrease in production of red blood cells when certain treatment fields (pelvis, sternum, proximal ends of long bones) are included (Clark et al., 1987). Anemia is indicated by a reduction in the hemoglobin and hematocrit values. The effects of anemia include fatigue and dyspnea during exertion, as well as headache, dizziness, and irritability. As the anemia becomes more severe, tachycardia, tachypnea, hypotension, and tissue hypoxia can occur (Maxwell, 1984; Goodman, 1989).

Transfusional needs may be reduced in patients undergoing nonmyeloablative preparative regimens. As an example, in a comparative retrospective analysis, red cell transfusions were required in 63% versus 96% of those undergoing nonmyeloablative or myeloablative transplants, respectively (p ≤ 0.0001 for both) (Weissinger et al., 2001).

The indications for transfusion of blood products vary from center to center. With respect to transfusion of red cells, most centers use a hematocrit threshold of 30%. This threshold may be influenced by a number of factors, including the number of days from the transplant, the clinical condition of the patient, or evidence of engraftment of other cell types including reticulocytes. Patients with GVHD or those being treated with immunosuppressive drugs such as cyclosporine may have continued blood product requirements from bleeding and/or microangiopathic hemolysis (Bernstein et al., 1998).

A variety of techniques, including RBC antigen phenotyping and cytogenetic analysis, have been used to distinguish between a host or donor source for erythrocyte repopulation following allogeneic BMT (Bar et al., 1989). This information can be useful when attempting to distinguish between engraftment of donor marrow and regeneration of host marrow. If the RBCs are of host origin, it may be due to an inadequate conditioning regimen, and disease relapse may result (Caudell and Whedon, 1991). Return of normal hematopoiesis is generally first evidenced by the appearance of reticulocytes in the circulation (Griffin, 1986).

The reticulocyte maturation index (RMI), which has been used to study erythropoiesis, is another measurement of engraftment in autologous transplants and has been shown to detect engraftment sooner than the reticulocyte or the erythrocyte count. The RMI is a proportional measurement of reticulocyte maturity determined by the content of reticulocyte RNA using flow cytometric reticulocyte quantification with thiazole orange (Caudell and Whedon, 1991).

Thrombocytopenia

Thrombocytopenia is an abnormal decrease in the number of circulating platelets, and usually results in bleeding or hemorrhage. Platelets are critical to the process of hemostasis. They ensure the continued maintenance of vascular integrity, the initial arrest of bleeding by platelet plug formation, and the stabilization of clot formation (Bennett and Shattil, 1990). When thrombocytopenia is present, the most frequent sites of bleeding are the mucous membranes, skin, gastrointestinal system, respiratory system, genitourinary system, and intracranial area. Thrombocytopenia results when there is a decrease in the production of megakaryocytes, which are precursors of platelets. This can occur in transplant patients as a result of the toxic effects of chemotherapy on stem cells. Radiation therapy to the active sites of bone marrow function (skull, ribs, sternum, vertebrae, pelvis, and ends of long bones) can also result in a decreased platelet count (Petursson, 1993).

When the platelet count falls below $20,000/mm^3$, spontaneous hemorrhaging is a major clinical concern, and bruising, petechiae, and mucosal bleeding may be detectable. There is a strong association between intracranial bleeding and a platelet count of less than $5000/mm^3$ (Rostad, 1991).

Immune System Effects

Recovery of the immune system following HSCT is slow. WBC engraftment occurs within the first 3 to 4 weeks posttransplant (Lewis, 2002). Recovery of humoral and cell-mediated immunity with full lymphocyte function takes much longer. Therefore, patients are susceptible to viral and opportunistic infections for several months after autologous transplant and for up to years after allogeneic transplant. The CD4/CD8 lymphocyte ratio decreases very quickly after transplant, but remains abnormal for approximately one year posttransplant (Steingrimsdottir et al., 2000). Patients who receive CD34+ selected autologous peripheral blood stem cell transplant (PBSCTs) experience more immune dysfunction than patients receiving unselected autologous PBSCTs (Sica et al., 2001). For allogeneic transplants, the decrease starts slightly later, at about 2 weeks posttransplant, nadirs at 2 months, and does not begin to show recovery until 3 months posttransplant (Marin et al., 1999). NK cells are elevated posttransplant. Once again, they are slower to drop and rise in the allogeneic setting than in the autologous setting (Marin et al., 1999). B cells are severely depressed posttransplant in both autologous and allogeneic settings. They do not recover until more than 3 months posttransplant (Marin et al., 1999). Many factors influence the length of time and severity of immune dysfunction posttransplant. Among them are T cell depletion to prevent GVHD, HLA mismatch between donor and recipient, immunosuppressive therapy, and GVHD (Marin et al., 1999).

Graft Failure

Graft failure is the lack of functional hematopoiesis after marrow transplantation. Primary graft failure is the failure to establish hematopoiesis, and the causes may be multifactorial. In autologous transplants, this may be due to inadequate volume or quality of stem cells, which may be related to prior treatment, damage during collection, or cryopreservation. In allogeneic transplants, graft failure is especially common with the use of HLA-mismatched donor marrow or with transplantation of T cell–depleted marrow (Klumpp, 1991). In the absence of myelosuppressive drug therapy or infectious drug complications, primary graft failure should be attributed to rejection of the marrow allograft by residual immunocompetent cells in the patient (Filipovich et al., 1990; Anasetti et al., 1989; Kernan et al., 1987).

Secondary graft failure or graft rejection is the failure of functional hematopoiesis after the occurrence of transient hematopoiesis. This can be due to myelosuppression from medications or infections but is often rejection mediated by immunological factors (Kernan, 1988). Classically, the transient hematopoiesis that characterizes graft rejection is of donor origin. This is followed by an increase in the number of lymphocytes from the cells of host origin and either failure of all hematopoietic activity or the return of host hematopoiesis (Quinones, 1993).

It is often not possible to distinguish true graft rejection from intrinsic graft failure since they are so closely related. Another clinically similar syndrome is post-BMT autoimmune pancytopenia. Although rare, the latter syndrome is important to recognize because it may respond well to treatment with corticosteroids (Klumpp et al., 1990).

Therapy for graft rejection is often limited by difficulty in recognizing the complication in its early stages, because delayed engraftment can also be caused by infection and drug toxicity. The fragility of the new marrow and the lack of effective agents to prevent rejection also complicate treatment (Quinones, 1993).

Bleeding

Bleeding and anemia also require prompt attention and skill in order to prevent life-threatening emergencies. The preparative regimen used in full myeloablative transplants often results in profound thrombocytopenia and anemia. Platelet engraftment is delayed in patients who develop GVHD (First et al., 1985), those on cyclosporine (Bensinger et al., 1989), and those whose marrow has been purged (Ball et al., 1990; Korbling et al., 1989). The administration of myelosuppressive medications such as methotrexate, trimethoprim-sulfamethoxazone, ganciclovir, and interferon also contributes to poor graft function and the resulting thrombocytopenia and anemia (Storb, 1989). Coagulation abnormalities resulting from hepatotoxicity, GVHD, disseminated intravascular coagulation (DIC), and/or sepsis may also contribute to abnormal bleeding (Oncology Nursing Society, 1994). Other risk factors include venoocclusive disease with impaired production of coagulation factors (Ballard, 1991), altered mucosal barriers (Vanacek, 1991), viral infections (Cahn et al., 1989), and ABO incompatible allogeneic BMT (Petz, 1989).

The nursing management of patients at risk for bleeding begins with a thorough assessment for signs and symptoms of bleeding. Laboratory data including red blood cell count, hemoglobin, hematocrit, platelet count, and coagulation studies are closely monitored at least daily. Bleeding episodes can be minimized by the avoidance of unnecessary invasive procedures such as enemas, rectal temperatures, suppositories, bladder catheterizations, venipunctures, finger sticks, nasogastric tubes, and intramuscular or subcutaneous injections. Medications that inhibit platelet function such as aspirin-containing products are also to be avoided (Oncology Nursing Society, 1994).

Blood Product Support

The administration of blood products to transplant recipients is another essential component of their daily care during the first few weeks after transplant. It is imperative that nurses possess a thorough understanding of the rationale behind the administration of each specific blood product, as well as the special considerations required for administration. Because viable lymphocytes, which are thought to be capable of triggering GVHD, are present in all cellular transfusion products, irradiation is recommended in order to inactivate T lymphocytes (Petz and Scott, 1983). Leukocyte-reduction filters are used for packed red blood cells (PRBCs) and platelets to reduce exposure to HLA antigens (Sniecinski et al., 1988) and prevent adverse reactions as a result of the transfusions (Caudell and Whedon, 1991). CMV serologically tested negative blood products are given to patients who are CMV serologically negative. Because the virus is carried on the granulocyte, the risk of CMV infection may increase if CMV-positive products are used (Bowden et al., 1991; Petz and Scott, 1983).

Red blood cells (RBCs) are administered over 2 to 4 hours to patients with symptomatic anemia due to blood loss. It is expected that one unit of packed RBCs will increase the patient's hemoglobin to 1 gm/dl above the pretransfusion hemoglobin. It is important for RBCs to be ABO compatible. Leukocyte-poor or filtered RBCs are given to patients at risk for febrile transfusion reactions.

Platelets from random donors are given over 5 to 10 minutes per unit for bleeding due to thrombocytopenia. ABO compatibility is not required for platelet transfusions. Random donor platelets are not usually effective for BMT recipients who have received many platelet transfusions.

Platelets from a single donor are given over 20 to 60 minutes in order to increase the platelet count to 40,000 per unit. Single-donor platelets are given to patients who are bleeding due to thrombocytopenia and who possess antiplatelet antibodies. Single-donor platelets may be random or HLA matched. HLA-matched platelet products are indicated if a patient's platelet count fails to increase after multiple transfusions. Patients who receive multiple transfusions may develop lymphocytotoxic anti-HLA antibodies and platelet refractoriness (Fuller, 1990).

Fresh, frozen plasma, which contains plasma and all coagulation factors and complements, is given over 10 to 15 minutes. Coagulation factors are increased by 5% to 10% per unit. It is given for a coagulation factor deficiency or for disseminated intravascular coagulation (DIC). ABO compatibility is necessary when transfusing fresh, frozen plasma.

Cryoprecipitate contains plasma and stable clotting factors. It is given over 15 to 30 minutes and increases factor VIII, factor XIII, and fibrinogen levels. It is given to treat deficiencies of stable clotting factors (II, VII, IX, X, XI) and disseminated intravascular coagulation. ABO compatibility is preferred (Hardaway and Adams, 1989; Jassak and Godwin, 1991; Snyder, 1987; Oncology Nursing Society, 1994).

It is important to monitor ABO titers in patients who received ABO-incompatible marrow. The recipient's ABO type will change to that of the donor approximately 3 to 4 months after transplant. The titers are followed to determine when the ABO type of the transfusion is changed from the recipient's to the donor's type.

Nursing interventions are aimed at closely monitoring patient symptomatology regarding the need for blood products. Essential nursing care also includes assessing for signs and symptoms of bleeding and intervening to stop or minimize bleeding when and if it does occur, as well as educating patients and families regarding bleeding precautions. Other specific interventions are:

- testing urine, stool, and emesis for occult blood
- encouraging the use of a soft toothbrush and discouraging flossing
- administering topical agents such as thrombin, adrenaline, and cocaine to stop bleeding
- administering H2 antagonists to prevent ulcers and estrogen to prevent menstruation
- administering bladder irrigations and IV hydration for prevention and management of hemorrhagic cystisis
- applying pressure to sites of invasive procedures when possible (ONS, 1994)

The actual transfusion of blood products necessitates careful monitoring for adverse reactions. Premedication with an antipyretic and antihistamine and possibly a steroid are usually a routine part of the transfusion administration. Close monitoring of vital signs and patient symptoms is essential, especially during the first hour of transfusion (ONS, 1994).

Management of the HSCT Patient with Myelosuppression

Neutropenia

Prevention, early detection, and prompt management of infections in patients with neutropenia are essential if sepsis and septic shock are to be avoided. Neutrophil recovery and engraftment varies depending on type of transplant and stem cell source. Peripheral stem cells that have been mobilized with hematopoietic growth factors improve hematologic recovery after transplant in both the autologous and allogeneic setting (Johnson and Quiett, 2004; Beyer et al., 1995; Pavletic et al., 1997). Neutrophil reconstitution is uniformly reported to occur faster after allogeneic PBSCT than after bone marrow transplant (BMT). Reaching a neutrophil count greater than $0.5 \times 10^9/L$ takes between 15 and 23 days for most BMT patients and between 12 and 19 days for most PBSCT recipients (Korbling and Anderlini, 2001). Neutrophil recovery has been shown to be more rapid after granulocyte-colony stimulating factor (rhG-CSF) primed peripheral blood stem cells (PBSC) in patients who have undergone allogeneic transplant than in historical steady-state PBSC controls (Korbling and Anderlini, 2002). Umbilical cord blood transplant has been shown to have a low yield of stem cells resulting in higher rates of engraftment failure and slower time to engraftment compared to BMT (Cohena and Nagler, 2003).

It is important to be aware of some of the factors that place HSCT patients at a particularly high risk for infections; these are shown in **Table 7-9** (Buchsel, 1990; Donowitz et al., 2001). A thorough assessment is vital when patients are at risk for infection. A comprehensive physical assessment is performed at least every 4 to 8 hours, with special attention to catheter sites, lungs, integument, oral mucosa, and the rectal areas. Special attention is given to signs and symptoms of infection at common sites of occurrence. Temperature and vital signs are assessed for trends and deviations from the normal at least every 4 hours during the immediate post-HSCT phase. A complete blood count and absolute neutrophil count is obtained daily (Caudell and Whedon, 1991).

One of the goals of care for the HSCT recipient is to prevent or minimize infectious complications. The Centers for Disease Control and Prevention, Infectious Diseases Society of America (IDSA), American Society of Blood and Marrow Transplantation and blood and marrow practice guidelines list interventions to achieve this goal (**Table 7-10**).

Table 7-9 RISK FACTORS FOR INFECTION IN HSCT RECIPIENTS.

1. Hematologic or lymphoid malignancy.
2. Previous treatment with high-dose chemotherapy and/or radiation
3. Type of preparative treatment (myeloablative versus nonmyeloablative).
4. Prolonged neutropenia and immune deficiency.
5. Graft-versus-host disease (GVHD) and immunosuppressive therapy to prevent and/or treat acute or chronic GVHD.
6. Altered mucosal barriers.
7. Microorganism colonization.
8. Prolonged use of antibiotics.

Source: Centers for Disease Control and Prevention et al. (2000). Guidelines for preventing opportunistic infections among hematopoietic stem cell transplant recipients. *Biol Blood Marrow Transplant,* 6(61), 695–713.

Table 7-10 Intervention to prevent or minimize infection in HSCT recipients.

---

1. Institute isolation and barrier precautions.
2. Perform appropriate hand hygiene.
3. Properly maintain and clean all equipment used for HSCT recipients.
4. Implement and enforce policies related to plants, play areas, and toys to protect HSCT recipients.
5. Develop infection control policies related to health-care workers and illness.
6. Develop written policies for screening visitors and visiting patients during the HSCT transplant process.

Source: Centers for Disease Control and Prevention et al. (2000). Guidelines for preventing opportunistic infections among hematopoietic stem cell transplant recipients. *Biol Blood Marrow Transplant,* 6(61), 695–713.

Protective Isolation

A variety of techniques have been employed to protect patients from nosocomial infections. Techniques range from simple protective precautions to total protective environments (Rostad, 1991). The type of isolation used differs among transplant centers. The CDC, IDSA, and American Society of Blood and Marrow Transplantation practice guidelines provide information on hospital infection control (see **Table 7-11**).

It is important to promote meticulous hygiene as part of infection control. HSCT recipients should take daily showers or baths during and after transplantation, using a mild soap. Skin care during neutropenia should also include daily inspection of skin sites likely to be portals of infection (e.g., the perineum and intravascular access sites). HSCT recipients should maintain good perineal hygiene to minimize loss of skin integrity and risk for infection. HSCT center personnel should develop protocols for patient perineal care, including recommendations for gentle but thorough perineal cleaning after each bowel movement and thorough drying of the perineum after urinating.

Table 7-11 Guidelines for hospital infection control using protective isolation.

---

1. Allogeneic stem cell recipients should be placed in rooms with HEPA filtration.
2. HEPA filtration is especially important in areas near construction and renovation.
3. HEPA-filtered rooms should be evaluated for autologous recipients if they experience prolonged neutropenia.
4. Use of LAF rooms, if available, is optional.
5. Generally, hospital rooms for HSCT recipients should have positive room air pressure when compared with any adjoining hallways or anterooms.

Source: Centers for Disease Control and Prevention et al. (2000). Guidelines for preventing opportunistic infections among hematopoietic stem cell transplant recipients. *Biol Blood Marrow Transplant,* 6(61), 695–713.

Females should be instructed to always wipe the perineum from front to back after using the toilet to prevent fecal contamination of the urethra and urinary tract. To prevent vaginal irritation, menstruating immunocompromised HSCT recipients should not use tampons. The use of rectal thermometers, enemas, suppositories, and rectal exams are contraindicated among HSCT recipients to avoid skin or mucosal breakdown (Centers for Disease Control and Prevention et al., 2000).

All HSCT candidates should receive a dental evaluation and relevant treatment before conditioning therapy begins. Likely sources of dental infection should be vigorously eliminated. Ideally, 10 to 14 days should elapse between the completion of tissue-invasive oral procedures and onset of conditioning therapy to allow for adequate healing and monitoring for postsurgical complications (Centers for Disease Control and Prevention et al., 2000).

Oral cavity assessment should be performed a minimum of once per shift. An assessment tool that measures the appearance as well as level of function of the oral cavity should be used (Beck, 1993; Eilers et al., 1988; Kolbinson et al., 1988; Western Consortium for Cancer Nursing Research, 1991). Mouth care should be planned daily on the basis of individual patient assessment (Miller and Kearney, 2001). All HSCT candidates and their caregivers should be educated regarding the importance of maintaining good oral and dental hygiene for at least the first year after HSCT to reduce the risk for oral and dental infections. HSCT recipients with mucositis and HSCT candidates undergoing conditioning therapy should maintain safe oral hygiene by performing oral rinses 4 to 6 times/day with normal saline, sterile water, or sodium bicarbonate solutions (Miller and Kearney, 2001;

Ransier et al., 1995). HSCT recipients should brush their teeth at least two times/day with a soft, regular toothbrush. Increasing the frequency of oral care has been shown to have a positive effect on the oral health of the patient (Miller and Kearney, 2001). Performing oral care every 4 to 6 hours can reduce the patient's potential for infection from microorganisms. Mouth care every 2 hours can reduce mouth care problems, and performing oral care hourly can be helpful for patients requiring oxygen therapy or those with severe mucositis (Miller and Kearney, 2001). Recipients who cannot tolerate a soft toothbrush may use an ultrasoft toothbrush or toothette. For patients who cannot tolerate brushing their teeth, a toothette soaked in chlorhexidine has been shown to reduce plaque and control gingivitis as effectively as tooth brushing (Miller and Kearney, 2001). Flossing may be done daily if it can be done without trauma to the gums. Routine dental supervision is advised to monitor and guide the patient's maintenance of oral and dental hygiene. To decrease the risk for mechanical trauma and infection of oral mucosa, fixed orthodontic appliances and space maintainers should not be worn from the start of conditioning therapy until preengraftment mucositis resolves, and these devices should not be worn during any subsequent periods of mucositis. Patients who wear removable dental prostheses might be able to wear them during conditioning therapy before HSCT and during mucositis after HSCT, depending on the degree of tissue integrity at the denture-bearing sites and the ability of the patient to maintain denture hygiene on a daily basis (Centers for Disease Control and Prevention et al., 2000).

Almost all HSCT recipients have a central venous catheter placed to receive fluids, medications, and blood products. Use of intravascular devices is complicated by local and systemic infections that increase morbidity and mortality (Zitella, 2003). The Centers for Disease Control and Prevention have developed *Guidelines for the Prevention of Intravascular Catheter-Related Infections*. The guidelines state dressing type is a matter of preference, but dry, sterile gauze dressings should be changed every 2 days and transparent dressings should be changed weekly. Chlorhexidine (2%) is strongly recommended for skin antisepsis of all intravascular catheters (Zitella, 2003, Centers for Disease Control and Prevention, 2002). Contact with tap water should be avoided at the CVC site. The CVC site should be covered when the patient showers. To prevent bloodstream infections associated with needleless intravenous access devices, HSCT recipients should cover and protect the catheter tip or end cap from tap water during bathing or showering. Needleless caps should be changed in accordance with manufacturers' recommendations. HSCT recipients and their caregivers should be educated regarding proper care of needleless intravenous access devices (Centers for Disease Control and Prevention et al., 2000).

Nursing care of the HSCT patient involves administering and monitoring the patient's response to medications and treatments, which may include antibacterial, antifungal, and antiviral prophylaxis. (See **Table 7-12**.)

Nurses caring for patients with absent WBCs or very low WBC counts play a vital role in their outcomes. Nursing interventions aimed at decreasing or eliminating the likelihood of infection must be an essential part of the daily care of the HSCT patient. Nurses providing care at the bedside are in a position to notice the first subtle signs of infection and can intervene as early as possible. Nursing assistance in obtaining diagnostic tests is helpful in ensuring their comple-

Table 7-12 IMPORTANT AREAS OF ASSESSMENT FOR HSCT RECIPIENTS.

Skin sites
Oral cavity
Indwelling catheters
Respiratory status
Gastrointestinal status
Genitourinary status
Neurologic status
Vital signs
Hematological status

Source: Oncology Nursing Society, 1994.

tion, as well as in adhering to precautions against infections. Patients and families must be educated about signs and symptoms of infection as well as prevention, prophylaxis, and treatment.

Summary

Opportunistic bacterial and fungal infections remain major complications after HSCT. Although prophylaxis and treatment strategies have been improved, infections still contribute significantly to morbidity and mortality among HSCT recipients (Junghanss et al., 2002). The infectious complications related to HSCT are changing with advances in the field of HSCT. The use of peripheral stem cells, alternative donors, and advances in treatment of GVHD, as well as nonmyeloablative transplants, are changing the patterns of infectious complications. The use of peripheral blood stem cells has led to quicker engraftment and shortened periods of neutropenia (Devine et al., 2003). Advances in treatment of GVHD lead to greater immunosuppression and increased risk of opportunistic infections. Nonmyeloablative transplants have allowed older and sicker patients to receive transplants (Spitzer and Anderlini, 2002). A study at Fred Hutchinson Cancer Research Center showed patients undergoing nonmyeloablative HSCT had decreased risk of early bacteremia, but risk of late fungal infection persists (Junghanss et al., 2002).

During the last several years, the use of blood stem cells as well as growth factors such as G-CSF, which affects granulocytes; granulocyte-macrophage colony-stimulating factor (GM-CSF), which affects both granulocytes and macrophages; and erythropoietin, which affects red blood cells, have all had a positive impact on bone marrow transplantation by minimizing the severity and duration of myelosuppression. Other growth factors that stimulate even more of the cell line continue to be investigated. Among them are macrophage, colony-stimulating factor (M-CSF), interleukin-3 (IL-3), stem cell factor (SCF), and GM-CSF and IL-3 (PIXY 321) (Abernathy, 1995). In addition, nonmyeloablative allogeneic transplants, a treatment using standard doses of chemotherapy followed by infusions of donor stem cells, has been developed in an effort to take advantage of the graft-versus-tumor effect while providing an effective, yet less toxic modality for performing allogeneic hematopoietic stem cell transplantation (Niess and Duffy, 2004). This has opened the possibility of hematopoietic stem cell transplantation to a broader population of patients.

Hematopoietic stem cell transplantation continues to grow as a challenging and rewarding subspecialty of nursing. The hematologic system is the system that first indicates the success of the transplant. Hematologic effects necessitate most of the care provided to patients during transplant. As a broader range of diseases continue to be treated with transplantation, and as the techniques continue to evolve and be refined, nursing care needs to progress in the same way and at the same pace. Nurses will continue to play key roles in the outcomes of patients' treatments through precision in assessing and caring for patients and through intensive education of patients in a variety of settings.

References

Abernathy, E. (1995). Role of hematopoietic growth factors in post-induction treatment. In Wujcik, D. (Ed.). *Nursing Care Issues in Adult Leukemia* (vol. 2, pp. 20–27). Huntington, NY: PRR Inc.

Anasetti, C., Amos, D., Beatty, P.G., Appelbaum, F.R., Bensinger, W., Buckner, C.D., et al. (1989). Effect of HLA compatibility on engraftment of bone marrow transplants in patients with leukemia or lymphoma. *New England Journal of Medicine.* 320(4):197–204.

Western Consortium for Cancer Nursing Research. (1991). Development of a staging system for chemotherapy-induced stomatitis. *Cancer Nursing.* 14(1): 6–12.

Antin, J.H. (2002). Long-term care after hematopoietic-cell transplantation in adults. *New England Journal of Medicine.* 347(1):36–42.

Atkinson, K. (1990). Reconstruction of the hemopoietic and immune systems after marrow transplantation. *Bone Marrow Transplantation.* 5(4):209–226.

Ball, E.D., Mills, L.E., Cornwell, G.G., 3rd, Davis, B.H., Coughlin, C.T., Howell, A.L., et al. (1990). Autologous bone marrow transplantation for acute myeloid leukemia using monoclonal antibody-purged bone marrow. *Blood.* 75(5):1199–1206.

Ballard, B. (1991). Renal and hepatic complications. In Whedon, M.B. (Ed.). *Bone Marrow Transplantation: Principles, Practice and Nursing Insights* (pp. 240–261). Boston: Jones and Bartlett.

Bar, B.M., Schattenberg, A., Van Dijk, B.A., De Man, A.J., Kunst, V.A., De Witte, T. (1989). Host and donor erythrocyte repopulation patterns after allogeneic bone marrow transplantation analysed with antibody-coated fluorescent microspheres. *British Journal of Haematology*. 72(2):239–245.

Beck, S. (1993). Prevention and management of oral complications in the cancer patient. In Hubbard, S.M., Greene, P.E., Knobf, M.T. (Eds.). *Current Issues in Cancer Nursing Practice Updates* (pp. 1–12). Philadelphia: Lippincott.

Bennett, J.S., Shattil, S.J. (1990). Platelet function. In Williams, W.J., et al. (Eds.). *Hematology* (pp. 1233–1242). New York: McGraw-Hill.

Bensinger, W., Petersen, F.B., Banaji, M., Buckner, C.D., Clift, R., Slichter, S.J., et al. (1989). Engraftment and transfusion requirements after allogeneic marrow transplantation for patients with acute non-lympho-cytic leukemia in first complete remission. *Bone Marrow Transplantation*. 4(4): 409–414.

Bernstein, S.H., Nademanee, A.P., Vose, J.M., Tricot, G., Fay, J.W., Negrin, R.S., et al. (1998). A multicenter study of platelet recovery and utilization in patients after myeloablative therapy and hematopoietic stem cell transplantation. *Blood*. 91(9):3509–3517.

Beyer, J., Schwella, N., Zingsem, J., Strohscheer, I., Schwaner, I., Oettle, H., et al. (1995). Hematopoietic rescue after high-dose chemotherapy using autologous peripheral-blood progenitor cells or bone marrow: A randomized comparison. *Journal of Clinical Oncology*. 13(6):1328–1335.

Boeckh, M. (2003). Pneumocystis carinii pneumonia: Current prevention and treatment strategies. *Blood and Marrow Transplantation Reviews*. 13(3):8–10.

Bowden, R.A., Slichter, S.J., Sayers, M.H., Mori, M., Cays, M.J., Meyers, J.D. (1991). Use of leukocyte-depleted platelets and cytomegalovirus-seronegative red blood cells for prevention of primary cytomegalovirus infection after marrow transplant. *Blood*. 78(1):246–250.

Brown, J. (2004). Fungal infections in bone marrow transplant patients. *Current Opinion in Infectious Diseases*. 17(4):347–352.

Buchsel, P.C. (1990). Bone marrow transplantation. In Groenwald, S.L., Frogge, M.H., Goodman, M., Yarboro, C.H. (Eds.). *Cancer Nursing: Principles and Practice* (2nd ed., pp. 307–337). Boston: Jones and Bartlett.

Cahn, J.Y, Chabot, J., Esperou, H., Flesch, M., Plouvier, E., Herve, P. (1989). Autoimmune-like thrombocy-topenia after bone marrow transplantation. *Blood*. 74(8):277.

Caudell, K.A., Whedon, M.B. (1991). Hematopoietic complications. In Whedon, M.B. (Ed.). *Bone Marrow*

Transplantation: Principles, Practice, and Nursing Insights (pp. 135–159). Boston: Jones and Bartlett.

Centers for Disease Control and Prevention. (2002). Guidelines for the prevention of intravascular catheter-related infections. *Morbidity and Mortality Weekly Report*. 51:1–32.

Centers for Disease Control and Prevention, Infectious Diseases Society of America, American Society of Blood and Marrow Transplantation. (2000). Guidelines for preventing opportunistic infections among hematopoietic stem cell transplant recipients. *Biology of Blood & Marrow Transplantation*. 6(6a): 659–713, 715, 717–727, quiz 729–733.

Clark, J., Landis, L., McGee, R. (1987). Nursing management of outcomes of disease, psychological response, treatment and complications. In Ziegfield, C.R. (Ed.). *Core Curriculum for Oncology Nursing* (pp. 272–274). Philadelphia: Saunders.

Cohena, Y., Nagler, A. (2003). Hematopoietic stem-cell transplantation using umbilical-cord blood. *Leukemia & Lymphoma*. 44(8):1287–1299.

Devine, S.M., Adkins, D.R., Khoury, H., Brown, R.A., Vij, R., Blum, W., et al. (2003). Recent advances in allogeneic hematopoietic stem-cell transplantation. *Journal of Laboratory Clinical Medicine*. 141(1):7–32.

DiPersio, J.F., Khoury, H., Haug, J., Vij, R., Adkins, D.R., Goodnough, L.T., et al. (2000). Innovations in allogeneic stem-cell transplantation. *Seminars in Hematology*. 37(Suppl 2):33–41.

Donowitz, G.R., Maki, D.G., Crnich, C.J., Pappas, P.G., Rolston, K.V. (2001). Infections in the neutropenic patient—new views of an old problem. *Hematology*. 1:113–139. Retrieved 5/5/05 from http://www.ash educationbook.org/cgi/reprint/2001/1/113.

Eilers, J., Berger, A.M., Petersen, M.C. (1988). Development, testing, and application of the oral assessment guide. *Oncology Nursing Forum*. 15(3):325–330.

Englund, J.A., Zimmerman, M.E., Swierkosz, E.M., Goodman, J.L., Scholl, D.R., Balfour, H.H. Jr. (1990). Herpes simplex virus resistant to acyclovir. A study in a tertiary care center. *Annals of Internal Medicine*. 112(6):416–422.

Filipovich, A.H., Vallera, D., McGlave, P., Polich, D., Gajl-Peczalska, K., Haake, R., et al. (1990). T cell depletion with anti-CD5 immunotoxin in histocompatible bone marrow transplantation. The correlation between residual CD5 negative T cells and subsequent graft-versus-host disease. *Transplantation*. 50(3): 410–415

First, L.R., Smith, B.R., Lipton, J., Nathan D.G., Parkman, R., Rappeport, J.M. (1985). Isolated thrombocytopenia after allogeneic bone marrow transplantation: Existence of transient and chronic thrombocytopenic syndromes. *Blood*. 65(2):368–374.

Ford, R., Eisenberg, S. (1990). Bone marrow transplant. Recent advances and nursing implications. *Nursing Clinics of North America*. 25(2):405–422.

Fuller, A.K. (1990). Platelet transfusion therapy for thrombocytopenia. *Seminars in Oncology Nursing*. 6(2): 123–128.

Goodman, M. (1989). Managing the side effects of chemotherapy. *Seminars in Oncology Nursing*. 5(2 Suppl 1):29–52.

Griffin, J.P. (1986). Physiology of the hematopoietic system. In Griffin J.P. (Ed.). *Hematology and Immunology: Concepts for Nursing* (pp. 19–40). Norwalk, CT: Appleton-Century-Crofts.

Hardaway, R.M., Adams, W.H. (1989). Blood clotting problems in acute care. *Acute Care*. 14–15:138–207.

Hughes, W.T., Armstrong, D., Bodey, G.P., Bow, E.J., Brows, A.E., Calandra, T., et al. (2002). 2002 guidelines for the use of antimicrobial agents in neutropenic patients with cancer. *Clinical Infectious Diseases*. 34(6):730–749.

Jassak, P.F., Godwin, J. (1991). Blood component therapy. In Baird, S.B., McCorkle, R., Grant, M. (Eds.). *Cancer Nursing: A Comprehensive Textbook* (pp. 370–384). Philadelphia: Saunders.

Johnson, G., Quiett, K. (2004). Hematologic effects. In Ezzone, S. (Ed.). *Hematopoietic Stem Cell Transplantation: A Manual for Nursing Practice* (pp. 133–145). Pittsburgh, PA: Oncology Nursing Society.

Junghanss, C., Marr, K., Carter, R., Sandmaier, B., Maris, M., Maloney, D., et al. (2002). Incidence and outcome of bacterial and fungal infections following nonmyeloablative compared with myeloablative allogeneic hematopoietic stem cell transplantation: A matched control study. *Biology of Blood and Marrow Transplantation*. 8(9): 512–520.

Kernan, N.A. (1988). Graft failure following transplantation of T-cell-depleted marrow. In Burakoff, S.J., Deeg, H.J., Ferrara, J.L.M., Atkinson, M.K. (Eds.). *Graft-vs- Host Disease: Immunology, Pathophysiology and Treatment* (p. 57). New York: Marcel Dekker.

Kernan, N.A., Flomenberg, N., Dupont, B., O'Reilly, R.J. (1987). Graft rejection in recipients of T-cell-depleted HLA-nonidentical marrow transplants for leukemia. Identification of host-derived antidonor allocytotoxic T lymphocytes. *Transplantation*. 43(6):842–847.

Klumpp, T.R. (1991). Immunohematologic complications of bone marrow transplantation. *Bone Marrow Transplantation*. 8(3):159–170.

Klumpp, T.R., Caligiuri, M.A., Rabinowe, S.N., Soiffer, R.J., Murray, C., Ritz, J. (1990). Autoimmune pancytopenia following allogeneic bone marrow transplantation. *Bone Marrow Transplantation*. 6(6):445–447.

Kolbinson, D.A., Schubert, M.M., Flournoy, N., Truelove, E.L. (1988). Early oral changes following bone marrow transplantation. *Oral Surgery, Oral Medicine, Oral Pathology*. 66(1):130–138.

Korbling, M., Anderlini, P. (2001). Peripheral blood stem cell versus bone marrow allotransplantation: Does the source of hematopoietic stem cells matter? *Blood*. 98(10):2900–2908.

Korbling, M., Hunstein, W., Fliedner, T.M., Cayeux, S., Dorken, B., Fehrentz, D., et al. (1989). Disease-free survival after autologous bone marrow transplantation in patients with acute myelogenous leukemia. *Blood*. 74(6):1898–1904.

Lewis, I.D. (2002). Clinical and experimental uses of umbilical cord blood. *Internal Medicine Journal*. 32: 601–609.

Lin, E.M., Tierney, D.K., Stadtmauer, E.A. (1993). Autologous bone marrow transplantation. A review of the principles and complications. *Cancer Nursing*. 16(3):204–213.

Marin, G.H., Mendez, M.C., Menna, M.E., Malacalza, J., Bergna, M.I., Klein, G., et al. (1999). Immune recovery after bone marrow and peripheral blood stem cells transplantation. *Transplantation Proceedings*. 31: 2582–2584.

Marr, K. (2001). Prevention of fungal infections after hematopoietic stem cell transplantation. *Blood and Marrow Transplant Reviews*. 11(1):4–6.

Marr, K. (2003). New approaches to invasive fungal infections. *Current Opinion in Hematology*. 10(6):445–450.

Maxwell, M.B. (1984). When the cancer patient becomes anemic. *Cancer Nursing*. 7(4):321–326.

McLaren, C., Chen, M.S., Ghazzouli, I., Saral, R., Burns, W.H. (1985). Drug resistance patterns of herpes simplex virus isolates from patients treated with acyclovir. *Antimicrobial Agents and Chemotherapy*. 28(6):740–744.

Miller, M., Kearney, N. (2001). Oral care for patients with cancer: A review of the literature. *Cancer Nursing*. 24(4):241–253.

Nash, R.A. (2003). Overview: Treatment settings and duration of risk for infections. *Blood and Marrow Transplant Reviews*. 13(3):4–8.

Niess, D., Duffy, K.M. (2004). Basic concepts of transplantation. In Ezzone, S. (Ed.). *Hematopoietic Stem Cell Transplantation: A Manual for Nursing Practice* (pp. 13–21). Pittsburgh: Oncology Nursing Society.

Oncology Nursing Society. (1994). *Manual for Bone Marrow Transplant Nursing*. Pittsburgh, PA: Oncology Nursing Press.

Pavletic, Z.S., Bishop, M.R., Tarantolo, S.R., Martin-Algarra, S., Bierman, P.J., Vose, J.M., et al. (1997). Hematopoietic recovery after allogeneic blood stem-cell transplantation compared with bone marrow transplantation in patients with hematologic malignancies. *Journal of Clinical Oncology*. 15(4):1608–1616.

Petursson, C. (1993). Bleeding due to thrombocytopenia. In Yasko, J.M. (Ed.). *Nursing Management of Symptoms Associated with Chemotherapy* (3rd ed., pp. 135–141). Philadelphia: Menicus Health Care Communications.

Petz, L.D. (1989). Bone marrow transplantation. In Petz, L.D., Svisher, S. (Eds.). *Clinical Practice of Transfusion Medicine* (pp. 485–508). New York: Churchill Livingstone.

Petz, L.D., Scott, E.P. (1983). Supportive care. In Blume, K.G., Petz, L.D., (Eds.). *Clinical Bone Marrow Transplant* (pp. 117–223). New York: Churchill Livingstone.

Prentice, A., Donnelly, P. (2001). Oral antifungals as prophylaxis in haematological malignancy. *Blood Reviews*. 15(1):1–8.

Quinones, R.R. (1993). Hematopoietic engraftment and graft failure after bone marrow transplantation. *American Journal of Pediatric Hematology-Oncology*. 15(1): 3–17.

Ransier. A.. Epstein. J.B., Lunn, R., Spinelli, J. (1995). A combined analysis of a toothbrush, foam brush, and a chlorhexidine-soaked foam brush in maintaining oral hygiene. *Cancer Nursing*. 18(5):393–396.

Rostad, M.E. (1991). Current strategies for managing myelosuppression in patients with cancer. *Oncology Nursing Forum*. 18(2 Suppl):7–15.

Schuening, F.G., Nemunaitis, J., Appelbaum, F.R., Storb, R. (1994). Hematopoietic growth factors after allogeneic marrow transplantation in animal studies and clinical trials. *Bone Marrow Transplantation*. 14(Suppl 4):S74–S77.

Shafer, S.L. (1993). Infection due to leukopenia. In Yasko, J.M. (Ed.). *Nursing Management of Symptoms Associated with Chemotherapy* (3rd ed., pp. 143–168). Philadelphia: Meniscus Health Care Communications.

Shaffer, S., Wilson, J.N. (1993). Bone marrow transplantation: Critical care implications. *Critical Care Nursing Clinics of North America*. 5(3):531–550.

Sica, S., Laurenti, L., Sora, F., Menichella, G., Rumi, C., Leone, G., et al. (2001). Immune reconstitution following transplantation of autologous peripheral CD 34+ cells. *Acta Haematologica*. 105:179–187.

Sniecinski, I., O'Donnell, M.R., Nowicki, B., Hill, L.R. (1988). Prevention of refractoriness and HLA-alloimmunization using filtered blood products. *Blood*. 71(5):1402–1407.

Snyder, E.L. (Ed.). (1987). *Blood Transfusion Therapy: A Physician's Handbook*. Arlington, VA: American Association of Blood Banks.

Spitzer, T. (2003). New strategies for the prevention of pneumocystis carinii pneumonia and other opportunistic infections following stem cell transplantation. *Blood and Marrow Transplant Reviews*. 13(3):10–14.

Spitzer, T., Anderlini, P. (2002). New strategies for the prevention of pneumocystis carinii pneumonia and other opportunistic infections after stem cell transplantation. *Blood and Marrow Transplantation Reviews*. 12(3): 4–10.

Steingrimsdottir, H., Gruber, A., Bjorkholm, M., Svensson, A., Hansson, M. (2000). Immune reconstitution after autologous hematopoietic stem cell transplantation in relation to underlying disease, type of high-dose therapy and infectious complications. *Haematologica*. 85:832–838.

Storb, R. (1989). Bone marrow transplantation. In DeVita, V.T., Hellman, S., Rosenberg, S. (Eds.). *Cancer Principles and Practice of Oncology* (pp. 2474–2489). Philadelphia: Lippincott.

Storb, R. (2003). Allogeneic hematopoietic stem cell transplantation—yesterday, today, and tomorrow. *Experimental Hematology*. 31(1):1–10.

Sullivan, K.M., Dykewicz, C.A., Longworth, D.L., Boeckh, M., Baden, L.R., Rubin, R.H., et al. (2001). Preventing opportunistic infections after hematopoietic stem cell transplantation: The Centers for Disease Control and Prevention, Infectious Diseases Society of America, and American Society for Blood and Marrow Transplantation Practice Guidelines and beyond. *Hematology*. Retrieved 5/5/05 from http://www.asheducationbook.org/cgi/reprint/2001/1/392.

Tabbara, I.A., Zimmerman, K., Morgan, C., Nahleh, Z. (2002). Allogeneic hematopoietic stem cell transplantation: Complications and results. *Archives of Internal Medicine*. 162(14):1558–1566.

Vanacek, K.S. (1991). Gastrointestinal complications of bone marrow transplantation. In Whedon, M.B. (Ed.). *Bone Marrow Transplantation: Principles, Practice and Nursing Insights* (pp. 206–239). Boston: Jones and Bartlett.

Van Burik, J.H., Weisdorf, D.J. (1999). Infections in recipients of blood and marrow transplantation. *Hematology/Oncology Clinics of North America.* 13(5): 1065–1089.

Walsh, T.J., Teppler, H., Donowitz, G.R., Maertens, J.A., Baden, L.R., Dmoszynska, A., et al. (2004). Caspofungin versus liposomal amphotericin B for empirical antifungal therapy in patients with persistent fever and neutropenia. *New England Journal of Medicine.* 351(14): 1391–1402.

Weissinger, F., Sandmaier, B.M., Maloney, D.G., Bensinger, W.I., Gooley, T., Storb, R. (2001). Decreased transfusion requirements for patients receiving nonmyeloablative compared with conventional peripheral blood stem cell transplants from HLA-identical siblings. *Blood.* 98(13):3584–3588.

Wingard, J.R. (1990). Management of infectious complications of bone marrow transplantation. *Oncology (Huntington).* 4(2):69–75, 76, 81–82.

Winston, D.J., Gale, R.P. (1991). Prevention and treatment of cytomegalovirus infection and disease after bone marrow transplantation in the 1990s. *Bone Marrow Transplantation.* 8(1)17–11.

Wujcik, D., Ballard, B., Camp-Sorrell, D. (1994). Selected complications of allogeneic bone marrow transplantation. *Seminars in Oncology Nursing.* 10(1):28–41.

Yeager, A. (2004). Reduced-intensity allogeneic hematopoietic cell transplantation: Shifting paradigms, new definitions, new challenges. *Current Opinion in Organ Transplantation.* 9(1):36–38.

Zitella, L. (2003). Central venous catheter site care for blood and marrow transplant recipients. *Clinical Journal of Oncology Nursing.* 7(3):289–298.

Chapter 8

Gastrointestinal Effects

Elizabeth
Warnick, RN,
MSN, CRNP, BC

Complications of the gastrointestinal (GI) tract are the first clinical problems experienced by patients undergoing all types of blood and marrow transplantation (BMT). They have also been cited as the most distressing complication of transplant (Bellm et al., 2000). Despite advances in symptom management, transplant-related GI complications continue to cause significant problems. Effective management of graft-versus-host-disease (GVHD) and antiviral agents has reduced the incidence of associated hepatic and intestinal complications (van Burik and Weisdorf, 1999). Similarly, the arrival of serotonin antagonists has helped control the emetogenicity of dose-intensive chemotherapy (Abbott et al., 2000; Spitzer et al., 2000). However, GI-associated morbidity and mortality remain high as a result of three factors: 1) venoocclusive disease (VOD); 2) increased incidence of GVHD as the number of matched, unrelated donor transplants grows (Mielcarek et al., 2003); and 3) delayed nausea, vomiting, and anorexia, which historically have not been well controlled. The impact that neurokinin-1 antagonists will have on delayed nausea and vomiting has yet to be fully explored.

Gastrointestinal sequelae associated with transplantation are generally attributed to one or more of the following causes: 1) dose-intensive preparative regimens; 2) GVHD; and 3) infections affecting any segment of the GI tract or liver (Vargas and Silverman, 2000). Dose-intensive cytoreductive regimens are especially implicated in the cause of acute GI toxicities that occur early in the transplant process. In contrast to standard-dose chemotherapy, high-dose regimens typically cause GI complications that are more severe in nature and of longer duration. The use of peripherally derived stem cells and nonmyeloablative therapies has shortened the timing of some GI effects (Mielcarek et al., 2003). Acute GI complications have not yet been fully described in the setting of nonmyeloablative transplants (Basara et al., 2002). However, three factors remain. First, the individual host response will have an impact on the intensity of symptoms and effect. Second, combining total body irradiation (TBI) and high-dose chemotherapy will both intensify and prolong GI damage more severely than either alone. Finally, prior treatment exposure may alter the incidence and severity of the individual response.

GI complications can range in character from mild, temporary disturbances to protracted, life-threatening clinical challenges. Many present only early in the transplant process; however, some can produce long-term problems. Continuous, specialized nursing management is critical to control and recovery. The most toxic effects include severe emetic responses, mucositis, diarrhea, hemorrhage, and liver damage. Compounding GI sequela are secondary effects, which include sepsis resulting from mucosal disruption, nutritional deficiencies, electrolyte and biochemical abnormalities, and irreversible end organ damage by GVHD. One study found patients reported, in order, mouth sores, nausea, vomiting, and diarrhea as the most distressing effects of transplant (Bellm et al., 2000). Nurses play a vital role in the early detection, monitoring, and delivery of therapeutic interventions aimed at managing GI problems and minimizing discomfort during the entire transplant process.

The Emetic Response

Nausea, vomiting, and anorexia comprise a symptom complex that is experienced almost universally by patients at some point during the transplant process (Bellm et al., 2000). Generally, the emetic response is the first significant GI problem to develop in patients undergoing BMT. The physiologic mechanisms associated with the emetic response involve central stimulation by the true vomiting center located in the fourth ventricle of the brain (e.g., cerebral cortex, chemoreceptor trigger zone) or are peripherally mediated by certain neurotransmitters including dopamine, serotonin, histamine, and acetylcholine. The regulatory peptide, substance P, has been found to be most influential in delayed nausea and vomiting. These mechanisms are described in depth elsewhere (Dando and Perry, 2004; Bremerkamp, 2000).

Anorexia often accompanies nausea and vomiting. The mechanism of anorexia is not well understood. However, it is felt that elevated levels of circulating lipids, peptides, and certain cytokines such as tumor necrosis factor and interleukin-1 may be contributing factors. Taste alterations and altered olfactory sense secondary to TBI, mucosal damage and mucositis, oral infections, and antibiotic therapy can also contribute to anorexia (Epstein et al., 2002; Strasser and McDonald, 1999).

Typically, nausea and vomiting occur in concert 24 hours after the initiation of the preparative regimen, lasting up to 14 days after therapy. These symptoms are generally accompanied by anorexia, which can be self-limiting once nausea and vomiting have stopped or be long lived during the entire transplant process, depending on individual experience and complications (Perez et al., 1999). Delayed nausea and vomiting are commonly experienced by those undergoing an allogeneic transplant and are related to the effects of concurrent therapies as well as disease states. Larsen and colleagues (2004) asked patients to rank symptoms commonly experienced by stem cell transplant (SCT) patients in order of intensity at various intervals during admission for transplant. They found more than half the patients reported loss of appetite as the second most intense and distressing symptom followed by dry mouth as the third and nausea as the fourth. Persistent symptoms beyond day 20 are most likely related to another etiology such as viral infection or GVHD (Wu et al., 1998).

Unremitting acute nausea and vomiting can lead to other treatment-related complications.

These include electrolyte imbalances, Mallory-Weiss tears, aspiration pneumonia, severe nutritional problems, extended hospital stays, and diminished quality of life. Uncontrolled nausea, vomiting, and anorexia can have a significant impact on family members and caregivers as well (Bellm et al., 2000).

The emetic response can be acute or chronic and is initiated by a variety of factors. **Table 8-1** outlines the causes of acute and chronic nausea, vomiting, and anorexia.

Certain chemotherapeutic agents and radiation, specifically including the abdominal region, entire brain, sacral, and lumbar regions in the treatment field, are known to initiate the emetic response by direct or indirect stimulation of the midbrain vomiting centers. The type of therapy used in the preparative regimen will dictate the risk for nausea and vomiting. Those regimens that contain platinum or TBI are considered more highly emetogenic, resulting in severe symptoms of earlier onset and of longer duration. Individual drugs that have a high emetogenic potential include carmustine, carboplatin, cyclophosphamide, and busulfan (Perez et al., 1999). In contrast, melphalan is considered to be only moderately emetogenic and short lived. High-dose etoposide and mitoxantrone are categorized as mild to moderate.

Table 8-1 CAUSES OF NAUSEA AND VOMITING.

Acute	Chronic
Preparative regimen	Chronic GVHD
Supportive medications	Infection
Acute GVHD	Supportive
Preexisting	medications
GI problems	TPN

Nonmyeloablative regimens have been reported to have less of an emetic effect when compared to myeloablative regimens (Basara et al., 2002). It is the authors' experience that nonmyeloablative regimens produce less nausea and vomiting **Table 8-2** outlines the more familiar chemotherapeutic agents and emetic potential.

The addition of TBI to the preparative regimen will enhance the emetic response. Nausea and vomiting will increase with each treatment and has been demonstrated in almost all patients receiving greater than 12 Gy of unfractionated radiation (Spitzer et al., 2000). Buchali and colleagues (2000) found the emetic response to increase with each daily dose of TBI with a plateau at day 4. They also found patients under the age of 30 were more likely to experience nausea, as well as those diagnosed with chronic myelogenous leukemia. Cyclosphosamide was also a component of the preparative regimen utilized in conjunction with TBI in this study.

A wide variety of pharmaceuticals are utilized during all phases of the transplant process to treat associated complications. Many of these agents affect appetite and have the capacity to cause nausea with or without vomiting. These include nonabsorbable antibiotics, antifungal agents, and opiates.

Additional pharmaceuticals include total parenteral nutrition (TPN), lipid infusions, and steroid therapy. These pharmaceuticals cause high serum glucose and amino acid levels, which can elicit nausea and vomiting. In addition, TPN can delay gastric emptying, causing appetite suppression for up to 3 weeks following the discontinuation of therapy (Strasser and McDonald, 1999). This can have a significant impact on posttransplant recovery.

Viral infections are the most common infectious process, causing anorexia, nausea, and

Table 8-2 Emetic potential of chemotherapy.

High

Carmustine (> 250 mg/m2)	Cisplatin
Cyclophosphamide (> 150 mg/m2)	Dacarbazine (> 500 mg/m2)
Lomustine (> 60 mg/m2)	
Pentostatin	Mechlorethamine
Dactinomycin	Streptozocin

Moderate

Cyclophosphamide (< 150 mg/m2)	Carmustine (< 250 mg/m2)
Doxorubicin	Cisplatin (< 50 mg/m2)
Epirubicin	Cytarabine (> 1 gm/m2)
Idarubicin	Irinotecan
Ifosfamide	Melphalan
Hexamethylamine (p.o.)	Procarbazine (p.o.)
Carboplatin	Mitoxantrone (> 12 mg/m2)
Cyclophosphamide (p.o.)	

Low

Aldesleukin (IL-2)	Doxorubicin (< 20 mg/m2)
Methotrexate (> 100 mg/m2)	Fluorouracil (< 1000 mg/m2)
Mitoxantrone (< 12 mg/m2)	Gemcitabine
Temozolomide	Mitomycin
Etoposide (p.o.)	Paclitaxel
Asparaginase	Thiotepa
Cytarabine (< 1gm/m2)	Topotecan
Docetacxel	

Minimal

Methotrexate (< 100 mg/m2)	Bleomycin
Capecitabine	Rituximab
Vincristine	Trastuzumab
Vinorelbine (i.v)	
Etoposide/teniposide (i.v.)	

Source: "Emetic Risk of Chemotherapy" from Koeller, J.M., et al. (2002). Antiemetic Guidelines: Creating a more practical approach.

vomiting. However, viral infections are more prevalent later in the transplant process, usually occurring after day 30. In the absence of prophylactic antiviral therapy, the incidence was as high as 70–80%. Vomiting is a major symptom of HSV esophagitis. Again, posttransplant viral infections are less common with the use of antiviral prophylaxis and pretransplant viral testing. Most infections are a result of reactivation in sero-positive patients and the early discontinuation of ganciclovir. Nausea is associated with active viral infections, gastrointestinal reflux, and GI ulceration (van Burik and Weisdorf, 1999). In contrast, fungal and bacterial infections are known to cause anorexia. Bacterial infections of the GI tract can develop in the presence of existing mucosal injury and loss of tissue integrity caused by the preparative regimen and prolonged immunocompromise. Typically, GI infections are caused by colonized oral microflora (Vargas and Silverman, 2000; Strasser and McDonald, 1999).

Emetic responses may be early indicators of acute gastrointestinal GVHD. The average onset of GVHD of the GI tract is about day 34 posttransplant. However, acute GVHD must be ruled out if emetic symptoms continue despite appropriate therapy after day 20 in the allogeneic population (Iqbal et al., 2000). Patients who are undergoing nonmyeloablative therapy have been found to develop acute GVHD of the GI tract later when compared to those who have a myeloablative transplant (Mielcarek et al., 2003). Initial symptoms include anorexia, followed by nausea, vomiting or retching, dyspepsia, and food intolerance (Iqbal et al., 2000). One study evaluated nausea, vomiting, and anorexia persisting beyond day 20 postallogeneic transplant and found 63 of 78 patients to have pathologic evidence of acute GVHD. Most patients received either a matched unrelated donation or marrow from a mismatched family member (Wu et al., 1998). Wakui and colleagues (1999) performed routine upper endoscopic examinations between day 20 and 50 postallogeneic transplant and found 46% of 26 patients to have evidence of acute GVHD.

Psychoneurologic factors may also influence nausea, vomiting, and anorexia. For unknown reasons, anticipatory or conditioned responses may have an impact on patient response to the preparative regimen, prolonging nausea and vomiting. It is speculated that this phenomenon is the result of previous treatment experience. Other psychological symptoms common to the transplant population include anxiety, depression, powerlessness, and exaggerated responses to pain, and these may also have an impact on the severity of the emetic response. This area is less explored and studied in the literature. Larsen and colleagues (2004) evaluated patient symptoms during admission for the preparative regimen. They found that those reporting higher anxiety levels at day 0 of therapy improved as treatment ensued. Those who reported less anxiety at admission were more likely to have anxiety prior to discharge.

Management

Important to management of the emetic response is comprehensive assessment in conjunction with preventive strategies. A thorough history and physical prior to treatment will assist in identifying those who may be at risk for prolonged nausea, vomiting, or anorexia. Continuous patient evaluation with focus on effectiveness of therapy will allow for modification to individualize the treatment plan. The timing as well as etiology of the emetic response is crucial in order to provide effective management. Both pharmacologic and nonpharmacologic interventions may be employed during all phases of the transplant process. Recent studies show improved control of acute nausea and vomiting; however, the phenomenon of delayed nausea and vomiting is not well described in the transplant literature. **Table 8-3** depicts the current National Cancer Institute (NCI) guidelines for grading GI toxicities, which will assist with evaluation and management.

Table 8-3 NCI TOXICITY GRADING GUIDELINES.

GASTROINTESTINAL

Adverse Event	Short Name	Grade				
		1	2	3	4	5
Anorexia	Anorexia	Loss of appetite without alterations in eating habits.	Oral intake altered without significant weight loss or malnutrition; oral nutritional supplements indicated.	Associated with significant weight loss or malnutrition (e.g., inadequate oral caloric and/or fluid intake); IV fluids or TPN indicated.	Life-threatening consequences	Death
Diarrhea	Diarrhea	< 4 stools per day over baseline; mild increase in ostomy output compared to baseline.	4–6 stools per day over baseline; IV fluids indicated, 24 hrs; moderate increase in ostomy output compared to baseline; not interfering with ADL.	≥ 7 stools per day over baseline; incontinence; IV fluids ≥ 24 hrs; hospitalization; severe increase in ostomy output compared to baseline; interfering with ADL.	Life-threatening consequences (e.g., hemodynamic collapse	Death
Dry mouth/ salivary gland (xerostomia)	Dry mouth	Symptomatic (dry or thick saliva) without significant dietary alterations; unstimulated saliva flow > 0.2 ml/min.	Symptomatic and significant oral intake alterations (e.g., copious water, other lubricants, diet limited to purees and/or soft, moist foods); unstimulated saliva 0.1 to 0.2 ml/min.	Symptoms leading to inability to adequately aliment orally, IV fluids, tube feedings, or TPN indicated; unstimulated saliva > 0.1 ml/min.		

Dysphagia (difficulty swallowing)	Symptomatic; able to eat regular diet.	Symptomatic and altered eating/swallowing (e.g., oral supplements); IV fluids indicated < 24 hrs.	Symptomatic and severely altered eating/swallowing (e.g., inadequate oral caloric or fluid intake); IV fluids or TPN indicated < 24 hrs.	Life-threatening consequences (e.g., obstruction, perforation)	Death
Esophagitis	Asymptomatic pathologic, radiographic, or endoscopic findings only.	Symptomatic; altered eating/swallowing (e.g., altered dietary habits, oral supplements); IV fluids indicated < 24 hrs.	Symptomatic and severely altered eating/swallowing (e.g., inadequate oral caloric or fluid intake); IV fluids, tube feedings, or TPN indicated ≥ 24 hrs.	Life-threatening consequences.	Death
Mucositis/stomatitis (clinical exam) –Select: –Anus –Esophagus –Large bowel –Larynx –Select: –Oral cavity –Pharynx –Rectum –Small bowel –Stomach –Trachea	Erythema of the mucosa.	Patchy ulcerations or pseudomembranes.	Confluent ulcerations or pseudomembranes; bleeding with minor trauma.	Tissue necrosis; significant spontaneous bleeding; life-threatening consequences.	Death

(continues)

Table 8-3 NCI TOXICITY GRADING GUIDELINES *continued.*

GASTROINTESTINAL

Adverse Event	Short Name	Grade 1	Grade 2	Grade 3	Grade 4	Grade 5
Mucositis/stomatitis (functional/ symptomatic) —*Select:* —Anus —Esophagus —Large bowel —Larynx —Oral cavity —Pharynx —Rectum —Small bowel —Stomach —Trachea	Mucositis (functional/ symptomatic)	*Upper aerodigestive tract sites:* Minimal symptoms, normal diet; minimal respiratory symptoms but not interfering with function. *Lower GI sites:* Minimal discomfort, intervention not indicated.	*Upper aerodigestive tract sites:* Symptomatic but can eat and swallow modified diet; respiratory symptoms interfering with function but not interfering with ADL. *Lower GI sites:* Symptomatic; medical intervention indicated but not interfering with ADL.	*Upper aerodigestive tract sites:* Symptomatic and unable to adequately aliment or hydrate orally; respiratory symptoms interfering with ADL. *Lower GI sites:* Stool incontinence or other symptoms interfering with ADL.	Symptoms associated with life-threatening consequences.	Death
Nausea	Nausea	Loss of appetite without alterations in eating habits.	Oral intake decreased without significant weight loss, dehydration, or malnutrition; IV fluids indicated < 24 hrs.	Inadequate oral caloric or fluid intake; IV fluids, tube feedings, or TPN indicated ≥ 24 hours.	Life-threatening consequences.	Death
Vomiting	Vomiting	1 episode in 24 hrs.	2–5 episodes in 24 hrs; IV fluids indicated < 24 hrs.	≥ 6 episodes in 24 hrs; IV fluids or TPN indicated ≥ 24 hr hrs.	Life-threatening consequences.	Death

Cancer Therapy Evaluation Program. (2003). Common Terminology Criteria for Adverse Events (Version 3.0). Retrieved December 12, 2003 from http://ctep.cancer.gov/forms/CTCAEv3.pdf

Pharmacologic approaches are the key to controlling preparative regimen–induced emetic responses. Available studies are now defining antiemetic regimens that manage chemo-irradiation nausea, vomiting, and anorexia more effectively. However, total emetic control has not been achieved because the management of the delayed response is still difficult. The issue of delayed nausea, vomiting, and anorexia has only recently been addressed and applied to conventional chemotherapy, and studies are ongoing with regard to the impact on symptoms associated with high-dose therapy.

Generally, prophylactic multiagent antiemetic therapy is initiated with the beginning of the preparative regimen and extends 24 to 48 hours after completion. Prior to the development of serotonin antagonists, drug combinations utilized were associated with many adverse side effects, including sedation, akathesias, and possibly cardiac effects (Perez et al., 1999). These drugs included metoclopramide, lorazepam, dexamethasone, diphenhydramine, prochlorperazine, thiethylperazine, and haloperidol. With the advent of serotonin antagonists, these drugs are commonly employed as second line agents.

The serotonin antagonists—ondansetron, granisetron, dolasetron, and palonosetron—are now important components of current antiemetic regimens. The success of these agents in controlling chemotherapy-induced emetic responses is based on their ability to block 5-HT3 receptors located in the GI tract. The efficacy of ondansetron was compared to perphenazine and diphenhydramine in 28 children undergoing transplant preparative regimens. Sixty-seven percent of the ondansetron arm achieved emetic control, compared to zero percent of the perphenazine/diphenhydramine arm (Mehta et al., 1997). This demonstrated the important role serotonin antagonists play in high-dose therapies. Another study compared bolus administration to continuous infusion ondansetron, finding bolus dosing more effective (Osowski et al., 1998). Dolasetron was found to be less efficacious in one study comparing patients receiving dolasetron, granisetron, or ondansetron (Bubalo et al., 2001).

One major advantage of these newer agents is their side effect profile when compared to traditional agents utilized in the past. The most frequently reported side effects of serotonin antagonists are headache, diarrhea, and constipation (Abbott et al., 2000; Spitzer et al., 2000). Cost is a concern. However, the oral route of administration does provide equal control at lower costs than intravenous administration (Abang et al, 2000). Combining a serotonin antagonist with a steroid such as dexamethasone has been demonstrated to produce better antiemetic control outcomes (Abbott et al., 2000; Spitzer et al., 2000). Serotonin antagonists not only provide better emetic control, but also decrease the number of medications required for effective prophylaxis. Traditional antiemetic drugs are typically employed to provide relief from breakthrough nausea and vomiting (Perez et al., 1999).

The phenomenon of delayed nausea and vomiting is of a different origin than that of the acute response. Delayed responses occur 48 hours after chemotherapy has been completed and do not respond well to intervention with serotonin antagonists. It is becoming apparent that delayed nausea and vomiting is mediated by different physiologic mechanisms and responds better to other pharmacologic approaches. Typically, drugs employed for delayed emetic responses include dopamine antagonists plus steroids and antihistamines. Again, they lack effectiveness and have the potential to produce unwanted side effects. **Table 8-4** lists current drugs utilized for management of the emetic response.

Aprepitant is a novel oral antagonist of substance P in the central nervous system. This agent binds with neurokinin-1 (NK-1) receptors in the brain, thus blocking the effects of substance P and ultimately preventing delayed nausea and vomiting. Major side effects include fatigue, anorexia, constipation, diarrhea, and hiccups. Nausea can occur, usually after day 5 of therapy (Dando and Perry, 2004). It has been found to be effective in controlling delayed nausea and vomiting experienced by patients receiving multiple cycles of cisplatin-based therapies (de Wit et al., 2003; Hesketh et al., 2003). Presently, studies incorporating aprepitant into the antiemetic regimen for patients receiving high-dose therapy in transplant are ongoing. The results should once again have a dramatic impact on symptom management. Aprepitant has been found to moderately inhibit CYP3A4 metabolism, and thus, may affect plasma levels of other drugs. One study did show that coadministration of dexamethasone or methylprednisolone increased the plasma levels of these drugs (Hesketh et al., 2003; McCrea et al., 2003). These findings may have a significant impact on emetic management of the transplant patient in the future.

Table 8-4 COMMONLY USED ANTIEMETICS.

Drug	Classification	Comments
Dolasetron Ganisetron Ondansetron Palonosetron	Serotonin antagonist	—Most effective for acute nausea and vomiting —Common side effects: headache and constipation —Dolasetron can increase QT interval
Dexamethasone	Corticosteroid	—Used for both acute and delayed nausea and vomiting —Common side effects: anxiety, insomnia, and euphoria
Aprepitant	Neurokinin-1 antagonist	—Effective for delayed nausea and vomiting —Increases plasma levels of corticosteroids
Lorazepam	Benzodiazepine	—Often helpful for anticipatory nausea and vomiting —Can cause sedation
Metoclopramide	Dopamine and serotonin antagonist	—Can cause extrapyramidal side effects —Diarrhea common
Diphenhydramine	Antihistamine	—Has sedative properties —Not a potent antiemetic —Prevents extrapyramidal side effects

Stevens, M. (2004). Gastrointestinal complications of hematopoietic stem cell transplantation. In S. Ezzone (ed.), *Hematopoietic stem cell transplantation: A manual of nursing practice* (pp. 147–165). Pittsburgh: ONS Publishing Division; and Koeller et al. (2002). Antiemetic guidelines: Creating a more practical treatment approach. *Support Care Center,* 10, 519–522.

Nonpharmacologic approaches to deal with the emetic response include dietary modifications, relaxation strategies, and distraction, utilizing a number of different methods. These approaches can serve as a valuable adjunct to antiemetic drug regimens. Recent research exploring these methods is sparse and includes small patient populations. Patients must be fully motivated to pursue them as part of antiemetic therapy.

It is difficult to manage emetic responses that are a result of infection or adjunctive drug therapy. Nausea, vomiting, and anorexia associated with supportive pharmaceuticals can be partially alleviated utilizing antiemetic agents. It is usually impossible to discontinue the offending agent, because it is important to manage or prevent life-threatening posttransplant complications. One option may be to replace one drug with a suitable substitute from the same class that will produce fewer side effects. Switching the route of administration form oral to parenteral may be another option in managing symptoms.

The management of the emetic response secondary to infection and GVHD involves successful treatment of the underlying etiology. More specific information on prevention and therapeutic approaches to GVHD was discussed in Chapter 6.

Mucosal Damage

Xerostomia

Normally, pairs of sublingual parotid and numerous minute buccal glands compose a network of salivary glands responsible for producing saliva. Saliva is a watery secretion responsible for cleaning the oral cavity and facilitating the passage of the food bolus along the alimentary tract. The cells of the salivary glands are highly susceptible to injury and subsequent altered function from radiation therapy. The effects can lead to a decrease in the amount of saliva production and changes in the character of secretions. Most often the saliva becomes tenacious and ropy. Alteration of the normal microbial flora and subsequent oral superinfection can result from the saliva becoming abnormally acidic (Duncan and Grant, 2003). Immunoglobulin A, normally secreted in the saliva, will be decreased. This will have a negative impact, possibly promoting infectious complications as well as the development of mucositis (Epstein et al., 2002).

Inflammation of the parotid glands, or parotitis, is commonly reported in those patients receiving TBI as part of the preparative regimen (Buchali et al., 2000). Parotitis associated with TBI is characterized as tender mumpslike neck swelling that occurs after the initiation of therapy and resolves spontaneously within 24 to 48 hours once completed. Acute neck and shoulder pain may accompany swelling. Xerostomia generally begins 7 to 10 days following completion of therapy and can be of long duration, never resolving. Alkylating agents and methotrexate have been known to cause xerostomia (Scully et al., 2003), as have anticholinergic drugs (Plevova, 1999).

Chronic oral GVHD, or oral sicca syndrome, can also cause significant xerostomia. This is a result of chronic fibrotic changes of the oral mucosa and adjacent salivary ducts. Symptoms include oral dryness, increased oral sensitivity, and pain (Sullivan, 1999; Sale et al., 1999). Dental caries and loss of tooth structure can develop, leading to tooth loss. Sicca syndrome can be a major transplant complication.

MANAGEMENT

Assessment and management of xerostomia overlap that of mucositis. Table 8-3 provides the NCI guidelines for assessment purposes. Goals include stimulation of existing salivary gland function, lubrication and hydration of the mucosa, prevention of infectious complications, pain control, and prevention of malnutrition. Meticulous oral hygiene is very important and will be described in more detail in the mucositis section of this chapter. Lubricants, frequent oral fluids, and artificial saliva products may be of benefit. One study utilized pilocarpine to manage sicca syndrome, reporting salivary flow rates returned to normal 2 weeks after initiation of therapy at 30 milligrams per day. If pilocarpine was discontinued, salivary flow rates returned to baseline. Side effects included sweating (Nagler and Nagler, 1999). Analgesics, either topical or systemic, will help control oral pain. Topical cold applications may help neck and shoulder pain as well as oral discomfort. Avoiding mechanically hard and spicy foods, alcohol, and cigarettes may help maintain oral integrity. A dietary evaluation may be helpful. Regular, ongoing professional dental exams posttransplant may assist in preventing long-term complications.

Mucositis/Espohagitis

The mucosal lining of the entire alimentary tract undergoes dramatic change in response to the effects of high-dose preparative regimens, GVHD, and infection. The mucosa of the mouth and esophagus is composed of stratified squamous epithelium. Recent research has demonstrated that mucositis occurs in four phases. First, there is epithelial damage from direct cellular destruction as a result of the offending agent. Second, tissue injury results in proinflammatory mediation resulting in the influx of cytokines such as interleukin-1, interleukin-6, tumor necrosis factor, and platelet-activating factor. Third, ulcerative lesions allow for easy microbial invasion, which can lead to extended infection, both local and systemic. Finally, healing does occur; however, the mucosal cells do not return to their normal state, allowing susceptibility to future injury (Sonis, 2004; Scully et al., 2003). Mucositis can also increase hospital costs because it has been shown to prolong the number of days patients have fever, increase the risk of infection, extend narcotic use and TPN, and ultimately prolong hospital stays (Sonis, 2004). Although mucositis secondary to treatment is generally temporary and self-limiting, it can pose a potential life-threatening complication of therapy. Mucosal damage secondary to GVHD tends to be chronic in nature and will be discussed elsewhere in this chapter and in Chapter 6 of the text.

Mucosal injury develops approximately 7 days after cytotoxic therapy is administered, with peak symptoms at about day 14 (Sonis, 2004). Patients with oral symptoms present with gingival edema and erythema, oral dryness, ulceration, and oral pain. Oral symptoms of longer duration are suggestive of another etiology. The most common sites of ulceration are the nonkeratinized mucosa of the floor of the mouth, tongue, buccal mucosa, soft palate, and sometimes labia (Schubert et al., 1999). It has also been suggested that nonmyeloablative regimens may reduce treatment-related toxicities, as the actual neutropenic period has been reduced (Champlin et al., 2001). Dysphagia, epigastric pain or burning, and reflux are typical symptoms of esophagitis. Whereas symptoms of mucositis are easily characterized and visually evaluable, those of the esophagus are more difficult, as direct visualization is almost impossible without endoscopic examination.

Bellm and colleagues (2000) found patients report mouth sores as the most debilitating effect of transplant. Oral complications affect patients following allogeneic transplant more often than after autologous or syngeneic transplant. Also, those who develop acute GVHD have fewer sequelae than those with chronic GVHD. Preparative regimens that incorporate TBI and methotrexate for GVHD prophylaxis tend to produce more severe mucositis than if these two are eliminated (Basara et al., 2002). The incidence of mucositis in transplant patients is quite high, occurring in 36–89% of patients after the preparative regimen (Sonis et al., 2001).

Some drugs utilized in the preparative regimens have been found to cause more toxicity to the GI mucosa than others. Mucositis is considered the dose-limiting toxicity of busulfan, cyclophosphamide, methotrexate, and thiotepa (Scully et al., 2003). Prior therapy has also been found to have an impact on the development of mucositis with future chemotherapy (Sonis, 2004). One study found mucositis was prolonged if etoposide was an agent utilized in the preparative regimen during stem cell mobilization in a group of patients receiving an autologous transplant. Prolonged mucositis was associated with prior radiation therapy (Bolwell et al., 2002).

Oral and esophageal infections are often difficult to distinguish from treatment-induced toxicity because they generally occur simultaneously. Clinical presentation of mucosal infections depends on the offending organism. Gram-negative bacterial infections usually present as creamy but nonprurulent, raised, shiny erosions on an erythematous foundation. In contrast, gram-positive staphylococcal and streptococcal infections appear as dry, raised, yellowish-brown, round plaques.

HSV Infections can develop within the first 30 days after transplant and are more common in sero-positive patients. It is typically manifested as multiple, discrete vesicular lesions on the lips or oral cavity. The incidence of HSV may be lower for those receiving autologous peripheral stem cell transplant, due to shorter periods of immunosuppression (Offidani et al., 1999). CMV infections typically present 4 weeks after transplant through week 12. CMV is less common in those receiving an autograft. Oral candidiasis presents as pinpoint lesions under yellowish or whitish curdlike plaques on the tongue and buccal mucosa. Most often, complaints of burning pain or dysgeusia accompany clinical findings. Standard prophylaxis with antivirals and antifungals has significantly reduced occurrence (van Burik and Weisdorf, 1999).

The presentation of acute oral GVHD is similar to that associated with other complications. Findings include painful desquamation, mucosal ulceration, erythema, plaques, and lichenoid keratosis. Acute oral GVHD is less common and is a diagnostic consideration if mucositis does not resolve after engraftment (Vargas and Silverman, 2000). In contrast, chronic oral GVHD differs significantly from other etiologies. Findings include gingival fibrosis and oral pain. Persistent oral dryness and sensitivity are typically reported. Symptoms usually develop 3 months after transplant (Sullivan, 1999; Sale et al., 1999). Existing oral HSV or candidiasis can confuse the diagnosis of oral GVHD (Sullivan, 1999).

There are specific findings associated with infectious complications of the esophagus. Esophagitis and subsequent infection develop when there is existing damage from mucositis and prolonged neutropenia (Iqbal et al., 2000). Bacterial infections usually accompany those caused by viral or fungal pathogens. Typically, organisms derived from oral flora are causative. Diagnostic findings include large numbers of bacterial colonies in esophageal biopsy specimens (Strasser and McDonald, 1999).

Esophageal findings associated with HSV include small vesicles in the squamous epithelium in the middle and distal regions. Sloughing of infected epithelial tissue produces ulcerations with raised erythematous borders. CMV will appear as shallow ulcerations with erythematous edges. Symptoms include nausea, vomiting, fever, dysphagia, retrosternal chest pain, diarrhea, and bleeding (Bashey, 2000; Strasser and McDonald, 1999). Fortunately, viral esophagitis is rare today since antiviral prophylaxis is not standard (van Burik and Weisdorf, 1999).

Fungal esophagitis is primarily due to candida and aspergillus but other species can cause infection. Most esophageal fungal infections develop during the neutropenic period following the preparative regimen and before engraftment. However, prolonged neutropenia, acute and chronic GVHD, CMV infections, and medications used to treat these syndromes can predispose one to develop fungal esophagitis. Clinical symptoms include nausea, vomiting, dysphagia, odynophagia, malaise, and fever. The onset of symptoms is gradual. Diagnosis relies on direct biopsy of lesions, which typically appear as white plaques. Progression to systemic disease can occur without appropriate treatment. The use of prophylactic antifungal agents has significantly reduced disease rates (De La Rosa et al., 2002; Vargas and Silverman, 2000; Strasser and McDonald, 1999; van Burik and Weisdorf, 1999).

Acute GVHD of the upper GI tract commonly presents with symptoms of anorexia, nausea, vomiting, epigastric pain, and food intolerance. Symptoms of chronic GVHD include retrosternal chest pain, dysphagia, odynophagia, and weight loss. Aspiration may be another finding. Visualization will demonstrate esophageal webbing and stricture formation. Again, nonspecific symptoms make biopsy an important tool for accurate diagnosis (Iqbal et al., 2000; Cruz-Correa et al., 2002; Vargas and Silverman, 2000; Strasser and McDonald, 1999).

MANAGEMENT

Important to the management is the timing with which symptoms and physical findings develop after transplant. Those that develop early post-stem cell infusion will most likely be secondary to the preparative regimen whereas those that occur after day 20 will usually be of another etiology, such as infections. Use of standardized grading systems such as that depicted in Table 8-2 will be most helpful in accurate communication of physical findings. Routine, thorough inspection of the oral cavity and careful attention to symptoms is the most important tool to develop effective interventions.

Multiple assessment guides that assist in characterizing oral mucositis are available. To date, no one guide has been evaluated as the most accurate or standardized to transplant in general. Patient self-assessment tools have been developed, as have health-care provider scales. Parulekar and colleagues (1998) reviewed a number of scales commonly used to describe oral toxicities for inter- and intra-user reliability. They found variations existing between the scales evaluated significant enough that they were difficult to accurately measure mucositis.

Although treatment-associated mucositis is self-limiting, it is still distressful enough that quick intervention can provide relief and comfort. Despite the plethora of recommendations and agents utilized, there is not one standard treatment. Variations also exist between institutions. Most often, frequent, gentle rinses with saline or sodium bicarbonate are utilized. Soft-bristled toothbrushes should be used, and flossing should be reserved for those with adequate platelet counts. Toothettes can be substituted when platelet counts are too low and bleeding is an issue. Electric brushes and electric irrigation should be reserved until after the patient has recovered from transplant. Dentures should be cleansed on a regular basis and soaking solution changed daily (MMWR, 2000; Barker, 1999). Posttransplant fluoride rinses may be prescribed to prevent dental caries (Barker, 1999). Chlorhexidine, an oral microbial, is also utilized in the transplant setting. It has been found to reduce microbial burden but does not prevent the development or decrease the severity of mucositis (Filicko et al., 2003; Barker, 1999).

Oral and esophageal pain can be managed either topically or systemically. Eliminating irritating foods and providing adequate fluids will help with mild mucositis. Topical anesthetics applied directly to the mucosal surface may provide short-term relief. Lidocaine, diphenhydramine, and kaolin pectin combinations have been utilized (Plevova, 1999). Care must be taken when using these items, as they have the potential to decrease the gag reflex. Opiate analgesics may be necessary, including continuous infusion. Side effects such as sedation and decreased mental acuity have been reported as incapacitating by patients (Bellm et al., 2000) and can cause other problems, including aspiration. In cases of severe mucositis, TPN may be required.

Although no one agent is recommended as empiric therapy, there are multiple agents that have been or are currently undergoing investigation to prevent or treat mucositis. These agents have not been applied to general practice. When reviewing prevention and treatment of mucositis, Plevova (1999) listed multiple agents that had been or were currently under investigation, including mesalazine, GM-GSF, beta transforming growth factors, epidermal growth factor, misoprostol, and prostaglandin E2. Other agents include glutamine, pentoxifylline, sucralfate, keratinocyte growth factor, interleukin-11, amifostine, iseganan, immunol oral rinse, and laser therapy (Filicko et al., 2003).

If infection is suspected, cultures of the visible lesions appearing in the oral cavity will define the offending organism(s), whether it be bacterial or viral. Direct visualization is necessary for diagnosis of any esophageal symptoms, as they often overlap. Culture of the lesions and biopsy will provide information regarding treatment. It is important to make prompt diagnosis because systemic disease may result (Strasser and McDonald, 1999). If oral GVHD is suspected, biopsy will make a definitive diagnosis. Chapter 6 provided more information regarding treatment of GVHD.

If bacteria are implicated as the cause, then appropriate antibiotic coverage will be necessary. HSV, either oral or esophageal, can be treated with acyclovir with good results. Resistant isolate may require alternative drug choices. CMV usually responds well to ganciclovir; however, resolution of symptoms is slow. Foscarnet may be an alternative, as may valacyclovir. Oral administration of valacyclovir makes it an attractive alternative to parenteral drugs (Winston et al., 2003). Fungal infections can be treated utilizing fluconazole. Newer antifungals are just now available and may be better tolerated. Cost, as well as efficacy, is always a concern. The impact new antifungals will have on transplant complications has not yet been fully documented.

Perirectal Lesions

The skin and surrounding tissues of the perirectal area are highly susceptible to breaks in integrity and ultimately infection in the transplant population. Preparative regimens can cause altered skin integrity of the perirectal area similar to that of the oral mucosa. TBI can cause acute skin reactions that include erythema, hyperpigmentation, and breakdown. Chemotherapy can cause a similar response or be additive if both modalities are utilized in the preparative regimen. Diarrheal illness can cause further impairment of the mucosal integrity. The result is an ideal environment for numerous preexisting skin floral and fecal organisms to flourish while impaired mucosa permits invasion of tissues and ultimate sepsis (Hainsfield-Wolfe and Rund, 1999). Organisms predominantly associated with rectal infections include *Pseudomonas aeruginosa*, *E. coli*, and *Klebsiella* species. Other causative organisms include group-D *Streptococcus, Staphulococcus areas, Hemophilus influenzae, Enterobacter cloacae, Candida albicans,* and *Bacteroides fragilis* (Strasser and McDonald, 1999). Vancomycin-resistant enterococci pose a more difficult challenge to the immunocompromised patient. *Clostridium difficile* infections as a result of multiple antibiotic therapies can cause considerable discomfort as well as become a recurring problem. Lastly, viral invasion may also cause perirectal infections (MMWR, 2000).

Fever with accompanying rectal pain may be the first sign of rectal abscess. Generally, fever and rectal pain precede diagnosis by 3 to 6 days. Pain presenting as point tenderness with visible areas of induration is an early clinical finding. Pain following bowel movements may be caused by hemorrhoids or fissure (Rubin, 2000). Vesicles will be visible on examination if infection is caused by HSV (Strasser and McDonald, 1999).

MANAGEMENT

Careful, regular assessment is most important in diagnosis and management of perirectal abscess. Ongoing, daily evaluation of the rectal area for breaks in integrity must be included in the nursing assessment during periods of neutropenia and if specific complaints develop. Table 8-2 gives an accurate grading system for perirectal abscess. Cultures of the area should be performed if there is any suspicion of infection, and appropriate antibiotics should be initiated. Routine, thorough perineal care should be performed on a daily basis and after each bowel movement. Gentle cleaning and drying of the area should be performed to prevent ulceration. Females should perform perianal care utilizing a front to back method and avoid using tampons if menstruation does occur. Sitz baths utilizing tepid water may not only clean the area, but also provide relief from discomfort. The immunocompromised patient should also avoid enemas and suppositories (MMWR, 2000).

Diarrhea

Diarrhea can be an acute, complex problem for those undergoing transplant, because it has a significant impact on quality of life as well as affecting physiologic functioning. The etiology can be multifactorial. Toxicity associated with the preparative regimen can cause diarrhea for the first 20 days posttransplant. Diarrhea that continues beyond day 20 most likely represents another etiology. GVHD is the most common cause of diarrhea in the allogeneic population, followed by viral, bacterial, and finally parasitic origin.

Medications can also cause diarrhea as a side effect of therapy. Most common are antibiotics, metoclopramide, oral magnesium, and antacids. In addition, preexisting GI disorders, such as irritable bowel syndrome or Crohn's disease, can have an impact on posttransplant diarrhea (Strasser and McDonald, 1999; Ippoliti, 1998). Diarrhea can lead to significant fluid and electrolyte imbalances, as well as malnutrition.

Diarrhea is caused by many factors in the transplant setting, so there are characteristics to each etiology that will assist in classification and ultimately treatment. Each type of diarrhea affects the intestinal mucosa differently. How the patient responds to diarrhea is individual, and treatment is dependent upon the etiology. Chemotherapy-induced diarrhea results from the inhibition of the mitotic activity of the crypt cells of the GI tract. These cells are rapidly dividing, thus damage affects the villous architecture, rendering them ineffective in nutritional absorption. These changes are seen 7 to 10 days following the completion of the preparative regimen and normalize about 15 days later, after healing has occurred. Diarrhea is described as watery with accompanying crampy abdominal pain and anorexia (Ippoliti, 1998). Blood may also be observed. Busulfan, cytarabine, paclitaxel, melphalan, thiotepa, and methotrexate are antineoplastic agents commonly utilized in the transplant setting associated with diarrhea. Mesna has also been known to cause diarrhea (Strasser and McDonald, 1999). TBI causes the same physiologic response, resulting in diarrhea lasting 1 to 2 weeks (Ippoliti, 1998).

Secretory-type diarrhea usually presents as large-volume, watery stool that persists despite limited or absent oral intake. It typically develops after day 30 posttransplant. Damage to the crypt cells will inhibit intestinal absorption of necessary fluid and electrolytes, resulting in diarrhea of greater than one liter per day. Primary etiologies include noninvasive infectious organisms that produce enterotoxin such as *Clostridium difficile*, astrovirus, adenovirus, CMV, and rotavirus (Iqbal et al., 2000; Williams, 1999; Ippoliti, 1998; Hurley, 1997).

The predominant feature of GVHD of the gut is secretory diarrhea. In the case of GVHD, stool volume can be as high as 10 to 15 liters per day, accompanied by severe dehydration and protein and electrolyte imbalances (Williams, 1999). The portions of the gut most often affected by GVHD are the ileum and cecum, which are also primarily responsible for fluid absorption (Przepiorka and Cleary, 2000; Strasser and McDonald, 1999). This is a direct result of localized cytokine release producing mucosal edema and increased vascular permeability, which enhances the movement of fluid across the intestinal wall, hence, liquid stools (Strasser and McDonald, 1999). Diarrheal stools typically appear greenish with ropy mucoid strands indicative of protein loss (Williams, 1999). Severe cases of GVHD can produce intestinal hemorrhage and accompanying blood loss (Przepiorka and Cleary, 2000).

Exudative diarrhea is caused by direct damage to the mucosa, resulting in loss of function. Vital nutrients are not absorbed, leading to protein loss. Unlike other types of diarrhea, stools are not necessarily large volume or liquid, but instead, presentation is high stool frequency. Most often stools number greater than 6 per day, leading to hypoalbuminemia and anemia. Exudative diarrhea is associated with actual radiation injury and infection with such organisms as *Shigella, Salmonella, Strongyloides, Giardia lamblia*, and rotavirus (Ippoliti, 1998; Strasser and McDonald, 1999).

Osmotic diarrhea is not associated with mucosal damage, but rather mechanical disturbances that affect the bowel wall. These substances retard fluid absorption, causing frequent stools (Ippoliti, 1998). Diarrhea is typically large volume, watery-appearing stools that resolve once the offending agent has been removed. Causative agents include magnesium-based antacids, intraluminal blood, and peristaltic stimulants.

One study evaluated causes of diarrhea in both autologous and allogeneic stem cell transplant patients. The study population was composed of 28 allogeneic and 19 autologous patients. Researchers found intestinal infection in 3 of 48 diarrheal episodes. Two cases of *Clostridium difficile* were isolated, and one stool sample was positive for *Cryptosporidium*. Viruses were isolated in the cultures. When looking at the total number of episodes between the two groups, allogeneic recipients developed more diarrhea than autologous patients (van Kraaij et al., 2000). In a retrospective study looking at frequency of *C. difficile* infections in allogeneic patients, only 13% (10 patients) were positive at a median of 38 days posttransplant. Infection was not associated with the onset of GVHD, but individuals were found to be positive after the onset of GVHD (Chakrabarti et al., 2000). Viral infections were found to be more common in those who developed *C. difficile*. Lastly, diarrhea was found to occur in 61 of 80 patients receiving an autologous peripheral stem cell transplant. Only 3 were positive for pathogens (Avery et al., 2000).

MANAGEMENT

It can be difficult to make a definitive diagnosis on presenting symptoms alone, as the underlying etiologies often overlap. Careful assessment focusing on stool character and pattern, any abdominal symptoms, and perianal skin integrity is important. Other concurrent symptoms, such as fever and pain, should be included in the assessment. Totaling stool volume will help with staging and grading of diarrhea if GVHD is suspected (Stevens, 2004). Table 8-3 will assist with assessment. Considering the actual onset of symptoms in relation to the posttransplant day will help differentiate chemotherapy-induced diarrhea from other etiologies. Electrolyte panels will provide information regarding abnormalities that require replacement. Changes in albumin level will guide possible nutritional supplementation. Finally, direct visualization of the intestinal wall may be required via colonoscopy to determine the degree of damage and to obtain cultures. Weekly stool surveillance for vancomycin-resistant enterococcal (VRE) infections is routinely performed in some transplant centers. Although VRE is typically a systemic disease not confined to the bowel, carrier states can be identified by stool sample. Currently, standard recommendations for routine surveillance do not exist, but each center has its own recommendations (MMWR, 2000; Kapur et al., 2000).

Management of diarrhea includes maintaining fluid balance as a result of losses in stool content, decreasing transit time, and promotion of fluid absorption in the actual lumen. If infection is the cause, treatment with antibiotics will be necessary. However, decreasing intestinal motility may inhibit removal of the offending organism, and antidiarrheal medications are not recommended (Ippoliti, 1998). Current guidelines recommend using metronidazole if *C. difficile* is the offending microbe and limiting the use of vancomycin, as it may promote the development of VRE (MMWR, 2000). Viral etiologies should be treated with the appropriate antiviral agent such as ganciclovir or foscarnet if CMV is detected. Diarrhea associated with GVHD will respond well to prednisone, mycophenolate mofetil, and cyclosporine (Flowers et al., 1999). Dietary modifications that eliminate stimulants or irritants will also normalize bowel patterns. A bland, low-residue diet is most appropriate. In severe cases, bowel rest and the initiation of TPN may be necessary.

If infection is not the cause, a variety of pharmaceutical agents are available to restore normal bowel patterns and provide symptomatic relief. Antidiarrheal agents can be classified as intestinal transit inhibitors, intraluminal agents, proabsorptive agents, or antisecretory drugs. Intestinal transit inhibitors are opiate agonist; however, they can cause toxic megacolon as a side effect to treatment. These drugs decrease intestinal transit time by interfering with the release of acetylcholine in the nerves, which regulate intestinal motility. Examples include loperamide and codeine. Intraluminal agents work by improving stool consistency, thus decreasing the number of stools. These drugs include cholestyramine, clay, and activated charcoal. Proabsorptive agents are alpha-adrenergic-receptor agonists that prevent secretion of intestinal fluid and stimulate absorption. Side effect profile includes hypotension. An example is clonidine. Lastly, antisecretory drugs control diarrhea by acting on somatostatin receptors. Octreotide has been found to be very effective in controlling diarrhea and is widely used for treatment of GVHD of the gut (Ippoliti, 1998). One study demonstrated effective management of patients who developed grade 2 or greater diarrhea during transplant. Twenty-four patients were enrolled in the study; 14 developed diar-

rhea posttransplant. Twelve patients maintained complete control, defined as no more than two stools per day (Wasserman et al., 1997). It has been suggested that timing of treatment and dosage is more influential for successful treatment using octreotide. Drugs that appear to be the most effective in controlling diarrhea are octreotide and opiate agonists (Ippoliti, 1998).

Ulceration and GI Bleeding

Patients undergoing stem cell transplant are at risk for actual or occult bleeding from any site within the GI tract where there is mucosal wall damage. Incidence of GI bleeding has decreased to less than 10% within the first 100 days posttransplant. This is a reflection of the utilization of viral and fungal prophylaxis, better treatment for acute GVHD (Strasser and McDonald, 1999), and the use of peripheral stem cells, which have been shown to decrease the time to platelet engraftment (Bensinger et al., 2001). The use of 5HT-3 antagonists has also decreased the incidence of esophageal bleeding; however, Mallory-Weiss tears and intramural hematoma may still cause significant problems when platelet counts are less than 35,000. Esophageal bleeding due to reflux can be controlled with proton pump inhibitors and platelet transfusions. Surgical intervention may be necessary if bleeding persists (Strasser and McDonald, 1999).

Acute GVHD of the GI tract has been shown to produce extensive ulceration and bleeding. Better management has decreased but not eliminated bleeding risk. It has been demonstrated that bleeding risk due to acute GVHD of the GI tract increased in those individuals receiving a graft from a matched, unrelated donor. It was felt that tissue injury from viral sources, drugs used to treat acute GVHD, inflammatory cytokines, and thrombocytopenia were factors contributing to bleeding risk in this population (Nevo et al., 1999).

Gastric antral vascular ectasia (GAVE) can be another cause of upper GI bleeding. The gastric antrum and proximal duodenum develop areas of diffuse hemorrhage; however, the underlying mucosa appears normal. Found by endoscopic exam, treatment is supportive. Risk factors may include use of growth factors, male gender, and VOD (Strasser and McDonald, 1999).

One study evaluated the difference in incidence, cause, and outcome of bleeding in hematopoietic stem cell transplant patients in 1987 and those in 1997. Bleeding rates decreased from 10.7% in 1987 to 2.4% in 1997. Mortality between the two groups decreased form 3.6% to 0.9%. The authors cite better viral and fungal control as a significant factor improving outcomes between the two groups, as well as better treatment of GVHD (Schwartz et al., 2001).

MANAGEMENT

Monitoring laboratory indices such as hematocrit, platelet counts, and coagulation studies will help identify those who are risk for or may develop bleeding. All stool and emesis should be tested for occult blood when there is suspicion of bleeding or if blood studies change abruptly to reflect abnormal values.

Treatment is mainly supportive. The addition of proton pump inhibitors to medical regimens when platelet counts are below 100,000 will prevent gastric irritation. Maintaining platelet counts above 50,000 when symptoms indicate active bleeding will help prevent complications. Red cell transfusions and volume-expanding agents will help maintain vascular status. It is also recommended that existing coagulopathy be corrected by administering vitamin K or fresh frozen plasma. Surgical intervention such as angiography and endoscopic exams must be performed with care in order to prevent doing undue harm to the patient (Schwartz et al., 2001; Strasser and McDonald, 1999).

Liver Injury

Liver damage occurs for a variety of reasons during transplant. The causes can also be determined by the point at which they occur during the transplant process. Liver toxicity secondary to drugs in the preparative regimen is usually seen within the first 30 days. This is the most common etiology of elevated liver function tests in the autologous population. Supportive medications utilized during transplant have the potential to cause liver dysfunction. These include cyclosporine, methotrexate, antihymocyte globulin, antimicrobial agents such as trimethoprim-sulfa, and antifungal agents such as fluconazole and voriconazole. Also, prednisolone has been found to elevate liver function tests. This list is not inclusive, however; because of the evolution of new drugs utilized in transplant, this list has the potential to grow. TPN has the potential to cause hepatitis and cholestasis. Iron overload may also be causative because frequent transfusions are common in treating transplantable diseases, especially aplastic anemia (Kim et al., 2000; Vinayek et al., 2000; Strasser and McDonald, 1999).

Infectious etiologies of liver injury include viral, bacterial, and fungal infiltration. Most often, bacterial and fungal infiltrate develop as a result of system infection. However, with the use of fungal prophylaxis, there has been a significant decrease in systemic infection. Typically, the liver may develop abscesses, large cysts, or granulomas as a result of infiltration. The biliary ducts may become involved, causing a picture similar to VOD. Bacterial abscesses and cholangitis are less frequent in the transplant setting. This is most likely related to better antibiotic utilization when systemic symptoms develop, as well as prophylaxis (Vinayek et al., 2000).

Viral etiologies of liver damage include hepatitis C (HCV), hepatitis B (HBV), CMV, HSV, varicella zoster, adenovirus, and Epstein-Barr virus (EBV). HCV poses a significant problem due to the transfusion requirements of transplanted patients; however, better screening techniques have decreased rates. Portal inflammation is a typical finding with HCV infections. Those who are HCV positive prior to transplant poses a potential problem. Patients with chronic HBV infections prior to transplant have been reported to develop active viral replication while on immunosuppressive therapy, particularly at the time of drug withdraw. Transplants are performed using sero-positive donors if no others are available. In this scenario, the risk of the recipient developing infection is very high (Ljungman, 2000, 2002; Vinayek et al., 2000; Strasser and McDonald, 1999). Because the pathogenesis and management of VOD and GVHD of the liver are detailed elsewhere, they will not be addressed in this chapter.

Management

Pretransplant liver function tests and serology testing will identify those who may be at risk or have existing viral infections or liver abnormalities. Frequent serum evaluation of alkaline phosphatase, bilirubin, alanine aminotransferase, and aspartate aminotransferase will help identify those with potential for liver dysfunction after transplant. Most often, liver imaging and direct biopsy are required for diagnosis.

Kim and colleagues (2000) studied liver disease during the first year posttransplant in both autologous and allogeneic recipients. Abnormal liver functions developed in 93 of 130 patients. This sample consisted of 101 allogeneic recipients and 29 autologous transplants. Of the 93, 85 had allogeneic transplants, and 13 had autologous transplants. They found the incidence of liver function abnormalities to be 71.5% in the study group, which was similar to previous studies. The main cause of liver toxicity in allogeneic patients was found to be secondary to GVHD and drug injury. Drug toxicity was found to be the primary cause of liver dysfunction in autologous patients.

Management varies depending on the etiology. If drugs or TPN are felt to be the offending agent, removal or substitution with a similar drug may resolve the problem. The addition of steroids will treat GVHD if this is felt to be the underlying cause. Appropriate antiviral therapy will be necessary if the etiology is the result of CMV, HSV, varicella zoster, adenovirus or EBV (Vinayek et al., 2000). However, if HBV or HCV is the causative agent, treatment can be a challenge. There are no standard recommendations with regard to treatment, and long-term risk for the development of cirrhosis years after transplant is high. Pretransplant immunoglobulin can be give to the recipient of HBV-positive marrow. Famciclovir and lamivudine have been given to small samples of sero-positive transplant patients, but additional studies are needed before this treatment can be considered a standard. Posttransplant HCV can be treated with interferon with or without ribavirin in long-term survivors. Those with active infection at the time of transplant are typically monitored. There is evidence that ribavirin can be safely utilized during the transplant phase; however, additional studies with larger sample sizes are needed to confirm safety (Ljungman, 2002).

Nutrition for the BMT Patient

Protein-calorie deficiency can occur rapidly and can continue during the posttransplant phase (Raynard et al., 2003). The nutritional support of patients experiencing GI and metabolic effects during the transplant process is an exceedingly important element of medical and nursing care. A variety of nutritional strategies that can be employed to manage specific GI complications have been addressed earlier in this chapter. The specific nutritional concerns that require attention for managing the transplant population are related to nutritional assessment, low-microbial diets, and the role of parenteral and enteral nutrition.

Nutritional Assessment

The primary goals of nutritional assessment of the bone and marrow transplant patient are to (1) identify risk factors, (2) determine nutritional requirements, and (3) evaluate the effectiveness of the nutritional support in maintaining a patient's nutritional status (Mitchell, 2001). Nutritional assessment begins prior to the transplant and continues until the patient is no longer taking medications. No standard of care has been established to provide guidelines to assess patients; however, assessment should be carried out before transplantation (Raynard et al., 2003).

The majority of bone and marrow transplantation patients have an acceptable nutritional status prior to treatment. In fact, patients with hematological malignancies are usually well nourished at the time of bone and marrow transplantation, whereas malnutrition is frequent in patients with solid tumors (Laviano & Meguid, 1996; Muscaritoli et al., 2002). It is best to evaluate the patient prior to the initiation of therapy; however, nutritional assessment is an ongoing process. During the pretransplant phase, an initial nutritional assessment and screening should be performed. Accurate measurements of height and weight are recorded for baseline information and for the calculation of chemotherapy drug doses. Body weight may not be an accurate indicator of a patient's nutritional status. Changes in body weight can be influenced by aggressive hydration, fluid shifts, TPN, vomiting, or diarrhea, although body composition or body mass may not change (Singh & McDonald, 1997).

The initial components of baseline assessment include the patient's nutritional practices: current nutritional intake, food allergies, factors that influence oral intake, activity level, special dietary likes and dislikes, identification of the food preparer, and medications.

Pretransplant assessment and counseling consist of an understanding of nutrition-related problems associated with transplantation and the concept of parenteral and/or enteral supplementation. Baseline nutritional assessment of the bone and marrow transplantation patient is of critical importance to determine the nature and extent of nutritional deficiencies in order to rapidly prepare for and intervene with nutritional strategies to prevent further deterioration during very stressful treatment. If the patient is well nourished prior to transplantation, then the goal of nutritional support is maintenance.

The nurse and dietitian should collaborate with the transplant team on a continual basis to promote optimum nutrition. Elements the nurse can use to evaluate nutrition of the bone and marrow transplant patient are outlined in **Table 8-5**.

Anthropometric measurements have been used to assess changes in the bone and marrow transplantation patient's body composition; however, the fluid and electrolyte abnormalities leading to overhydration or dehydration limit their usefulness. A number of serum markers have been traditionally used for nutritional assessment. The total lymphocyte count is affected

---

Table 8-5 NUTRITIONAL ASSESSMENT OF THE BMT PATIENT.

General history
Medical history
  Illnesses example: diabetes mellitus
  Educational level
  Insurance coverage
Energy/activity level and exercise tolerance
Gastrointestinal review of symptoms
  Anorexia/nausea/vomiting, dysphagia, heartburn, reflux, hematemesis, xerostomia, bowel habits:
  diarrhea, constipation
Psychiatric review of systems
  Anxiety, depression, attention, drug abuse history
Dietary history
  Current appetite
  Previous treatment and nutritional side effects
  Food allergies
  Food aversion and preferences
  Dietary practices at home
    Meal patterns
    Food preparation assistance
    Timing of meals
    Grocery shopping assistance
  Ethnic preferences
Physical exam
  Height and weight
  Age and gender
  Hydration status
  Oral cavity and dental status
  Current medications
  Vitamin therapy
Laboratory data
  CBC: WBC, hemoglobin, hematocrit, platelet
  PT, PTT
  Electrolytes: sodium, chloride, potassium, carbon dioxide, glucose
  BUN, creatinine
  Calcium, magnesium, phosphorus
  Total bilirubin, SGOT, SGPT, alkaline phosphatase, LDH
  Plasma proteins: albumin, serum transferrin

by treatment-induced neutropenia and immunosuppression, which can limit its usefulness for nutritional assessment. Additionally, biochemical markers such as plasma proteins (e.g., albumin, transferrin, and prealbumin) have been shown to inaccurately reflect changes in nutritional status of bone and marrow transplantation patients (Muscaritoli et al., 1995).

Patients undergoing transplant can have an alteration in their metabolic functioning related to the current or previous treatment they received or their diseases. A thorough understanding of the metabolic alterations is essential in order to provide adequate nutritional support for these patients. Bone and marrow transplantation can be divided into three phases, each presenting distinct metabolic challenges: (1) conditioning period with therapies causing tissue damage, (2) neutropenic period with tissue repair, and (3) engraftment, which can be complicated by GVHD, graft failure, or sepsis.

The acute treatment-related effects from the conditioning regimens both from chemotherapy and total body radiation have an impact on two major systems: the GI mucosa and the central nervous system. This can decrease intake of nutrients, placing the patient on the path to malnutrition. The normal growth and repair of the GI mucosa is disrupted (Raynard et al., 2003; Muscaritoli et al., 2002). With the loss of functioning intestinal epithelium, malabsorption, mucositis, and taste alterations develop, resulting in diarrhea and protein loss. Additionally, the effects on the central nervous system result in severe vomiting, setting up another barrier to oral nutrition. Intestinal dysmotility due to narcotic analgesics can exacerbate vomiting. Many of the GI complications, such as mucositis, GVHD, fever, infection, enteritis, diarrhea, and nausea, make the nutritional requirements of a transplant patient paramount.

Following the conditioning regimen, the bone and marrow transplant patient is profoundly neutropenic. This places the patient at risk for bacterial infections. The loss of GI mucosal barrier function due to damaged intestine serves as a portal of entry for bacteria. Additionally, narcotic analgesia can cause intestinal stasis, predisposing the mucosa to bacterial overgrowth, which in turn leads to further intestinal damage or translocation of gut bacteria into the bloodstream. This can cause an infection having a significant appetite-suppressant effect leading to weight loss (Bush, 1999). Tissue damage and nitrogen mobilization from protein breakdown also are exacerbated by infection. During the neutropenic period, tissue repair is also occurring, thus increasing nutrient requirements.

After engraftment, mucosal lesions heal and patients are often able to resume some oral intake. With the absence of enteral nutrients, which stimulate the intestine, absorption can be affected, delaying epithelial cell repair and regeneration. Diarrhea can occur during this time, caused by GVHD or infection. This can once again lead to mucosal cell breakdown or tissue necrosis. Clinically, GVHD diarrhea is similar to that during the conditioning regimen but is more severe and prolonged. It can cause massive protein loss and a profound decrease in nitrogen balance (Bush, 1999).

Several nutritional effects result from GVHD prophylaxis and treatment with high-dose corticosteroids. Corticosteroids promote muscle breakdown, increasing the urea cycle and causing a loss of nitrogen. With this loss of protein, fluid overload can result from the IV fluids and nephrotoxic agents, including cyclosporine and antibiotics.

In spite of interventions aimed at improving oral intake, changes in oral metabolism may further contribute to weight loss and malnutrition. A thorough understanding of both the generalized and specific metabolic alterations is essential in providing effective nutritional support.

The transplant procedure has a dramatic effect on the recipient, affecting energy and metabolism. Initially, negative nitrogen balance or nitrogen deficiency is common in bone and marrow transplant patients as a consequence of both intestinal losses with diarrhea and catabolic effects on skeletal muscle. Initially, negative nitrogen balance is exerted by the underlying disease, then by the conditioning regimens, and subsequently by bone and marrow transplant complications such as sepsis and GVHD. Nitrogen balance is a measure of protein metabolism and is largely influenced by calories, so protein may improve both total body weight and nitrogen balance (referred to as anabolism). Protein catabolism or the destruction of body protein such as muscle leads to negative nitrogen balance, even with the provision of adequate calories (Raynard et al., 2003). Despite adequate caloric and protein intake, protein catabolism may not be preventable. If the protein needs of the bone and marrow transplant patient are not met, skeletal and visceral muscle mass may be depleted. What is observed clinically includes loss of respiratory muscle mass, which increases the potential for complications such as pneumonia or loss of skeletal muscle, which leads to decreased mobility. Finally, without adequate protein, lymphocyte production is decreased, causing prolonged immunosuppression.

Measurement of protein loss must be quantified (e.g., diarrhea, urine, pleural effusion). This will allow for replacement of exogenous protein. To meet nitrogen needs, dietary protein must be provided in adequate daily amounts (Rust and Kogut, 2001). The protein requirements of a bone and marrow transplant patient range from 1.4 to 1.5 g/kg body weight per day, which is double the requirements of a healthy adult. Protein needs increase in bone and marrow transplant patients with severe stress such as GVHD, sepsis, and diarrhea (Muscaritoli et al., 1998).

Energy needs in the initial 30 to 50 days posttransplant have been estimated to be 170% of the basal energy expenditure and approximately 130% and 150% at the time of discharge. Protein requirements at the recommended daily allowance for the bone and marrow transplant patient can be estimated by the Harris Benedict equation (Apovian et al., 1998). Many investigators have proved that 30 to 35 kcal/kg per day are needed for the adult bone and marrow transplant patient; however, Szeluga and colleagues (1985) found that up to 50 kcal/day are needed for most adult patients with acute GVHD. Others have demonstrated the energy requirements of bone and marrow transplant patients to be 130% to 150% times their predicted basal energy expenditure (Muscaritoli et al., 2002; Raynard et al., 2003).

Treatments associated with BMT may have a significant effect on metabolism of carbohydrates. Human metabolism depends on carbohydrates or glucose. Carbohydrates, a primary energy source, provide 50% to 60% of required daily calories. When carbohydrate intake is inadequate, gluconeogenesis occurs and glucose is obtained from protein and fat. Anaerobic metabolism is the breakdown of glucose without oxygen. It yields less energy, produces lactic acid, and leads to poor tissue perfusion. In the bone and marrow transplant patient, steroids, often used in conjunction with immunosuppressive therapy, can precipitate hyperglycemia. Specific antineoplastic agents used in conditioning regimens also can cause alterations in carbohydrate metabolism. For example,

L-asparaginase can precipitate insulin-dependent diabetes whereas bulsulfan can cause direct damage to the pancreatic beta cells (Herrmann and Petruska, 1993).

Ingested fat is used for energy if inadequate amounts of carbohydrates are ingested. If the amount and type of food eaten are more than the body's current needs, the food will be stored in the adipose tissue. The normal process does not occur in the patient with cancer, because the cancer patient's ability to store fat is limited. Therefore, wasting of stored body fat and increased levels of serum lipids in transplant patients may occur (Kern and Norton, 1988). Lipids can inhibit the immune system's functioning. Exogenously administered essential lipids or fatty acids interfere with synthesis of biological effector cells and inflammation such as prostaglandins by incorporating into the cell membrane, and may therefore play an additional role in affecting outcomes of BMT patients (Muscaritoli et al., 2002). This can further compromise a neutropenic transplant patient, especially since many of the interventions employed to increase caloric intake use lipids in the diet. Immunosuppressive therapy, specifically cyclosporine, also has been associated with altered lipid metabolism.

Low-Microbial Diets

Although controversial (Smith and Besser, 2000), most transplant centers provide food selection guidelines to follow in the first weeks after transplant until white cell recovery occurs. Recommendations regarding the use of low-microbial diets have been based on the theory of reducing the risk of contracting infections from pathogens in foods that may colonize and seed the blood through the GI tract that has been damaged by the conditioning regimen. It was believed that the GI tract serves as an important barrier, preventing the migration of pathogenic microorganisms into the systematic circulation. The absence of nutrients in the gut results in atrophy of the mucosal villi, which leads to decreased activity of the gut enzymes and affects gut-associated lymphoid tissue, which are essential to maintaining the integrity of the intestinal barrier (Muscaritoli et al., 2002; Smith and Besser, 2000). When the mucosal integrity is disrupted, this can lead to decreased nutrient absorption.

Other factors that reduce the efficiency of the gut barrier include decreased gastric motility secondary to narcotics analgesia, increased gastric pH, and disrupted GI flora. Therefore, malnutrition, ileus, acid-sequestering drugs, and antibiotic therapy can interfere with the protective mechanism of the gut. This interference can lead to transmission of bacteria into the intestines and also the systemic circulation, resulting in sepsis.

The type of food restrictions used with patients undergoing BMT include sterile diet, low microbial diet, cooked food, and modified hospital diet; however, there is no research that exists on the relative benefit of these diets. The principles of these diets in general are that all foods must be well cleaned and prepared following sanitary practices (**Table 8-6**). Allogeneic transplant patient are usually advised to avoid foods such as aged cheese, commercially prepared meats, vegetable salads, delicatessen foods, raw eggs, and uncooked meat or seafood. In general, foods high in fiber, highly spiced, caffeinated, or lactose-based are eliminated from the diet (Mitchell, 2001). Foods are gradually added to the patient's diet based on tolerance.

A variety of methods can prevent cross-contamination of high-risk foods, specifically

Table 8-6 FOOD GUIDELINES FOR THE IMMUNOCOMPROMISED PATIENT.

Meats and proteins	Avoid raw foods.
	Meat should be cooked.
Beef	Cooking temperature should be 160°F (71°C).
	Rare pink meat should not be eaten.
	Avoid cooked meats that have been in contact with raw meats or juice.
Eggs	Yolks and whites should be firm.
	Suggest hard-boiled.
	Consider egg substitutes.
	Avoid dishes prepared with uncooked eggs (examples: Caesar salad, custard).
Poultry	Cooking temperature should be 180°F (74°C).
Seafood	Cook until flesh is firm.
	Ingest seafood from clean waters.
Dairy products	Drink only pasteurized milk.
	Avoid flavored milks: chocolate, strawberry.
Fruits and vegetables	Wash fruits and vegetables by using a scrub brush with chlorinated water.
	Peel raw fruits and vegetables if consumed raw.
Water	Have private water supply checked for bacterial contamination or use bottled water.
Food preparation and handling	Avoid cross-contamination.
	Thaw foods by refrigeration versus room temperature.
	Maintain proper hygiene prior to and during food preparation (example: wash hands before meal preparation).
	Discard outdated foods and unused leftovers after 2 days.

raw meats, poultry, and seafood. One method is to designate separate cutting boards for meats and other foods. Cutting boards should be washed and sanitized. Plastic boards with knife grooves provide an environment for the transmission of organisms. Separate utensils should be used when preparing meats. Food preparers should thoroughly wash their hands, lathering for at least 20 seconds. Marinades, gravies, and sauces should be brought to boiling if they contain meat juices or if they have been in contact with raw meat. Meats should be thawed on the bottom shelf of the refrigerator, in a dish with sides to prevent the meat juices from coming in contact with other foods. At the grocery store,

meats should be wrapped and packaged separately from the nonmeat foods

Patients with private water supplies such as septic tanks or wells should be instructed to have their water checked when a change in taste, odor, or color is noted. Water should be checked quarterly thereafter. In the event of substantial rainfall or flooding, water should be checked for bacteria. Patients with a public water supply do not need to have their water checked for bacteria, because the Safe Drinking Water Act regulates strict community standards established by the Environmental Protection Agency and/or state (Cabelof, 1994; Centers for Disease Control, 2004).

Methods of preventing transmission of food-borne pathogens are strict guidelines intended for the BMT patient at high risk for developing foodborne infections. Assessment of the patient's risk for infection and specific teaching by the nurse are necessary. Clinical decision making should determine which guidelines would be most beneficial for each patient based on risk of infection, lifestyle, and level of malnutrition.

Research may be defining the optimal low-microbial dietary practices for BMT patients. Cost in relationship to the therapeutic outcome should also be examined. The collaborative relationship of the nurses and dieticians is critical for effective implementation of any strategies. Patients and family members require education in the rationale and importance of the selected dietary practice, both during and after hospitalization.

In practice, there is no consensus among health-care professionals about the best policy to increase oral intake and promote recovery in the posthospital phase. Some consider eating problems in this phase transient and pay little attention to them whereas others choose invasive procedures such as home parenteral nutrition (Iestra et al., 2002). Oral intake is usually initiated when mucositis subsides and narcotic therapy is reduced. Narcotic weaning as mucositis improves and pain subsides allows for reintroduction of oral intake. In order to enhance nutritional value food selection should involve choosing foods that are either high protein or energy dense, or using oral supplements (Iestra et al., 2002). Since oral intake is often severely decreased during the 20 to 30 days after transplant, oral intake should be neither forced nor overemphasized (Hopman et al., 2003). It could severely discourage the patient who has a fear of eating and create a negative atmosphere,

thus preventing successful refeeding. During this period, many patients consume only water or ice chips.

When the patient becomes clinically stable, teaching can be initiated to suggest foods and fluids that are appealing and easily tolerated. Taste is altered, with a decreased threshold for sweet and salt that can last for more than one year. As appetite improves, previously rejected foods may become more acceptable; the patient should be encouraged to retry foods.

Oral intake can become a major nursing strategy, particularly when the patient is approaching discharge. Patients usually consume 60% of their oral intake on the day prior to discharge. A food plan must be designated to provide a variety of foods at frequent intervals to meet patients' needs and therefore reduce dependence on TPN. It is critical that the patient be able to maintain an adequate oral intake, and is especially crucial for patients receiving cyclosporin. This will prevent dehydration, thereby minimizing the need for hospital readmission or intravenous fluid hydration in the home setting.

The role of the nurse in enhancing oral intake is critical throughout the treatment process. Nurses can identify barriers to eating such as refractory nausea, food aversions, depression, medications causing GI disturbances, and other GI complications that plague the BMT patient. They can coordinate a plan of care that includes monitoring of daily oral food and fluid intake, nutritional strategies to manage GI symptoms and patient/family education and support. Families frequently find support from hearing that patients other than their family member have difficulty eating.

Nutrition classes and support groups may be helpful, not only for education, but also for motivation. It has been noted that oral intake frequently improves when patients are able to eat familiar food, such as home-cooked or ethnic foods rather than hospital food. Nurses, physicians, and dieticians should collaborate to mobilize all resources available to enhance oral intake by the BMT patient.

Enteral and Parenteral Nutrition

Poor oral intake with a poor performance and a debilitated nutritional status is a central concern in the BMT patients. All of the GI complications such as mucositis, GVHD, fever, infection, enteritis diarrhea, xerostomia, dysgeusia, nausea with or without vomiting, and organ damage predispose the transplant patient to severe metabolic disorders, catabolism, and almost certainly the inability to meet nutritional requirements both during and frequently after discharge. Nutritional consequences are compounded by the fact that many transplant candidates were nutritionally compromised pretransplant from their disease, previous treatment, psychological stress, or underlying GI complaints.

ENTERAL NUTRITION

Controlled trials of the effects of enteral nutrition in BMT patients to date are still sparse and not a common practice. Artificial nutrition should be given to patients with malnutrition defined as more than 10% loss of body weight irrespective of the type of transplant. The summary of standards and recommendations for nutritional support in patients undergoing bone marrow transplant indicates that enteral nutrition rather than parenteral nutrition should be the preferred line of treatment for patients undergoing BMT (Raynard et al., 2003). In recent years indications for TPN have markedly decreased in favor of

enteral nutrition (Muscaritoli et al., 2002; Raynard et al., 2003). Prior to this shift, enteral nutrition was not typically used in BMT patients because GI side effects associated with BMT result in poor tolerance of enteral feedings.

Research, however, showing benefits of feeding via the GI tract and the focus on cost in health care has caused some centers to consider enteral feedings of BMT patients (Hopman et al., 2003). There have been several studies comparing enteral and parenteral nutrition support in these patients. Both the Szeluga (1985) and Mulder (1989) groups demonstrated that enteral feedings were an acceptable alternative to TPN. Enteral nutrition has been clearly demonstrated to help maintain intestinal mucosal integrity and support the barrier function of the gut; this protective effect of enteral feeding is not realized with TPN.

Factors to be considered when initiating enteral feedings are disease status, marrow function, control of GI symptoms, estimated duration of enteral feedings, availability of caregivers, and insurance. Allogeneic BMT patients who fail to thrive may benefit from placement of a percutaneous endoscopic gastrostomy (PEG) tube for long-term nutritional support.

PARENTERAL NUTRITION

Total parenteral nutrition is frequently a supportive care strategy for the BMT patient; however, recently published nutritional support standards indicate that TPN should be reserved for patients who have an intolerance to oral or enteral nutrition, obstruction, severe mucositis, or oral intake less than 50% of estimated needs (Raynard et al., 2003; Scolapio et al., 2002). The studies done to date have been aimed at evaluating the effects of TPN on the outcome of BMT. Parenteral nutrition can result in more intact nutritional status; however, it has not proven to have an impact on the length of stay or survival when compared to oral dietary intake (Roberts et al., 2003). In instances where severe GI side effects of myeloablative conditioning regimens in conjunction with fever, infection, organ dysfunction, and GVHD often preclude oral diets or enteral feedings, TPN has been utilized. TPN has not strictly been "total" because patients have been allowed oral intake. The transplant procedure has been associated with prolonged negative nitrogen balance and loss of muscle mass in the BMT patient. Literature indicates that if parenteral nutrition is delayed in these patients, it is difficult to "catch up," particularly as organ failure develops after treatment, impeding the tolerance of fluids and high concentrations of proteins, carbohydrates, and fats (Herrmann and Petruska, 1993).

TPN Administration

The primary clinical goals of TPN administration include the prevention of nitrogen imbalance and loss of lean body mass while not overloading patients with excessive fluids and nutrients. The availability of different concentrations of amino acids, dextrose, and lipid substrates allows the dietician, TPN pharmacist, and physician to specify a TPN regimen based on the nutritional needs of the transplant patient (Roberts et al., 2003; Ezzone & Mirtallo, 2000). The role of the nurse in caring for the transplant patient receiving TPN includes the administration of the TPN solution and monitoring for adverse complications.

Meticulous care must be exercised to maintain aseptic technique when caring for a patient receiving TPN via central venous catheter. Institutional policies and procedures should reflect current literature related to infection control in TPN administration including the changing of TPN tubing every 24 to 48 hours, maintaining a closed system, and avoiding collection of blood specimens through the TPN tubing except in an emergency, when changing the tubing, or when discontinuation of tubing is planned. When parenteral nutrition lumens are used for multiple purposes in the transplant patient, careful maintenance and care should be used to minimize risk of infection.

Other complications of TPN administration to BMT patients are varied because of the possible impact of concomitant metabolic disturbances from organ system dysfunction and other medications. Hyperglycemia, for example, may result because of the TPN and concurrent steroid therapy and/or sepsis. Hypoglycemia may result from abruptly stopping the solution or from excess insulin administration. Hypokalemia and hypomagnesemia may result despite supplementation of these electrolytes because of the effects of parenteral antibiotics, amphotericin B, and diarrhea. Hypermagnesemia, hyperkalemia, and hyperphosphatemia may result from renal failure. Sudden weight gain may reflect impending venoocclusive disease or volume overload, whereas significant volume depletion may occur because of prolonged vomiting or diarrhea. Fluid overload is also a frequent complication of intensive nutritional therapy in chronically undernourished patients (Muscaritoli et al., 2002; Ezzone & Mirtallo, 2000).

The nurse must be aware of all possible etiologies for the metabolic disturbances in BMT patients on TPN. Routine chemistries, careful assessment of fluid volume status, and electrolyte supplementation are all necessary interventions when caring for these patients. Certain laboratory studies are indicated to anticipate and correct potential metabolic problems that can be caused by parenteral nutrition. Hyperglycemia may require management of frequent serum-glucose testing with the addition of insulin to the TPN or sliding-scale insulin coverage. Hypoglycemia can be avoided by properly tapering solutions as ordered (Cetin et al., 2002; Muscaritoli et al., 2002).

TPN allows for better modulation of fluid, electrolytes, and nutrients, which is of pivotal importance when complications occur such as acute GVHD or VOD. For example, the onset of VOD complications by hepatic encephalopathy may suggest the need for fluid-restricted TPN enriched with branch chain amino acids. This underscores the need for personalized nutritional support for BMT patients. Management of fluid overload may require diuresis and concentration of medications (antibiotics) to the minimum permissible volume of the drug (Muscaritoli et al., 2002; Raynard et al., 2003). Some researchers indicate that a shift of fluid from the intracellular compartment occurs during the first 4 weeks after marrow engraftment; TPN can result in such fluid shifts. Strict intake and output and daily weights need to be monitored. Weight is assessed primarily to judge hydration status, which is reflected by electrolytes, BUN, creatinine, and albumin levels. Constant weight fluctuations often reflect difficulty in managing fluids, rather than actual gains and losses in body mass.

Cycling of TPN (i.e., 10- to 18-hour administration) can be successful in the BMT patient in order to create a daily infusion-free period. In this way, the catheter is available for administration of other medications and blood products. The nurse may encounter difficulty with the timely administration of drugs and blood products when continuous TPN is infused into one lumen. Cycling may allow the patient some freedom by temporarily being disconnected from intravenous infusion lines.

The use of lipid substrates and glutamine deserve careful consideration in BMT patients. A variety of specialized nutritional support therapies may improve the ability to nourish the transplant patient effectively. This trend in nutritional support was to prevent and mitigate treatment-induced GI. Several novel therapies being investigated for the BMT patient are the use of glutamine, lipid substrates, and fatty acids.

Supplemental glutamine has been studied to determine its effects on prevention of GI toxicity. The rationale for administering glutamine was based on the concept that glutamine is a primary fuel for enterocytes and for gut-associated lymphoid tissue. Several studies have been performed to evaluate the effect of glutamine administration on GI toxicity in BMT (Anderson et al., 1998; Pytlik et al., 2002; Schloerb and Skikne, 1999; Zeigler, 2001, 2002). These trials failed to show a clear preventive or curative effect of glutamine on intestinal mucositis. Of note, these studies were performed in nonhomogenous patients undergoing either allo or auto BMT for solid tumors or hematologic malignancies, which renders these studies rather difficult to interpret. Future randomized studies would be of value in homogenous patient populations.

Glutamine administration after BMT is directed at the inflammatory, epithelial, ulcerative, and healing phases of the mucous membrane. Glutamine has indeed been shown to exert a positive effect on nitrogen balance; however, intravenous or oral glutamine did not reduce the incidence of infectious complications, indicate survival, or shorten the duration of hospital stay (Wilmore, 1991; Anderson et al., 1998).

Another area of glutamine investigation is the prevention and treatment of VOD. Preliminary analysis (Goringe et al., 1998; Zeigler, 2001) suggests that glutamine maintained hepatic function by preserving albumin and plasma protein C; however, further studies are needed to determine whether glutamine and vitamin E or use of other antioxidants reduces the incidence of posttransplant venoocclusive disease.

LIPID SUBSTRATES

The administration of lipid substrates may interfere with immune effector cells and inflammation such as prostaglandins by incorporating into the membrane of these cells, and might therefore play a role in affecting the outcome for BMT patients. Lipid-based TPN solution is associated with a lower incidence of acute GVHD in allogeneic BMT patients (Muscaritoli et al., 2002). The mechanism of action is hypothesized that prostaglandin metabolites decrease interleukin-1 and tumor necrosis factor macrophage production and increase T suppressor activity. The recent availability of intravenous admixtures containing fish oil–derived fatty acids has set the stage to investigate the effects of lipid compounds in the role of managing the complications of VOD and GVHD, specifically to investigate their role in inflammation and modulation of the immune response since initial studies of fatty acids have been shown to reduce vascoconstriction and platelet clumping or aggregation (Roulet et al., 1997).

Summary

Numerous GI complications can plague the patient undergoing transplant procedures, both during and after the actual transplant process. A spectrum of etiologies is responsible for these complications and involves the combined impact of various therapeutic interventions and their sequelae. Nurses caring for this population of patients are faced with formidable challenges because the management of these complications profoundly affects the patient's nutritional status. It is likely that consensus regarding assessment of GI complications will emerge as transplant technology continues to evolve; the current lack of uniformity in assessment approaches limits multicenter trials describing the character and efficacy of managing stomatitis, esophagitis, enteritis, and ulcerative pathologies. However, additional nursing research is necessary to provide information on the most efficacious ways to manage GI difficulties and to enhance nutritional intake throughout the process.

References

Abang, A.M., Takemoto, M.H., Pham, T., Mandanas, R.A., Roy, V., Selby, G.B., et al. (2000). Efficacy and safety of oral granisetron versus i.v. granisetron in patients undergoing peripheral blood progenitor cell and bone marrow transplantation. *Anti-Cancer Drugs, 11,* 137–142.

Abbott, B., Ippoliti, C., Hecth, D., Bruton, J., Whaley, B., & Champlin, R. (2000). Ganisetron (kytril) plus dexamethasone for antiemetic control in bone marrow transplant patients receiving highly emetogenic chemotherapy with or without total body irradiation. *Bone Marrow Transplantation, 25,* 1279–1283.

Anderson, P.M., Ramsay, N.K., Shu, X.O., et al. (1998). Effect of low dose oral glutamine supplemented on painful stomatitis during bone marrow transplantation. *Bone Marrow Transplantation, 22,* 339–344.

Apovian, C.M., Still, C.D., & Blackburn, G.L. (1998). Nutrition support. In A.M. Berger, R.K. Portenoy,

& D.E. Weissman (Eds.), *Principles and practice of supportive oncology* (pp. 571–588). Philadelphia: Lippincott-Raven.

Avery, R., Pohlman, B., Adal, K., Bolwell, B., Goldman, M., Kalaycio, M., et al. (2000). High prevalence of diarrhea but infrequency of documented *Clostridium difficile* in autologous peripheral blood progenitor cell transplant recipients. *Bone Marrow Transplantation, 25*, 67–69.

Barker, G.J. (1999). Current practices in the oral management of the patient undergoing chemotherapy or bone marrow transplant. *Support Care Cancer, 7,* 17–20.

Basara, N., Roemer, E., Kraut, L., Guenzelmann, S., Schmetzer, B., Kiehl, M.G., et al. (2002). Reduced intensity preparative regimens for allogeneic hematopoietic stem cell transplantation: A single center experience. *Bone Marrow Transplantation, 30,* 651–659.

Bashey, A. (2000). Infection. In E.D. Ball, J. Lister, & P. Law (Eds.), *Hematopoietic stem cell therapy* (pp. 510–520). Philadelphia: Churchill Livingstone.

Bellm, L.A., Epstein, J.B., Rose-Ped, A., Martin, P., & Fuchs, H.J. (2000). Patient reports of complications of bone marrow transplant. *Support Care Cancer, 8,* 33–39.

Bensinger, W.I, Martin, P.J., Storer, B., Clift, R., Forman, S.J., Steven, J., et al. (2001). Transplantation of bone marrow as compared with peripheral-blood cells from HLA-identical relatives in patients with hematologic cancers. *New England Journal of Medicine, 344*(3), 175–181.

Bolwell, B.J., Kalaycio, M., Sobecks, R., Andresen, S., Kuczkowski, E., Bernhard, L., et al. (2002). *Bone Marrow Transplantation, 30,* 587–591.

Bremerkamp, M. (2000). Mechanism of action of 5-HT3 receptor antagonists: Clinical overview and nursing implications. *Clinical Journal of Oncology Nursing, 4*(5), 201–207.

Bubalo, J., Seelig, F., Karbowicz, S., & Maziarz, R.T. (2001). Ramdomized open-label trial of dolasetron for the control of nausea and vomiting associated with high-dose chemotherapy with hematopoietic stem cell transplantation. *Biology of Blood and Marrow Transplant, 7*(8), 439–445.

Buchali, A., Feyr, P., Groll, J., Massenkeil, G., Arnold, R., & Budach, V. (2000). Immediate toxicity during fractioned total body irradiation as conditioning for bone marrow transplantation. *Radiotherapy and Oncology, 54,* 157–162.

Bush, W.W. (1999). Overview of transplantation immunology and the pharmacology of adult solid organ transplant recipients: Focus on immunosuppression. *AACN Clinical Issues, 10*(2), 253–269.

Cabelof, D.C. (1994). Preventing infection from food borne pathogens in liver transplant patients. *Journal of the American Dietetic Association, 94*(10), 1140–1144.

Cetin, T., Arpaci, F., Dere, Y., Turan, M., Ozturk, B., Komurcu, S., et al. (2002). Total parenteral nutrition delays platelet engraftment in patients who undergo autologous hematopoietic stem cell transplantation. *Nutrition, 18*(7–8), 599–603.

Chakrabarti, S., Lees, A., Jones, S.G., & Milligan, D.W. (2000). *Clostridium difficile* infection in allogeneic stem cell transplant recipients is associated with severe graft-versus-host disease and non-relapse mortality. *Bone Marrow Transplantation, 26,* 871–876.

Champlin, R., Khouri, I., Anderlini, P., Gajewski, J., Kornblau, S., Molldrem, J., et al. (2001). Nonmyeloablative preparative regimens for allogeneic hematopoietic transplantation. *Bone Marrow Transplantation, 27*(Suppl. 2), S13–S22.

Cruz-Correa, M., Ponnawala, A., Abraham, S.C., Wu, T.T., Zahruak, M., Vogelsang, G., et al. (2002). Endoscopic findings predict the histologic diagnosis of gastrointestinal graft-versus-host disease. *Endoscopy, 34*(10), 808–813.

Dando, T.M., & Perry, C.M. (2004). Aprepitant: A review of its use in the prevention of chemotherapy-induced nausea and vomiting. *Drugs, 64*(7), 777–794.

De La Rosa, G.R., Champlin, R.E., & Kontoyiannis, D.P. (2002). Risk factors for the development of invasive fungal infections in allogeneic blood and marrow transplant recipients. *Transplant Infectious Disease, 4,* 3–9.

de Wit, R., Herrstedt, J., Rapoport, B., Carides, A.D., Carides, G., Elmer, M., et al. (2003). Addition of the oral NK1 antagonist aprepitant to standard antiemetics provides protection against nausea and vomiting during multiple cycles of cisplatin-based chemotherapy. *Journal of Clinical Oncology, 22*(15), 4105–4111.

Duncan, M., & Grant, G. (2003). Review article: Oral and intestinal mucositis—causes and possible treatments. *Alimentary Pharmacology Therapy, 18,* 853–874.

Epstein, J.B., Phillips, N., Parry, J., Epstein, M.S., Nevill, T., & Stevenson-Moore, P. (2002). Quality of life, olfactory and oral function following high-dose chemotherapy and allogeneic hematopoietic cell transplantation. *Bone Marrow Transplantation, 30*(11), 785–792.

Ezzone, S.A., & Mirtallo, J.M. (2000). Total parenteral nutrition: Ordering and monitoring. In D. Camp Sorrell & R.A. Hawkins (Eds.), *Clinical manual for the oncology advanced practice nurse* (pp. 947–951). Pittsburgh: Oncology Nursing Press.

Filicko, J., Lazarus, H.M., & Flomenberg, N. (2003). Mucosal injury in patients undergoing hematopoietic progenitor cell transplantation: New approaches to prophylaxis and treatment. *Bone Marrow Transplantation, 31*, 1–10.

Flowers, M.E., Kansu, E., & Sullivan, K.M. (1999). Pathophysiology and treatment of graft-versus-host disease. *Hematology/Oncology Clinics of North America, 19*(5), 1091–1112.

Hainsfield-Wolfe, M.E., & Rund, C. (1999). A nursing protocol of the management of perineal-rectal skin alterations. *Clinical Journal of Oncology Nursing, 4*(1), 15–21.

Herrmann, V.M., & Petruska, P.J. (1993). Nutrition support in bone marrow transplant recipients. *Nutrition in Clinical Practice, 8*, 19–27.

Hesketh, P.J., Grunberg, S.M., Gralla, R.J.,Warr, D.G., Roila, F., de Wit, R., et al. (2003). The oral neurokinin-1 antagonist aprepitant for the prevention of chemotherapy-induced nausea and vomiting: A multinational, randomized, double-blind, placebo-controlled trial in patients receiving high-dose cisplatin: The aprepitant protocol 052 study group. *Journal of Clinical Oncology, 22*(15), 4112–4119.

Hopman, G.D., Pena, E.G., le Cessie, S., et al. (2003). Tube feeding and bone marrow transplantation. *Medical Pediatric Oncology, 40*, 375–379.

Hurley, C. (1997). Ambulatory care after bone marrow or peripheral blood stem cell transplantation. *Clinical Journal of Oncology Nursing, 1*(1), 19–21.

Iestra, J.A., Fibbe, W.E., Zwinderman, A.H., Van Staveren, W.A., & Kromhout, D. (2002). Body weight recovery, eating difficulties and compliance with dietary advice in the first year after stem cell transplantation: A prospective study. *Bone Marrow Transplantation, 29*, 417–424.

Ippoliti, C. (1998). Antidiarrheal agents for the management of treatment-related diarrhea in cancer patients. *American Journal of Health-System Pharmacy, 55*(15), 1573–1580.

Iqbal, N., Salzman, D., Lazenby, A.J., & Wilcox, C.M. (2000). Diagnosis of gastrointestinal graft-versus-host disease. *The American Journal of Gastroenterology, 95*(11), 3034–3038.

Kapur, D., Dorsky, D., Feingold, J.M., Bona, R.D., Edwards, R.L., Aslanzadeh, J., et al. (2000). Incidence and outcome of vancomycin-resistant enterococcal bacteremia following autologous peripheral blood stem cell transplantation. *Bone Marrow Transplantation, 25*, 147–152.

Kern, K.A., & Norton, J.A. (1988). Cancer cachexia. *Journal of Parenteral and Enteral Nutrition, 12*, 286–298.

Kim, B.K., Chung, K.W., Sun, H.S., Suh, J.G., Min, W.S., Kang, C.S., et al. (2000). Liver disease during the first post-transplant year in bone marrow transplantation recipients: Retrospective study. *Bone Marrow Transplantation, 26*, 193–197.

Koeller, J.M., Aapro, M.S., Gralla, R.J., Grunberg, S.M., Hesketh, P.J., Kris, M.G., & Clark-Snow, R.A. (2002). Antiemetic guidelines: Creating a more practical treatment approach. *Support Care Cancer, 10*, 519–522.

Larsen, J., Nordstrom, G., Ljungman, P., & Gardulf, A. (2004). Symptom occurrence, symptom intensity, and symptom distress in patients undergoing high-dose chemotherapy with stem-cell transplantation. *Cancer Nursing, 27*, 55–64.

Laviano, A., & Meguid, M.M. (1996). Nutritional issues in cancer management. *Nutrition, 12*, 358–371.

Ljungman, P. (2000). Viral infections. In E.D. Ball, J. Lister, & P. Law (Eds.), *Hematopoietic stem cell therapy* (pp. 414–423). Philadelphia: Churchill Livingstone.

Ljungman, P. (2002). Review: Prevention and treatment of viral infections in stem cell transplant recipients. *British Journal of Haematology, 118*, 44–57.

McCrea, J.B., Majumdar, A.K., Goldberg, M.R., Iwamoto, M., Gargano, C., Panebianco, D.L., et al. (2003). Effects of neurokinin1 receptor antagonist aprepitant on the pharmacokinetics of dexamethasone and methylprednisolone. *Clinical Pharmacology & Therapeutics, 7*, 17–24.

Mehta, N.H., Reed, C.M., Kuhlman, C., Weinstein, H.J., & Parsons, S.K. (1997). Controlling conditioning-related emesis in children undergoing bone marrow transplantation. *Oncology Nursing Forum, 24*(9), 1539–1544.

Mielcarek, M., Martin, P.J., Leisenring, W., Flowers, M.E.D., Maloney, D.G., Sandmaier, B.M., et al. (2003). Graft-versus-host disease after nonmyeloablative versus conventional hematopoietic stem cell transplantation. *Blood, 102*(2), 756–762.

Mitchell, S.A. (2001). Hematopoietic stem cell transplantation. In E.M. Lin (Ed.), *Advanced practice in oncology nursing* (pp. 51–212). Philadelphia: WB Saunders.

Morbidity and Mortality Weekly Report. (2000). *49*(RR-10), 1–128.

Mulder, P.O., et al. (1989). Hyperalimentation in autologous bone marrow transplantation for solid tumors: Comparison of total parenteral versus partial parenteral plus enteral nutrition. *Cancer, 64,* 2045–2052.

Muscaritoli, M., et al. (2002). Nutritional and metabolic support in patients undergoing bone marrow transplantation. *American Journal of Clinical Nutrition, 75,* 183–190.

Muscaritoli, M., Conversano, L., Cangiano, C., et al. (1995). Biochemical indices may not accurately reflect changes in nutritional status after allogeneic bone marrow transplantation. *Nutrition, 11,* 433–436.

Muscaritoli, M., Conversano, L., Torelli, G.F., et al. (1998). Clinical and metabolic effects of different parenteral nutrition regimens in patients undergoing allogeneic bone marrow transplantation. *Transplantation, 66,* 610–616.

Nagler, R.M., & Nagler, A. (1999). Pilocarpine hydrochloride relieves xerostomia in chronic graft-versus-host disease: A sialometrical study. *Bone Marrow Transplantation, 23,* 1007–1011.

Nevo, S., Enger, C., Swan, V., Wojno, K.J., Fuller, A.K., Altomonte, V., et al. (1999). Acute bleeding after allogeneic bone marrow transplantation: Association with graft versus host disease and effect on survival. *Transplantation, 67*(5), 681–689.

Offidani, M., Corvatta, L., Olivieri, A., Rupoli, S., Frayfer, J., Mele, A., et al. (1999). Infectious complications after autologous peripheral blood progenitor cell transplantation followed by G-CSF. *Bone Marrow Transplantation, 24,* 1079–1087.

Osowski, C.L., Dix, S.P., Lynn, M., Davidson, T., Cohen, L., Miyahara, T., et al. (1998). An open-label dose comparison study of ondansetron for the prevention of emesis associated with chemotherapy prior to bone marrow transplantation. *Support Care Cancer, 6,* 511–517.

Parulekar, W., Mackenzie, R., Bjarnason, G., & Jordan, R.C.K. (1998). Scoring oral mucositis. *Oral Oncology, 34,* 63–71.

Perez, E.A., Tiemeier, T., & Solberg, L.A. (1999). Antiemetic therapy for high-dose chemotherapy with transplantation: Report of a retrospective analysis of a 5-HT3 regimen and literature review. *Support Care Cancer, 7,* 413–424.

Plevova, P. (1999). Prevention and treatment of chemotherapy- and radiotherapy-induced oral mucositis: A review. *Oral Oncology, 35,* 453–470.

Przepiorka, D., & Cleary, K. (2000). Therapy of acute graft-vs-host disease. In E.D. Ball, J. Lister, & P. Law (Eds.), *Hematopoietic stem cell therapy* (pp. 531–540). Philadelphia: Churchill Livingstone.

Pytlik R., Benes P., Patrokova M., Chocenska E , Gregora E. Prochazka B., & Kozak, T. 2002. Standardized parenteral alanyl-glutamine dipeptide supplementation is not beneficial in autologous transplant patients: A randomized double blind placebo controlled study. *Bone Marrow Transplant, 30*(12) 953–961.

Raynard, B., Nitenberg, G., Gory-Delabaere, G., Bourgis, J.H, Bachmann, P., Bensadoun, R.J., et al. (2003). Summary of the standards, options and recommendations for nutritional support in patients undergoing bone marrow transplantation. *British Journal of Cancer, 89,* S101–S105.

Roberts, S., Miller, J., Pineiro, L., & Jennings, L. (2003). Total parenteral nutrition vs. oral diet in autologous hematopoietic cell transplant recipients. *Bone Marrow Transplantation, 32*(7), 715–721.

Roulet, M., Frascarolo, P., & Pilet, M. (1997). Effects of intravenously infused fish oil on platelet fatty acid phospholipids composition on platelet function in postoperative trauma. *Journal of Parenteral and Enteral Nutrition, 21,* 296–300.

Rubin, J. (2000). Surgical emergencies. In E.D. Ball, J. Lister, & P. Law, *Hematopoietic stem cell therapy* (pp. 599–602). Philadelphia: Churchill Livingstone.

Rust, D.M., & Kogut, V.J. (2001). Anorexia and cachexia. In J.M. Yasko (Ed.), *Management of symptoms associated with chemotherapy* (pp. 41–62). West Conshohocken, PA: Pharmacia.

Sale, G.E., Shulman, H.M., & Hackman, R.C. (1999). Pathology of hematopoietic cell transplantation. In E.D. Thomas, K.G. Blume, & S.J. Forman (Eds.), *Hematopoietic cell transplantation* (2nd ed., pp. 248–263). Malden, MA: Blackwell Science, Inc.

Schloerb, P.R., & Skikne, B.S. (1999). Oral and parenteral glutamine in bone marrow transplantation: A randomized, double blind study. *Journal of Parenteral and Enteral Nutrition, 23,* 117–122.

Schubert, M.M, Peterson, D.E., & Lloid, M.E. (1999). In E.D. Thomas, K.G. Blume, & S.J. Forman (Eds.), *Hematopoietic cell transplantation* (2nd ed., pp. 751–763). Malden, MA: Blackwell Science, Inc.

Schwartz, J.M., Wolford, J.L., Tornquist, M.D., Hockenbery, D.M., Marakami, C.S., Drennan, F., et al. (2001). Severe gastrointestinal bleeding after hematopoietic cell transplantation, 1897–1999: Incidence, causes, and outcome. *The American Journal of Gastrointerology, 86*(2), 386–393.

Scolapio, J.S., Tarrosa, V.B., Stoner, G.L., Moreno-Aspitia, A., Solberg, L.A., & Atkinson, E.J. (2002). Audit of nutrition support for hematopoietic stem cell transplantation at a single institution. *Mayo Clinical Proceedings, 77*(7), 654–659.

Scully, C., Epstein, J., & Sonis, S. (2003). Oral mucositis: A challenging complication of radiotherapy, chemotherapy, and radiochemotherapy: Part 1, pathogenesis and prophylaxis of mucositis. *Head & Neck, 25*, 1057–1070.

Singh C., & McDonald, G.B. (1997). Intestinal and hepatic complications of bone marrow and stem cell transplantation. In M.B. Taylor, J.L. Gollan, M.A. Peppercorn, et al. (Eds.), *Gastrointestinal emergencies.* (pp. 1–21). Baltimore: Williams and Wilkins.

Smith, L.H., & Besser, S.G. (2000). Dietary restrictions for patients with neutropenia: A survey of institutional practices. *Oncology Nursing Forum, 27*(3), 515–520.

Sonis, S.T. (2004). A biological approach to mucositis. *The Journal of Supportive Oncology, 2*(1), 21–32.

Sonis, S.T., Oster, G., Fuchs, H., Bellm, L., Bradford, W.Z., Edelsberg, J., et al. (2001). Oral mucositis and the clinical and economic outcomes of hematopoietic stem-cell transplantation. *Transplantation, 19*(8), 2201–2205.

Spitzer, T.R., Friedman, C.J., Bushnell, W., Frankel, S.R., & Raschko, J. (2000). Double-blind, randomized, parallel-group study on the efficacy and safety of oral granisetron and oral ondansetron in the prophylaxis of nausea and vomiting in patients receiving hyperfractionated total body irradiation. *Bone Marrow Transplantation, 26*, 203–210.

Stevens, M. (2004). Gastrointestinal complications of hematopoietic stem cell transplantation. In S. Ezzone (Ed.), *Hematopoietic stem cell transplantation: A manual of nursing practice* (pp. 147–165) Pittsburgh: ONS Publishing Division.

Strasser, S.I., & McDonald, G.B. (1999). Gastrointestinal and hepatic complications. In E.D. Thomas, K.G. Blume, & S.J. Forman (Eds.), *Hematopoietic cell transplantation* (2nd ed., pp. 627–658). Malden, MA: Blackwell Science, Inc.

Sullivan, K.M. (1999). Graft-versus-host disease. In E.D. Thomas, K.G. Blume, & S.J. Forman (Eds.), *Hematopoietic cell transplantation* (2nd ed., pp. 515–536). Malden, MA: Blackwell Science, Inc.

Szeluga, D.J., et al. (1985). Energy requirements of parenterally fed bone marrow transplant recipients: A prospective, randomized clinical trial comparing total parenteral nutrition to an enteral feeding program. *Cancer Research, 47*, 3309–3316.

van Burik, J.H., & Weisdorf, D.J. (1999). Infections in recipients of blood and marrow transplant. *Hematology/Oncology Clinics of North America, 19*(5), 1065–1087.

van Kraaij, M.G.J., Dekker, A.W., Verdonck, L.F., van Loon, A.M., Vinjé, J., Koopmans, M.P.G., et al. (2000). Infectious gastro-enteritis: An uncommon cause of diarrhea in adult allogeneic and autologous stem cell transplant recipients. *Bone Marrow Transplantation, 26*, 299–303.

Vargas, H.E., & Silverman, W.B. (2000). Mucositis and other gastrointestinal complications. In E.D. Ball, J. Lister, & P. Law (Eds.), *Hematopoietic stem cell therapy* (pp. 5557–5561). Philadelphia: Churchill Livingstone.

Vinayek, R., Demetris, J., & Rakela, J. (2000). Liver disease in hematopoietic stem cell transplant recipients. In E.D. Ball, J. Lister, & P. Law (Eds.), *Hematopoietic stem cell therapy* (pp. 554–556). Philadelphia: Churchill Livingstone.

Wakui, M., Okamoto, S., Ishida, A., Kobayashi, H., Watanabe, R., Yajima, T., et al. (1999). Prospective evaluation for upper gastrointestinal tract acute graft-versus-host disease after hematopoietic stem cell transplantation. *Bone Marrow Transplantation, 23*, 573–578.

Wasserman, E.L., Hidalgo, M., Hornedo, J., & Cortes-Funes, H. (1997). Octreotide (SMS 201-995) for hematopoietic support-dependent high-dose chemotherapy (HSD-HDC)-related diarrhea: Dose finding study and evaluation of efficacy. *Bone Marrow Transplantation, 20*, 711–714.

Williams, M. (1999). Gastrointestinal manifestations of graft-versus-host disease: Diagnosis and management. *Advanced Practice in Acute Critical Care, 10*(4), 500–506.

Wilmore, D.W. (1991). Catabolic illness: Strategies for enhancing recovery. *New England Journal of Medicine, 325*, 695–702.

Winston, D.J., Yeager, A.M., Pranatharthi, C.H., Snydman, D.R., Peterson, F.B., Territo, M.C., & the Valacyclovir Cytomegalovirus Study Group. (2003). Randomized comparison of oral valacyclovir and intravenous ganciclovir for prevention of cytomegalovirus disease after allogeneic bone marrow transplant. *CID, 36*, 749–758.

Wu, D., Hockenbery, D.M., Brentnall, T.A., Baehr, P.H., Ponec, R.J., Kuver, R., et al. (1998). Persistent nausea and anorexia after marrow transplantation: A prospective study of 78 patients. *Transplantation, 66*(10), 1319–1324.

Zeigler, T.R. (2001). Glutamine supplementation in cancer patients receiving bone marrow transplantation and high dose chemotherapy. *Journal of Nutrition, 131,* 2378S–2584S.

Zeigler, T.R. (2002). Glutamine supplementation in bone marrow transplantation. *British Journal of Nutrition, 878*(Suppl 1), S9–S15.

Chapter 9

Pulmonary and Cardiac Effects

Mary Reilly
Burgunder, MS,
BSN, RN, OCN®

Introduction

Pulmonary complications pose a major clinical problem after blood and marrow transplantation (BMT). Pulmonary dysfunction of various forms occurs in up to 55% of transplant recipients and can account for as much as 50% of BMT-related mortality. Patients requiring mechanical ventilation for respiratory failure have a particularly dismal prognosis, with a mortality rate that approaches 100% (Kreit, 2000).

The respiratory complications of BMT can be divided into two broad categories, infectious and noninfectious, and can be further classified as early or late depending on when they occur. They are listed in **Table 9-1.**

All patients who undergo BMT are routinely screened pretransplant for underlying pulmonary disease; however, the pretransplant evaluation is limited in its ability to prospectively identify patients who will experience respiratory failure. The primary screening tools are a chest x-ray and a pulmonary function test, which includes a measurement of diffusion capacity. Poor pulmonary function often indicates underlying pul-

monary disease and may either preclude a patient from receiving a BMT or require further evaluation with a pulmonologist.

Significant cardiotoxicity has been estimated at between 5% and 10% of patients who undergo BMT (Snowden, 2000). In a retrospective study from the University of Minnesota of 2821 BMT patients between 1977 and 1997, 26 patients were identified as having suffered major or fatal cardiotoxicity. Rapidly progressing heart failure resulted in death in 11 patients, one patient had fatal cardiac tamponade, and one had an acute ventricular fibrillation arrest. The remaining 13 patients (50%) had life-threatening cardiotoxicity, including 4 patients with pericardial tamponade and 9 patients with cardiac arrhythmias. Overall, they observed that acute, major cardiotoxic events attributable to BMT are uncommon and occurred with a frequency of < 1% (Murdych and Weisdorf, 2001).

Nursing plays a vital role in the prevention of, detection of, and intervention in cardiopulmonary complications of BMT. This necessitates that nurses caring for these patients have a strong medical knowledge base. This chapter discusses most cardiopulmonary complications that occur following BMT and their medical and nursing management.

Table 9-1 PULMONARY COMPLICATIONS OF BLOOD AND MARROW TRANSPLANT.

Noninfectious

Airway
  Mucositis
Parenchyma
  Idiopathic pneumonia syndrome (IPS)
  Diffuse alveolar hemorrhage (DAH)
  Pulmonary edema
Pulmonary vascular disease
  Pulmonary venoocclusive disease
  Pulmonary embolism

Infectious

Bacterial
Viral
  Cytomegalovirus (CMV)
  Herpes simplex virus (HSV)
  Respiratory syncytial virus (RSV)
  Others
Fungal
  Aspergillus
  Candida
  Others
Protozoal
  Pneumocystis carinii
Mycobacterial

Source: Reprinted from Kreit, J.W. (2000). Respiratory complications. In E.D. Ball, J. Lister, & P. Law (Eds.), *Hematopoietic stem cell therapy* (pp. 563–577). New York: Churchill Livingstone. Adapted with permission from Elsevier.

Noninfectious Pulmonary Complications

Airway Disease

Chemotherapy and radiation-induced injury to the mucosa of the nose, mouth, and pharynx is common following BMT and occurs early in the transplant course. Mucositis causes dysphagia and odynophagia, and if it becomes severe, mucositis may lead to aspiration. Involvement of laryngeal structures may cause upper airway obstruction that may require translaryngeal intubation or tracheostomy to maintain airway patency. Mucositis may also be prolonged due to the presence of infection such as the herpes simplex viral infection (Kreit, 2000).

Parenchymal Disease

IDIOPATHIC PNEUMONIA SYNDROME

Idiopathic pneumonia syndrome (IPS) is used to define post-BMT acute lung injury for which no infectious agent can be identified (Veys and Owens, 2002). Previously called idiopathic interstitial pneumonia, the term *idiopathic pneumonia syndrome* was suggested at a workshop sponsored by the National Institutes of Health and more accurately reflects the variability of the etiology and radiographic and histologic appearance of IPS. Idiopathic pneumonia syndrome occurs in approximately 15% of all patients who undergo BMT and is more common in patients with an underlying hematologic malignancy than those with nonmalignant disease. The incidence of IPS is also higher in patients receiving an allogeneic

BMT. The onset is usually around 50 days posttransplant, with most cases occurring within 100 days (Veys and Owens, 2002). Risk factors associated with IPS include total body irradiation (TBI), the presence of graft-versus-host disease (GVHD), and methotrexate for GVHD prophylaxis (Crawford, 1999).

IPS is characterized by the presence of fever, dyspnea, a nonproductive cough, and hypoxemia, and progression to respiratory failure is common. Chest radiography and computed tomography (CT) typically demonstrate diffuse or multilobular interstitial or alveolar infiltrates, diffuse patchy opacities, thickened deep and superficial interlobular septa, and nodules of varying sizes (Crawford, 1999; Veys and Owens, 2002). The diagnosis of IPS is based on the presence of compatible clinical and radiographic features and the exclusion of infection by diagnostic tests such as bronchoscopy and open lung biopsy. Histology may reveal a wide variety of nonspecific findings, ranging from interstitial inflammation and fibrosis to diffuse alveolar damage (Kreit, 2000).

Therapy is primarily supportive. There are some reports of improvement after corticosteroid therapy, but there is not sufficient evidence to support this treatment. The use of corticosteroids may actually increase the risk of infection. Reported mortality rates are as high as 60–70% in biopsy-proven IPS. Survivors of IPS eventually will return to near normal pulmonary function (Crawford, 1999).

DIFFUSE ALVEOLAR HEMORRHAGE

The syndrome of diffuse alveolar hemorrhage (DAH) occurs in up to 21% of BMT patients and occurs equally with allogeneic and autologous recipients (Lewis et al., 2000; Kreit, 2000). DAH occurs very early in the posttransplant period, usually around the time of engraftment. This syndrome is characterized by a sudden onset of cough, dyspnea, and respiratory compromise. Hemoptysis may occur but is infrequent.

Reported risk factors for DAH include radiation prior to transplantation, age greater than 40 years, solid tumors, severe mucositis, granulocyte recovery, fever, renal insufficiency, and acute GVHD (Lewis et al., 2000; Kreit, 2000). The majority of patients have normal bleeding factors, and although patients typically have a marked thrombocytopenia, no difference between the platelet counts of patients with DAH and without DAH has been demonstrated (Kreit, 2000; Keller, 2004).

Diagnostic studies to evaluate DAH include a chest radiograph (or chest x-ray) and bronchoscopy. The chest x-ray shows unilateral or bilateral infiltrates, commonly involving the central and lower lungs, in a predominantly diffuse alveolar pattern (Crawford, 1999). Bronchoscopy examination with bronchial alveolar lavage (BAL) shows progressively bloodier fluid with each instillation of saline and often contains hemosiderin-laden macrophages. Histological exam reveals intraalveolar hemorrhage, usually associated with diffuse alveolar damage.

DAH has a very poor prognosis, with mortality nearly 100% (Lewis et al., 2000). Treatment of DAH includes correcting thrombocytopenia, treating renal failure, and providing supportive management, including mechanical ventilation. High-dose corticosteroid therapy (1.0 g/day of methylprednisolone) may reduce the need for mechanical ventilation and mortality in patients with DAH (Crawford, 1999). The successful use of activated factor VII to treat 3 cases of DAH was reported in the March 6, 2004, *Annals of Internal Medicine* by Henke and colleagues.

DRUG-INDUCED PULMONARY TOXICITY

Several agents used in the preparative regimens for both autologous and allogeneic BMT may induce lung injury without evidence of infection. Risk factors for chemotherapy-induced pulmonary toxicity include total cumulative dose, increased age, radiation history, oxygen therapy, smoking, and preexisting pulmonary disease (Keller, 2004). Chemotherapeutic agents that have been implicated include carmustine (BCNU), busulfan, bleomycin, cyclophosphamide (CY), melphalan, and cytarabine (Fassas et al., 2001; Keller, 2004).

BCNU causes toxic lung reactions characterized by chronic interstitial fibrosis, cough, dyspnea, and decrease in lung-diffusing capacity (Allesandrino et al., 2000). Combinations of various agents may potentially lead to lung injury due to drug interactions. Allesandrino and colleagues (2000) completed a retrospective study of 65 patients with hematological malignancies who received a carmustine-based regimen followed by autologous BMT. There was a higher incidence of noninfectious pulmonary complications in patients who received a conditioning regimen with BCNU, etoposide, and cyclophosphamide (35%) than in patients who received a conditioning regimen with BCNU, etoposide, and melphalan (12%).

In addition, host–drug interactions may contribute to the unrecognized development of pulmonary toxicity. This is supported by the lack of correlation between severity of pulmonary toxicity or baseline pulmonary function in cases of BCNU-based high-dose chemotherapy with age or tobacco use, suggesting other factors play

a role in pulmonary toxicity in addition to chemotherapy exposure (Fassas et al., 2001). Several studies have also found an association between pulmonary toxicity and the use of methotrexate to prevent acute GVHD (Kreit, 2000; Ho et al., 2001).

The pathology of chemotherapy-induced pulmonary toxicity is characterized by alveolar septal thickening with fibrosis, fibroblast proliferation, fibrin deposition, and pulmonary epithelial cell injury (McGaughey et al., 2001).

Definitive diagnosis is made with a lung tissue biopsy, but as this procedure is not well tolerated by BMT recipients, the diagnosis is typically made by the exclusion of other possible causes. The most sensitive noninvasive method of diagnosis is the measurement of diffusing capacity for carbon monoxide (DLCO) on pulmonary function tests. Diagnosis is made based on a drop in DLCO to less than 60% of predicted value in the presence of dyspnea; nonproductive cough, with or without fever; or a drop in the DLCO of less than 50% without symptoms (McGaughey et al., 2001).

Drug-induced pulmonary toxicity may occur between 5 weeks and 12 months following BMT, and typical treatment involves the administration of intravenous corticosteroids; however, the optimal dose and duration of treatment are unknown (Fassas et al., 2001). Lung injury induced by BCNU can be reversed by steroids, which may reduce symptoms and improve DLCO (Allesandrino et al., 2000). Some clinical trials have been performed to evaluate the effectiveness of inhaled steroids to prevent pulmonary toxicity. The mechanism of action of inhaled steroids is not clear, although they may reduce the amount of inflammatory cytokines present in the lungs following high-dose chemotherapy and help preserve pulmonary function (McGaughey et al., 2001).

RADIATION-INDUCED PULMONARY TOXICITY

Total body irradiation (TBI) has been implicated as a major cause of pulmonary toxicity in both the allogeneic and autologous settings (Chen et al., 2001). Chen and colleagues reported a 31% incidence of radiation-induced pulmonary toxicity in patients receiving a regimen with TBI compared to patients treated with a non-TBI-containing regimen. Cumulative chemotherapy toxicity in conjunction with TBI may contribute to lung damage. Shielding the lungs, reducing the total exposure of TBI to 600 cGy or less, fractionating the TBI over several days, and decreasing the dose delivery rate all seem to decrease the incidence of radiation pneumonitis (Kreit, 2000; Chen et al., 2001).

Acute radiation pneumonitis usually may occur between 2 and 12 weeks following completion of radiation. Chen and colleagues reported a median interval of 9.4 weeks from transplant to development of symptoms. The clinical syndrome presents most commonly with dyspnea and nonproductive cough, plus or minus hypoxemia with occasional hemoptysis, tachypnea, and fatigue (Chen et al., 2001). Radiologic evidence includes nonlobar pulmonary infiltrates without evidence of congestive heart failure. Chest x-ray may be normal initially but will reveal interstitial and alveolar infiltrates as radiation pneumonitis progresses. Pulmonary infiltrates may be present on CT scan prior to appearing on a chest x-ray (Keller, 2004; Chen et al., 2001).

Treatment includes corticosteroids and oxygen therapy. Steroids may need to be continued for months and symptoms may reappear with tapering of steroids. Progression to refractory hypoxemia will require mechanical ventilation (Crawford, 1999).

Radiation fibrosis can develop with or without a history of radiation pneumonitis and is a more chronic reaction. The symptoms are more insidious, and the patient may notice a gradual increase in dyspnea and a decrease in exercise tolerance. Late symptoms include cyanosis, clubbing of the nails, orthopnea, and chronic cor pulmonale (Shapiro, 1997). The chest x-ray reveals ground glass appearance and hazy pulmonary markings. As with acute radiation pneumonitis, the treatment of choice is corticosteroids; however, there is no evidence that the fibrosis is reversed with this treatment (Crawford, 1999).

PULMONARY EDEMA

Pulmonary edema develops early after BMT and in most cases the onset is rapid within the first 2 to 3 weeks following BMT. The incidence is reported in 11–65% of patients (Winer-Muram et al., 1996).

Pulmonary edema is usually associated with volume overload resulting from the pretransplant conditioning regimen, stem cell infusion, and large volumes of intravenous fluids commonly given during the pretransplant and immediate posttransplant period. There may also be other potential etiologic factors. Systolic or diastolic heart failure precipitated by myocardial ischemia or dysrhythmias, and severe myopericarditis have been described after high-dose cyclophosphamide therapy (Shapiro, 1997).

Pulmonary edema due to increased capillary permeability may be produced by radiation and chemotherapeutic agents or by extrathoracic sepsis (Kreit, 2000). Symptoms include dyspnea, tachypnea, cough, significant weight gain, bibasilar rales, and hypoxemia. A chest x-ray reveals cardiac enlargement and vascular redistribution (Shapiro, 1997).

Nursing management of the patient with pulmonary edema includes fluid restriction, diuretic therapy, strict monitoring of intake and output, and management of oxygen therapy. For severe cases in patients who experience true congestive heart failure, management may include digitalis and nitroglycerin (Shapiro, 1997).

A disorder consisting of noncardiogenic pulmonary edema, fever, and multiorgan dysfunction with azotemia and impaired hepatic function following HCT has been described and is believed to be a result of diffuse capillary endothelial injury (Kreit, 2000). Because this develops within a few days of engraftment, cytokine release may be important in its pathogenesis. This is also known as engraftment syndrome.

Ravenel and colleagues (2000) reviewed the medical records of 50 patients who underwent autologous BMT. Engraftment syndrome was diagnosed if the expected clinical findings occurred at the time of engraftment of neutrophils and no other cause was identified. Chest radiographs were correlated with the clinical course. Sixteen patients (32%) were found to have engraftment syndrome. Of these, eight had abnormal radiographs. Radiographic findings consisted of pleural effusions and interstitial pulmonary edema and were observed in association with clinical history such as fever, skin rash, weight gain, capillary leak, diminished oxygen saturation, and neutrophil recovery (Ravenel et al., 2000).

Pulmonary Vascular Disease

PULMONARY VENOOCCLUSIVE DISEASE

Pulmonary venoocclusive disease (PVOD) is a rare disorder characterized by pulmonary hypertension with narrowing or obstruction of the pulmonary venules and veins by fibrous tissue (Trobaugh-Lotrario et al., 2003). Symptoms include dyspnea on exertion, hypoxemia, signs of pulmonary hypertension, and right ventricular failure (Crawford, 1999).

The cause of PVOD is unknown, although chemotherapy, viral infection, and malignancy have been implicated. PVOD occurs in BMT patients in the presence of hepatic venoocclusive disease and IPS (Crawford, 1999). It is difficult to diagnose antemortem secondary to the patient's instability (Trobaugh-Lotrario et al., 2003).

Diagnosis is based on right heart catheterization with pulmonary angiogram. Angiography allows for thrombi to be excluded as the cause for pulmonary hypertension (Crawford, 1999). PVOD is also diagnosed by histology with lung tissue obtained during open lung biopsy or autopsy.

There is no definitive treatment, and although vasodilators, immunosuppressants, and anticoagulants have been used with some success, the mortality remains high (Crawford, 1999).

PULMONARY EMBOLISM

Although small pulmonary emboli are commonly found at autopsy, patients undergoing BMT do not appear to be at disproportionate risk for clinically significant thromboembolic disease (Kreit, 2000). Possible causes include fat or bone spicules from poorly filtered marrow, deep vein thrombosis, coagulation disorder, or congestive heart failure (Keller, 2004).

Symptoms may include hypoxia, pulmonary edema, and hypotension. A chest x-ray is not definitive for diagnosis; a perfusion scan reveals the venous circulation of the lungs. Treatment includes anticoagulant therapy, which may be difficult to manage in the BMT patient (Keller, 2004).

BRONCHIOLITIS OBLITERANS

Bronchiolitis obliterans (BO) is an obstructive airway disease with an intraluminal accumulation of inflammatory cells and granulation tissue, which lead to partial or complete occlusion of the bronchioles (Marcellus and Vogelsang, 2000). BO is considered a severe manifestation of chronic graft-versus-host disease, and it occurs after day 100 posttransplantation.

Symptoms include progressive dyspnea, wheezing, and nonproductive cough. Chest radiographs may be normal or may show signs of hyperinflation, bleb formation, pneumatosis, pneumothorax, or pneumomediastinum (Marcellus and Vogelsang, 2000). Pulmonary function testing reveals airflow obstruction as evidenced by a marked decrease in FEV1, reduced vital capacity, increased residual lung volume, and a normal DLCO (Keller, 2004; Marcellus and Vogelsang, 2000).

Although typically treated with corticosteroids, no therapy has been proven to improve survival, and BO carries a very poor prognosis. An adequate biopsy of lung tissue is necessary to distinguish BO from bronchiolitis obliterans with organizing pneumonia (BOOP). BOOP results from the formation of granulation tissue plugs within the lumens of the small airways with occasional obstruction of these airways that extends into the alveolar ducts and alveoli (Keller, 2004). PFTs reveal a restrictive ventilatory defect with a normal FEV1 and a reduced DLCO. A chest x-ray reveals patchy areas of consolidation and a ground glass appearance. BOOP is rare in the BMT population, and unlike BO, is usually successfully treated with corticosteroids (Keller, 2004; Marcellus and Vogelsang, 2000).

ACUTE RESPIRATORY DISTRESS SYNDROME

Acute respiratory distress syndrome (ARDS) is defined as a clinical syndrome of acute lung injury that can occur in adults or children; in BMT patients, the most common causes are sepsis and pneumonia (Keller, 2004). ARDS typically has an acute onset that can rapidly lead to respiratory failure and require mechanical ventilation.

Treatment involves supportive care and treatment of the underlying cause of ARDS. Mortality rates vary from 40–60%, with the majority of deaths the result of sepsis or multiorgan failure (Keller, 2004).

Infectious Complications

Immunosuppression

A sequence of pre- and posttransplant events contribute to the severe, immunosuppressed state and leave the patient vulnerable to infection. Typically, neutrophil recovery occurs within 2 to 3 weeks, but may be delayed by the presence of acute GVHD and the administration of myelosuppresssive medications such as methotrexate, trimethoprim-sulfamethoxazole, and ganciclovir (Veys and Owens, 2002). Although the total lymphocyte count usually approaches the normal range by 12 weeks after BMT, T cell response does not return to normal until at least 6 months posttransplant. The number of B cells usually returns to normal within 1 month, although immunoglobulin production may be completely absent for up to 3 months after BMT, and IgA levels may remain decreased for years (Veys and Owens, 2002).

The sequence of immunologic recovery determines the predisposition of the BMT recipient to respiratory infections at any given time. The posttransplant period can be divided into two risk periods. During the preengraftment period, patients are most susceptible to bacterial infections and specific viral infections. After neutrophil recovery, T and B cell immunity remains impaired, predisposing the patient to infection with viruses, fungi, mycobacteria, and parasites (Veys and Owens, 2002). In addition, impaired synthesis of immunoglobulins, including secretory IgA, results in persistent susceptibility to bacterial pneumonia. See **Figure 9-1**.

Bacterial Pneumonia

Bacterial pneumonia commonly occurs within the first 3 months after BMT and is most frequently seen in patients with GVHD. Risk factors include prolonged neutropenia, B cell immune deficiency, impaired splenic function, and IgA deficiency. In normal individuals, the flora of the upper respiratory tract are primarily gram-positive organisms, which are relatively nonvirulent and sensitive to antibiotics. Because

of a special interaction between these bacteria and the specialized receptors on the surface of the upper respiratory tract, colonization with gram-negative bacilli is prevented. In the immunocompromised BMT patient, this ecological system is disturbed, resulting in a high rate of colonization of the respiratory tract by gram-negative organisms. Bacterial pneumonias usually take the form of consolidation of the alveolar sacs in the lungs (Veys and Owens, 2002).

Both gram-positive organisms, such as *Staphylococcus aureus, Staph. epidermidis,* and *Streptococcus pneumoniae* and gram-negative organisms like *Klebsiella* and the *Pseudomonas* species are the common causative pathogens. In addition, patients with chronic GVHD have a higher incidence of pneumococcal pneumonia. *Legionella, Chlamydia,*

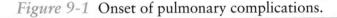

Figure 9-1 Onset of pulmonary complications.

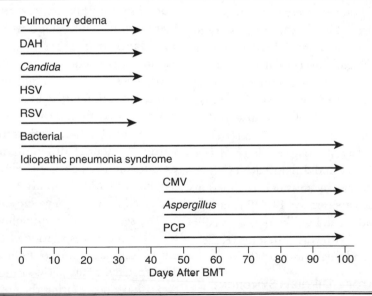

Source: Reprinted from Kreit, J.W. (2000). Respiratory complications. In E.D. Ball, J. Lister, & P. Law (Eds.), *Hematopoietic stem cell therapy* (pp. 563–577). New York: Churchill Livingstone. Adapted with permission from Elsevier.

Mycobacteria, and *Mycoplasma* are also being seen more frequently late in the BMT course (Veys and Owens, 2002).

Clinical manifestations of bacterial pneumonia include cough, fever, dyspnea, and hypoxemia. The approach to therapy for pulmonary bacterial infections is antibiotic treatment tailored according to the culture and sensitivity reports, if a pathogen is identified. Frequently, blood and sputum cultures are negative. Therefore, therapy is often empirical and must provide coverage against gram-negative bacilli and gram-positive organisms. Combination therapy with an aminoglycoside and an antipseudomonal penicillin with or without vancomycin is typically used (Veys and Owens, 2002). Patients who are being treated for chronic GVHD should receive prophylactic antibiotic coverage against encapsulated bacteria such as *Streptococcus pneumoniae* and *Haemophilus influenza* for the duration of their immunosuppression (Dykewicz et al., 2000).

Viral Pneumonia

CYTOMEGALOVIRUS

Pulmonary infection with cytomegalovirus (CMV) accounts for up to 20% of all pneumonias occurring after BMT (Veys and Owens, 2002). CMV occurs more often in allogeneic (10–20%) than autologous (1–5%) BMT recipients. Most cases occur within the first 100 days after BMT, and the peak of incidences is 21 to 80 days (Kreit, 2000).

Risk factors for CMV include total dose and dose rate of total body irradiation and severity of GVHD. Prior exposure to the virus is the major risk factor. As a result of the profound immunosuppression required for BMT, there is a risk for CMV reactivation. Antiviral prophylaxis has reduced the rate of CMV reactivation among CMV seropositive allogeneic patients from a high of about 70% to between 20% and 40% (van Burik and Weisdorf, 1999).

Symptoms of CMV pulmonary infection include fever, nonproductive cough, and progressive dyspnea and hypoxemia. A chest x-ray typically demonstrates diffuse interstitial or alveolar infiltrates, and numerous small nodules may be evident on a CT scan (Veys and Owens, 2002).

CMV pneumonia can be diagnosed by bronchoscopy or open lung biopsy, and several techniques are used to detect the virus in bronchial alveolar lavage (BAL) or tissue samples.

The mortality rate from untreated CMV pneumonia is about 85%, and single-drug therapy does not result in improved survival rates. Combination therapy with intravenous ganciclovir and immune globulin has been shown to significantly decrease patient mortality and is currently the treatment of choice (Veys and Owens, 2002). However, response rates can be low, and the mortality rate in patients requiring mechanical ventilation is nearly 100% (Veys and Owens, 2002).

Most centers perform routine surveillance with weekly throat, blood, and urine cultures. If patients have evidence of viral infection without clinical or radiographic signs of pneumonia, they are treated with ganciclovir. This has significantly reduced the incidence of CMV pneumonia (Kreit, 2000). In the event of severe neutropenia or resistance, foscarnet may be substituted for ganciclovir. Foscarnet is nephrotoxic and generally not recommended for first-line treatment (Keller, 2004).

RESPIRATORY SYNCYTIAL VIRUS

Respiratory syncytial virus (RSV) is a common cause of respiratory tract infections in infants and children and may cause mild rhinitis and pharyngitis in adults. In BMT patients, RSV can lead to a devastating viral pneumonia. The incidence of RSV is unknown and has been estimated as high as 11% (Veys and Owens, 2002). RSV pneumonia usually occurs early posttransplant and is most common in the spring and winter months.

Symptoms include rhinitis, fever, cough, and nasal congestion, which can rapidly lead to pneumonia (Keller, 2004). A chest x-ray initially shows diffuse infiltrates, and progression to diffuse air space disease is common. Therapy consists of nebulized, plus or minus intravenous ribavirin and intravenous immunoglobulin. Despite antiviral therapy, RSV pneumonia is associated with a mortality rate around 50% (Veys and Owens, 2002). RSV is highly contagious and may spread rapidly through the transplant unit. Aggressive policies for prevention of nosocomial infection may reduce the incidence of RSV during the winter months (Veys and Owens, 2002).

Other Viruses

Adenovirus, parainfluenza virus, influenza virus, and human herpes virus 6 have all been reported to cause pneumonia in patients undergoing BMT, typically during the postengraftment period (Kreit, 2000). Respiratory viral infections may occur in as many as 20% of transplant recipients during the winter months (Bowden, 1999). Pneumonia caused by adenovirus, parainfluenza virus, or influenza virus is often preceded by symptoms of upper respiratory tract infection. Standard treatment of respiratory viral pneumonia is supportive care. The use of aerosolized ribavirin has not been shown to be of benefit in clearing respiratory viruses or decreasing mortality (Bowden, 1999).

Patients who develop respiratory viral pneumonia prior to engraftment have poorer outcomes.

During the respiratory virus season, all patients should have nasopharyngeal washings tested for respiratory viruses. Transplantation in a patient with nasopharyngeal washings that are positive for one of the respiratory viruses should be delayed until the infection has resolved (Keller, 2004). Nurses are vital in providing education to the patient and family in order to prevent the spread of respiratory viruses. Education should include the rationale for the restriction of sick friends or family members from visiting BMT patients and emphasizing good hand-washing practices. Family members and medical staff should consider vaccination against influenza to help limit exposure to the patient (Keller, 2004).

Parasitic Pneumonia

Pneumocystis carinii is an opportunistic parasite capable of producing pneumonia in immunocompromised patients. Due to the routine use of prophylactic therapy, *Pneumocystis carinii* pneumonia (PCP) is uncommon in patients undergoing BMT, with an incidence of about 1% (Veys and Owens, 2002). The most effective prophylaxis is trimethoprim-sulfamethoxazole (TMP-SMZ), beginning at time of engraftment and continuing for 6 months posttransplant. Dapsone-pyrimethamine can be used in patients who cannot tolerate TMP-SMZ due to allergy or bone marrow suppression. Dapsone should be used with caution in patients who are allergic to TMP-SMZ since there are reports of a cross-reactivity between dapsone and TMP-SMZ. Pentamadine administered intravenously or by inhalation is also effective prophylaxis for patients who have poor compliance in taking oral TMP-SMZ or in patients with an allergy to TMP-SMZ or dapsone. Although PCP rarely develops in patients who are receiving prophylaxis, there is a 30% mortality rate.

Clinical manifestations of PCP include non-productive cough, rapid progressive dyspnea, and hypoxia often resulting in respiratory failure (Veys and Owens, 2002). A chest x-ray and CT scan typically show diffuse interstitial alveolar infiltrates, and a CT scan may demonstrate areas of ground glass attenuation and multiple small nodules (Veys and Owens, 2002). Median onset is two months post-BMT (Keller, 2004).

Definitive diagnosis is made by microbiological identification of *Pneumocystis carinii* based on positive staining of sputum, BAL fluid, or tissue from open lung biopsy (Veys and Owens, 2002; Keller, 2004). Intravenous TMP-SMZ is the drug of choice for initial treatment (Veys and Owens, 2002).

Fungal Pneumonia

Opportunistic fungal infection is a common cause of serious morbidity and mortality in immunocompromised patients. These infections occur primarily in patients with chemotherapy-induced neutropenia or immunosuppression after BMSCT (Connolly et al., 1999). The most frequently seen fungal pathogens include *Aspergillus, Candida,* and *Cryptococcus neoformans.* Opportunistic pneumonia caused by previously unrecognized pathogens, such as *Fusarium, Penicillium,* and the dematiaceous fungi, are increasingly reported (Connolly et al., 1999).

Aspergillus

Aspergillus spores are ubiquitous and, because of their small size, are commonly inhaled and reach the alveoli. Under normal circumstances, the spores are eradicated by alveolar macrophages and, if fungal hyphae are formed, neutrophils enter the lungs and destroy them (Veys and Owens, 2002).

Risk factors for invasive aspergillosis include prolonged neutropenia, the presence of GVHD, and prolonged immunosuppression. Construction in or near the hospital or patient's living environment may pose a risk. Patients and caregivers should be taught early ways to prevent possible exposure to *Aspergillus,* such as avoiding areas with high concentration of dust, food that contains molds, fresh plants, dried plants, and moss (Keller, 2004).

Incidence of aspergillosis is estimated to be about 4% with a high mortality rate (Kreit, 2000). Clinical symptoms of *Aspergillus* pneumonia may be nonspecific and include fever, cough, pleuritic chest pain, and hemoptysis (Veys and Owens, 2002). Fungal infections should be suspected in patients who are persistently febrile despite receiving 3 to 5 days of broad-spectrum antibiotics (Keller, 2004). Disseminated infection may be present and symptoms of sinusitis, meningitis, and cerebral lesions may precede or accompany pulmonary infection (Veys and Owens, 2002).

A chest x-ray typically shows solitary or multiple pulmonary nodules, nonspecific infiltrates, and cavitations. A CT scan often reveals ground glass opacities, consolidations, and cavitations not appearing on a chest x-ray (Heussel et al., 1999). A classic sign of *Aspergillus* pneumonia on CT scan is the presence of a crescent-shaped area of cavitation at the periphery of a lung nodule or infiltrate called a halo sign. *Aspergillus* is best diagnosed by tissue culture but the patient's clinical condition may prohibit an open lung biopsy. Sputum and BLA fluid is sensitive only 50% of the time (Veys and Owens, 2002). The best current approach for treatment of suspected or confirmed *Aspergillus* pneumonia includes high-dose liposomal amphotericin (e.g., liposomal amphotericin 5–10mg/kg/day) (Veys and Owens, 2002).

Candida

Candida is a common pathogen in the immediate posttransplant period, and invasive infections (fungemia or visceral organ involvement) occur in 11–16% of BMT patients (Veys and Owens, 2002). Infection is most commonly caused by *C. albicans* and *C. tropicalis* and is most common in the preengraftment period. The risk of infection increases with the duration of neutropenia and the severity of acute graft-versus-host disease. Candidal pneumonia is rare and may result from aspiration from the oral pharynx or hematogenous dissemination (Veys and Owens, 2002). Most SCT centers use fungal prophylaxis with fluconazole or itraconazole, and if patients develop candidemia they treat with liposomal amphotericin (Veys and Owens, 2002).

OTHER FUNGI

Pneumonia due to *Trichosporon, Fusarium,* and *Micorales* organisms has only been occasionally reported in patients undergoing BMT, but the incidence of the infections may be increasing (Veys and Owens, 2002). As with other fungal infections, major risk factors include prolonged neutropenia and steroid therapy.

Nursing Care

All patients who undergo BMT are at risk for pulmonary complications. The transplant nurse plays a key role in the prevention, detection, and treatment of patients who develop acute pulmonary complications.

PREVENTION

An important preventive measure by the nurse is encouraging patients to exercise. Many transplant centers use a variety of exercise equipment such as exercise bikes and treadmills. Physical therapists may be consulted to assist in individualizing an exercise plan for each patient. These types of activities may also improve the patients' state of mind and may increase their motivation to participate in their own care. Patients should also be encouraged to perform good pulmonary toilet. Coughing and deep breathing every 2 to 4 hours, as well as the use of incentive spirometry, are effective in preventing atelectasis and facilitating gas exchange (Keller, 2004). The nurse will also administer prophylactic antibiotic, antifungal, and antiviral therapy as indicated and will educate the patient and family appropriately. Other preventive measures include the appropriate environmental restrictions such as the use of laminar airflow rooms or HEPA filtration rooms. The nurse should educate the patient and family regarding the limiting of visitors and good hand-washing.

As the use of BMT in the outpatient setting increases, patient and family education is critical, because the patients are no longer in an environment the health-care team controls. Instruction should also include stressing the avoidance of fresh fruits and vegetables; areas with high concentration of dust; food that contains molds; and fresh or dried plants and moss that may contain bacteria, mold, or fungus.

ASSESSMENT

Nursing assessment is an essential component of the patients' care. Patients' lungs should be auscultated at least every 8 hours. Oxygen saturation should be assessed with any sign of respiratory distress. Prompt reporting of changes can ensure proper and timely medical intervention and improved outcomes.

BMT patients with respiratory problems should be monitored frequently, at least every 4 hours. Oxygen therapy with saturation should be monitored closely. Antianxiety medications may assist patients with relaxation, causing less energy expenditure.

The nurse will also assist with preparing the patient for diagnostic testing and accompany the patient if necessary. Diagnostic tests may include arterial blood gases, pulmonary function testing, chest x-ray, CT scan, bronchoscopy, and surgical biopsy (such as open lung biopsy or transbronchial needle biopsy).

BMT recipients can deteriorate rapidly, and if they do, they might quickly require mechanical ventilation. The nurse should be prepared for transfer to the ICU as indicated, or if patients remain on the BMT unit, staffing should be adjusted to allow for close monitoring of such patients.

TREATMENT

The likelihood that BMT recipients will be admitted to the ICU varies from 20–40%. In the majority of the cases, ICU transfer is indicated for respiratory insufficiency (Kreit, 2000).

The outcome of patients requiring admission to the ICU is poor, with only about 20% surviving to hospital discharge, and patients requiring ventilator support experience a mortality rate of 95% (Kreit, 2000). Transfer to the ICU is a frightening experience for both patients and families. Ongoing support and involvement from the transplant team is important so the patient and family do not feel abandoned.

Care in the ICU may include mechanical ventilation, dialysis, Swan-Ganz catheter placement, and multiple medications to support organ function. Once the patient is stabilized, specific therapy should commence if the causative organism is known or suspected. If the causative organism is not known, empiric therapy should be instituted. Empiric therapy usually includes broad-spectrum antibiotics, liposomal amphotericin, and/or ganciclovir if CMV is suspected.

Nurses play an important role in both directly caring for the patient and supporting and educating the family about the care. If withdrawal of life support is discussed, the nurse's role is vital. The transplant team should be involved in discussions with the patient and family, along with the ICU team. It is hoped that aggressive approaches to the diagnosis and management of patients with pulmonary complications will favorably affect patient outcomes.

Cardiac Complications

Cardiac complications of BMT are not uncommon but are rarely the cause of death in this patient population. Overall incidence has been reported as 25%. Acute, major cardiotoxic events attributable to BMT are uncommon and occur with a frequency of < 1% (Murdych and Weisdorf, 2001). Murdych and Weisdorf reviewed the records of 2821 patients who received a blood or marrow transplant at the University of Minnesota between January 1, 1977 and September 1, 1997. These 2821 patients (1631 males, 58%) were a median of 22 years old (range 0.6 to 67) at transplant and 1257 (45%) received a related donor allograft; 592 (21%) an unrelated donor graft; and 972 (34%) an autograft. Two hundred and five (7%) received total body irradiation; 111 (4%) received total lymphoid irradiation in their conditioning regimen; and 659 (23%) received chemotherapy agents only. Patients with circulatory events ($n = 842$) were identified, and 628 events occurring within the first 100 days posttransplant were evaluated (Murdych and Weisdorf, 2001). Only 26 patients suffered life threatening or lethal cardiac toxicity (0.9%) during the first 100 days post-transplant. The majority of fatal events were secondary to acute, decompensated heart failure. Cardiac tamponade and cardiac arrhythmias were the most common life-threatening, but reversible events. Cardiac complications of high-dose cyclophosphamide and total body irradiation have been well documented. Several other cytotoxic drugs may cause significant cardiotoxicity (Murdych and Weisdorf, 2001).

The challenge for pretransplantation evaluation is to identify patients at highest risk for cardiac complication. The history, physical examination, electrocardiogram (EKG), and radionuclide scan are the principle screening tools. The two broad categories of heart disease are electrical and structural abnormalities. If any cardiac abnormalities are identified as part of the pretransplantation evaluation, further studies may be needed. This may include 24-hour continuous heart monitoring and electrophysiologic studies. A diminished left ventricular ejection fraction (< 45%) may not preclude a patient from transplant. However, a history of clinically documented congestive heart failure has a strong association with cardiac toxicity (Oblon, 2000).

Murdych and Weisdorf (2001) concluded that there is not a clear association among pretransplant cardiotoxic drugs, prior use of mediastinal irradiation, pretransplant left ventricular function, and the development of BMSCT-related cardiac toxicity.

Cardiac Arrhythmias

An arrhythmia is defined as an alteration in the rhythm or rate of the heart. The clinical significance of arrhythmias in BMT recipients varies. Patients may experience mild arrhythmias without symptoms; however, more severe arrhythmias are characterized by the presence of palpitations; chest discomfort; anxiety; a weak, thready pulse; abnormal heart sounds; or hypotension (Camp-Sorrell, 1999). Arrhythmias are diagnosed with a 12-lead EKG, which will show the rate, regularity, and pattern of the heart rhythm. Of the nine patients in the University of Minnesota retrospective study with reported arrhythmias, six had symptomatic and/or hemodynamically significant atrial-fibrillation/flutter requiring electrical cardioversion. One patient arrested secondary to ventricular fibrillation and two other patients developed cardiac arrest with asystole responding to cardiopulmonary resuscitation (Murdych and Weisdorf, 2001). Treatment is based upon the diagnosed arrhythmia and the patient's clinical condition.

Treatment-Induced Cardiac Damage

Regimen-related toxicity accounts for the majority of cardiac complications. Previous exposure to anthracyclines such as doxorubicin hydrocloride and daunorubicin can contribute to cardiac damage. The heart damage caused by anthracyclines is from a loss of myocardial fibrils, mitochondrial changes, and cellular degeneration. Necrosis of the cardiac fibers of the heart can be seen on autopsy (Shapiro, 1997).

Cyclophosphamide is also known to cause cardiac complications and is a mainstay in transplant conditioning regimens. Cardiac damage may be worse if the patient is also treated with TBI. Cyclophosphamide causes hemorrhagic myocardial necrosis, thickening of the left ventricular wall, serosanguineous pericardial effusions, and a fibrinous pericarditis. Clinical signs occur 1 to 10 days following cyclophosphamide administration and include pulmonary edema, cardiomegaly, poor peripheral perfusion, and systemic edema. Decreased voltage may be noted on the patient's EKG (Shapiro, 1997).

Symptoms may progress to hemorrhagic myocarditis and cardiac tamponade, and death might occur. At the first indication of cardiac symptoms, the patient should have a cardiac ejection fraction measured to compare to the pretransplant baseline study. If symptoms occur prior to the completion of the patient's course of cyclophosphamide, the drug may be stopped and replaced with another chemotherapeutic agent. Like the toxicity suffered with anthracyclines, little can be done to treat cyclophosphamide-induced cardiac damage.

Supportive care involves precise fluid management and the judicious use of diuretics and digitalis. Pericardiocentesis and placement of a pericardial window are sometimes performed on patients who suffer from pericardial effusions, since cardiac tamponade is a threat with cyclophosphamide-induced cardiac damage (Shapiro, 1997).

Pure radiation-induced cardiac toxicity is unlikely; however, there does seem to be a synergistic effect between chemotherapy and radiation therapy. Cardiac irradiation has been associated with the development of pericardial effusions and constrictive pericarditis, which predisposes the patient to pulmonary edema. Supportive measures for radiation-induced cardiac toxicity are the same as those for cyclophosphamide toxicity (Shapiro, 1997).

Transplant patients at highest risk for radiation-induced cardiac damage are those who have received radiation to the chest prior to the transplant conditioning regimen (Shapiro, 1997). The cardiac damage seen with regimen-related toxicity has similar results regardless of the causative factors. Although only fatal in about 10% of cases, little can be done to reverse the cardiac damage that results from high-dose chemotherapy and radiation therapy.

Many patients suffer from mild and often undetected cardiac toxicity. Long-term follow-up of patients who received cyclophosphamide and TBI as conditioning has shown that 23% suffer a decrease of their resting ejection fraction (Shapiro, 1997).

Cardiac Infections

Cardiac infections in the BMT recipient are rare, and if they do occur, they affect the pericardium, endocardium, and myocardium. Among the most common causative organisms are *Candida albicans, Aspergillus, Pseudomonas, Clostridia, Streptococcus,* and *Staphylococcus* (Shapiro, 1997). The pathogenesis of acute infectious endocarditis is related to the presence of a bacteremia caused by a highly virulent organism. The rate of acute infections occurring in patients without previous valvular deformities is 50–60%. Valvular vegetations can break off and become emboli. Bacterial infections of the heart may also result from central venous catheter infections. *Aspergillus* is associated with endocarditis and pericarditis secondary to extrapulmonary spread (Keller, 2004).

The diagnosis of cardiac infections is difficult, because the symptoms are nonspecific and include fever, chills, cough, malaise, and night sweats (Ellerhorst-Ryan, 1997). Other indications of possible cardiac infection may be clinical manifestations that may include new or changing murmurs, a pericardial friction rub, thromboemboli, unexplained heart failure, and arrhythmias (Ellerhorst-Ryan, 1997). The EKG may show conduction or rhythm disturbances, or myocardial ischemic changes. An echocardiogram may reveal vegetations and decreased ventricular function on the patient's heart valves. Treatment should include broad-spectrum antibiotics (antifungal therapy fever persists after several days of antibiotics). Other supportive nursing care should include careful management of fluids and diuretics, administration of digitalis and nitroglycerin as indicated, and monitoring adequate oxygenation (Ellerhorst-Ryan, 1997; Keller, 2004).

Cardiac Tamponade

Cardiac tamponade is characterized by impaired hemodynamic function due to increased intrapericardial pressure that overcomes normal compensatory mechanisms. This occurs when fluid in the pericardial space compresses the heart and results in a decrease of cardiac output. Cardiac tamponade is the most severe symptom complex of pericardial effusion, is considered an oncological emergency, and is seen in about 16% of patients who are symptomatic for pericardial effusion (Maxwell, 1997). As fluid accumulates in the pericardial space, right ventricular filling is impaired and may result in the collapse of the right ventricle during diastole (Keller, 2004).

Symptoms of cardiac tamponade may include elevated central venous pressure, distant heart sounds, dyspnea, tachypnea, hypotension, and pulsus paradoxus. Pulsus paradoxus is present when the pulse is weaker or absent during inspiration or when the systolic blood pressure is more than 10 mmHg lower during inspiration than expiration (Keller, 2004).

An echocardiogram is the most accurate test for diagnosing cardiac tamponade. Pericardiocentesis is the treatment of choice. This removal of fluid may produce dramatic symptom relief. It may also be necessary to place a pericardial window; this procedure removes a small section of the pericardium to allow the fluid to drain (Murdych and Weisdorf, 2001).

Nursing interventions for cardiac tamponade include frequent monitoring of vital signs, including assessment for pulsus parodoxus, cardiac monitoring, and precise measurement of intake and output. Administration of oxygen and medication to relieve anxiety and pain, as well as the administration of diuretics and vasopressors, may also be necessary (Maxwell, 1997).

Nursing Care

Assessment and identification of BMT patients at risk for cardiac complications should be included in the nursing history prior to the start of the conditioning regimen. Pretransplant evaluation should include baseline cardiac function to identify patients at highest risk for cardiac complication.

During the conditioning regimen, the nursing assessment should include daily weights, intake, and output. Following BMT, nursing assessment for murmurs, friction rubs, and breath sounds are key in the early detection of infective endocarditis. Frequent assessment for cardiac tamponade includes tachypnea, pleuritic chest pain, distended neck veins, and a positive pulsus paradoxus. Detection of these symptoms should result in prompt medical intervention.

For the patient with cardiac-induced pulmonary edema and/or congestive heart failure, the nursing focus should be on maintaining oxygenation and resolution or reduction of edema. It is important to stress the patient's heart as little as possible. Rest periods between procedures may be helpful. Strict intake and output, close monitoring of the patient's electrolytes, weighing the patient at least daily, and administering diuretics are essential to managing the patient's fluid balance. Cardiac complications occur infrequently, thus cardiology consultations may be helpful in managing these patients.

Conclusion

Nursing care is a critical component in identifying, assessing, and treating cardiopulmonary complications following BMT. The advent of newer regimens such as the nonmyeloablative strategies may reduce the cardiac risks. However, the greater use of immunosuppressive medications (such as fludarabine) as part of some nonmyeloablative regimens may increase the risk for opportunistic pulmonary infections. An important component of nursing care is patient education. Patients and caregivers must be educated on the risk factors and symptoms of cardiopulmonary complications and how to report these to the health-care team. Astute nursing care can contribute to rapid identification and early medical treatment, thus contributing to a decrease in the morbidity and mortality of these complications.

References

Allesandrino, E.P., Bernasconi, P., Colombo, A., Cladera, D., Martinelli, G., Vitulo, P., et al. (2000). Pulmonary toxicity following carmustine-based preparative regimens and autologous peripheral blood progenitor cell transplantation in hematological malignancies. *Bone Marrow Transplantation, 25,* 309–313.

Bowden, R.A. (1999). Other viruses after hematopoietic cell transplantation. In E.D. Thomas, K.G. Blume, & S.J. Forman (Eds.), *Hematopoietic Cell Transplantation* (pp. 618–626). Boston: Blackwell Science.

Camp-Sorrell, D. (1999). Surviving the cancer, surviving the treatment; acute cardiac and pulmonary toxicity. *Oncology Nursing Forum, 26,* 983–990.

Chen, C.I., Abraham, R., Tsang, R., Crump, M., Keating, A., Stewart, A.K. (2001). Radiation-associated pneumonitis following autologous stem cell transplantation: predictive factors, disease characteristics and treatment outcomes. *Bone Marrow Transplantation, 27,* 177–182.

Connolly, J.E., McAdams, H.P., Erasmus, J.J., Rosado-deChristenson, M.L. (1999). Opportunistic fungal infection. *Journal of Thoracic Imaging, 14,* 51–62.

Crawford, S.W. (1999). Noninfectious lung disease in the immunocompromised host. *Respiration, 66,* 385–395.

Dykewicz, C.A., Jaffe, H.W., Kaplan, J.E. (2004). Guidelines for preventing opportunistic infections among hematopoietic stem cell transplant recipients: Recommendations of the CDC, Infectious Diseases Society of America, and the American Society of Blood and Marrow Transplantation. *Biology of Blood and Marrow Transplantation, 6,* 659–727.

Ellerhorst-Ryan, J.M. (1997). Infection. In S.L. Grioenwald, M. Godoman, M.H. Frogge, & C.H. Yarbro (Eds.), *Cancer nursing: Principles and practice* (pp. 585–603). Sudbury, MA: Jones and Bartlett.

Fassas, A., Gojo, I., Rapoport, A., Cottler-Fox, M., Meisenberg, B., Papadimitriou, J.C., et al. (2001). Pulmonary toxicity syndrome following CDEP (cyclophosphamide, dexamaethasone, etoposide, cisplatin) chemotherapy. *Bone Marrow Transplantation, 28,* 399–403.

Henke, D., Flak, R.J., Gabriel, D.A. (2004). Successful treatment of diffuse alveolar hemorrhage with activated factor VII. *Annals of Internal Medicine, 140,* 493–494.

Heussel, C.P., Kauczor, H., Heussel, G.E., Fischer, B., Begrich, M., Mildenberger, P., et al. (1999). Pneumonia in febrile neutropenic patients and in bone marrow and blood stem cell transplant recipients: Use of high resolution computed tomography. *Journal of Clinical Oncology, 17,* 796–805.

Ho, V.T., Weller, E., Lee, S.J., Alyea, E.P., Antin, J.H., Soiffer, R.J. (2001). Prognostic factors for early severe pulmonary complications after hematopoietic stem cell transplantation. *Biology of Blood and Marrow Transplantation, 7,* 223–229.

Keller, C.A. (2004). Cardiopulmonary effects. In S. Ezzone (Ed.), *Hematopoietic stem cell transplantation* (pp. 177–189). Pittsburgh, PA: Oncology Nursing Society.

Kreit, J.W. (2000). Respiratory complications. In E.D. Ball, J. Lister, & P. Law (Eds.), *Hematopoietic stem cell therapy* (pp. 563–577). New York: Churchill Livingstone.

Lewis, I.D., DeFor, T., Weisdorf, D.J. (2000). Increasing incidence of diffuse alveolar hemorrhage following allogeneic bone marrow transplantation; Cryptic etiology and uncertain therapy. *Bone Marrow Transplantation, 26,* 539–543.

Marcellus, D.C., Vogelsang, G.B. (2000). Chronic graft versus host disease. In E.D. Ball, J. Lister, & P. Law (Eds.), *Hematopoietic stem cell therapy* (pp. 614–624). New York: Churchill Livingstone.

Maxwell, M.B. (1997). Malignant effusions and edemas. In S.L. Grioenwald, M. Godoman, M.H. Frogge, & C.H. Yarbro (Eds.), *Cancer nursing: Principles and practice* (pp. 721–741). Sudbury, MA: Jones and Bartlett.

McGaughey, D.S., Nikevich, D.A., Long, G.D., Vredenburgh, J.F., Rizzieri, D., Smith, C.A., et al. (2001). Inhaled steroids as prophylaxis for delayed pulmonary toxicity syndrome in breast cancer patients undergoing high dose chemotherapy and autologous stem cell transplantation. *Biology of Blood and Marrow Transplantation, 7,* 274–278.

Murdych, T., Weisdorf, D.J. (2001). Serious cardiac complications during bone marrow transplantation at the University of Minnesota, 1977–1997. *Bone Marrow Transplantation, 28,* 283–287.

Oblon, D.J. (2000). Evaluation of patients before hematopoietic stem cell transplantation. In E.D. Ball, J. Lister, & P. Law (Eds.), *Hematopoietic stem cell therapy* (pp. 225–232). New York: Churchill Livingstone.

Ravenel, J.G., Scalzetti, E.M., Zamkoff, K.W. (2000). Chest radiographic features of engraftment syndrome. *Journal of Thoracic Imaging, 15,* 56–60.

Shapiro, T.W. (1997). Pulmonary and cardiac effects. In M.B. Whedon & D. Wujcik (Eds.), *Blood and marrow stem cell transplantation: Principles, practice, and nursing insights* (pp. 266–297). Sudbury, MA: Jones and Bartlett.

Snowden, J.A., Hill, G.R., Hunt, P., Camoutsos, S., Spearing, R.C., Espiner E., et al. (2000). Assessment of cardiotoxicity during haemopoietic stem cell transplantation with plasma brain natriuretic peptide. *Bone Marrow Transplant, 26,* 309–313.

Trobaugh-Lotrario, A.D., Greffe, B., Deterding, R., Deutsch, G., Qiunones, R. (2003). Pulmonary veno-occlusive disease after autologous bone marrow transplant in a child with stage IV neuroblastoma; case report and literature review. *Journal of Pediatric Hematology Oncology, 25,* 405–408.

Van Burik, J.H., Weisdorf, D.J. (1999). Infections in recipients of blood and marrow transplantation. *Hematology/Oncology Clinics of North America, 13,* 1065–1089.

Veys, P., Owens, C. (2002). Respiratory infections following haemopoietic stem cell transplantation in children. *British Medical Bulletin, 61,* 151–174.

Winer-Muram, H.T., Gurney, J.W., Bozeman, P.M., Krance, R.A. (1996). Pulmonary complications after bone marrow transplant. *Radiologic Clinics of North America, 34,* 97–118.

Chapter 10

Renal and Hepatic Effects

Tracy T. Douglas, RN, MSN, OCN®

Brenda K. Shelton, MS, RN, CCRN, AOCN®

The kidneys and liver are organs vital to the body's homeostasis. Complications of the renal and hepatic systems from high-dose radiation and/or chemotherapy and stem cell transplantation cause interrelated disruptions in this homeostasis and present unique challenges to the nurse managing a transplant patient.

Renal Failure

Basic renal function can be summarized as the attempt to maintain homeostasis in body water and electrolytes and to distribute them within the body's various fluid compartments. The renal regulation of acid–base balance and hormonal functions are but some of these actions. The clearance of the metabolic waste products of cellular metabolism and the removal of therapeutic drugs are the body's attempt to maintain balance.

Renal compromise can cause or exacerbate other organ system complications as well. Pulmonary compromise from fluid overload; cardiac compromise from excess fluid or renal hypertension; neurological symptoms from increased cir-

culating waste products; and electrolyte imbalances, which can lead to seizures or other organ malfunction, all contribute to the morbidity and mortality of this patient population. Clinicians often wrestle with the paradox of striving to optimize their patient's renal function while continuing therapies that impair renal function.

Renal insufficiency is a significant complication of blood cell and bone marrow transplant. It is a doubling of the baseline creatinine. Renal insufficiency is a dynamic pathological process and exists on a continuum ranging from mild to severe. Although most cases are mild, the problem is still of consequence because it can compromise administration of optimal therapies required for the transplant patient. Even a subtle decrease in renal function can herald a more complicated clinical course involving renal failure, fluid and electrolyte imbalance, and multiorgan failure. *Acute renal failure* (ARF) is a sudden onset of oligura (< 500 ml urine in 24 hours or < 0.5 ml/kg per hr) (Price, 1994). *Chronic renal failure* (CRF) is prolonged ARF of more than a few months. The time period is arbitrary.

Impact of Renal Insufficiency and Failure in Transplant

Renal compromise can have a great impact on the care and treatment of the transplant patient. Hematopoietic stem cell transplant is associated with ARF and CRF (Cohen, 2001). Renal insufficiency occurs in approximately 40–50% of transplant patients during the first 3 weeks after hematopoietic cell transplantation (HCT) (Zager, 1994; Parikh et al., 2002). ARF occurs in approximately 50% of patients with renal insufficiency, primarily due to circulatory problems, drug-induced toxicities, and infection (Deeg et al., 1988; Zager, 1994). For the patient receiving allogeneic bone marrow transplant (BMT), treatment of graft-versus-host disease (GVHD) may be impaired due to the need to decrease or withhold cyclosporine or FK506. In one study, allogeneic stem cell recipients who had ARF had an 83% mortality rate as compared to a 58% mortality rate overall for allogeneic stem cell recipients (Parikh et al., 2002). Other drugs, such as methotrexate, antibiotics, and biological response modifiers, depend in part on adequate renal function for the best therapeutic response. Any alteration in the ability to use these agents to their full measure is challenging and could compromise the long-term health of the patient.

Renal Physiology

Normal kidney function requires four processes to be carried on continuously by the nephrons: 1) creation of an ultrafiltrate of whole blood; 2) absorption of electrolytes, bicarbonate, glucose, and essential amino acids; 3) secretion of electrolytes, medications, and other waste products; and 4) excretion of the urine (Price, 1994) (see **Figure 10-1**).

Figure 10-1 Illustration of the nephron and its associated blood supply.

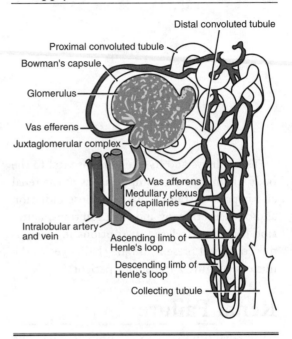

Source: From Schottelius, B.A., & Schottelius, D.D. (1973). *Textbook of Physiology* (17th ed.). St. Louis: C.V. Mosby Co.

The first step is filtration, which occurs at the glomerulus and Bowman's capsule of each nephron. Renal arterial blood branches down into the capillary tuft of the glomerulus. Filtering in this section occurs based on molecular size, as substances small enough move through the porous capillary walls. Blood cells, plasma proteins, and any substances bound to protein are not normally cleared by this filtration. Water, electrolytes, blood urea nitrogen (BUN), and creatinine filter easily and become part of the filtrate that moves out of the glomerulus and into the space surrounded by Bowman's capsule. The rate at which this filtrate is produced is the glomerular filtration rate (GFR), normally about 100 ml per minute in the adult. All fluid and materials not filtered at the glomerulus are passed downstream into the network of capillaries that surround the renal tubules.

From Bowman's capsule, the filtrate solution travels to the renal tubules; the purpose of the proximal and distal tubules and/or the collecting duct of the nephron is to modify the filtrate by absorption and secretion of electrolytes and water (Price, 1994). The inner lumen of each tubule is lined with epithelial cells, which perform these functions. As the filtrate passes through the renal tubules, materials and water are reabsorbed into the bloodstream via the capillaries surrounding the tubules. At the same time, secretion is occurring, with the transport of the substances from the capillaries into the lumen of the tubule. Additionally, aldosterone, antidiuretic hormone, and the prostaglandins have specific functions to assist in the control of total body fluids, electrolytes, and vascular pressures (Price, 1994).

The collecting tubules continue the processes of absorption and secretion and pass the urine to the ureters, bladder, and urethra for excretion. Average urine output is 2 ml to 3 ml per minute. A decrease in urine output is one of the first signs of renal compromise. Absorption and secretion are active processes that substantially alter the character and composition of the urine. These activities provide the body with the proper balance of water, electrolytes, and acid–base.

Determinants of Renal Function

For the kidneys to fulfill their function, they must be able to perform each of the processes outlined above. If any determinant of renal function is impaired, renal insufficiency results (see **Table 10-1**). Good renal perfusion is necessary

Table 10-1 Determinants of renal function.

Renal perfusion—filtration
    Intravascular volume
    Cardiac output
    Renal vasculature

Tubular function—secretion, absorption
    Tubular epithelial cells
    Tubular lumen

Postrenal structure—excretion
    Ureters
    Bladder
    Urethra

to allow enough blood to reach the glomerulus with enough force to allow filtration to occur. An adequate number of tubular epithelial cells and a tubular lumen free from obstructive debris must be present for secretion and absorption. For excretion to occur, the postrenal structures of the ureters and bladder must be patent and unobstructed.

Acute Renal Failure

Acute renal failure is generally classed into three types based on the etiology of the failure (Stark, 1988). The first is termed *prerenal*. Prerenal failure has as its etiology inadequate glomerular filtration due to inadequate delivery of blood to the nephron or lack of the proper pressure differential across the capillary wall. The causes include clinical states common in transplantation such as hypovolemia, congestive heart failure, and septic shock. *Intrarenal* failure originates at the level of the nephron and is caused by clogged or damaged tubules, a toxic injury to the tubular epithelial secretion, and at times filtration capacity. Nephrotoxicity secondary to aminoglycosides is a prime example. *Postrenal* failure originates below the level of the kidney. If obstruction, there is an increase in hydrostatic pressure in the renal pelvis and a decreased glomerular filtration rate and hydronephorosis, and renal failure is the result. Tumor masses may be a factor in this type of renal failure.

Etiology in the Transplant Patient

In BMT patients ARF usually develops 10–21 days after BMT. ARF is often multifactorial and may be caused by sepsis, hypotension, the use of aminoglycosides, and amphotericin. Patients are at increased risk of ARF if there is liver compromise with a total bilirubin greater than 7 mg/dl. This combination of hepatic failure and renal failure is called hepatorenal syndrome (Zager, 1994). Hepatorenal syndrome in BMT has a 75% mortality rate (Noel, et al., 1998). Renal insufficiency in the transplant patient can arise from any of the types of renal failure discussed above (see **Table 10-2**). Considering the clinical problems that predominate in this population, it is not surprising that the majority of renal problems have prerenal and intrarenal etiologies (Zager et al., 1989). Disruption of a normal fluid distribution in the body's compartments is a common problem, and it is exacerbated by sensible and insensible losses from the body. Also, nephrotoxic drugs (antibiotics, cyclosporine, and tacrolimus) are common therapy for these patients, predisposing them to acute tubular necrosis, an intrarenal class of renal failure.

Other intrarenal problems possible for this group are syndromes secondary to massive cell lyses such as tumor lyses syndrome, rhabdomyolysis, and hemolysis from administration of

Table 10-2 ETIOLOGY OF RENAL FAILURE IN BMT PATIENTS.

PRERENAL CONDITIONS
Hypovolemia
Dehydration
Third-spaced fluid
Venoocclusive disease (VOD)
Hemorrhage

Impaired Circulation of Blood Volume
Septic shock
Congestive heart failure
Cardiotoxic effects

Renal Vascular Constriction
Pressor drugs

INTRARENAL CONDITIONS
Acute Tubular Necrosis
Nephrotoxic drugs
Prolonged ischemia

Tumor Lysis Syndrome
Massive tumor lysis

Postrenal Obstruction
Hemorrhagic cystitis

blood components or reinfusion of cryopreserved autologous or ABO incompatible stem cells (Smith et al., 1987). Each of these problems involves the obstruction of renal tubules by the products of the cell lyses (Hou and Cohen, 1985).

Prerenal Failure

The most common type of renal insufficiency seen in the patient who receives high-dose therapy is prerenal failure (Zager et al., 1989). The etiology of the prerenal state is usually multifactorial and complex to assess and diagnose. As a rule, it arises from one of the following: hypovolemia, impaired circulation of blood volume, or coexisting vascular constriction caused by several processes.

Hypovolemia

Hypovolemia results from dehydration, when body losses are greater than intake. Common etiologies of hypovolemia in this population are fever, diuresis, and gastrointestinal losses from severe mucositis, diarrhea, or hemorrhage. Another cause of hypovolemia is *third spacing* of fluid. This is the shift of fluid from the vascular system to other body compartments that occurs commonly with the problems of septic shock, capillary leak syndrome, and venoocclusive disease.

Impaired Circulation of Blood Volume

A prerenal failure can arise from impaired circulation of the blood, even if an adequate volume exists. This is a common problem in septic shock resulting from profound neutropenia, where the mean arterial pressure is too low for adequate perfusion of the nephron. Congestive heart failure, which can result from myocardiotoxic drugs, is another situation in which the blood volume is more than adequate, but the ability of the heart to pump enough of it to perfuse the kidneys is impaired.

Renal Vascular Constriction

Lastly, during acute crises, transplant patients may be on pressor doses of drugs such as dopamine, so that the vasoconstriction of the renal arteries restricts the flow of blood to the nephron. Renal artery vasoconstriction is also seen to a lesser but significant degree with other drugs such as cyclosporine and amphotericin,

both commonly administered to this group of patients. Cyclosporine causes renal artery vasoconstriction and is synergistic with amphotericin in causing renal insufficiency (Zager, 1994). Renal impairment occurs in 5–80% of cases receiving amphotericin (Bates et al., 2001). Tacrolimus has equal or more renal vasoconstriction than cyclosporine, with less systemic vasoconstriction or hypertension (U.S. Multicenter FK506 Liver Study Group, 1994). Concurrent use of CSA or other nephrotoxins increases risk of renal failure and causes vasoconstriction and elevation of baseline creatinine (Harbarth et al., 2001).

The commonality among these problems is an insufficient blood volume delivered to the nephron or filtered at the glomerulus. Without adequate GFR, the blood-altering work of the kidney cannot be accomplished.

Determining the etiology of prerenal problems is the key to appropriate intervention. Prerenal problems are generally reversible by correcting the underlying cause. In contrast, intrarenal problems exacerbated by a profound or prolonged prerenal state result in a more severe course, both in recovery time and in the restriction of therapies necessary for these patients.

Syndrome of Inappropriate Antidiuretic Hormone

Although not a type of renal failure, syndrome of inappropriate antidiuretic hormone (SIADH) is addressed here due to its common occurrence with administration of high-dose cyclophosphamide and its implications for fluid management. A transitory release of antidiuretic hormone is common immediatlely following cyclophosphamide therapy (Pharmacia and Upjohn, 2001). Fluid retention at this time of vigorous hydration is common. Careful evaluation of patients' weight gains, intake and output, and evaluation of pulmonary compromise is required. Furosemide or other diuretics can be administered only after completion of mesna doses. Overdiuresis is possible, resulting in a prerenal vascular depletion state.

Acute Tubular Necrosis

Acute tubular necrosis (ATN) is the most common type of intrarenal failure seen in the transplant patient. ATN is caused by damage or destruction of the renal tubules. If the injury is limited to the tubular epithelial cell layer, without damage to the underlying tissues, recovery is possible in time. Generally, the epithelial cell layer regenerates and begins functioning sufficiently in 1 to 5 weeks to carry out the demands placed on it.

Etiology of ATN in the Transplant Patient

In the transplant population, the most common cause of ATN is the use of nephrotoxic drugs. These include amphotericin B, cyclosporine, cisplatin, aminoglycosides, and acyclovir (Cooper et al., 1993; Deeg et al., 1988; Yee et al., 1985). Each of these drugs, in addition to causing renal artery constriction, causes damage to the tubular cells and/or tends to crystallize in a concentrated filtrate and deposit in the tissues. The tubular lumens become clogged due to the debris of tubular cell destruction and the swelling of the tubular wall caused by the insulting agent. Filtrate cannot pass through the tubule. With no movement of filtrate, GFR is reduced or stopped. Even if the healing process clears the debris, it takes time for new tubular cells to become established and functional. Until this occurs, the renal functions of absorption and secretion cannot take place, necessitating therapies such as hemodialysis.

A second cause of ATN is an ischemic insult to the tubule. Since the oxygen supply to the renal tissue also supplies the glomerulus, if impairment of the blood supply is profound and prolonged, renal tissues become anoxic. Severe anoxia may cause a necrosis of nephrons and their associated vasculature. The transplant patient commonly experiences fever and is often on steroidal drugs, both of which increase metabolism and, therefore, oxygen demand. Increased oxygen demand at a time of decreased supply predisposes tissue to anoxic insult. If the anoxic insult is severe, changes to recovering renal function are severely reduced. The use of calcium channel blockers decreases vasoconstriction but not tubulointerstitial injury (Rahn et al., 1999). ATN is associated with venoocclusive disease (VOD) and sepsis. ATN results in urinary potassium wasting, resulting in hypokalemia, urinary magnesium wasting, metabolic acidosis from type 1 renal tubular acidosis, and polyuria from nephrogenic diabetes insipidus (Branch, 1988).

Phases of ATN

Acute tubular necrosis has three phases: oliguric, diuretic, and recovery (Stark, 1988). During the oliguric phase, little if any urine is produced because the edematous epithelial cell lining and debris from cell destruction generally clog the tubules. During the diuretic phase, diluted urine is increasingly produced as a result of the clearance of the tubular lumen. This clearance allows GFR to occur at a time of impaired tubular function. Concentration of the filtrate is a function of the tubules and collection ducts. Until they are functioning properly, filtration proceeds without the required reabsorbtion of water. This explains why the quantity of urine may seem sufficient while the quality is poor. Epithelial cells are required for the task of secretion, which is vital for the clearance of metabolic waste products and the removal of metabolized drugs. The last phase of ATN, recovery, is characterized by the ability of the nephron to concentrate the dilutent via absorption and to clear waste products and drugs out of the blood via secretion.

Within this classification for the phases of ATN, there is variability in both timing and severity of each phase. It is not unusual for the oliguric phase to be absent. This is common for cases of ATN caused by nephrotoxic drugs. Nonoliguric ATN is often called *high output renal failure* due to the typical clinical picture of profuse urine volume at a time of poor waste product clearance (Dixon and Anderson, 1985). High output ATN occurs due to less damage and has a better prognosis than oliguric ATN (Rose, 2004).

Radiation Nephritis

A syndrome of late (3 to 13 months posttransplant) radiation nephritis that may result from radiation damage has become evident in recent years. A clinical and pathological process affecting the kidneys has been characterized by increased serum creatinine and BUN, and decreased GFR, along with anemia and hypertension (Lawton et al., 1992; Lonnerholm et al., 1991; Guinan et al., 1988; Cohen and Robbins, 2003). Kidney biopsy in these patients shows tubular atrophy and tubular interstitial scarring (Cohen and Robbins, 2003). The multiagent conditioning regimens combined with total body irradiation (TBI) in these patients are suspected as possible synergizers of the radiation

effects to the kidneys resulting in this clinical syndrome. Lawton and colleagues (1992) found that partial renal shielding reduced the incidence of late nephropathy. However, mild chronic renal insufficiency is still often associated with TBI (Borg et al., 2002).

Acute Hemolytic Reaction

Rapid-onset acute renal failure has occurred following infusion of autologous marrow or peripheral blood stem cells. Investigation of this problem has centered on both the condition of the patient at the time of reinfusion and the marrow processing and storage materials such as dimethylsulfoxide (DMSO) (Smith et al., 1987). Much is still unclear about this situation, but management is similar to other forms of hemolysis. Administration of mannitol during and after the cell reinfusion, coupled with preinfusion hydration with sodium bicarbonate, seems to prevent most of these occurrences.

The nurse should be alert for signs of hemolytic reactions by testing the urine for blood. If there is a sudden onset of hematuria and significant change in urine volume in the hours after reinfusion, prompt action must be taken. If hemolysis is determined, rapid hydration and the use of mannitol are necessary to allow the movement of hemoglobin through the renal tubules and out of the body.

Hemolytic Uremic Syndrome (HUS)

Hemolytic uremic syndrome (HUS) is associated with the high-dose therapy used prior to bone marrow transplantation and usually occurs as a late complication months after transplant. HUS is characterized by slowly progressive renal failure, hypertension, and bland urine sediment (Roy et al., 2001). Cyclosporine and tacrolymus rarely cause a reversible thrombocytic thrombocytopenic purpura hemolytic uremic syndrome (TTP-HUS) that is related to endothelial injury caused by these drugs (Trimarchi, et al., 1999). TTP-HUS is most common as a subacute chronic process that occurs around 3 to 12 months after transplantation (Fuge et al., 2001).

In summary, the following characteristics of renal failure are common after bone marrow or blood cell transplant. Renal failure is generally acute in nature. On resolution of the problems that produced the renal insufficiency, kidney function should recover. Mild impairment is common, especially that of prerenal failure etiology. ATN is the most common type of intrarenal failure and is often of the nonoliguric type. It is the most common insufficiency to occur in the first 3 weeks after transplant, but it can occur at any time.

Nursing Assessment of Renal Function

Renal insufficiency rarely exists in isolation from other clinical problems. It tends to arise at a time of multiorgan failure. If renal insufficiency is the only major clinical problem, it is generally easy to support the patient through its course. Unfortunately, this is seldom the case.

Renal insufficiency is not usually a primary toxicity of the high-dose therapy. **Figure 10-2** illustrates the interrelationships of some of the toxicities and shows that the major problem in keeping the kidneys functioning properly is keeping the other organs at optimum perfor- mance. Lines from each of the toxicities may be drawn to factors that affect some element of renal function discussed here. It is the task of the nurse to understand the implications of each and to use the appropriate assessment tools to assist in the management of the patient whose renal system is impaired.

The assessment of the renal patient (see **Table 10-3**) includes five areas:

1. blood chemistries, which help determine the fluid and electrolyte balance, the level of vital organ functions, and the acid–base balance;
2. urine assessment, which helps determine the level of renal tubular function and/or damage;
3. fluid balance assessment, which determines the compartmental distribution of fluid in the body;
4. pharmacologic agents, to examine the contributors to renal dysfunction, and peak and trough levels of drugs renally metabolized and excreted; and
5. mental status assessment, which elucidates neurological effects of renal impairment.

Blood Chemistries

Assessment of serum sodium helps calculate the patient's free water balance. Appropriate therapy of fluid quantity and quality is based on this calculation.

Assessment of serum CO_2 helps estimate the acid–base balance and determine the existence of the anion gap. If the CO_2 is low, it indicates a metabolic acidosis. If the calculated anion gap is high, it can indicate sepsis, ketoacidosis, or uremia. An acidosis without a significant anion gap is indicative of renal tubular acidosis (RTA).

Figure 10-2 Interrelationships of posttransplant patient problems and potential contributors to renal failure.

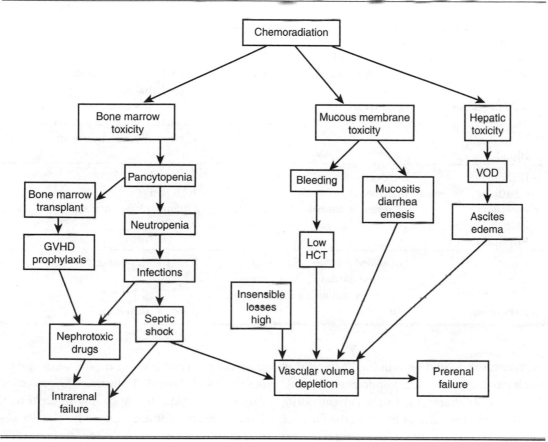

This is common in patients receiving cyclosporine or amphotericin B, and it is easily treatable by changing the amphotericin B product or changing the immune suppression from cyclosporine.

Assessment of potassium is important. In renal insufficiency, hyperkalemia would be expected, but in the marrow transplant patient receiving cyclosporine or amphotericin B, potassium wasting in the urine is common. Potassium wasting results in hypokalemia, which often requires aggressive intravenous potassium replacement.

Renal magnesium wasting is common in CSA due to change in magnesium reabsorption (Miura et al., 2002). Hypophosphatemia, hyperuricemia, and metabolic acidosis are also associated with the use of amphotericin.

Serum blood urea nitrogen is a complex value to interpret from these patients. Because the rate of BUN production is a function of several factors, the patient's metabolic rate, the patient's

Table 10-3 DIFFERENTIAL FINDINGS IN ACUTE RENAL FAILURE.

Test	Prerenal Findings	Intrarenal Findings Typical to ATN
Urine		
Specific gravity	> 1.015	< 1.010
Sodium	< 10 to 20 mEq/l	> 20 to 40 mEq/l
Sediment	MOD hyaline and finely granular casts	Dirty brown granular casts and epithelial cells
Volume output	Oliguria and anuria	Nonoliguria most common, but oliguria or anuria possible, especially if also prerenal
Blood		
BUN	Increased	Increased
Creatinine	Increased	Increased
Potassium	Increased or normal	Oliguric phase: increased
BUN/creatinine	> 10/1	< 10/1
Physical Exam		
Blood pressure	Low blood pressure, often with orthostatic drop in systolic blood pressure and increase in heart rate	Varies with volume
Neck veins	Flat	Varies with volume

hydration status, and protein intake levels may be elevated with even a slight decrease in GFR. The addition of steroids to the patient's drug profile or the presence of blood in the GI tract can significantly increase the production of BUN without any significant alteration in kidney function.

Serum creatinine is a better gauge of kidney function than is BUN. It can indicate a change in GFR, yet is not diagnostic of the etiology of the renal insufficiency.

The first important aspect of serum creatinine and BUN is the baseline measurement for that patient compared with the degree and rate of change from the baseline. A doubling of the creatinine level means a 50% decline in renal functioning. This is an important concept. Con-sider the patient whose creatinine on the previous day was 1.2 mg/dl. If the morning creatinine rises to 1.5 mg/dl, the response is different than if that same patient had a creatinine the day before of 0.07 mg/dl.

Urine Assessment

VOLUME

Examination of the urine's quantity and quality indicates the adequacy of renal tubular function and the type of renal insufficiency. Assessment should include the measurement of urine volume for a single shift plus the previous 24-hour period. A decrease in this volume along with an increase in serum creatinine suggests renal insufficiency. However, other assessments are needed to determine a prerenal or intrarenal etiology of the failure.

Specific Gravity

Since the tubular functions of secretion and absorption alter the filtrate character, abnormal values can be expected for urine electrolytes and specific gravity (McCance and Huether, 1998). Values typical of particular types of renal failure may be found. Also, urine sediment, determined by urinalysis, can be diagnostic of tubular damage. A healthy tubule has the ability to concentrate urine if it senses inadequate intravascular volume. It does this by reabsorbing filtered water into capillaries, surrounding the tubules and creating concentrated urine. Typically, the specific gravity is greater than 1.020. If the tubules have been sufficiently damaged, as in ATN, this ability is lost and the urine's specific gravity tends to be similar to that of the blood it filters. The specific gravity of blood is about 1.010.

As an example, consider how one might distinguish between a prerenal condition and intrarenal damage in the patient whose urine volume is decreased and the morning serum creatinine is elevated. A routine specific gravity measurement in the high range indicates that the tubules are working well and a prerenal condition would be suspected. We know this because it takes the tubular function of absorption to accomplish this state. A damaged tubule cannot concentrate urine.

Urine Sodium

In a prerenal state, the kidneys attempt to increase blood volume by resorbing sodium as well as water. This tends to deplete the tubular filtrate of sodium, yielding low urine sodium, typically less than 20 mEq/liter. If the tubules are damaged, as in ATN, resorption of sodium is less efficient and urine sodium levels are high, typically greater than 50 mEq/liter (Lam and Kaufman, 1985).

Urine Sediment

Epithelial casts are also diagnostic of tubular damage. If large amounts of renal tubular epithelial cell casts are passed out of the tubules, they can be seen in the urine under microscopic examination.

Fluid Balance

Fluid balance should be considered from two perspectives—the total body fluid and the distribution of that fluid in the body. Change in total body fluid is easily determined from changes in the patient's weight. For example, an overnight change in body weight is not a change in the amount of muscle or fat; it is a change in the amount of fluid in the body. Explanations for changes in weight may be found in the intake and output records and by taking into consideration insensible losses, which may be profuse in a febrile patient. Other less obvious factors causing a disturbance in fluid balance may be depletion due to the decreased intake when mucositis is present or loss due to high volume of emesis. These are significant factors in the early posttransplant period.

Each of these assessments helps explain the amount of, or changes in, the body fluid. They do not describe how that fluid is distributed in the body. From the kidney's standpoint, it is vital to determine whether the intravascular volume is sufficient. This determination guides therapy to prevent or reverse prerenal failure and to reestablish homeostasis. It may be that the replacement of an adequate blood volume is the quickest and easiest intervention for the patient. Physical assessment is the key in this evaluation.

Significant depletion of the patient's intravascular volume produces significant orthostatic changes in blood pressure and heart rate. Even a patient who spends a major portion of the day in bed should be able to compensate for postural changes in vital signs within 60 to 90 seconds. Measurement of orthostatic vital signs is significant in confirming a prerenal state due to hypovolemia. A finding of significant postural changes in blood pressure and heart rate, in addition to the other findings discussed in this chapter, is generally definitive of hypovolemia, without the need for invasive monitoring.

The level of intravascular fluid can be determined by assessing the presence of distended neck veins when the patient is in Trendelenburg position, and by a cardiac exam listening for signs of fluid overload. Pulmonary edema, as a result of fluid overload, may be manifested as rales in the lungs, or if severe, by frothy sputum, respiratory distress, signs of fluid on the chest x-ray, or a drop in oxygen saturation. Each of these signs supports the case that fluid has left the vascular space and gone to the interstitial spaces in the lungs.

The bone marrow transplant patient, especially one who has venoocclusive disease (discussed later), can sequester enormous amounts of fluid in the abdominal cavity, which will result in engorged organs and, at times, ascites (McDonald et al., 1986). Changes in abdominal girth and sudden weight gain indicate fluid that is not available for renal perfusion. An increase in abdominal girth without a concomitant rise in weight usually indicates a decrease in intravascular volume.

Pharmacological Considerations

Impaired renal functions can be a result of drugs. In turn, the drugs we give can be affected by impaired renal function. If a change in renal function is noted, it is important to look at the patient's drug profile and make appropriate adjustments. The adjustments are aimed at preventing toxic side effects of drugs that will be poorly excreted.

Assessments of the drug profile may also disclose a potential etiology of the renal insufficiency. If diuretics were aggressively used around the time of onset of renal insufficiency, assessment for signs of hypovolemia should occur. An elevation in BUN may reflect the increased metabolic rate seen with steroids. High-dose vasopressors such as dopamine constrict the renal arteries, causing prerenal condition. Salt loading with a liter of normal saline has been shown to decrease renal impairment associated with amphotericin B (Llanos et al., 1991; Girmenia et al., 2002). Not all offending medications can be stopped. Some may be necessary to sustain life, but due to the presence of renal insufficiency, adjustments in drugs or doses to avoid compounding the problem may be required.

Mental Status

The patient suffering severe renal impairment often exhibits changes in mental status that must be monitored. BUN and other waste products can build up in the blood and cause uremic encephalopathy. Nonrenal etiologies for changes of mental status are common, so other causes must also be evaluated. For instance, since the kidneys metabolize many drugs, a review of the drug profile may reveal the source of mental changes. This may be true for some drugs even if the kidney is not the major site of that drug's metabolism. The liver metabolizes many narcotics, yet the kidney clears the metabolites. It is often the case, especially if both renal and hepatic functions are impaired, that the metabolites cause the changes in mental status.

Management of Renal Insufficiency

The management of renal insufficiency in the bone marrow or blood cell transplant patient requires a multidisciplinary approach that involves at least the nurse, doctor, pharmacist, and nutritionist. The goal of management is to improve or maintain renal function while allowing the other organs to function properly.

Assessment

The first step in this management is assessment. Proper diagnosis directs proper treatment. The concepts and actions discussed previously give the physician the information necessary to establish the proper treatment. The nurse is often first to have the information because the nursing assessment involves the collection of weight, intake and output, abdominal girth, postural blood pressure and heart rate, lung exam, urine specific gravity, and the other indices vital to therapeutic decisions.

Correcting Vascular Volume Disequilibrium

The next management step involves the correction of any vascular volume disequilibrium. This may require diuretics or volume replacement. Whether replacement takes the form of crystalloid or colloid is determined by concurrent problems and the unique needs of the patient.

Correcting Electrolyte Imbalance

Along with this intravascular volume correction, electrolyte imbalances are corrected as well. This involves the correction of free water excess or deficit and adjustment of electrolytes in the intravenous fluids to match calculated losses and correction of any deficit or excess.

Minimizing Nephrotoxins

Adjustment or removal of nephrotoxic drugs must be attempted. This is often easier said than done in this population, given the requirements for such essential drugs as amphotericin B and cyclosporine. The decision to reduce or to maintain such therapy is based on the unique needs of the patient.

Treating Infections

To manage the renal problems that often arise in the transplant patient, infections must be adequately treated. This may seem to contradict the previous paragraph. Yet the most severely malfunctioning kidneys are those of the patient suffering septic shock and receiving pressor doses of dopamine.

Hemorrhagic Cystitis

Incidence

Hemorrhagic cystitis (HC) is reported to occur in up to 50% of BMT patients (Sencer et al., 1993; Efros et al., 1994; Miyamura et al., 1989). It is frequently a primary toxicity from the high-dose regimen due mainly to the use of cyclophosphamide. Fortunately, it is usually preventable and/or responsive to conservative treatment.

Etiology

The etiology of HC is twofold, depending on its time of occurrence. Risk factors include the use of busulfan during the preparative regimen, allogeneic BMT, and GVHD (Leung et al., 2002; Seber et al., 1999).

Early HC, within 48 hours of cyclophosphamide administration, is felt to result from acrolein, a metabolite of cyclophosphamide that is toxic to the transitional epithelium of the bladder mucosal tissue. Small vessels in the underlying tissue hemorrhage into the bladder (Champlin and Gale, 1984; Sale and Shulman, 1984). Later development of HC, up to several months post-transplant, is felt to involve a superimposed infectious agent. HC associated with adenovirus, cytomegalovirus, and BK virus is common in this late onset group (Akiyama et al., 2001; Leung et al., 2002; Bedi et al., 1995). BK virus is found in 77–90% of adult BMT patients, and therefore patients with a higher viral load may be more likely to have HC (Priftakis et al., 2003).

Presentation and Clinical Course

Hemorrhagic cystitis may present immediately with the administration of cyclophosphamide or be delayed, sometimes for months after the cyclophosphamide course. It is most commonly seen at the time of cyclophosphamide administration and presents as hematuria with or without blood clots. It may also present as dysuria or frequency. HC is generally responsive to the treatment measures instituted and is generally resolved within 1 or 2 days of the end of the administration of cyclophosphamide (Champlin and Gale, 1984). Late HC is more truculent to treatment with an average duration of 40 days (Akiyama et al., 2001).

In this severe form, larger and more deeply invasive ulcerations extend into the vascular tissue underlying the bladder mucosa (Sale and Shulman, 1984). Bleeding may develop into a severe, life-threatening problem. Also, because the blood often clots in the bladder, painful obstruction of bladder outflow may result.

Prevention

The prevention of HC involves measures to decrease the toxicity of the metabolite. Three-way irrigation catheters are placed, and 100–500 ml/hr of fluid continuously irrigates the bladder from the start of cyclophosphamide until at least 24 hours after the last dose or until the urine shows no evidence of blood. The goal of this intervention is to dilute and remove as fast as possible the toxic substance from contact with the sensitive bladder tissue (Turkeri et al., 1995; Meisenberg et al., 1994).

Another preventive measure is the use of aggressive intravenous hydration with fluids at twice the usual maintenance rate (Meisenberg et al., 1994). This aggressive hydration causes a rapid and dilute filtrate to pass through the ureters, thus preventing prolonged contact of the metabolite with epithelium. Vigorous hydration requires monitoring of the patient's fluid. It is common for the patient to develop either an overhydrated state or, if diuretics are used to force diuresis, a prerenal state. Measures discussed in the previous section of this chapter are useful in determining the appropriate therapies for the patient's situation.

The use of drugs to prevent HC is becoming more common. Mesna is an example of a drug that binds acrolein to form a nontoxic compound and prevent damage (Vose et al., 1993; Shepherd et al., 1991). With the prevalence of outpatient chemotherapy, mesna is often used as a replacement to continuous bladder irrigation.

Treatment

Since mesna acts at the time of the cyclophosphamide administration, there is no benefit for its use once HC has occurred. Treatment of HC involves many of the same therapies used for prevention. Continuous bladder irrigation at 500 ml to 2 liters per hour is generally sufficient to clear developing clots and prevent obstruction. Infusing platelets to maintain high platelet levels is also very important. At times, cystoscopy is required, and cautery of bleeding ulcerative areas may be attempted. Unfortunately this is usually not a long-term solution due to the diffuse, widespread pathology associated with the problem. The instillation of chemicals, such as acetylcystene, into the bladder is also used and may benefit the patient.

Hepatic Complications

Major causes of liver dysfunction in BMT are infections, drugs, hepatic venoocclusive disease (VOD), portal hypertension, graft-versus-host disease (GVHD), viral hepatitis, and relapse (McDonald et al., 1987). Cyclosporine toxicity causes a rise in bilirubin, other liver function test abnormalities, fluid retention, hypertension, and renal impairment at increased drug levels (Baldwin et al., 2000). Tacrolimus causes similar toxicities.

For information on liver infection, see Chapter 7. For a discussion of liver GVHD, see Chapter 6.

Incidence of Hepatic Complications

In one study, 77–84.2% of allogeneic patients and 44.8–52% of autologous patients had liver dysfunction in the first year after transplant (Kim et al., 2000; Ozdogan et al., 2003). In another study, fulminant hepatic failure occurred in 7% of patients (Ozdogan et al., 2003). Studies to determine whether there is increased risk of liver failure after BMT in patients with mildly elevated liver function tests (LFTs), or in patients that are hepatitis B surface antigen and

hepatitis C antibody positive are conflicting (Kim et al., 2000), although it is generally thought that elevated liver function tests increase the risk of liver toxicity. Mortality from hepatic failure is 4–15% in most studies (Locasciulli et al., 1994).

Hepatic Physiology

The liver is composed of a series of lobules. These lobules are composed of capillaries or sinusoids surrounded by endothelium and then sheets of hepatocytes. Hepatocytes have a canalicular surface, and when they are adjacent to each other there are small channels called *bile canaliculi*. These bile canaliculi run together to form bile ducts, which combine to make up the common bile duct, which opens into the duodenum. Production of bile salts is one of the liver's main functions. Kupffer cells, which are macrophages, line the sinusoids and remove bacteria, which usually originate in the intestine. The liver is a very vascular organ and contains 25% of the cardiac output. The blood arrives via the hepatic artery and the portal vein, which drains to smaller and smaller vessels to the sinusoids, and then the blood is processed by the hepatocytes in the sinusoids, moves across, and leaves the liver via hepatic venules to the hepatic vein and into the inferior vena cava (see **Figure 10-3**). If cardiac output drops, the liver can shunt blood out of the liver into the main vasculature to support blood pressure. The liver synthesizes coagulation factors, prothrombin, fibrinogen, and factors I, II, VII, IX, and X, and it synthesizes proteins such as aspartate aminotransferase (AST), aloacetate transaminase (ALT), lactate dehydrogenase (LDH), and alkaline phosphatase. The liver releases glucose during states of hypoglycemia and stores glucose as glycogen when there is ex-

Figure 10-3 Basic structure of a liver lobule.

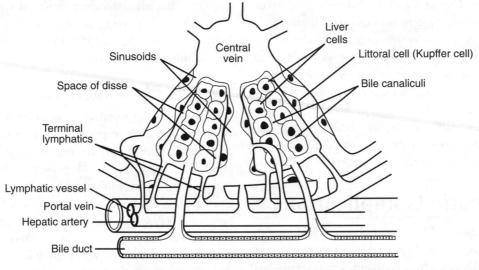

Source: Reprinted from Guyton, A.C. (1986). *Textbook of Medical Physiology.* Philadelphia: W.B. Saunders, p. 88, with permission.

cess. The Glisson's capsule that contains blood vessels, lymphatics, and nerves covers the liver (Huether, 1998).

Venoocclusive Disease of the Liver

Venoocclusive disease (VOD) of the liver is a life-threatening complication that arises after bone marrow transplant, usually within the first 3 weeks of BMT (Arai et al., 2002). It is intimately involved with the disruption of normal renal function and the fluid and electrolyte balance (hypernatremia) of the patient. VOD is a distinct disease involving the blood vessels of the liver. This disease has a specific syndrome that manifests clinically with great variation in severity, affects several other organ systems, requires close attention, and alters the clinical management of the patient. In addition, it is associated with significant mortality.

If a patient is jaundiced, encephalopathic, has a distended abdomen, and is experiencing complex fluid and electrolyte problems, the clinician should consider VOD.

Incidence and Risk Factors

The incidence of VOD in the BMT population is reported as being between 10% and 60%. This variation is due to the variability of the populations studied, the variability of diagnostic criteria, and the differing intensity of conditioning therapies (Bearman, 1995; McDonald et al., 1984; Jones et al., 1987). VOD ranges from mild, reversible disease to severe and life-threatening. McDonald and colleagues (1993) found 12% with mild disease, 26% with moderate disease, and 15% with severe disease.

Ablative therapy preparative regimens that include busulfan or cytarabine, carmustine, mitomycin, 6-mercaptopurine, and dacarbazine have been implicated in VOD (Arai et al., 2002). Total body irradiation, especially when receiving single, daily-dose TBI, increases a patient's risk of VOD (Girinsky et al., 2000).

The following known factors predispose a patient to VOD:

- Pretransplant liver enzyme elevation
- Higher intensity cytoreductive therapy
- Mismatched or unrelated donor
- Previous radiation therapy to the abdomen
- Cyclosporine and methotrexate GVHD prophylaxis

The most significant risk factor is the presence of liver abnormalities at the time of conditioning therapy. Whether the cause of abnormalities is viral hepatitis, tumor infiltrates, or infections, the finding of elevated bilirubin and/or liver enzymes predicts an increased risk for VOD. This is such a significant finding that, if at all possible, the transplant should be postponed until liver function tests return to normal. Of the other risk factors for developing VOD, a higher intensity of the conditioning regimen and the presence of the infection anywhere in the body are the most significant (McDonald et al., 1993; McDonald et al., 1984; Jones et al., 1987).

Although the clinical symptoms of VOD arise in the time period shown in **Figure 10-4**, the liver insult actually occurs well before the clinical symptoms.

Etiology of VOD

Interestingly, using a single conditioning agent generally does not bring on the disease. Yet given in combination, there seems to be a syn-

Figure 10-4 Time of occurrence of acute complications after bone marrow transplantation.

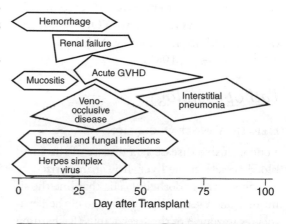

Source: From Ford, R., & Ballard, B. (1998). Acute complications after bone marrow transplantation. *Seminars in Oncology Nursing*, 4(1), 15–24.

ergistic effect producing hepatic damage well beyond that produced by any single agent (McDonald et al., 1986). Inflammatory cytokines seem to play a role in the development and severity of the disease (McDonald et al., 1993). The finding that a higher number of febrile days during conditioning therapy results in an increased occurrence of severe VOD suggest that inflammatory crytokines participate in the liver damage caused by cytoreductive therapy (Bearman, 1995).

Onset and Resolution

Venoocclusive disease clinically appears at any time after the start of conditioning, with its peak onset in the second week after transplant. Recovery occurs about 3 weeks after the onset of jaundice (McDonald et al., 1985). Mild disease is defined by no apparent adverse effect from liver dysfunction and then resolution of symptoms.

Moderate disease conveys adverse effects of liver dysfunction including fluid retention and pain, but eventually resolves. Severe VOD is essentially fatal (Richardson and Guinan, 2001). Overall, about half of the patients with VOD recover. In those who have VOD at death, VOD is the direct cause of death in the majority (McDonald et al., 1985; Jones et al., 1987).

Pathophysiology

HEPATIC VENULE OCCLUSION

Venoocclusive disease is a disease of the small blood vessels in the liver. It is characterized by damage to the endothelial cells that line the sinusoids and eventually by damage of the hepatocytes in zone 3 of the liver acinus (Richardson and Guinan, 2001). The two areas of hepatic injury from VOD are the hepatic venules and the hepatocytes that line the sinusoids. As the hepatocytes metabolize and process the chemotherapeutic agents passing through the liver, the by-products, which tend to be toxic, are dumped into these small vessels. The endothelial linings of the sinuses and hepatic veins are damaged by the toxicity of these metabolites. Cellular damage in the sinusoids leads to collagen and fibrin deposition in the sinusoids, leading to occlusion in the venous outflow tract of the liver, hence its name. The eventual result is impaired blood flow through the sinuses secondary to obstruction (Storek et al., 1993; McDonald et al., 1993; McDonald et al., 1986).

During the pathogenesis the tissue is swollen from the chemo/radiation insult. The hepatocytes release cytokines, like tumor necrosis factor-alpha, resulting in hypercoagulability followed by perivascular deposition of coagulation factors with gradual occlusion of the vessels (Storek et al., 1993; Shulman and Hinterberger, 1992).

Fibrin is deposited in the injured area in an attempt to stabilize the area. This fibrin presents an impediment to the passage of cellular debris and exfoliated hepatocytes that have died from the conditioning toxicities. The process becomes self-perpetuating as the blood flow becomes impaired and the tissue is deprived of the oxygen necessary to support the tissue. The entire liver becomes engorged as venous outflow becomes more and more occluded. Anoxia leads to further injury and necrosis of hepatic tissue with the result that hepatic blood flow and function is even more impaired. The liver damage produces low levels of antithrombin III, protein C, factor VII, and platelet refractoriness (Scrobahaci et al., 1991). The clinical syndrome is a logical extension of the pathophysiological changes that occur. It is from this occluded flow that all the resultant clinical problems stem (McDonald et al., 1986).

Clinical Diagnosis of VOD

The clinical diagnosis of VOD can be based on as few as four criteria. Jones and colleagues (1987) and McDonald and colleagues (1984) showed that the presence of hyperbilirubinemia (bilirubin < 2.0 mg/dl), hepatomegaly (usually painful), ascites, and significant weight gain (greater than 5%), correlated highly with the presence of VOD as confirmed by biopsy. In fact, they showed that if the patient was in the first 3 weeks after bone marrow transplant, and if these signs could not be explained by other mechanisms, the finding of any two of the four criteria was sufficient to confirm the diagnosis 89% of the time. McDonald and colleagues (1984) also showed that in the absence of two of the three, there was a 92% chance that VOD did not exist. Other studies have used much the same criteria and had similar results. More recent work by Shulman confirmed a correlation of the clinical and histologic findings (Shulman et al., 1994). This seems valid when one constructs a frequency chart (see **Figure 10-5**) of signs and symptoms in patients with VOD. The four most frequent symptoms are the ones used in the clinical diagnosis and occur in the majority of patients with the disease. Doppler ultrasound may demonstrate reversal of flow in the portal vein, but this is not an early sign of VOD and therefore is not a good diagnostic tool (Herbetko et al., 1992). Transvenous liver biopsy allows both tissue diagnosis and measurement of hepatic venous pressure gradient, which is specific for VOD (Shulman et al., 1995).

Other diagnostic studies also can contribute to the diagnosis of VOD:

- *CAT scans*—demonstrate hepatomegaly, absence of lesions that could be disease or infection, ascites, hepatic vein or biliary dilation.
- *Doppler ultrasound*—reversal of portal venous flow, measurement of hepatic artery resistive index.
- *Transvenous liver biopsy*—tissue diagnosis and hepatic venous pressure gradient (> 10 mmHg is > 90% specific).

The severity of the disease may be predicted by the degree of weight gain and serum bilirubin for a given day posttransplant (Bearman et al., 1993). Greater weight gain and bilirubin early in the course indicated a more severe course and worse outcome. The most definitive diagnosis is by tissue biopsy, but this presents risks to the thrombocytopenic patient. It is necessary and appropriate to make the diagnosis based on clinical signs and symptoms.

MEASUREMENT OF THE AREA UNDER THE CURVE

Oral high-dose busulfan has an unpredictable absorption in the gastrointestinal tract. Studies have shown a correlation between the area under the curve (AUC) and VOD. Busulfan kinetics can be done to predict the AUC. An AUC of 800–1400 micromoles/minute/liter is considered therapeutic (Growchow et al., 1989). Intravenous busulfan, which is now available, has

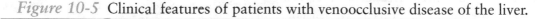

Figure 10-5 Clinical features of patients with venoocclusive disease of the liver.

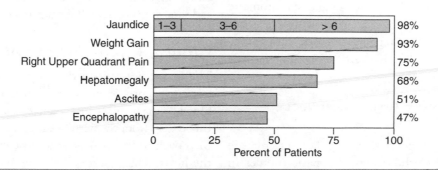

Source: From G. McDonald et al. (1985). The clinical course of 53 patients with venoocclusive disease of the liver after bone marrow transplantation. *Transplantation, 39*(6), 604. © Williams & Wilkins, 1985. Used with permission.

much less variable absorption (Vaughan et al., 2002). However, some institutions continue to do kinetics with intravenous busulfan due to the variability of drug metabolism (Vaughan et al., 2002).

HEPARIN

Prophylactic medications to prevent the occurrence of VOD have been proposed and used with contradictory results. Heparin given as a continuous infusion, in low doses (100–150 U/kg per day), fractionated heparin, or low molecular weight heparin have been used. Prophylactic heparin is not recommended (Arai et al., 2002).

URSODEOXYCHOLIC ACID

Ursodeoxycholic acid (ursodiol), a nonhuman bile acid, protects hepatocytes from the damage caused by cholestasis by virtue of its ability to replace the more toxic bile acids (Bearman, 1995). Pilot data from Essell and colleagues (1992) suggest that ursodiol may decrease the incidence of VOD. Some BMT centers use ursodiol for prevention of VOD (Arai et al., 2002).

Treatment of VOD

There is no definitive treatment to reverse VOD. At present, the clinical effort is generally directed toward supportive and symptomatic management of the patient until VOD has run its course and the regenerative capabilities of the liver have had a chance to repair the damage from the disease.

RECOMBINANT TISSUE PLASMINOGEN ACTIVATOR

Given the evidence that coagulation factors are deposited in the damaged hepatic tubules in VOD patients, thrombolytic therapy has been proposed. Recombinant human tissue plasminogen activator (rh-tPA) is being used in

cases of severe VOD where the benefit is worth the risk. Fatal hemorrhage is a significant potential, but pilot data support that rh-tPA can alter the natural course of severe VOD if treated early in the course (Yu et al., 1994; Bearman et al., 1992, Kulkarni, et al., 1999).

DEFIBROTIDE

Defibrotide has antithrombotic, anti-ischemic, anti-inflammatory, and thrombolytic properties without systemic anticoagulation (Palmer and Goa, 1993). A study of 19 patients with severe VOD revealed no toxicities or hemorrhage was related to the drug, and resolution of VOD was seen in 42% of patients (Richardson et al., 1998; Chopra et al., 2000). Randomized trials are now under way.

ANTITHROMBIN III

Antithrombin III concentrate was given to patients with VOD and a documented deficiency. In this study, all patients achieved clinical improvement (Morris et al., 1997).

ANTIOXIDANT THERAPY

Glutamine infusions have been tried in a few case studies to reduce the free radical damage that occurs to the endothelial cells in VOD. Two patients were successfully treated with glutamine and vitamin E therapy (Goringe et al., 1998).

Clinical Complications of VOD

The majority of blood that enters the liver is from the portal vein system, which delivers blood from the intestines, pancreas, and spleen. Blood goes from the portal vein to the sinusoids, then back to the inferior vena cava and back to the heart. This system allows the liver to metabolize and detoxify substances such as drugs from the gastric organs. Portal hypertension occurs when there is an obstruction by thrombus, inflammation, or fibrosis of the sinusoids (this happens in cirrhosis, VOD, and viral hepatitis). Portal hypertension can lead to splenomegaly, ascites, and other signs of liver failure as shown in **Table 10-4**. The liver becomes swollen. As the pressure in the hepatic vasculature exceeds its ability to keep the fluid inside the capillary bed, sodium and protein-rich fluid drip off the surface of the liver into the peritoneal cavity. In many patients, this fluid is absorbed by the lymphatic system at the rate it is produced. If it becomes too profuse, this compensatory maneuver is inadequate, and ascetic fluid accumulates.

Restricted blood flow through the liver also causes pressure in the portal system, engorging the mucosal lining of the small intestine. A further consequence of poor flow is strong reabsorption of sodium and water by the renal tubules (Cade et al., 1987; McDonald et al., 1985).

Each of these conditions presents its own set of problems, yet the primary effect is to shunt the vital blood away from the liver. This consequence has the most serious implications because the shunting of blood, if severe and pro-longed, can prevent the delivery of oxygen to the hepatic tissue. Without oxygen and the ability to carry off the hepatically metabolized substances, liver cells start to die, tissue necroses occur, and this destruction adds to the problems already existent. Liver enzymes start to reflect hepatic dysfunction, and the overall metabolic capability of the liver can become severely impaired (Shulman et al., 1980).

Managing VOD Complications

The management of VOD entails preventing the extremes of the optimal vital organ function. The key is a thorough assessment that includes the knowledge of the patient's baseline information and the degree of change from this baseline. From this knowledge base comes the plan to manage the clinical problems.

The management of VOD symptoms entails efforts to:

1. maintain fluid and electrolyte balance,
2. minimize the adverse effects of ascites,
3. adjust drugs to reflect impaired hepatic and renal function,

Table 10-4 CONSEQUENCES OF IMPAIRED HEPATIC BLOOD FLOW AND FUNCTION.

Pathology	Clinical Symptoms/Results
Hepatic, splenic, and GI mucosal congestion	Abdominal distention, pain, respiratory compromise, third-space fluid
Accumulation of ascites	Abdominal distention, intravascular volume loss
Sodium/water retention by renal tubules	Total body fluid gain, edema
Serum proteins weep off liver into peritoneum	Hypoalbuminemia, edema, ascites
Ischemia, hepatocyte death, tissue necrosis	Elevated liver enzymes, impaired hepatic functions
Impaired bilirubin handling	Jaundice
Altered drug metabolism	Increased serum levels, narcotics, CSA, MTX
Impaired handling of metabolic waste production	Hepatic encephalopathy
Poor synthetic functions	Coagulopathy

4. avoid compounding encephalopathy with drugs that alter mental status, and

5. attend to coagulopathy.

The overall goals of these tasks are to:

1. improve the impaired flow of blood through the liver and kidneys,

2. redistribute body fluids appropriately,

3. assist the body's compensatory efforts, and

4. counter inappropriate compensatory actions that the body institutes.

Hepatitis B

There are an estimated 350 million individuals chronically infected with hepatitis B worldwide, and 2 billion have hepatitis positive markers. In the United States there are an estimated 140,000–320,000 acute infection cases of hepatitis B (HBV) per year (Centers for Disease Control, 2004). The onset of hepatitis B is insidious, and the incubation period is from 45 to 185 days (see **Figure 10-6**). Often, patients or donors are unaware that they have been exposed to the virus. Therefore, testing for hepatitis B prior to transplantation is imperative. **Table 10-5** lists hepatitis B markers and their clinical significance. Most transplant centers test donors for HbsAg and anti-HBc to rule out infection of the donor or patient with hepatitis B.

Hepatitis B and Bone Marrow Transplant

HBV develops in transplant recipients via progression of pretransplant infection, reactivation of HBV, or acquisition of HBV from infected donors. HBV infection is not a contraindication to BMT, but liver damage due to cirrhosis and fibrosis in these patients does increase the risk of

---

Figure 10-6 Acute HBV infection with recovery—typical serologic course.

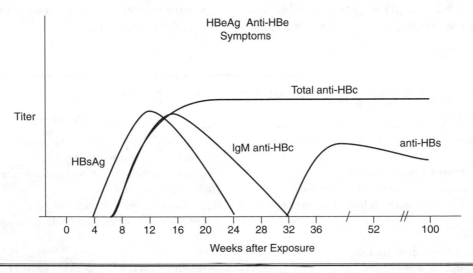

Source: Centers for Disease Control, Center for Infectious Disease. Hepatitis B and refugees. Retrieved February 18, 2004, from http://www.cdc.gov/ncidod/diseases/hepatitis/slideset/refugee/slide_28.htm

Table 10-5 HEPATITIS B MARKERS.

Abbreviation	Virus Marker	Comments
HBV	Viral culture	Takes 2–3 weeks to grow
HbsAg	Hepatitis B surface antigen	Evidence of viral coat, marker of infectivity
Anti-HBs	Antibody to hepatitis B surface antigen	Marker of immunity to disease from vaccine
Anti-HBc	Antibody to hepatitis B core viral material	Marker of antibody of past or current infection
IgM anti-HBc	Early antibody subclass to anti-HBc	Indicates recent infection (< 4–6 mos)
HbeAg	Hepatitis B "e" antigen	Sign of viral replication, marker of infectivity
Anti-Hbe	Antibody to hepatitis B "e"	Marker of present or past infection with hepatitis B

organ toxicity to BMT (Strasser and McDonald, 1999). Patients with latent hepatitis B who are treated with corticosteroids are at an increased risk of reactivation of the virus due to a glucocorticoid responsive element on the virus. Patients are at increased risk for transplant-related mortality due to liver failure if they have any history of splenic or hepatic enlargement associated with the virus (Bain, 2000). Hepatitis B infection is also related to an increased incidence of GVHD (Lau et al., 1997). The increased incidence of liver GVHD makes death from liver failure more common in allogeneic bone marrow transplant recipients (Chen, 1999).

Fewer than 30% of recipients become infected with hepatitis B virus (HBV) from donors who are HBV surface antigen positive. Of those who become infected, only 5–15% develop severe hepatitis after transplant (Strasser and McDonald, 1999). Immunity to HBV can also be transferred from donor to recipient (Arai et al., 2002). If the patient is HbsAg positive, the amount of viral load must be determined by sending HbeAg, anti-Hbe, and quantitated HBV DNA. Posttransplant during immune suppression HBV replicates; however, there is no inflammation of the liver (Bain, 2000). The higher levels of virus are cytotoxic and can cause cholestasis and periportal fibrosis (Bain, 2000). Patients who were anti-HBs positive only have had reactivation after transplant (Dhedin et al., 1998; Lau et al., 1997).

Once cellular immunity is restored, generally at the time of the withdrawal of immune suppression, clinical hepatitis can be seen (Pariente et al., 1988). HBV DNA should be monitored posttransplant, and those who have increasing viral load should be preemptively treated with antiviral drugs. Unfortunately, how long and which antiviral drug is under discussion. Ganciclovir does not always work, and resistant strains of HBV have been known to develop with the use of famciclovir and lamivudine (Arai et al., 2002).

Hepatitis C and Bone Marrow Transplant

Hepatitis C virus (HCV) infection is transmitted to the recipient from a hepatitis C positive donor 100% of the time. One study demonstrated the use of interferon alpha (stopped one week prior to donation) to reduce the transmission of HCV to recipients (Vance et al., 1996). The viral load of these recipients becomes very high; however, there is usually no clinical hepatitis; fulminant immune-rebound hepatitis has occurred on rare occasions (Maruta et al., 1994). Cirrhosis in recipients who have hepatitis C is a late complication that occurs in the second or third decade after transplant (Strasser and McDonald, 1999). All donors and recipients should be tested for hepatitis C using a hepatitis C polymerase chain reaction (PCR) test. All BMT recipients who were positive for the hepatitis C virus or had a hepatitis C positive donor must be monitored frequently.

Iron Overload

Hemosiderosis of the liver happens in 90% of BMT patients with hematological malignancies (Arai et al., 2002). Serum ferritin levels are measurements of iron stores in stable patients (Jenson et al., 1995). There is an increased risk of infections in patients with iron overload and

worsening of the natural history of hepatitis C (Arai et al., 2002). Phlebotomy or chelation therapy should be considered (Curry et al., 1996). It is important to monitor ferritin levels in BMT patients during follow-up after the first 100 days.

Gallbladder Disease

Oral antibiotics, cyclosporine, amphotericin, mycophenolate mofetil, timethoprim-sulfamethoxazole, and high-dose opioids can cause drug-induced cholestasis. Total parenteral nutrition and fasting are also associated with hepatobiliary disease. This disorder is reversible by stopping the causative drug, or if associated with TPN, the patient increases his or her oral intake (Teffey et al., 1994).

Consequences of Impaired Hepatic Function

As hepatic function fails, the ability to remove drugs and metabolic wastes becomes impaired. The patient becomes jaundiced, as bilirubin is not processed out of the body. Impaired pro-

Table 10-6 SYMPTOMS OF LIVER FAILURE.

Normal Metabolic Functions	Symptoms of Failure
Synthesis of plasma proteins, albumin, and globulins	Low plasma levels of total protein and albumin leading to edema
Storage of glycogen and release of glucose in stress	Loss of glycemic control—hypoglycemia
Deamination to allow ammonia to be excreted by the kidneys	Increased levels of ammonia in the blood
Immune function of Kupffer cells	Loss of Kupffer cells; increased risk of infections
Synthesis of prothrombin, fibrinogen, and factors I, II, VII, IX, and X	Increased risk of bleeding related to increased partial thromboplastin time and prothrombin time ratios, as well as loss of vitamin K_1
Production of bile	Loss of bile, leading to malabsorption of fats
Metabolic detoxification	Increased toxicity of many drugs

duction of coagulation factors can also develop with a resultant coagulopathy. See **Table 10-6** for symptoms of hepatic failure.

Nursing Implications of Liver Failure

NEUROLOGICAL ASSESSMENT

Nurses should assess for subtle changes in personality, memory loss, irritability, and lethargy. These symptoms can lead to confusion, flapping tremor of hands, stupor, convulsions, coma, and death. It is important to decrease the amount of toxins that are introduced into the liver circulation, including acetaminophen, narcotics, and benzodiazepines. Decrease NH_3 by providing a protein-restricted diet and eliminating intestinal bacteria. Lactulose should be administered as ordered. Lactulose goes to the intestines, changes NH_3 to NH_4, and makes it not absorbable.

FLUID ASSESSMENT

Assessment for ascites should be completed by daily measurement of abdominal girth, weight gains, and refractoriness to diuresis. Fluid shifts should be treated by dietary salt restrictions, use of potassium-sparing diuretics, and use of paracentesis; however, the fluid usually reaccumulates quickly, and if too much is removed, there is a risk of hypotension and shock.

RESPIRATORY ASSESSMENT

Displacement of the diaphragm by the enlarged liver and ascites causes dyspnea and shallow breathing. This displacement may lead to the need for intubation. Ventilation may also be affected by the accumulation of medications, especially narcotics used for pain control of the hepatomegaly.

SKIN ASSESSMENT

Nurses should assess for jaundice, which occurs with a bilirubin > 1.2 mg/dl, pruritis from hyperbilirubinemia, and uremia.

RENAL ASSESSMENT

Hepato-renal syndrome can occur, causing an increased creatinine, oliguria, and sodium retention. Potassium levels do not rise until terminal stages. BUN increases, followed by increased creatinine. Often the BUN is much higher in proportion to the creatinine due to dehydration in the vascular space. Circulation of blood to the vital organs of the abdominal cavity can be impaired if the intraperitoneal pressure becomes too great and impairs renal function, which is common in patients with VOD (McDonald et al., 1985).

CARDIOVASCULAR ASSESSMENT

Changes in circulation with liver failure decrease blood pressure. Nurses should assess for bleeding due to coagulopathy. Fresh frozen plasma, platelets, and cryoprecipitate should be administered as ordered. Bleeding precautions must be taken.

ABDOMINAL DISTENTION

In addition to findings used in the clinical diagnosis, a vast array of other common abdominal findings are associated with VOD. The congested GI mucosa, liver, spleen, and ascites all lead to abdominal distention. Severe enlargement of the abdomen can impair respiratory efforts; for example, full ventilatory movement might be painful.

HYPONATREMIA, HYPOALBUMINEMIA, EDEMA

Water reabsorption by the renal tubules tends to produce a free-water excess. This is compounded by the renal reabsorption of sodium, increasing total body sodium. The result of too much total body sodium is too much free water (which dilutes the serum sodium concentration to hyponatremic levels). In addition, the leak of serum proteins into the peritoneal space produces hypoalbuminemia, reducing the oncotic pressure, forcing water out of the capillaries into the interstitial space, or edema.

ENCEPHALOPATHY

The shunting of blood away from the liver, coupled with a loss of hepatic cells, often causes the liver to inadequately metabolize waste products and the metabolites of drugs. These materials can build up in the blood and cause hepatic encephalopathy, which is clinically manifested as lethargy, confusion, and disorientation.

RENAL INSUFFICIENCY

Several forces operate against proper renal function in the patient suffering from VOD. Although many patients with VOD never show impaired renal function, some have concomitant renal insufficiency. VOD can lead to hepatorenal syndrome, often with hyponatremia due to decreased renal perfusion (Bearman, 1995). Prerenal factors, as discussed earlier in this chapter, and the impairment of the liver's metabolism of nephrotoxic drugs seem to be the etiology of the concurrent renal failure. For instance, several prerenal factors are common to patients with VOD (see **Figure 10-7**). Most important is the loss of fluid from effective circulation due to an engorged liver, GI mucosa, and spleen. Ascites and edema rob the kidneys of needed intravascular volume. The use of diuretics and the restriction of IV or oral fluids, while often necessary actions, may overshoot the intended target and deplete the already tenuous intravascular status. If the intraperitoneal pressure becomes too great, venous return becomes im-

paired and further restricts the already poor hepatic and renal blood flow.

The kidneys' response to these conditions is, in effect, to add fuel to the fire. Filtered sodium and water are reabsorbed at the renal tubules, urine output drops, clearance of metabolic waste products decreases still further, and weight gain continues. In addition to the prerenal conditions is the potential that the kidneys may fall victim to nephrotoxic levels of hepatically metabolized drugs. Chief among these is cyclosporine, which is so commonly used in this population (Yee et al., 1984). This close relationship between the kidneys and liver is a major concern and the focus of much of the clinical intervention directed at VOD.

MAINTAINING FLUID AND ELECTROLYTE BALANCE

Maintenance of fluid and electrolyte balance requires a good assessment of total fluid through evaluation of weight, intake and output, and estimated insensible losses. The next task is to assess the distribution of that fluid in the body. Nursing assessment plays an essential role in this task. The performance of postural blood pressure and heart rate, abdominal girth, lung exam, estimation of changes in peripheral edema, and the collection of urine for analysis are vital in determining the distribution of fluid in the body. With this information, one can determine the effect of the fluid distribution on the renal, pulmonary, and cardiac status of the patient.

OPTIMIZING INTRAVASCULAR FLUID

Though not a universal finding, it is common for the patient with VOD to be intravascularly depleted. Much of the crystalloid intravenous fluid given to the patient has an end point outside the vascular space. For this reason, judicious

Figure 10-7 Impact of venoocclusive disease on renal function.

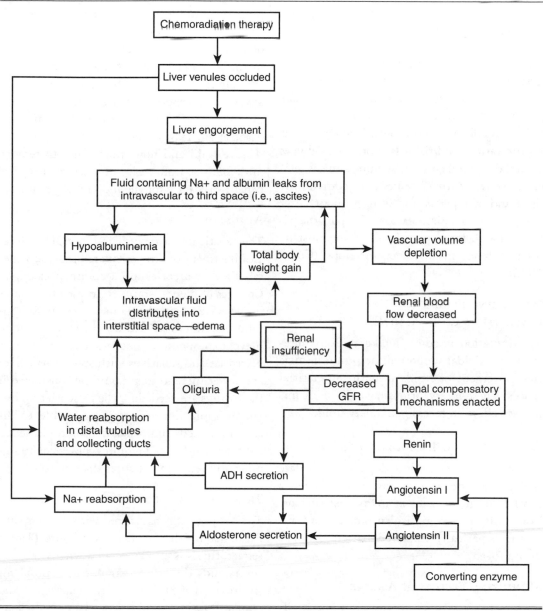

use of red blood cells and/or salt-poor albumin are often recommended to maintain the volume of intravascular fluid. The infusion of these col- loids is generally indicated when the patient ex- hibits signs of volume depletion, such as ortho- static hypotension. Salt-poor albumin is used to increase the oncotic pressure in the vascular space and to replace serum proteins that are lost into the peritoneal cavity with ascites (McDonald et al., 1985).

TREATING SODIUM IMBALANCE

The treatment of elevated total body sodium levels requires a restriction of sodium intake plus the initiation of sodium diuresis. Spironolactone is effective in this regard, though it has its limitations and risks. It is only available as an oral drug, and effective sodium diuresis generally starts 36 to 72 hours after starting the drug and may persist for 24 to 36 hours after stopping doses. Spironolactone also puts the patient at risk for hyperkalemia. Care must be used if renal insufficiency develops (Conn, 1972).

MINIMIZING FLUIDS IN INTERSTITIAL COMPARTMENTS

The limitation of sodium intake, sodium diuresis, and colloidal support all help to minimize the movement of fluids into the interstitial spaces. These interventions have the most important effect on excess pulmonary fluid.

ALTERING RENAL HEMODYNAMICS

The use of low, renal-dose dopamine to dilate the renal arteries and improve renal efficiency has fallen out of favor at many institutions. The ability to accomplish an increase in GFR in the hepatically impaired patient has not been proven.

MINIMIZING EFFECTS OF ASCITES

In those cases of VOD where ascites is a significant problem, it is often the intent of clinicians to reduce ascitic fluid or to reduce the amount of fluid that has become sequestered in the abdominal organs. The removal of fluid by the aggressive use of diuretics, dialysis, or directly tapping the fluid via serial paracentesis are all effective. Yet whatever method is used, the underlying process that allowed the ascites to form in the first place persists, and the ascites inevitably reaccumulate. This reaccumulation is always at the expense of the intravascular volume and invariably leads to renal impairment (Cade et al., 1987). The decision of whether to remove fluid and how much fluid to remove must be based on a careful assessment of the benefit–risk ratio for the individual situation.

ADJUSTING DRUGS

The hepatic impairment found in VOD requires an adjustment of drugs that are hepatically metabolized. Narcotics are a common example. Changes of mental status from use of narcotics in the patient with VOD may necessitate stopping or reducing the drugs in an attempt to prevent compounding hepatic encephalopathy. Narcotics and sedatives with shorter half-lives and fewer metabolites should be considered if these drugs are needed for the patient's comfort. For example, lorazepam is preferable to diazepam for sedation. Also, hydromorphone has a shorter half-life and requires conversion to significantly fewer metabolites than morphine.

TREATING COAGULOPATHY

The coagulopathy associated with VOD is similar to that of other causes of liver failure. Platelet refractoriness is also associated with VOD and compounds the other coagulopathic problems (Bearman, 1995). Vitamin K replacement and regular infusions of platelets when required are generally sufficient to prevent severe bleeding. If severe coagulopathy exists, strict attention to the prevention of bleeding is required.

Summary

The clinical issues discussed in this chapter are complex and present a challenge to the nurse caring for the bone marrow and blood cell transplant patient. Much of the required nursing assessment and action goes beyond that typical for the usual oncology patient. There is often some element of critical-care nursing required for these patients, especially those who are experiencing severe renal or hepatic dysfunction. It has been the focus of this chapter to impress upon caregivers the significance of the nursing process in the overall management of these critical issues in order to improve the quality of complex care required by the transplant patient. Non-myeloablative bone marrow transplants are being done with increasing frequency. However, literature about the timing and incidence of liver and kidney dysfunction is slow in coming. Liver and kidney dysfunction in this setting is dependent on the preparative regimen used, comorbid conditions, infections, and the use of cyclosporine or tacrolimus.

References

Akiyama, H., Kurosu, T., Sakashita, C., Inoue, T., Mori, S., Ohashi, K., et al. (2001). Adenovirus is a key pathogen in hemorrhagic cystitis associated with bone marrow transplant. *Clinical Infectious Diseases, 32,* 1325–1330.

Arai, S., Lee, L., & Vogelsang, G. (2002). A systematic approach to hepatic complications in hematopoietic stem cell transplantation. *Journal of Hematotherapeudic Stem Cell Research, 11*(2), 215–229.

Bain, V. (2000). Hepatitis B in transplantation. *Transplant Infectious Disease, 2,* 153–165.

Baldwin, A., Kingman, H., Darville, M., Foot, A., Greier, D., Cornish, J., et al. (2000). Outcome and clinical course of 100 patients with adenovirus infection following bone marrow transplantation. *Bone Marrow Transplantation, 26,* 1333–1338.

Bates, D., Su, L., Yu, D., et al. (2001). Correlates of acute renal failure in patients receiving parenteral amphotericin B. *Kidney International, 60,* 1452.

Bearman, S. (1995). The syndrome of hepatic venoocclusive disease after marrow transplantation. *Blood, 85,* 3005.

Bearman, S., Anderson, G., Mori, M., et al. (1993). Venoocclusive disease of the liver: Development of a model for predicting fatal outcome after marrow transplantation. *Journal of Clinical Oncology, 11*(9), 1729–1736.

Bearman, S., Shuhart, M., Hinds, M., et al. (1992). Recombinant human tissue plaminogen activator for the treatment of established venoocclusive disease of the liver after bone marrow transplantation. *Blood, 80*(10) 2458–2462.

Bedi, A., Miller, C., Hanson, J., Goodman, S., Ambinder, R., Charache, P., et al. (1995). Association of BK virus with failure of prophylaxis against hemorrhagic cystitis following bone marrow transplantation. *Journal of Clinical Oncology, 13*(5), 1103–1109.

Borg, M., Hughes, T., Hovarth, N,, et al. (2002). Renal toxicity after rotal body irradiation. *International Journal of Radiation Oncology, Biology Physics, 54,* 1165.

Branch, R. (1988). Prevention of amphotericin B-induced renal impairment: A review on the use of sodium supplementation. *Archives of Internal Medicine, 148,* 2389.

Cade, R., et al. (1987). Hepatorenal syndrome. *American Journal of Medicine, 82,* 427–438.

Centers for Disease Control. (2004). Prevalence of HBV markers in adults throughout the world. Retrieved February 18, 2004, from http://www.cdc.gov/ncidod/diseases/hepatitis/slideset/hep_b/hep_b.ppt

Champlin, R., & Gale, R. (1984). The early complications of bone marrow transplantation. *Seminars in Hematology, 21*(2), 101–108.

Chen, P. (1999). Fulminent hepatitis is significantly increased in hepatitis B carriers after allogeneic bone marrow transplantation. *Transplantation, 67,* 1425–1433.

Chopra, R., Eaton, J., Grassi, A., Potter, M., Shaw, B., Salat, C., et al. (2000). Defibritide for the treatment of hepatic veno-occlusive: Results of the European Compassionate-Use study. *British Journal of Haematology, 111,* 1122–1129.

Cohen, E. (2001). Renal failure after bone-marrow transplantation. *Lancet, 357,* 6.

Cohen, E.P., & Robbins, M.E. (2003). Radiation nephropathy. *Seminars in Nephrology, 23*(5), 486–499.

Conn, H. (1972). The rational management of ascites. *Progress in Liver Disease, 4,* 269–288.

Cooper, B., Creger, R., Soegiarso, W., et al. (1993). Renal dysfunction during high-dose cisplatin therapy and autologous hematopoetic stem cell transplantation: Effect of aminoglycoside therapy. *American Journal of Medicine, 94,* 497–504.

Curry, G., Gould, J., Ferrier, R., Halls, D., McNeil, D., & Beatie, A. (1996). Clinically significant transfusional iron overload in survivors of hematological malignancies. *Gastroenterology, 110,* A1176.

Deeg, H., et al. (1988). In Klingeman, H.; Phillips, G.L. (Eds.). *A guide to bone marrow transplantation* (pp. 123–139). New York: Springer-Verlag.

Dhedin, N., et al. (1998). Reverse seroconversion of hepatitis B after allogeneic bone marrow transplantation: A retrospective study of 37 patients with pretransplant anti-HBs and anti-HBc. *Transplantation, 66,* 616–619.

Dixon, B., & Anderson, R. (1985). Nonoliguric acute renal failure. *American Journal of Kidney Disease, 6,* 71.

Efros, M., Ahmed, T., Coombe, N., et al. (1994). Urologic complications of high-dose chemotherapy and bone marrow transplantation. *Urology, 43*(3), 355–360.

Essell, J., Thomson, J., Harman, G., Halvorson, R., Snyder, M., Callander, N., & Clement, D. (1992). Pilot trial of prophylactic ursodiol to decrease the incidence of veno-occlusive disease of the liver in allogeneic bone marrow transplant patients. *Bone Marrow Transplantation, 10*(4), 367–372.

Fuge, R., Bird, J., Fraser, A., et al. (2001).The clinical features, risk factors and outcomes of thrombotic, thrombocytopenic purpura occurring after bone marrow transplantation. *British Journal of Haematology, 113,* 58.

Girinsky, T., Benhamou, E., Bourhis, J., Dhermain, F., Guillot-Valls., D., Ganasia, V., et al. (2000). Prospective randomized comparison of single-dose versus hyperfractionated total-body irradiation in patients with hematologic malignancies. *Journal of Clinical Oncology, 18,* 981.

Girmenia, C., Cimino, G., Micozzi, A., Gentile, G., & Martino, P. (2002). Risk factors for nephrotoxicity associated with conventional amphotericin B therapy. *American Journal of Medicine, 113,* 351,

Goringe, A., Brown, S., O'Callaghan, U., Rees, J., Jebb, S., Elia, M., et al. (1998). Glutamine and vitamin E in the treatment of hepatic veno-occlusive disease of

following high-dose chemotherapy. *Bone Marrow Transplant, 21,* 829.

Growchow, L., Jones, R., & Brundrett, R. (1989). Pharmokinetics of busulfan: Correlation with veno-occlusive disease in patients undergoing bone marrow transplantation. *Cancer Chemotherapy Pharmacology, 25,* 55–61.

Guinan, E., et al. (1988). Intravascular hemolysis and renal insufficiency after bone marrow transplantation. *Blood, 72*(2), 451–455.

Harbarth, S., Pestotnik, S., Lloyd, J., et al. (2001). The epidemiology of nephrotoxicity associated with conventional amphotericin B. *American Journal of Medicine, 111,* 528.

Herbetko, J., Grigg, A., Buckly, A., & Philips, G. (1992). Venoocclusive liver disease after bone marrow transplantation: Findings at duplex sonography. *American Journal of Roentgenology, 158,* 1001–1005.

Hou, S., & Cohen, J. (1985). Diagnosis and management of acute renal failure. *Acute Care, 11,* 59–84.

Huether, S. (1998). Structure and function of the digestive system In McCance, K., & Huether, S. (Eds.), *Pathophysiology: The biologic basis for disease in adults and children* (3rd ed., pp. 1307–1317). St. Louis: Mosby.

Jenson, P., Jenson, T., Christensen, T., & Ellegaard, J. (1995). Evaluation of transfusional iron overload before and during iron chelation by magnetic resonance imaging of the liver and determination of serum ferritin in adult non-thalassaemic patients. *British Journal of Haematology, 89,* 880–890.

Jones, R., Lee, K., Beschorner, W., Vogel, V., Groschow, L., Braine, H., et al. (1987). Venoocclusive disease of the liver following bone marrow transplantation. *Transplantation, 44,* 778–783.

Kim, B., Chung, K., Sun, H., Suh, J., Min, W., Kang, C., et al. (2000). Liver disease during the first post-transplant year in bone marrow transplantation recipients: Retrospective study. *Bone Marrow Transplantation, 26,* 193–197.

Kulkarni, S., Rodriguez, M., Lafuente, A., Mateos, P., Mehta, J., Singhal, S., et al. (1999). Recombinant tissue plasminogen activator (rtPA) for the treatment of hepatic veno-occlusive disease (VOD). *Bone Marrow Transplantation, 23,* 803–807.

Lam, M., & Kaufman, C. (1985). Fractional excretion of sodium as a guide to volume depletion during recovery from acute renal failure. *American Journal of Kidney Disease, 6*(1), 18–21.

Lau, G., Liang, R., Chiu, E., Lee, C., & Lam, S. (1997). Hepatic events after bone marrow transplantation in patients with hepatitis B infection: A case controlled study. *Bone Marrow Transplantation, 19,* 795–799.

Lawton, C., Barbar-Derus, S., Murray, D., et al. (1992). Influence of renal shielding on the incidence of late renal dysfunction associated with T-lymphocyte-depleted bone marrow transplantation in adult patients. *International Journal of Radiation Oncology Biological Physiology, 23,* 381–686.

Leung, A., Mak, R., Lie, A., Yuen, K., Cheng, V., Liang, R., et al. (2002). Clinicopathological features and risk factors of clinically overt haemorrhagic cystitis complicating bone marrow transplantation. *Bone Marrow Transplantation, 29,* 509–513.

Llanos, A., Cieza, J., Bernardo, J., et al. (1991). Effect of salt supplementation on amphotericin B nephrotoxicity. *Kidney International, 40,* 302.

Locasciulli, A., Alberti, A., De Bock, R., et al. (1994). Impact of liver disease and hepatitis infections on allogeneic bone marrow transplantation in Europe: A survey from the European Bone Marrow Transplant (EBMT) Group-Infectious Diseases Working Party. *Bone Marrow Transplantation, 14,* 833–837.

Lonnerholm, G., Carlson, K., Brattby, L., et al. (1991). Renal function after autologous bone marrow transplantation. *Bone Marrow Transplantation, 8,* 129–137.

Maruta, A., Kanamori, H., Fukawa, H., Harano, II., Matsuzaki, M., Miyashita, H., et al. (1994). Liver function tests of recipients with hepatitis C virus infection after bone marrow transplantation. *Bone Marrow Transplant, 13,* 417–422.

McCance, K., & Heuther, S. (1998). *Pathophysiology: The biologic basis for disease in adults and children* (3rd ed.). St Louis: Mosby.

McDonald, G., Hinds, M., Fisher, L., et al. (1993). Venoocclusive disease of the liver and multiorgan failure after bone marrow transplantation: A cohort study of 355 patients. *Annals of Internal Medicine, 118,* 255–267.

McDonald, G., Sharma, P., Mathews, D., Shulman, H., & Thomas, E. (1984). Venoocclusive disease of the liver after bone marrow transplantation: Diagnosis, incidence, and predisposing factors. *Hepatology, 4,* 116.

McDonald, G., Shulman, H., Wolford, J., & Spencer, G. (1987). Liver disease after human marrow transplantation. *Seminars in Liver Disease, 7,* 210–229.

McDonald, G., et al. (1985). The clinical course of 53 patients with veno-occlusive disease of the liver after marrow transplantation. *Transplantation, 39*(6), 603–608.

McDonald, G., et al. (1986). Intestinal and hepatic complications of human bone marrow transplantation, part I. *Gastroenterology, 90,* 460–477.

McEvoy, G., Miller, J., Snow, E., & Welsh, O. (Eds.). (2005). *AHFS Drug Information,* Bethesda, MD: American Society of Health Systems Pharmacists, Inc.

Meisenberg, B., Lassiter, M., Hussein, A., et al. (1994). Prevention of hemorrhagic cystitis after high-dose alkylating agent chemotherapy and autologous bone marrow support. *Bone Marrow Transplantation, 14,* 287–291.

Miura, K., Nakatani, T., Asai, T., et al. (2002). Role of hypomagnesemia in chronic cyclosporine nephropathy. *Transplantation, 73,* 340.

Miyamura, K., et al. (1989). Hemorrhagic cystitis associated with urinary excretion of adenovirus type II following allogeneic bone marrow transplantation. *Bone Marrow Transplantation, 5,* 533–535.

Morris, J., Harris, R., Hashmi, R., Sambrano, J., Gruppo, R., Becker, A., et al. (1997). Antithrombin III for the treatment of chemotherapy-induced organ dysfunction following bone marrow transplantation. *Bone Marrow Transplantation, 17,* 443.

Noel, C., Hazzan, M., Noel, M.P., & Jouet, J.P. (1998). Renal failure and bone marrow transplantation. *Nephrology Dialysis and Transplant, 13,* 2464–2466.

Ozdogan, O., Ratip, S., Al Ahdab, Y., Dane, F., Al Ahdab, H., Imeryuz, N., et al. (2003). Causes and risk factors for liver injury following bone marrow transplantation. *Journal of Clinical Gastroenterology, 36*(4), 421–428.

Palmer, K., & Goa, K. (1993). Defibrotide: A review of its pharmacodynamic and pharmakinetic properties, and therapeutic use in vascular disorders. *Drugs, 45,* 25.

Pariente, E., Goudeau, A., Dubois, F., Degott, C., Gluckman, E., Devergie, A., et al. (1988). Fulminant hepatitis due to reactivation of chronic hepatitis B infection after allogeneic bone marrow transplantation. *Digestive Diseases and Sciences, 33,* 1185–1191.

Parikh, C., McSweeney, P., Korular, D., Ecder, T., Merourani, A., Taylor, J., et al. (2002). Renal dysfunction in allogeneic hematopoietic cell transplantation. *Kidney International, 62,* 566.

Pharmacia & Upjohn. (2001). *Neosar® (cyclophosphamide for injection) prescribing information.* Kalamazoo, MI: Author.

Price, C. (1994). Acute renal failure: A sequela of sepsis. *Critical Care Nursing Clinics of North America, 6*(2), 359–371.

Priftakis, P., Bogdanovic, G., Kokhaei, P., Mellstedt, H., & Dalianis, T. (2003). BK virus (BKV) quantification in urine samples of bone marrow transplanted patients is helpful for diagnosis of hemorrhagic cystitis, although wide individual variations exist. *Journal of Clinical Virology, 26*(1), 71–77.

Rahn, K., Barenbrock, M., Fritschka, E., et al. (1999). Effect of nitrendipine on renal function in renal transplant patients treated with cyclosporine: A randomized trial. *Lancet, 354,* 1415.

Richardson, P., Eilias, A., Krishnan, A., Wheeler, C., Nath, R., Hoppensteadt, D., et al. (1998). Treatment of severe veno-occlusive disease with defibrotide: Compassionate use results in response without significant toxicity in a high risk population. *Blood, 92,* 737–744.

Richardson, P., & Guinan, E. (2001). Hepatic veno-occlusive disease following hematopoietic stem cell transplantation. *Acta Haematology, 106,* 57–68.

Rose, B. (September 11, 2004). Nonoliguric versus oliguric acute tubular necrosis. Retrieved November 21, 2004, from patients.uptodate.com/topic.asp?file=renlfail/10642.

Roy, V., Rizvi., M., Vesely, S., & George, J. (2001). Thrombotic thrombocytic purpura-like syndromes following bone marrow transplantation: An analysis of associated conditions and clinical outcomes. *Bone Marrow Transplantation, 27,* 641.

Sale, G., & Shulman, H. (1984). Pathology of other organs. In Sale, G., & Shulman, H. (Eds.), *The pathology of bone marrow transplantation* (pp. 192–198). New York: Mason.

Scrobahaci, M., Drouet, A., Monem-Mansi, A., Devergie, A., Baudin, B., D'Agay, M., et al. (1991). Liver veno-occlusive disease after bone marrow transplantation changes in coagulation parameters and endothelial markers. *Thrombin Research, 63,* 509.

Seber, A., Shu, X., Defor, T., et al. (1999). Risk factors for severe hemorrhagic cystitis following BMT. *Bone Marrow Transplantation, 23,* 35–40.

Sencer, S., Haake, R., & Weisdorf, D. (1993). Hemorrhagic cystitis after bone marrow transplantation. *Transplantation, 56,* 875–879.

Shepherd, J., Pringle, L., Barnett, M., et al. (1991). Mesna versus hyperhydration for the prevention of cyclophosphamide-induced hemorrhagic cystitis in bone marrow transplantation. *Journal of Clinical Oncology, 9*(11), 2016–2020.

Shulman, H., Fisher, L., Schoch, G., et al. (1994). Veno-occlusive disease of the liver after marrow transplantation: Histological correlates of clinical signs and symptoms. *Hepatology, 19*(52), 1171–1181.

Shulman, H., Gooley, T., Dudley, M., Kofler, T., Feldman, R., Dwyer, D., et al. (1995). Utility of transvenous liver biopsies and wedged hepatic venous pressure measurements in sixty marrow transplantation recipients. *Transplantation, 59,* 1015–1022.

Shulman, H., & Hinterberger, W. (1992). Hepatic veno-occlusive disease—liver toxicity syndrome after bone marrow transplantation. *Bone Marrow Transplantation, 10,* 197–214.

Shulman, H.M, McDonald, G.B., Matthews, D., Doney, K.C., Kopecky, K.I., Gauvreau, J.M., et al. (1980). An analysis of hepatic veno-occlusive disease and centrilobular hepatic degeneration following bone marrow transplantation. *Gastroenterology, 79,* 1178–1191.

Smith, D., Weisenburger, D., Bierman, P., Kessinger, A., Vaughan, W., & Armitage, J. (1987). Acute renal failure associated with autologous bone marrow transplantation. *Bone Marrow Transplantation, 2,* 195–201.

Stark, J. (1988). Renal anatomy and physiology. In Kinney, M., Dunbar, S.B., & Packa, D.R. (Eds.), *AACN'S clinical reference for critical care nursing* (pp. 843–859). New York: McGraw-Hill.

Storek, J., Gale, R., & Goldstein, L. (1993). Analysing early liver dysfunction after bone marrow transplantation. *Transplant Immunology, 1,* 163–171.

Strasser, S., & McDonald, G. (1999). Hepatitis viruses and hematopoietic cell transplantation: A guide to patient and donor management. *Blood, 93,* 1127–1136.

Teffey, S., Hollister, M., Lee, S., Jacobsen, A., Higano, C., Bianco, J., et al. (1994). Gallbladder sludge formation after bone marrow transplant: Sonographic observations. *Abdominial Imaging, 19,* 57–60.

Trimarchi, H., Truong, L., Brennan, S., et al. (1999). FK506-associated thrombotic microangiopathy. *Transplantation, 67,* 539.

Turkeri, L., Lun, L., Uberti, J., et al. (1995). Prevention of hemorrhagic cystitis following allogeneic bone marrow transplant preparative regimens with cyclophosphamide and busulfan: Role of continuous bladder irrigation. *Journal of Urology, 153,* 637–640.

U.S. Multicenter FK506 Liver Study Group. (1994). A comparison of tacrolimus (FK 506) and cyclosporine for immunosuppression in liver transplantation. *New England Journal of Medicine, 331*(17), 1110–1115.

Vance, E., Stoiffer, R., McDonald, G., Meyerson, D., Fingeroth, J., & Ritz, J. (1996). Prevention of transmission of hepatitis C virus in bone marrow transplantation by treating the donor with alpha-interferon. *Transplantation, 62,* 1358–1360.

Vaughan, W.P., Carey, D., Perry, S., Westfall, A.O., & Salzman, D.E. (2002). A limited sampling study for pharmacokinetic directed therapy with intravenous busulfan. *Biology of Blood and Marrow Transplantation, 8*(11), 619–624.

Vose, J., Reed, E., Pippert, G., et al. (1993). Mesna compared with continuous bladder irrigation as uroprotection during high-dose chemotherapy and transplantation: A randomized trial. *Journal of Clinical Oncology, 11*(7), 1306–1310.

Yee, G., et al. (1984). Effect of hepatic dysfunction on oral cyclosporine pharmacokinetics in marrow transplant patients. *Blood, 64*(6), 1277–1279.

Yee, G., et al. (1985). Cyclosporin-associated renal dysfunction in marrow transplant recipients. *Transplantation Proceedings, 17*(4), 196–201.

Yu, L., Malkani, I., Regueriera, O., et al. (1994). Recombinant tissue plasminogen activator (r-tPA) for veno-occlusive liver disease in pediatric autologous bone marrow transplant patients. *American Journal of Hematology, 46,* 194–198.

Zager, R. (1994). Acute renal failure in the setting of bone marrow transplantation. *Kidney International, 46,* 1443.

Zager, R., et al. (1989). Acute renal failure following bone marrow transplantation: A retrospective study of 272 patients. *American Journal of Kidney Disease, 13,* 210–216.

Chapter 11

Neurologic Complications of Hematopoietic Stem Cell Transplantation

Brenda K. Shelton
MS, RN, CCRN,
AOCN®

Neurologic and neuromuscular complications occur in 11–39% of patients who undergo autologous hematopoietic stem cell transplantation (HSCT) (Guerrero et al., 1999; Graus et al., 1996), and 46–70% of those having allogeneic HSCT (Wiznitzer et al., 1984; Patchell et al., 1985, Graus et al., 1996; Antonini et al., 1998). In the past two decades, mortality from these complications has decreased from a reported 6% to approximately 2.4% (Guerrero et al., 1999; Antonini et al., 1998; Graus et al., 1996). The nature and severity of neurologic complications within the setting of HSCT is widely variable and dependent upon many host and treatment-related factors. Clearly the decreased incidence, morbidity, and mortality over the past two decades are attributable to our better understanding of these complications and how they can be prevented. As HSCT has been developed and refined, we have reduced the toxicity of conditioning regimens and immunosuppressive therapies, which have been the primary etiology of these complications (Guerrero et al., 1999). When evaluating patients with neurologic symptoms in the setting of HSCT, it is essential to consider how these variables influence the differential diagnosis or empirical treatment. A listing of potential risk factors for neurologic symptoms in the patient undergoing HSCT and their importance to the clinical evaluation of patients is described in Table 11-1.

For the purpose of clarification, neurologic complications in this text are organized by their physiologic mechanism. Disorders are first grouped as primarily physiologic or behavioral. Clearly these two groupings may overlap in signs, symptoms, or etiologies, but are distinct in their manifestations and treatment plan. Secondarily, the physiologic disorders are further subdivided according to the mechanism of injury. The most common neurologic complications in HSCT are cranio-cerebral disorders, followed by infectious and inflammatory conditions, and third are cerebrovascular disorders. Medication toxicities often overlap physiologic and neuropsychiatric effects, and so are addressed in a separate section. Nursing priorities are addressed within each section.

Table 11-1 VARIABLES INFLUENCING RISK FOR NEUROLOGIC COMPLICATIONS IN HSCT.

Clinical Variable	Implications for Neurologic Complications
Type of transplant (allogeneic versus autologous)	• Preparative regimens have similar toxicities. • Immunosuppressive regimens in allogeneic HSCT represent predisposition to additional neurologic complications. • Length of aplasia and degree of lymphocyte suppression differ between allogeneic and autologous HSCT, causing differing risk for neurologic infection.
Temporal relationship to the transplant itself	• Neurologic complications that occur temporally related to the preparative regimen, or a change in immunsuppressive medications (or doses) provide clues about the etiologies of complications.
Patient's specific preparative regimen	• Specific chemotherapy, radiotherapy, and biological therapy predispose to different complications. • Multimodality therapy may induce additive toxic effects.
Preexisting medical problems with neurologic symptoms	• Concomitant medical disorders may induce additive risk for neurologic complications. • Other medical problems may compromise clearance of neurotoxic therapies used in transplant. • The medications used to treat other medical problems may exacerbate the risk of specific neurologic complications.
Substance use at present and in past Medication profile	• Preexisting alcohol use increases the risk of certain neurologic complications, such as tremors and seizures. • Medications used to treat nausea and vomiting, diarrhea, depression, or infections may exacerbate neurologic complications in HSCT.

Sources: Abboud et al., 1996; Antonini et al., 1998; Armstrong et al., 2004; Bartynski et al., 2004; Davis and Patchell, 1988; Furlong and Gallucci, 1994; Gallardo et al., 1996; Guerrero et al., 1999; Krouwer and Wijdicks, 2003; Ljubisavljevic and Kelly, 2003; Patchell et al., 1985; Solaro et al., 2001; Sostak et al., 2003; Verstappen et al., 2003.

Neurologic Complications with Physiologic Origins

The neurologic system is composed of two major subsystems: the central nervous system (also called cranio-cerebral), and the peripheral nervous system. Although distinctively separate in their actions, there is integration of activities between the two systems. Specific neurological disease states associated with HSCT that can be described (e.g., leukoencephalopathy) and non-specific symptoms that are likely to be from multifactorial etiologic mechanisms (e.g., neuropathies) are discussed in this section.

Cranio-Cerebral Disorders

Disorders of the cranio-cerebrum involve the central nervous system. Some of these disorders are the most symptom producing and require the greatest level of expertise in assessment and management. Probability of survival 90 days after transplant directly correlates to the presence of serious cranio-cerebral complications (Antonini et al., 1998).

METABOLIC ENCEPHALOPATHY

Metabolic encephalopathy, or coma, occurred historically in approximately 26–37% of patients undergoing HSCT (Davis and Patchell, 1988; Furlong and Gallucci, 1994), but the incidence of this complication today in the setting of HSCT is less than 25% (Antonini et al., 1998). Encephalopathy is most frequently caused by hypoxia with organ ischemia, followed by multiorgan failure characterized most commonly by hepato-renal failure (Davis and Patchell, 1988; Snider et al., 1994). When patients present with confusion, somnolence, and other signs of metabolic encephalopathy, they will be further evaluated for treatable disorders such as hyperglycemia or hypoglycemia, drug intoxication, delirium, and large bowel obstruction. The characteristic feature of metabolic encephalopathy is the elevated serum ammonia level. It is standard to evaluate these symptoms with a brain computed tomography (CT) with contrast. If signs of central brain dysfunction, such as changes in respiratory pattern, coma, or posturing, are present, this may be followed with a magnetic resonance imaging (MRI) test (Inoha et al., 2002). If meningeal signs are present, a lumbar puncture may be considered but is not performed until the CT or MRI has proven the absence of increased intracranial pressure or bleeding (Tahsildar et al., 1996).

Idiopathic hyperammonemia is a rare encephalopathic disorder associated with high-dose chemotherapy. Its origins are unclear, but it is characterized by its abrupt onset during the period of aplasia following the conditioning regimen and is associated with a poor prognosis (Mitchell et al., 1988; Tse et al., 1991; Davies

et al., 1996; Conn, 2000). There are no clearly identifiable risk factors, perhaps only because it is of such low incidence that trends have not yet been elucidated. The condition is characterized by a severe, sudden alteration in mental status, lethargy, confusion, cerebellar dysfunction, seizures, and respiratory alkalosis associated with markedly elevated serum ammonia in the absence of hepatic failure (Tse et al., 1991, Davies et al., 1996). Due to this atypical presentation, it may be missed in the differential diagnosis of mental status changes. Untreated, patients can progress to coma and subsequent death (Mitchell et al., 1988; Davies et al., 1996). If diagnosed early, dialysis and ammonia-trapping agents may decrease the serum ammonia and prevent brain damage (Tse et al., 1991).

Patients with encephalopathy most prominently present with altered mental status with associated safety risks such as risk for injury or aspiration risk. In every case of encephalopathy, astute neurologic assessment is essential to ascertain if treatable causes are present and to detect signs of increased intracranial pressure. The most common causes of death in these patients are cerebral herniation and pulmonary aspiration (Conn, 2000). All patients with encephalopathy should have the head of their bed elevated to reduce the risk of these two complications (Watanabe, 2000). Laboratory values and intake-output measurements are monitored, and fluids and electrolytes are carefully replaced as needed.

SEIZURE DISORDERS

Seizure activity has long been associated with the conditioning regimens and complications of HSCT. Although most seizures in patients with cancer are partial in nature, many associated with HSCT are generalized. The most prominent risk factors are cranial irradiation, intrathecal chemotherapy, busulfan, and immunosuppressive agents such as cyclosporine, tacrolimus, and methotrexate (Azuno et al., 1998; Steg et al., 1999; Graus et al., 1996; Krouwer and Wijdicks, 2003). The onset of seizures is often acute, occurring within the first 2 weeks of transplant, and is related to the conditioning regimen or immunosuppressive agent. Seizures occurring later in the transplant process are more likely to be associated with encephalopathy or infectious complications. Patients at risk for seizures should be observed frequently and carefully assessed for altered mental status, speech, or motor signs indicative of seizures or a postictal state. Safety measures and accompanying the patient off the unit may also be implemented. In some cases, prophylactic anticonvulsants have been administered, but recognizing the contribution of drug blood levels and modified dosing of busulfan, methotrexate, cyclosporine, and tacrolimus have made this less necessary (Bleyer, 1977; deMagalhaes-Silverman et al., 1996; La Morgia et al., 2004).

Cognitive Dysfunction

Impairment of intellectual function is the definition of cognitive dysfunction. This syndrome of fuzzy thinking, altered reasoning, and decreased intelligence has only recently been described in the literature (Syrjala, 2004; Benke et al., 2004; Costello et al., 2004; Tannock et al., 2004; Schagen et al., 2002). It can range from mild variations in calculating ability to severe growth and developmental disorders. It has been postulated that the primary pathophysiologic mechanism is direct injury to the cells of the brain by chemotherapy or irradiation. The condition can be exacerbated by other manifestations of illness such as hypoxemia, glucose abnormalities, or anemia. In HSCT, there are two

clear cognitive dysfunction syndromes. One acute dysfunctional state, where the patient is out of touch with reality and displaying symptoms similar to psychosis, is called delirium. The second is a syndrome of chronic, impaired cognition that interferes with concentration, memory, and learning ability. In both disorders, other medical conditions and medications must be considered in the differential diagnosis. Conditions and medications that can cause altered mentation that mimics cognitive dysfunction associated with HSCT include antiretrovirals, antivirals, benzodiazepines, carbapenams, diabetes-induced glucose abnormalities (high or low), hyperammonemia, hypercalcemia, thyrotoxicosis, opiates, phenothiazines, or syndrome of inappropriate antidiuretic hormone excretion.

Delirium is an acute confusional state that is precipitated by a variety of metabolic and chemical risk factors (Slavney, 1998). It occurs in many hospitalized patients, and is present in 8–85% of patients with cancer throughout their continuum of care (Ljubisavljevic and Kelly, 2003). Patients who are elderly, frail, seriously ill, sleep deprived, and receiving polypharmacy are among those at highest risk for the disorder (Ljubisavljevic and Kelly, 2003). It is usually abrupt in onset, and patients display a wide range of symptoms that wax and wane. They at times have totally normal mentation, and alternatively are completely disoriented and hallucinating. The characteristic features of this disorder are altered wakefulness, clouded consciousness, disorientation, fears, irritability, and misperception of sensory stimuli, causing delusions and visual hallucinations. HSCT patients are at particular risk for delirium because of the frequent administration of narcotics and steroids, and the incidence of metabolic encephalopathy (Slavney, 1998). Patients can be screened for altered mentation and sleep disturbances, then more comprehensive evaluation can be done with an instrument such as the mini mental state examination (Chuurmans et al., 2003). The first treatment strategy for delirium is to eliminate potential etiologic factors such as medical problems (e.g., hypoxemia, hyperglycemia), then to examine the medication profile for additional etiologies. Safety measures are implemented to prevent the patients from injuring themselves or attempting to perform activities for which they are too weak or uncoordinated. Delirium is often the result of multiple factors interacting with one another. The administration of a medication known to cause delirium may cause additive symptoms when patients are also hyperglycemic or sleep deprived. Delirium is self-limiting, and will resolve with correction of the underlying cause and symptomatic support. Neuroleptic medications such as haloperidol may be required to address neuropsychiatric symptoms while discontinuing other causative medications. References for the administration of these agents can be found in the general literature.

Long-term cognitive dysfunction has been described most extensively in children who have received HSCT. Children undergoing HSCT during crucial growth periods have demonstrated clear diminishment of intellect with cranial irradiation (Armstrong et al., 2004; Moore et al., 2000). Chemotherapy administered intrathecally has also been closely associated with cognitive impairment (Tannock et al., 2004; Moore et al., 2000). High-dose alkylating agents and antimetabolites are also believed to cause at least temporary impairment such as short-term memory loss, difficulty concentrating, and insomnia (Tannock et al., 2004; Schagen et al., 2002; Kramer et al., 1997). Asking the patient and significant others about

their perceptions of changes in mentation can often reveal symptoms they attribute to other problems, such as therapy-induced fatigue, which can indeed be difficult to differentiate. A series of screening questions to be used to assess for basic changes in cognition are listed in **Table 11-2**. A yes answer to any of these questions should trigger administration of the mini mental state examination. Abnormal findings in this instrument constitute an indication for evaluation by a neurologic and/or mental health professional. Patients and their significant others who are prepared for these symptoms can make modifications in their lifestyle and home environment to lessen the impact of these changes. Developing routines and consistent places for items like car keys, or memory aids or check-off to-do lists, such as chore charts used by children, can be helpful. It is important that patients be assisted with taking their medications, for they may easily become confused about what they are taking or whether they have taken a specific dose of a medication. Our scientific knowledge

---

Table 11-2 SCREENING FOR COGNITIVE DYSFUNCTION.

- Do you have difficulty remembering where you put things?
- Do you forget to do things?
- Do people say they told you things you can't recall them saying?
- Do you have trouble focusing on a task?
- Do you feel unable to make decisions?
- Have you sensed changes in your ability to solve problems?
- Is it more difficult for you to learn new tasks?

Sources: Broers et al., 2000; Costello et al., 2004; Ljubisavljevic and Kelly, 2003; Schagen et al., 2002; Syrjala, 2004; Tannock et al., 2004.

of these complications in HSCT is limited at this time, but a growing body of research suggests that these changes are temporary in most patients (Tannock et al., 2004).

Leukoencephalopathy

Leukoencephalopathy (LEC) is a degenerative lesion occurring in the white matter of the CNS in up to 17% of patients who receive cranial irradiation and intrathecal chemotherapy (Antunes et al., 1999; Teive et al., 2001; Moore, 2003). The onset may be within days or months of HSCT. A JC polyomavirus is the suspected cause of the demyelination in immunosuppressed patients (Boerman et al., 1993; Kitamura et al., 1994). Oncologic medications reported to cause leukoencephalopathy include 5-fluorouracil, cisplatin, cladribine, corticosteroids (high dose), cyclosporine, cytarabine, fludarabine, interferon-alpha, interleukin-2, L-asparaginase, methotrexate, pentostatin, tacrolimus, and thiotepa (Moore, 2003; Filley and Kleinschmidt-DeMasters, 2001; Rathi et al., 2002; Vidarsson et al., 2002). Several of these agents are commonly used in conditioning regimens.

Although the pathophysiologic mechanisms of this disorder are still unclear, it is thought to arise from inflammatory capillary permeability. The propensity for injury in the posterior region correlates to the reduced autoregulatory capabilities and tendency toward vasodilation seen in these vessels (Moore, 2003). Leukoencephalopathy is characterized by severe neurologic degeneration that may be reversible, but often causes permanent neurologic disability or death. (Sakami et al., 1993). Clinically, LEC presents as lethargy, slurred speech, visual disturbances, ataxia, seizures, confusion, dysphagia, akinetic mutism, spasticity, aphasia, decerebrate posturing, and coma (Filley and Kleinschmidt-

DeMasters, 2001). A concomitant parkinsonian syndrome has also been described (Antunes et al., 1999; Halperin et al., 2005).

The development of LEC is most closely associated with prophylactic and/or therapeutic CNS treatment both before and after transplant. The treatment usually involves cranial irradiation in combination with intrathecal MTX and/or high-dose intravenous MTX pretransplant, and usually intrathecal MTX posttransplant (Chan et al., 2003; Halperin et al., 2005; Mohrmann et al., 1990). Administration of MTX after total body irradiation increases the risk of LEC (Johnson et al., 1987). In addition, cerebrospinal clearance of MTX may be altered in patients with acute lymphoblastic leukemia (ALL) who have CNS involvement, thus increasing the risk of injury (Halperin et al., 2005). The development of LEC is also related to HSCT patients who have acute lymphoblastic leukemia as the underlying disease, and age under 15 years, presumably due to brain immaturity at the time of radiation treatment (Fernandez-Bouzas et al., 1992). LEC in the patient with acute nonlymphoblastic leukemia is rare. Progressive multifocal LEC has also been reported in association with disseminated varicella-zoster infection (Hooper et al., 1982).

LEC is best diagnosed with an MRI. White matter lesions are usually symmetrical and located in the posterior cerebral hemispheres. The most common locations are the occipital region and the posterior parietal and temporal lobes (Filley and Kleinschmidt-DeMasters, 2001). Some reports have identified involvement of the frontal and thalamus regions, as well as the cerebellum (Reddick et al., 2002).

Once LEC is suspected, any potential risk factor is eliminated if possible. Corticosteroids and anticoagulation may be implemented to ameliorate the symptoms. Serial neurologic examinations will detect clinical changes indicative of LEC. Informed clinical staff will assess fluid balance, blood pressure, and mental status to detect the presence of LEC.

Although benzyl alcohol and chlorhexidine have not been proven neurotoxic, their use as cleansing agents when reconstituting MTX should be avoided (Conrad, 1986; Norrell et al., 1974). Combining MTX with hydrocortisone (Humphrey et al., 1979) and using a standard dose in patients 3 years and older may help decrease the risk of LEC (Bleyer, 1977). An MTX dose based upon body surface area is discouraged in persons older than 3 years because cerebrospinal fluid volume is constant after that age. Additionally, judicious use of radiation therapy is essential to prevent relapse and minimize the potential for development of devastating LEC (Thompson et al., 1986).

Infectious Complications Involving the Neurologic System

Central nervous system infection is a common neurologic complication of bone marrow transplantation. Heightened susceptibility is evident during two periods of time following transplant when there is high risk of infection. The first period of risk occurs 1 month posttransplant and corresponds to the period of granulocytopenia. During this time, bacterial, fungal, and viral infections predominate. The second period lasts from 1 month until 1 year after transplant, correlating with prolonged immunosuppression, usually the result of treatment for GVHD. Viral and protozoal infections are more likely to occur at this time (Anderlini et al., 1994; Hoyle and Goldman, 1994; Sable and Donowitz, 1994). Herpesvirus 6 and herpesvirus 7 are emerging significant pathogens that are similar to CMV

that have been implicated in development of this disorder (Clark, 2002; Yoshikawa, 2003; Fischmeister et al., 2000; Singh and Paterson, 2000; Lombardini et al., 1998; Mookerjee and Vogelsang, 1997). An overview of the clinical features of the most common infectious complications involving the neurologic system are included in **Table 11-3**.

Myelosuppression related to the transplant or immunosuppressive medications render the body unable to mount an inflammatory response to invading pathogens. Therefore, the typical signs and symptoms of inflammation are not commonly seen (Callaham, 1989). Most patients present with fever and headache, yet a substantial number may be without symptoms of CNS infection (Callaham, 1989). Most bacterial, and some fungal infections represent contiguous spread from the paranasal and paratympanic areas (Hoyle and Goldman, 1994). When present, signs of meningitis include changes in mental status, meningismus, lethargy, nuchal rigidity, increasing confusion, positive Kernig and Brudzinski signs, and seizures. Encephalitis has similar symptoms with more severe abnormalities in sensorium with a higher risk for coma, seizures, and behavioral disorders. Brain abscesses usually present first with altered consciousness, but focal neurologic findings like sudden hemiparesis, pupillary changes, and partial seizures are the common features differentiating this from other neurologic infectious complications.

Fungal infections account for approximately half of CNS infections in BMT recipients, and are by far most frequently caused by *Aspergillus fumigatus* (Denning et al., 1994). CNS infections are treated with traditional medications, but with conscientious attention to prescribing agents that will cross the blood–brain barrier or

Table 11-3 NEUROLOGIC INFECTIONS IN HSCT PATIENTS.

Microorganism	Site(s) of Infection	Nursing Care Issues
Listeria monocytogenes	Meningitis	Patients and families should be made aware that *Listeria* can contaminate milk, soft cheese, and pate, and should cook and chill prepared foods (Long et al., 1993).
Streptococcus pneumoniae	Meningitis	Neurologic changes after a sore throat are an ominous sign that the infection has spread to the brain.
Klebsiella pneumoniae	Meningitis	Usually only occurs in patients who have preexisting immune compromise, such as substance abuse.
Nocardia	Brain abscesses Encephalitis Pneumonitis	Nodular abscess lesions that can compress and erode normal tissues. Bradycardia may be a sign of widespread or intracranial disease.
Escherichia coli	Meningitis Encephalitis	Colonization with resistant strains of this organism increases the risk of infection in HSCT patients.
Aspergillus	Hematogenous spread by direct extension from the cranial sinuses, causing brain abscesses (Denning et al., 1994)	Necrotizing, cavitating lesions that present with symptoms similar to tumor. Bleeding into cavitating lesion most likely to occur several weeks into therapy as lesion begins to heal.
Candida	Meningitis Encephalitis Brain abscesses (Hiemenez and Greene, 1993; Hoyle and Goldman, 1994)	Colonization increases risk of infection. Prone to present with embolization of organism.
Cryptococcus	Hepatitis Meningitis Encephalitis	Risk increased with prolonged lymphocyte depletion as seen with HIV infection, prior myelodysplasia.
Cytomegalovirus (CMV)	Encephalitis	CMV-negative blood products are administered to HSCT recipients who are antibody negative and at high risk of CMV infection transmitted via transfusion. Ganciclovir prophylaxis is administered if the donor is CMV positive and the recipient is CMV negative.

Table 11-3 NEUROLOGIC INFECTIONS IN HSCT PATIENTS *continued.*

Microorganism	Site(s) of Infection	Nursing Care Issues
Varicella-zoster/ varicella virus (VZV)	Encephalitis Neuropathy	Risk factors for VZV infection include leukemia, age greater than 10 years, VZV seropositive, and pretransplant radiation (Han et al., 1994). Characteristically occurs along the dermatomes and may cause severe neuralgias.
Herpes simplex virus (HSV)	Encephalitis	Herpes encephalitis is associated with systemic viral dissemination and is fatal in 70% of cases, with long-term neurologic impairment evident in more than 90% of survivors (Whitley et al., 1992).
Toxoplasma gondii	Encephalitis Brain abscesses	Progressive neurologic deterioration occurs if untreated. Bradycardia signals severe brain abscesses. Since toxoplasmosis is a late infection, often occurring after discharge from the hospital, teaching should focus on avoiding possible sources of the pathogen. —Fruits and vegetables, which may be contaminated with toxoplasma gondii, should be washed carefully. —Contact with cat feces or litter boxes is to be avoided because parasite eggs can develop in the intestines of cats.

Sources: Lombardini et al., 1998; Krouwer and Wijdicks, 2003; Koc et al., 2000; Guerrero et al., 1999; Graus et al 1996; Gallardo et al., 1996; Fischmeister et al., 2000, Clark et al., 2002; Fireman et al., 2004; Long et al., 1992; Denning et al., 1994; Hiemenez & Greene, 1993; Han et al., 1994; Whitley et al., 1992; Long et al., 1993; Denning et al., 1994; Hiemanez and Greene, 1993; Han et al., 1994; Whitley et al., 1992; Clark, 2002; Lombardini et al., 1998; Koc et al., 2000; Krouwer and Wijdicks, 2003; Graus et al., 1996; Guerrero et al., 1999; Gallardo et al., 1996; Fischmeister et al., 2000; Fireman et al., 2004; Roemer et al., 2001; Hooper et al., 1982; Hoyle and Goldman, 1994.

dosing appropriate for crossing into the CNS. Patients at risk for CNS infections are frequently monitored for fever, mental status changes, and clinical manifestations of increased intracranial pressure. Focal changes such as papillary in equality of unilateral weakness are promptly reported. Nuccal rigidity and severe headache—typical meningeal signs—are rapidly evaluated. Early recognition of subtle neurologic changes and definitive therapy that crosses the blood–brain barrier may greatly affect outcomes.

Cerebrovascular Disorders

Cerebrovascular complications, the third most common neurologic complication, were reported as high as 28% in patients undergoing allogeneic HSCT several years ago (Mohrmann et al., 1990); however, the current incidence is as low as 2–6% in allogeneic HSCT, and even lower with autologous HSCT (Guerrero et al., 1999; Antonini et al., 1998; Gonzales et al., 2001). The incidence of vascular cerebral events in relation to HSCT has historically been of high concern due to the presence of other neurotoxicities and the known risk of bleeding with thrombocytopenia. Although the incidence of cerebrovascular events is low, the potential for high morbidity necessitates a high level of suspicion be maintained when central nervous system symptoms are present. Patients who have received cranial irradiation or intrathecal chemotherapy are at high risk for these complications, as are patients with coagulation abnormalities.

MINERALIZING MICROANGIOPATHY

Mineralizing microangiopathy causes dystrophic calcification of CNS gray matter (Mulhearn et al., 1992). This degeneration is usually apparent approximately 10 months after radiation and chemotherapy, and occurs much more frequently than LEC. Identified risk factors for the development of this dystrophy include a young age (less than 10 years at the time of radiation), duration of survival after chemo- and radiotherapy, and the number of CNS leukemic relapses after radiation therapy (Price, 1979). The clinical manifestations include focal seizures, poor muscle coordination, perceptual motor disabilities, and behavioral disorders (Packer et al., 1987).

Mineralizing microangiopathy causes permanent destructive changes in the brain, affecting neuropsychological functioning. Use of MTX and cranial radiation in various combinations seems to impair short-term memory, the speed of mental processing, and the acquisition of new knowledge. IQ test scores tend to be below the mean (Mulhearn et al., 1992), and as the posttreatment time interval increases, drops in IQ scores may become more severe, particularly in very young children (Halperin et al., 2005).

Risk for neuropsychological impairment is increased for younger children or if whole brain irradiation is employed (Halperin et al., 2005). Because mineralizing microangiopathy is not easily controlled, baseline and frequent neurologic examinations are important for all patients who receive radiation therapy and chemotherapy. The disorder is best detected by MRI, but early diagnosis does not confer a better prognosis since there are no known treatments.

CEREBROVASCULAR ACCIDENTS (HEMORRHAGE AND INFARCTION)

Hemorrhagic and ischemic cerebrovascular events occur infrequently in patients receiving HSCT, but with a higher incidence than most patients with cancer (van der Lelie et al., 1996). The rationale for this increased incidence is probably multifactorial. Severe and prolonged thrombocytopenia and long-term indwelling central venous catheters are common, and procoagulant disorders such as protein S and protein C deficiency occur with some frequency (Nevo and Vogelsang, 2001; Antonini et al., 1998). Subarachnoid hemorrhages and infarcts occur with equal frequency, and since arterial in origin, are more likely related to preexisting neurologic disease (Nevo and Vogelsang, 2001; Bashir, 2001). Subdural hemorrhages can occur with relatively minor injury such as bumping the head, but are usually detectable and treatable due to the slower onset of symptoms and sensitive diagnostic tests such as the CT scan.

Interestingly, parenchymal intracerebral hemorrhages are rare, despite extremely low platelet counts in all transplant patients, but are often lethal (Davis and Patchell, 1988; Pomeranz et al., 1994). Subarachnoid hemorrhages require rapid diagnosis with immediate neurosurgical intervention, whereas subdural hemorrhages may be managed medically until the patient's coagulation parameters can be supported adequately to enhance a safe surgical intervention. Most intracerebral bleeds are inoperable, so the goal of therapy is to reduce injury from intracranial pressure and contain the bleeding.

Cerebral infarcts are most commonly associated with endocarditis (Patchell et al., 1985). HSCT recipients have a higher incidence of developing endocarditis than those with similar diseases who do not undergo HSCT, most likely resulting from the additive effects of prior chemotherapy and radiotherapy (Wiznitzer et al., 1984).

Cerebrovascular accidents due to nonbacterial thrombotic endocarditis (NBTE) are an important cause of morbidity in HSCT recipients. They may be related to atrial dysrhythmias, immobility, or transplant-related hypercoagulability. Emboli to the CNS and heart may also manifest as seizures and focal neurologic or myocardial dysfunction. Monitoring for disseminated intravascular coagulation (DIC), especially fibrinogen and fibrin degradation products, may aid in the diagnosis and treatment with anticoagulation that may prevent the associated morbidity.

Patients with cerebrovascular disorders usually present with focal neurologic signs such as asymmetrical pupillary changes or paresis. The presence of one-sided symptoms should signal to the nurse that immediate neurologic evaluation by clinical experts is essential for rapid diagnosis and intervention. Daily evaluation of mentation and bilateral head-to-toe muscle strength can serve as first-line assessments that can trigger more advanced assessment as needed. Central blindness and visual field cuts also signal cerebrovascular events, and they can only be detected if asking patients about changes in their vision. In the presence of focal symptoms, a brain CT will always be ordered and will detect most vascular abnormalities. However, several case reports of sinus venous thrombosis only detectable on MRI suggest that a negative CT scan should be followed with an MRI to rule out other central brain disorders (Bertz et al., 1998; Harvey et al., 2000). Patients with suspected intracranial bleeding or infarctions should be treated with stroke standards as outlined by the American Heart Association (AHA). Clinical evaluation should be completed within 20 minutes of the onset of symptoms; a CT scan should be performed within 40 minutes of evaluation, and a radiologist should have interpreted this study within 2 hours of the onset of symptoms (American Heart Association, 2001). Treatment of increased intracranial pressure with diuretics and hyperventilation may be implemented while neurologists and neurosurgeons determine the best treatment plan. Most hospitals have stroke attack teams that are activated at the onset of symptoms so these national standards can be met. This is particularly important in the HSCT patient who is often being treated with curative intent.

Neuropathy

Neuropathy is defined as direct or indirect interruption in the nerve pathway resulting in disruption of the nerve's specific function. It can occur at any location within the nervous system and be patchy or continuous along the nerve fiber. Although frequently described as a complication of HSCT, the actual incidence is not reported. Neuropathies are classified as central or peripheral, based upon the nerves affected. Peripheral neuropathy is the most common syndrome, affecting motor fibers three times more commonly than sensory or autonomic nerves (Openshaw, 1997; Furlong & Gallucci, 1994). Neuropathies may be temporary or permanent. Dendritic damage is more indicative of extensive involvement, and is more permanent in nature. A summary of the common etiologic factors of neurologic syndromes is included in **Table 11-4** (Chaudry et al., 2002; Nagarajan et al., 2000; Kelly et al., 1996; Rabinstein et al., 2003; Koc et al., 2000).

Neuropathies of the peripheral nerves create pain, paresthesias, and difficulty with fine motor tasks. Since the longest fibers are usually affected first, symptoms usually begin peripherally and extend proximally. Intermittent paresthesia, tingling, or sensations of warmth or cold are the earliest symptoms of a beginning neuropathy. Sweating and circulatory impairment (e.g., Raynaud's syndrome) are later symptoms. The degree of pain associated with neuropathy is dependent upon the extent and mechanism of injury. Toxic nerve damage (e.g., taxane- or platinol-related) is more likely to produce pain than autoimmune or inflammatory etiologic factors (e.g., monoclonal antibodies or infections). Polyneuropathies related to graft-versus-host disease are immunologic in origin and often responsive to plasmapheresis (Nagashima et al., 2002; Montagna, 2000). If neuropathy occurs in a ganglion plexus (e.g., brachial plexus neuropathy involving shoulder, chest, and arm), pain is more prevalent and associated with radiation across a larger area. Neuropathy-related pain is often continuous and severely affects quality of life (Smith et al., 2002). Management of neuropathic pain with anti-inflammatory agents, anticonvulsants, and antidepressants has been helpful in abrogating these symptoms (Sommer, 2003). Refractory pain may also be treated with interventional therapies such as nerve blocks and transcutaneous nerve stimulation (TENS). Massage therapy and acupuncture have also been used to reduce the spasticity and neuropathic pain associated with this complication (Ahles et al., 1999; Sommer, 2003). One study described a structured exercise program that reduces gait disturbances due to neuropathies and enhances patients' ability to walk (Richardson et al., 2001).

Nurses should routinely assess motor and sensory function in patients receiving HSCT (Openshaw, 1997). The symptoms are often latent and occur after all therapy has been given. Questions to ask the patient that may signal the presence of peripheral neuropathy are included in **Table 11-5**. One easy method to assess for neuropathy is to have the patient attempt to differentiate fine touch from pressure or hot from cold. It is important to have the patient close her eyes while you randomly touch areas, starting from the most distal (e.g., toes) and progressively moving up the limb. Another test of both sensory impairment and cognitive recognition is to place a common item in the patient's hand and ask her to identify it while her eyes are closed. Altered sensory and motor function often occur in the same area. Nurses must provide for patient safety with altered activities of daily living such as walking assistance devices, or testing shower and bath water with a thermometer rather than a hand to reduce the risk of secondary complications. Assistance with eating and dressing may also be necessary. Patients are advised to avoid clothing with small buttons to close or zippers to put into track (Aventis, 2002). Motor abnormalities may include slowed responses, weakness, and possible flaccidity of muscles. Patients often com-

Table 11-4 RISK FACTORS FOR NEUROPATHIES.

	Peripheral	Central	Mixed or Unknown
Antineoplastic therapies	Arsenic trioxide Bortezomib Doxorubicin Etoposide Gemcitabine Interferon alpha Purine analogues Suramin Taxanes—paclitaxel, docetaxel Thalidomide	Asparaginase 5-FU Ifosfamide Methotrexate Procarbazine Tumor necrosis factor	Cytarabine (peripheral with bolus, high dose; central with continuous infusion) Platinols—cisplatin, carboplatin, oxaliplatin Vinca drugs—vinblastine, vincristine, vinorelbine
Other medications	Amiodarone Aminoglycoside antibiotics Antiemetics Chloramphenicol Colchicine Dapsone Disulfirim Diuretics Neuromuscular blocking agents Procainamide		Antidepressants Antiretrovirals Corticosteroids Ethambutol Hydralazine Isoniazid Metronidazole Nucleosides Pain medications Phenytoin
Comorbid health conditions	Sarcoidosis		Atheroslerotic heart disease Chronic use of alcohol Diabetes mellitus Herpes zoster HIV infection/treatment with antiretroviral agents Multiple myeloma with significant immunoglobulin elevations Thyroid disorder Wernicke's syndrome

Sources: Chaudhry et al., 2002; Nagarajan et al., 2000; Kelly et al., 1996; Rabinstein et al., 2003; Koc et al., 2000.

pensate for their altered sensation by using their whole foot to walk, producing a stepping or flat-footed gait. A special type of progressive ascending neuropathy that can lead to paralysis is Guillain-Barré syndrome (Bulsara et al., 2001). This is more likely associated with autoimmune reactions (e.g., graft-versus-host disease, post-transplant autoimmune hemolytic anemia) or

---

Table 11-5 SCREENING FOR PERIPHERAL NEUROPATHIES.

- Do you have difficulty walking or problems with balance?
- Do you have to hug the walker when you walk?
- Do you drop things?
- Do you have difficulty buttoning a shirt or blouse?
- Do you have difficulty closing a zipper?
- Do you have numbness in your fingers and toes?
- Do you have the feeling of pins and needles or tingling in your fingers and toes?

Source: Aventis, 2002; Openshaw, 1997; Richardson et al., 2001; Burns et al., 2003; Huebscher, 2000.

viral infection (e.g., cytomegalovirus) (Wen et al., 1997). This syndrome can cause progressive weakness with near paralysis and require mechanical ventilatory support.

Autonomic neuropathies are characterized by inconsistent function of the autonomic nerves that control involuntary functions. Manifestations of autonomic neuropathy include heart rate variations (e.g., tachycardia, bradycardia), orthostatic hypotension, constipation, urinary retention, uterine cramping, and impotence related to erection difficulties (Rabinstein et al., 2003). Treatments for these complications must include therapies that do not rely upon neurologic manipulation. For example, autonomic neuropathy-induced tachycardia should not be treated with beta-blockers, and bradycardia may be unresponsive to atropine. Bowel stimulants of peristalsis (e.g., metoclopramide) may not effectively treat constipation for these patients, and bulking agents may be more effective (Burns et al., 2003).

Central neuropathies may be cerebral or cerebellar in origin. They are less common than peripheral neuropathies and represent a greater risk for permanent neurologic dysfunction (Solaro et al., 2001). Cerebellar neuropathy presents as altered proprioception, nausea, nystagmus, and unsteady gait. This has been reported most often with intermittent high-dose cytosine arabinoside (Conrad, 1986). This is tested by having the patient stand with his feet together and arms straight out to the sides while his eyes are closed. If proprioception is impaired he will have a difficult time maintaining balance. Cerebral neuropathy is characterized by acute changes in mental status with varying degrees of sensory and motor involvement as well. This is often difficult to differentiate from other disorders such as delirium; however, the mixed symptomatology with changes in orientation, cranial nerves, and motor activity is a strong clue that cerebral neuropathies are present (Solaro et al., 2001). This is also clearly an early consideration when high-risk medications such as ifosphamide or cytosine arabinoside have been administered. Central nervous system neuropathies have the potential for more life-threatening complications than peripheral neuropathies and require aggressive treatment of symptoms. When a possible antidote, such as methylene blue administration for ifosphamide toxicity, is available, this is the treatment of choice (Pelgrims et al., 2000). Supportive treatment with anxiolytic medications or patient restraint may be necessary in some circumstances. In severe cases, airway support with mechanical ventilation may be necessary to prevent aspiration or respiratory arrest (Openshaw, 1997).

Definitive treatment of neuropathies often entails manipulation of the treatment plan (dose reduction or delay of therapy) when they are related to antineoplastic therapy. Some antineoplastic agents (most often taxanes) are given in conjunction with an agent called amifostine that has been shown to reduce the associated peripheral neuropathies (Yalcin et al., 2003). Ongoing studies validating its effects with other neuropathy-producing therapies are currently under way (Burns et al., 2003). There is also evidence to support that the addition of complementary therapy, such as vitamin B supplementation, may be effective in reducing the incidence or severity of neuropathies (Rabenstein et al., 2003; Huebscher, 2000).

TREMORS

The exact mechanism or etiology of tremors in the patient after HSCT is not known (Padovan et al., 2003). Tremors are a reported adverse effect of many of the supportive medications these patients receive, such as antiemetics, diphenhydramine, antidepressants, butyrophenones, cyclosporine, and tacrolimus (Wasserstein and Honig, 1996; Guerrero et al., 1999, Krouwer and Wijdicks, 2003). The contribution of metabolic factors such as hypomagnesemia or hypocalcemia is also not understood. It is advisable to prepare patients for the experience of involuntary tremors, assuring them that they are reported to be self-limiting, with resolution by discharge from the transplant clinic.

Behavioral and Psychologic Adjustment Disorders

Patients undergoing HSCT are challenged both physiologically and emotionally (Neitzert et al., 1998; Gunter et al., 1999; Illescas-Rico et al., 2002). They have often experienced a rapid progression from diagnosis to time of transplant and have been prepared to believe that their risk of death due to their illness is so high that a hematopoietic stem cell transplant is necessary to achieve a reasonable survival and quality of life (Baile, 1996). The transplant experience often proves to be more than many patients are prepared to handle. Therapy is intensive and causes many adverse effects, making it difficult to remain focused on positive outcomes. Maladaptive coping usually manifests as anxiety or depression (Baile, 1996; Syrjala et al., 2004; Illescas-Rico et al., 2002). These may be exacerbations of preexisting tendencies or reactional in nature. True psychoses are unusual, and psychotic symptoms are more often organic in nature, and hence discussed as a physiologic problem. Issues of survivorship and coping with late effects of HSCT must also be considered in care of these patients. Reintegration into the mainstream activities of daily living may be both physically and mentally challenging (Baker et al., 1999; Broers et al., 2000; Fife et al., 2000; Gunter et al., 1999).

Anxiety

Anxiety is defined as a tendency for excessive worry. Anxiety can be precipitated by a situation that is uncertain or when there are unpredictable outcomes. It is not surprising that patients undergoing HSCT may have exacerbation of preexisting anxiety disorders or develop a profound sense of worry. The process of HSCT is lengthy and complicated, and often involves many interactions with a multitude of healthcare providers. The preparation process is complex, requires many diagnostic tests, and may necessitate negotiation with the health insurance company. After these obstacles are overcome, patients must plan for several weeks of continuous therapy, either hospitalized the entire time, or coming to the hospital daily. HSCT regimens often involve multiple steps, several caregivers, and consent forms listing many potential complications. Although most HSCT therapies are targeted to achieving long-term remission or cure, it is natural for patients to worry about the risk of relapse or rejection syndrome. Information sharing is one of the best treatment strategies for anxiety. Well-informed patients and patients directly involved in decision making related to their health care report less worry and anxiety (Fife et al., 2000). It is also helpful to plan specific decisions that the patient can make without restriction. Direct involvement in decision making and problem solving makes patients feel more involved and in control of their own health. When anxiety continues to be problematic, distraction therapy, relaxation therapy, or anxiolytic medications may be used to abrogate symptoms (Neitzert et al., 1998).

Depression

Depression is defined as a sense of extreme sadness and feeling that there is nothing that can bring joy and fulfillment to an individual. Depression can be a psychiatric diagnosis or reactionary to a situation. Depression is common in the setting of HSCT. The prolonged therapy plan combined with significant physical adverse effects make some patients feel overwhelmed and unable to feel hopeful. Helping patients cope with side effects and feel hopeful about successful outcomes can reduce feelings of depression. Patients are also encouraged to remain physically active and engaged in their care. This sense of empowerment offers strong psychologic support that is important for long-term survival posttransplant (Neitzert et al., 1998; Hoodin

and Weber, 2003). Symptoms such as fatigue and pain exacerbate depression tendencies, so resolving these symptoms may decrease the patient's depressive symptoms. Medications such as corticosteroids may also increase the risk for depressive tendencies (Ito et al., 2003). There are still many institutions that exercise some level of protective environment or isolation, and patients are advised to avoid crowds to prevent infection. These measures, however effective at reducing infection, have been reported to increase depressive symptoms (Sasaki et al., 2000).

Neurotoxicity of Medications and Radiotherapy

Neurotoxic medications are used in preparative regimens and immunosuppressive therapies and for supportive care. The spectrum of toxicity will vary with agent, dose, schedule, and individual host factors. Multiple risk factors often produce an additive effect. A summary of the neurotoxicities associated with HSCT are summarized in Table 11-6.

Chemotherapy used in the conditioning process places the patient at risk for neurologic injury (Verstappen et al., 2003). Commonly used drugs with neurotoxic potential include etoposide, with associated peripheral neuropathy in approximately 4% of cases (Imrie et al., 1994); carmustine (BCNU), with rare instances of neuroretinitis and inflammatory peripheral neuropathy (Bashir et al., 1992); and busulfan, with the possible development of hallucinations, tremors, or seizures (Srivastava et al., 1993) and myasthenia gravis. Methotrexate is associated with the development of leukoencephalopathy (Land et al., 1994; Ozon et al., 1994).

Intrathecal and standard doses of cytosine arabinoside are associated with myelopathy and peripheral neuropathy (Kornblau et al., 1993; Ozon et al., 1994; Resar et al., 1993). High-dose regimens of cytosine arabinoside (Ara-C) may cause a range of neurotoxicities, which include headache, somnolence, personality changes, memory loss, intellectual impairment, confusion, slurred speech, stupor, coma, and seizures. Other cytosine arabinoside–related neurotoxicities include cerebellar dysfunction, hearing loss, visual loss, anosmia, encephalopathy, and severe expressive aphasia (Hoffman et al., 1993; Resar et al., 1993; Vogel and Horoupian, 1993).

Total body irradiation (TBI) may cause a somnolence syndrome, characterized by headache, fatigue, nausea, anorexia (Goldberg et al., 1992), weakness, and confusion. It is also associated with impaired cognitive function, particularly in children (Christie et al., 1994). The onset is usually 4 to 8 weeks after treatment and is thought to be related to transient brain edema following irradiation (Halperin et al., 2005). Irradiation has been identified as an important contributor to the development of retinopathy (Bernauer and Gratwohl, 1992), and selective autonomic neuropathy has a suspected link to fractionated TBI (Roscrow et al., 1992). Other effects of TBI (e.g., vascular complications and leukoencephalopathy), which occur as a result of its use in combination with other treatments or as late effects, are discussed elsewhere in this chapter.

Total body irradiation appears to be associated with a high incidence of late onset cataracts, which are usually correctable by surgery (Fife et al., 1994; Leisner et al., 1994). It is unclear whether other factors, such as the use of steroids, actually cause or greatly contribute to the development of cataracts (Dunn et al., 1993; Hamon et al., 1993). Superfractionated TBI appears to be more strongly associated with cataract formation than fractionated TBI, and cataract severity appears to be decreased with fractionated rather than single-dose TBI (Locatelli et al., 1993; Tichelli et al., 1993). The risk of cataract formation appears to be increased in patients who received cranial radiotherapy prior to TBI, those receiving a higher skull dose, those who receive a TBI dose rate greater than 3.5 cGy/min, and those who receive steroids after BMT (Fife et al., 1994; Tichelli et al., 1993).

Some late-onset neurological complications are thought to be due to a combination of factors, including pretransplant chemoradiotherapy. Lhermitte's sign (Wen et al., 1992) is high-grade pyrexia with accompanying neurological dysfunction (Murphy et al., 1994). The predisposition toward neurologic complications may also be enhanced by prior chemotherapy (for example, vincristine), which may have caused subclinical nerve damage that is magnified by the transplant and the conditioning regimen (Imrie et al., 1994).

Immunosuppressive Agents

Immunosuppressive therapies are an integral part of BMT. Their role is in prevention of graft rejection and in the prophylaxis and treatment of graft-versus-host disease (Walker and Brochstein, 1988). Neurotoxic effects may be the direct effect of the immunosuppressants or the sequelae of CNS infection resulting from prolonged immunosuppression. Common agents include cyclosporine, methotrexate, the corticosteroids, antithymocyte globulin, OKT3 antibody, azathioprine, thalidomide, and tacrolimus. Table 11-6 summarizes the drugs, their actions, uses in BMT, and most common neurological complications.

Cyclosporine

Cyclosporine (CyA) is a potent immunosuppressant, with little myelocytic toxicity, used in BMT to decrease the incidence and severity of GVHD (Furlong, 1993). CyA enhances the host tolerance of the allograft by selective inhibition of the resting T helper cells, and may secondarily also inhibit T suppressor cells. Therapy begins prior to transplant and continues for several weeks until recovery from chemoradiotherapy-induced gastrointestinal toxicity. At that time, an oral form can be given, with the dosage being tapered during the 6 months following transplant. The dosage of CyA may vary considerably across BMT centers, affecting the incidence rate of neurologic complications.

Neurologic complications occur in 8–29% of patients receiving this drug (Shah, 1999). Tremors, a reversible side effect that often appears within days of therapy initiation, occur in about one third of patients (Shah, 1999). Seizures can occur in up to 19% of patients; grand mal seizures have been reported in 5.5% of patients (Furlong, 1993; Shah, 1999). In addition, paresthesias have been documented in 29% of patients receiving CyA (McGuire et al., 1988), as have quadriparesis, cerebellar ataxia, and coma (Vogelsang and Morris, 1993). Burning dysesthesias of the palms of the hands and soles of the feet have also been documented. Mental status changes attributable to CyA include anxiety, confusion, amnesia, and visual hallucinations (Palmer and Toto, 1991; Katirji, 1987).

The mechanism of CyA-induced neurotoxicity is unclear, although MRI scans show abnormal metabolism (Shah, 1999; Trullemans et al., 2001). Factors thought to predispose to neurological symptoms, particularly seizures, include previous chemotherapy and irradiation, simultaneous administration of methylprednisolone, magnesium deficiency, concomitant hypertension, low cholesterol, and aluminum overload (Reece et al., 1991; Palmer and Toto, 1991). BMT patients receiving CyA are at risk for seizures related to chemotherapy and irradiation, which may lower their seizure threshold (Walker and Brochstein, 1988; Fireman et al., 2004).

Hypomagnesemia has been reported to be strongly associated with CyA neurotoxicity. CyA disrupts the tubular function, which results in renal magnesium wasting (June et al., 1985). The occurrence of grand mal seizures in patients on CyA is strongly associated with magnesium levels two standard deviations below normal values (Adams et al., 1987). Low magnesium levels are also associated with higher cyclosporine levels. Normalization of the magnesium levels usually results in cessation of the seizures and consistency in cyclosporine levels.

Tacrolimus

Tacrolimus is a polypeptide antibiotic immunosuppressive similar in action and toxicity to cyclosporine. It is used in both prevention and treatment of graft-versus-host disease. Neurologic toxicities occur in 49–86% of patients, with a higher reported frequency than neurotoxicity related to cyclosporine (Veroux et al., 2002; Wong et al., 2004). The majority are minor symptoms such as headache or myalgias, that although persistent, do not usually interfere with activities of daily living (Veroux et al., 2002). Other common non-life-threatening symptoms include tremors, hyperesthesias,

Table 11-6 NEUROLOGIC TOXICITIES OF MEDICATIONS COMMONLY USED FOR HSCT PATIENTS.

Medication	Sedation/ Somnolence	Seizures	Poor Coordination	Neuropathy	Tremors
Alkylating agents (cyclophosphamide, busulfan, melphalan)		X		X	X
Antiemetics, phenothiazines	X		X		X
Antiemetics, neurokinin antagonists serotonin	X	X			X
Antiemetics, antagonists	X	X	X		X
Antidepressants					X
Antimicrobial agents, aminoglycosides		X		X	X
Antimicrobial agents; agents, carbapenams		X			X
Anti-TNF monoclonal antibody (Infliximab)				X	
Antiviral agents, acyclovir, ganciclovir		X		X	X
Anxiolytics	X		X		X
Benzodiazepines	X		X		
Butyrphenomes, e.g., haloperidol			X		
Carmustine (BCNU)		X			X
Corticosteroids				X	X
Cytosine arabinoside		X	X	X	
Methotrexate		X			X
Polypeptide antibiotic immunosuppressives (cyclosporine, tacrolimus)		X		X	X
Thalidomide	X	X		X	

Sources: Abboud et al., 1996; Antonini et al., 1998; Aventis, 2002; Balis and Poplack, 1989; Bartynski et al., 2004; Bulsara et al., 2001; Chaudhry et al., 2002; DeMagalhaes-Silverman et al., 1996; Fireman et al., 2004; Johnson et al., 1987; Kramer et al., 1997; La Morgia et al., 2004; Nagarajan et al., 2000; Onose et al., 2002; Openshaw, 1997; Padovan et al., 2005; Pelgrims et al., 2000; Rabinstein et al., 2003; Shah, 1999; Steg et al., 1999; Verstappen et al., 2003; Wasserstein, 1996; Prescott et al., 2004.

insomnia, itching, photophobia, and mood changes (Veroux et al., 2002; Wong et al., 2004). Severe, potentially life-threatening neurotoxicities including seizures, encephalopathy, and coma occur in 5–8% of patients (Veroux et al., 2002; Wong et al., 2004). Proposed pathophysiologic mechanisms suggest that the agent crosses the blood–brain barrier and attaches to the lipid-rich myelin of the glial cells, permitting toxic injury (Veroux et al., 2002). This is followed by edema and vasogenic constriction that worsens clinical symptoms (Veroux et al., 2002). Factors shown to increase the risk of tacrolimus-related neurotoxicities are hypertension and hypomagnesemia (Veroux et al., 2002; Wong et al., 2004). Studies have shown that dose reduction is effective at abrogating minor symptoms, but is ineffective for management of severe symptoms (Steg et al., 1999). Serum blood levels have not been congruent with the degree or perceived severity of symptoms, although lower serum blood levels have reduced minor symptoms in about half of patients. One study administered tacrolimus in three divided daily doses instead of twice per day and showed that adequate therapeutic levels could be achieved while reducing the total daily dose by 27% (Khalaf et al., 2003). Others describe reduction in neurotoxicity by normalization of serum magnesium levels (Veroux et al., 2002; Wong et al., 2004). A case report also demonstrates the importance of drug–drug interactions in the case of a patient who developed excessive serum blood levels of tacrolimus while receiving concomitant metoclopromide for nausea. The proposed mechanism was believed to be enhanced absorption caused by improved bowel motility (Prescott et al., 2004).

A unique neurotoxicity associated with tacrolimus and cyclosporine is a syndrome of brain lesions called recurrent posterior reversible encephalopathy syndrome (PRES). This syndrome is characterized by acute alterations in mental status, cortical blindness, seizures, and coma (Veroux et al., 2002; Hagemann et al., 2004). The symptom cluster occurs in 1.6–7.7% of HSCT patients, with highest prevalence in unrelated or mismatched donor allogeneic transplant patients (Veroux et al., 2002). These symptoms must be differentiated from other neurologic crises such as cerebrovascular accident and delirium. The diagnosis is confirmed by characteristic lesions on CT or MRI scan. The most common findings are merging confluent lesions in the subcortical white matter of the occipital or parietal lobes, with highest prevalence near the middle cerebral artery (Hagemann et al., 2004; Shimono et al., 2003; Reinohs et al., 2002). A less common presentation, thought to be related to complex preparative regimens and a poorer prognosis, includes discrete lesions in a watershed pattern located in the deep cortical matter (Bartynski et al., 2001; Bartynski et al., 2004). This newer symptomatology has been identified since clinicians in HSCT have developed more varied and multitiered preparative regimens.

Corticosteroids

Glucocorticoids, including prednisone, methylprednisolone, and dexamethasone, are used to prevent and treat GVHD. Direct adverse neurologic effects are primarily mental status changes. Indirect effects include CNS infection or superinfection and cardiovascular accidents (CVAs) related to steroid-induced hypertension.

These drugs are also associated with neuropsychiatric side effects, with prednisone being most frequently implicated. The neuropsychiatric picture can range from mild euphoria to frank psychosis. The incidence of steroid-related major mental disturbances in patients without cancer ranges from 6% to 62% with severe psychiatric reactions occurring only in about 5% of patients (Furlong, 1993). The most common clinically significant disturbance encountered is affective disorders, such as depression (40%) and mania (28%). Delirium occurs in 10% of cancer patients with a typical picture of global cognitive impairment that may include hallucinations and delusions (Furlong, 1993). Symptoms such as anxiety, insomnia, tremor, nervousness, agitation, and euphoria/dysphoria are probably experienced by many patients and can go unnoticed by the medical and nursing team or be mistaken for another clinical problem.

Steroid psychoses, when present, correlate with the total dose, usually greater than 40 mg of prednisone daily (Greeves, 1984; Fireman et al., 2004). Females are slightly more susceptible. Age, previous psychiatric illness, or previous steroid use do not predispose the patient to increased risk for mental status changes or psychoses (Walker and Brochstein, 1988). These clinical manifestations can occur at any time during steroid treatment (Greeves, 1984). Withdrawal of the drug is the most effective way to treat these side effects, although the condition for which the steroids are being administered and the necessity for a gradual tapering of the dose may make this difficult. Side effects usually resolve rapidly with cessation of the steroids. If the drug must be continued or a taper is in progress, symptoms can be treated with low-dose neuroleptics with a response usually occurring within a few days.

Steroid myopathy is characterized by symmetrical involvement of proximal muscles. Although a mild degree of weakness is seen in all patients receiving steroidal therapy for 2 to 3 weeks, prolonged administration is directly related to the severity of myopathy (Owczarek et al., 2005). Patients may be unable to rise from a chair, brush their hair, or climb stairs, and the myopathy may progress to involve respiratory muscles.

Monoclonal Antibodies (Basiliximab, Daclizumab, Infliximab, Muromonab CD-3)

Monoclonal antibodies may bind to postthymic T lymphocytes or tumor necrosis factor, removing them from circulation. They are used in both the prophylaxis and treatment of rejection. Adverse effects are primarily related to immune responses—hypersensitivity during administration and immune compromise after extended therapy. General neurologic side effects include headache, tremors, and myalgia, occurring in fewer than half of patients. Premedication with a corticosteroid, acetaminophen, and an antihistamine has been administered in an attempt to abrogate these early adverse effects by blocking the mediators that are released from T lymphocyte lysis.

A CNS syndrome specifically associated with the monoclonal antibody muromonab has been identified as a form of aseptic meningitis that can occur 2 to 7 days after initiation of therapy (Hooks et al., 1991). Symptoms include fever, headache, photophobia, and meningismus. Generalized seizures have been reported. This clinical syndrome resolves without residual effects or treatment in 2 to 3 days, and does not require the cessation of octhoclone muromonab therapy. The pathogenesis of the meningitis after the administration of orthoclone muromonab is uncertain (Hooks et al., 1991), and it is extremely important that it be distinguished from any serious CNS infection.

Thalidomide

Another approach to the treatment of acute and chronic GVHD has been the use of thalidomide. Sedation is a common side effect of thalidomide; however, patients report adjusting to their sedation, with only a small number requiring dosage adjustment or withdrawal of the drug (Altomonte, 1993). Other neurotoxic side effects reported include peripheral neuropathy, paresthesias, and nocturnal muscle cramps (Chaudhry, 2002; Lopez et al., 1993).

Transplant patients are at substantial risk for the development of neurotoxic effects from immunosuppressive agents. These effects are magnified when the patient is receiving two or more of these therapies simultaneously. Fortunately, the majority of these complications are reversible and respond to drug withdrawal or dosage modification. Early recognition of these neurologic toxicities is paramount if unneeded physical and emotional discomfort for the patient is to be prevented or ameliorated.

Summary

Because neurologic deficits can render individuals incapable of self-care to varying degrees, either temporarily or permanently, the impact of neurologic and neuromuscular deficits on the patient, family, and health team and resources is significant. Therefore, early assessment for signs and symptoms of complications, which includes an understanding of the patient's baseline level of neurologic functioning and risk factors, may help prevent or ameliorate potentially severe neurologic impairment.

References

Abboud MR, Jackson SM, Barredo J, Holden KR, Cure J, Laver J. Neurologic complications following bone marrow transplantation for sickle cell disease. *Bone Marrow Transplantation*, 1996;17(3):405–407.

Adams DH, Ponsford S, Gunson B, Boon A, Honigsberger L, Williams A, et al. Neurological complications following liver transplantation. *Lancet*, 1987;1:949–951.

Ahles TA, Tope DM, Pinkson B, Walch S, Hann D, Whedon M, et al. Massage therapy for patients undergoing autologous bone marrow transplantation. *Journal of Pain and Symptom Management*, 1999;18(3):157–163.

Altomonte V. Use of thalidomide for CGVHD defended. *Oncology Nursing Forum*, 1993;20(3):428.

American Heart Association. *ACLS Provider Manual*. Dallas: American Heart Association; 2001. American Heart Association Publication #70-25-2.

Anderlini P, Przepiorka D, Luna M, Langford L, Andreeff M, et al. Acanthamoeba meningoencephalitis after bone marrow transplantation. *Bone Marrow Transplantation*, 1994;14:459–461.

Antonini G, Ceschin V, Morino S, Fiorelli M, Gragnani F, Mengarelli A, et al. Early neurologic complications following allogeneic bone marrow transplant for leukemia: a prospective study. *Neurology*, 1998;50(5):1441–1445.

Antunes NL, Small TN, George D, Boulad F, Lis E. Posterior leukoencephalopathy syndrome may not be reversible. *Pediatric Neurology*, 1999;20(3):241–243.

Armstrong CL, Gyato K, Awadalla AW, Lustig R, Tochner ZA. A critical review of the clinical effects of therapeutic radiation damage to the brain: the roots of controversy. *Neuropsychologic Review*, 2004;14(1):65–86.

Aventis Pharmaceuticals, Inc. How do I know if I have peripheral neuropathy? A common side effect of some anticancer treatments, Patient Information and Weekly Diary. Bridgewater, NJ: Aventis Pharmaceuticals; 2002.

Azuno Y, Yaga K, Kaneko T, Kaku K, Oka Y. Chronic graft-versus-host-disease and seizures. *Blood*, 1998;91(7):2626–2628.

Baile WF. Neuropsychiatric disorders in cancer patients. *Current Opinions in Oncology*, 1996;8(3):182–187.

Baker F, Zabora J, Polland A, Wingard J. Reintegration after bone marrow transplantation. *Cancer Practice*, 1999;7(4):190–197.

Balis FM, Poplack DG. Central nervous system pharmacology of antileukemic drugs. *American Journal of Hematology-Oncology*, 1989;11(1):74–86.

Bartynski WS, Zeigler ZR, Shadduck RK, Lister J. Pretransplantation conditioning influence on the occurrence of cyclosporine or FK-506 neurotoxicity in allogeneic bone marrow transplantation. *American Journal of Neuroradiology*, 2004;25:261–269.

Bartynski WS, Zeigler Z, Spearman MP, Lin L, Shadduck K, Lister J. Etiology of cortical and white matter lesions in cyclosporine-A and FK-506 neurotoxicity. *American Journal of Neuroradiology*, 2001;22:1901–1914.

Bashir RM. Neurologic complications of organ transplantation. *Current Treatment Options in Neurology*, 2001; 3(6):543–554.

Bashir RM, Bierman P, McComb R. Inflammatory peripheral neuropathy following high-dose chemotherapy and autologous bone marrow transplantation. *Bone Marrow Transplantation*, 1992;10:305–306.

Benke T, Wagner M, Pallua AK, Muigg A, Stockhammer G. Long-term cognitive and MRI findings in a patient with a paraneoplastic limbic encephalitis. *Journal of Neuro-oncology,* 2004;66(1–2):217–224.

Bernauer W, Gratwohl A. Bone marrow retinitis [letter]. *American Journal of Ophthalmology*, 1992;113(5);604.

Bertz H, Laubenberger J, Steinfurth G, Finke J. Sinus venous thrombosis: an unusual cause for neurologic symptoms after bone marrow transplantation under immunosuppression. *Transplantation*, 1998;66(2):241–244.

Bleyer WA. Clinical pharmacology of intrathecal methotrexate, II: an improved dosage regimen derived from age-related pharmacokinetics. *Cancer Treatment Reports*, 1977;61:1419–1425.

Boerman RH, Bax JJ, Beekhuis-Brussee JA. JC virus and multiple sclerosis: a refutation? *Acta Neurologica Scandinavia*, 1993;87(5):353–355.

Broers S, Kapstein AA, LeCessie S, Fibbe W, Hengeveld MW. Psychological functioning and quality of life following bone marrow transplantation: a 3-year follow-up. *Journal of Psychosomatic Research*, 2000;48(1): 11–21.

Bulsara KR, Baron PW, Tuttle-Newhall JE, Clavien PA, Morgenlander J. Guillain-Barre syndrome in organ and bone marrow transplant patients. *Transplantation*, 2001;71(8):1169–1172.

Burns TM, Ryan MM, Darras B, Jones HR Jr. Current therapeutic strategies for patients with polyneuropathies secondary to inherited metabolic disorders. *Mayo Clinic Proceedings*, 2003;78(7):858–868.

Callaham M. Fulminant bacterial meningitis without meningeal sign. *Annals of Emergency Medicine*, 1989; 8(1):90–93.

Chan AK, Bhargava R, Desai S, Joffe A. Reversible posterior leukoencephalopathy syndrome in a child with cerebral X-linked adrenoleukodystrophy treated with cyclosporine after bone marrow transplantation. *Journal of Inherited Metabolic Diseases*, 2003;26(6):527–536.

Chaudhry V, Cornblath DR, Corse A, Freimer M, Simmon-O'Brien E, Vogelsang G. Thalidomide-induced neuropathy. *Neurology*, 2002;59(12):1872–1875.

Christie D, Battin M, Leiper AD, Chessells J, Vargha-Khadem F, Neville BG. Neuropsychological and neurological outcome after relapse of lymphoblastic leukemia. *Archives Diseases in Childhood*, 1994;70(4): 275–280.

Chuurmans MJ, Deschamps PI, Markham SW, Shortridge-Baggett LM, Duursma SA. The measurement of delirium: review of scales. *Theory of Nursing Practice*, 2003;17(3):207–224.

Clark DA. Human herpesvirus 6 and human herpesvirus 7: emerging pathogens in transplant patients. *International Journal of Hematology*, 2002;76(Suppl 2): 246–252.

Conn HO. Hyperammonemia and intracranial hypertension: lying in wait for patients with hepatic disorders? *American Journal of Gastroenterology*, 2000;95(3): 814–816.

Conrad KJ. Cerebellar toxicities associated with cytosine arabinoside: a nursing perspective. *Oncology Nursing Forum*, 1986;13:57–59.

Costello A, Shallice T, Gullan R, Beaney R. The early effects of radiotherapy on intellectual and cognitive functioning in patients with frontal brain tumours: the use of a new neuropsychological methodology. *Journal of Neuro-oncology,* 2004;67(3):351–359.

Davies SM, Szabo E, Wagner JE, Ramsay NK, Weisdorf DJ. Idiopathic hyperammonemia: a frequently lethal complication of bone marrow transplantation. *Bone Marrow Transplantation*, 1996;17(6):1119–1125.

Davis D, Patchell RA. Neurologic complications of bone marrow transplantation. *Neurology Clinics*, 1988;6: 377–387.

deMagalhaes-Silverman M, Bloom EJ, Donnenberg A, Lister J, Pincus S, Rybka WB, et al. Toxicity of busulfan and cyclophosphamide (BU/CY2) in patients with hematologic malignancies. *Bone Marrow Transplantation*, 1996;17(3):329–333.

Denning DW, Lee JY, Hostetler JS, Pappas P, Kauffman CA, Dewsnup DH, et al. NIAID Mycoses study group multicenter trial of oral itraconazole therapy for invasive aspergillosis. *American Journal of Medicine*, 1994; 97(2):135–144.

Dunn JP, Jabs DA, Wingard J, Enger C, Vogelsang G, Santos G. Bone marrow transplantation and cataract development. *Archives Ophthalmology*, 1993;111:1367–1373.

Fernandez-Bouzas A, Ramirez Jimenez A, Vazques Zamudio J, Alonso-Vanegas M, Mendizabal Guerra R. Brain calcifications and dementia in children treated with radiotherapy and intrathecal methotrexate. *Journal of Neurosurgical Science*, 1992;36(4):211–214.

Fife BL, Huster GA, Cornettea KG, Kennedy VN, Akard LP, Brown ER. Longitudinal study of adaptation to the stress of bone marrow transplantation. *Journal of Clinical Oncology*, 2000;18(7):1539–1549.

Fife K, Milan S, Westbrook K, Powles R, Tait D. Risk factors for requiring cataract surgery following total body irradiation. *Radiotherapy and Oncology*, 1994; 33(2):93–98.

Filley CM, Kleinschmidt-DeMasters BK. Toxic leukoencephalopathy. *New England Journal of Medicine*, 2001; 345:425–432.

Fireman M, DiMartini AF, Armstrong SC, Cozza KL. Immunosuppressants. *Psychosomatics*, 2004;45:354–360.

Fischmeister G, Wiesbauer P, Holzmann HM, Peters C, Eibl M, Gadner H. Enteroviral meningoencephalitis in immunocompromised children after matched unrelated donor bone marrow transplantation. *Pediatric Hematology and Oncology*, 2000;17(5):393–399.

Furlong T. Neurologic complications of immunosuppressive cancer therapy. *Oncology Nursing Forum*, 1993; 20(9):1337–1354.

Furlong TG, Gallucci BB. Pattern of occurrence and clinical presentation of neurological complications in bone marrow transplant patients. *Cancer Nursing*, 1994;7(1):27–36.

Gallardo D, Ferra C, Berlanga JJ, Banda ED, Ponce C, Salar A, et al. Neurologic complications after allogeneic bone marrow transplantation. *Bone Marrow Transplantation*, 1996;18(6):1135–1139.

Goldberg SL, Tefferi A, Rummans TA, Chen MG, Solberg LA, Noel P. Post-irradiation somnolence syndrome in an adult patient following allogeneic bone marrow transplantation. *Bone Marrow Transplantation*, 1992;9: 499–501.

Gonzalez Vicent M, Diaz MA, Madero L. Pseudotumor cerebri following bone marrow transplantation (BMT). *Annals of Hematology*, 2001;80:236–237.

Gopal AK, Thorning DR, Back AL. Fatal outcome due to cyclosporine neurotoxicity with associated pathological findings. *Bone Marrow Transplantation*, 1999;23: 191–193.

Graus F, Saiz A, Sierra J, Arbaiza D, Rovira M, Carreras E, et al. Neurologic complications of autologous and allogeneic bone marrow transplantation in patients with leukemia: a comparative study. *Neurology*, 1996; 46:1004–1009.

Greeves JA. Rapid-onset steroid psychoses with very low dosage of prednisolone [letter]. *Lancet*, 1984; 1:1119–1120.

Guerrero A, Perez-Simon JA, Gutierrez N, Caballero D, Ortin F, Gomez-Sanchez JC, et al. Neurological complications after autologous stem cell transplantation. *European Neurology*, 1999;41:48–50.

Gunter M, Karle M, Werning A, Klingebiel T. Emotional adaptation of children undergoing bone marrow transplantation. *Candian Journal of Psychiatry*, 1999;44(1): 77–81.

Hagemann G, Ugur T, Witte OW, Fitzek C. Recurrent posterior reversible encephalopathy syndrome (PRES). *Journal of Human Hypertension*, 2004;18:287–289.

Halperin EC, Constine LS, Tarbell NJ. Late effects of cancer treatment. In: Halperin EC ed. *Pediatric Radiation Oncology*, 4th ed. New York: Raven Press; 2005: 515–520.

Hamon MD, Gale RF, MacDonald ID, Smith OP, Collis CH, Skeggs DB, et al. Incidence of cataracts after single fraction total body irradiation: the role of steroids and graft versus host disease. *Bone Marrow Transplantation*, 1993;1:233–236.

Han CS, Miller W, Haake R, Weisdorf D. Varicella zoster infection after bone marrow transplantation: incidence, risk factors, and complication. *Bone Marrow Transplantation*, 1994;13(3):277–283.

Harvey CJ, Peniket AJ, Miszkiel K, Patterson K, Goldstone AH, MacKinnon S, et al. MR angiographic diagnosis of cerebral venous sinus thrombosis following allogeneic bone marrow transplantation. *Bone Marrow Transplantation*, 2000;25(7):791–795.

Hiemenez JW, Greene JN. Special considerations for the patient undergoing allogeneic or autologous bone marrow transplantation. *Hematology Oncology Clinics of North America*, 1993;7(5);961–1002.

Hoffman DL, Howard JR Jr, Sarma R, Riggs JE. Encephalopathy, myelopathy, optic neuropathy and anosmia associated with intravenous cytosine arabinoside. *Clinicas of Neuropharmacology*, 1993;16(3): 258–262.

Hoodin F, Weber S. A systematic review of psychosocial factors affecting survival after bone marrow transplantation. *Psychosomatics*, 2003;44(3):181–195.

Hooks M, Wade C, Millikan W. Muromonab CD-3: a review of its pharmacology, pharmacokinetics, and clinical use in transplantation. *Pharmacotherapy*, 1991; 11(1):26–37.

Hooper DC, Pruitt AA, Rubin RH. Central nervous system infections in the chronically immunosuppressed. *Medicine*, 1982;61(3):166–188.

Hoyle C, Goldman JH. Life-threatening infections occurring more than 3 months after BMT. *Bone Marrow Transplantation*, 1994;14:247–252.

Huebscher, R. Peripheral neuropathy: alternative and complementary options. *Nurse Practitioner Forum*, 2000;11: 73–77.

Humphrey GB, Krous HF, Filler J, Maxwell JD, VanHoutte JJ. Treatment of CNS leukemia. *American Journal of Pediatric Hematology Oncology*, 1979;1:37–47.

Illescas-Rico R, Amaya-Ayala F, Jimenez-Lopez JL, Caballero-Mendez ME, Gonzalez-Llaven J. Increased Incidence of Anxiety and Depression During Bone Marrow Transplantation. *Archives of Medical Research*, 2002;33(2):144–147.

Imrie KR, Couture F, Turner CC, Sutcliffe SB, Keating A. Peripheral neuropathy following high-dose etoposide and autologous bone marrow transplantation. *Bone Marrow Transplantation*, 1994;13:77–79.

Inoha S, Inamura T, Nakamizo A, Ikezaki K, Amano T, Fukui M. Magnetic resonance imaging in cases with encephalopathy secondary to immunosuppressive agents. *Journal of Clincal Neuroscience*, 2002;9(3):305–307.

Ito M, Onose M, Yamada T, Onishi H, Fujisawa S, Kanamori H. Successful lithium carbonate treatment for steroid-induced depression following bone marrow transplantation: a case report. *Japanese Clinical Journal of Oncology*, 2003;33(10):538–540.

Jarosz JM, Howlett DC, Cox TC, Bingham JB. Cyclosporine-related reversible posterior leukoencephalopathy: MRL. *Neuroradiology*, 1997;39(10): 711–715.

Johnson NT, Crawford SW, Sargur M. Acute acquired demyelinating polyneuropathy with respiratory failure following high-dose systemic cytosine arabinoside and marrow transplantation. *Bone Marrow Transplantation*, 1987;2:203–207.

June CH, Thompson CB, Kennedy MS, Nims J, Thomas ED. Profound hypomagnesemia and renal magnesium wasting associated with the use of cyclosporine for marrow transplantation. *Transplantation*, 1985;39: 620–624.

Katirji MB. Visual hallucinations and cyclosporine. *Transplantation*, 1987;43(5):768–769.

Kelly P, Staunton H, Lawler M, Brennan P, Jennings S, Unger ER, Sung ER, et al. Multifocal remitting-relapsing cerebral demyelination twenty years following allogeneic bone marrow transplantation. *Journal of Experimental Neurology*, 1996;55(9):992–998.

Khalaf H, Al-Asseri A, Bhulyan J, Nafea O, Al-Sebayel M. Tacrolimus (FK 506) given three times daily after liver transplantation for minimizing nephrotoxicity and neurotoxicity. *Transplantation Proceedings*, 2003; 35:2787–2788.

Kitamura T, Satoh K, Tominaga T, Taguchi F, Tajama A, et al. Alteration in the JC polyomavirus genome is enhanced in immunosuppressed renal transplant patients. *Virology*, 1994;198(1):341–345.

Koc Y, Miller KB, Schenkein DP, Griffith J, Akhtar M, DesJardin J, et al. Varicella zoster virus infections following allogeneic bone marrow transplantation: frequency, risk factors, and clinical outcomes. *Biology of Blood and Marrow Transplantation*, 2000;6(1):44–49.

Kornblau SM, Cortes-Franco J, Estey E. Neurotoxicity associated with fludarabine and cytosine arabinoside chemotherapy for acute leukemia and myelodysplasia. *Leukemia*, 1993;7(3):378–383.

Kramer ED, Packer RJ, Ginsberg J, Goldman S, Thompson S, Bayer LA, et al. Acute neurologic dysfunction associated with high-dose chemotherapy and autologous bone marrow rescue for primary malignant brain tumors. *Pediatric Neurosurgery*, 1997; 27(5): 230–237.

Krouwer HG, Wijdicks EF. Neurologic complications of bone marrow transplantation. *Neurologic Clinics*, 2003;21(1):19–52.

La Morgia C, Mondini S, Guarino M, Bonifazi F, Cirignotta F. Busulfan neurotoxicity and EEG abnormalities: a case report. *Neurology Science*, 2004;25(2): 95–97.

Land VJ, Shuster JJ, Crist WM, Ravindranath Y, Harris NB, Krance RA, et al. Comparison of two schedules of intermediate-dose methotrexate and cytarabine consolidation therapy for childhood B-precursor cell acute lymphoblastic leukemia. *Journal of Clinical Oncology*, 1994;12(9):1939–1945.

Lee SJ, Vogelsang G, Flowers ME. Chronic graft-versus-host disease. *Biology of Blood and Marrow Transplantation*, 2003;9(4):215–233.

Leisner RJ, Leiper AD, Hann IM, Chessells JM. Late effects of intensive treatment for acute myeloid leukemia and myelodysplasia in children. *Journal of Clinical Oncology*, 1994;12(5):916–924.

Ljubisavljevic V, Kelly B. Risk factors for development of delirium among oncology patients. *General Hospital Psychiatry*, 2003;25(5):345–352.

Locatelli F, Giorgiani G, Pession A, Bozzala M. Late effects in children after bone marrow transplantation: a review. *Hematologica*, 1993;78(5):319–328.

Lockman LA, Sung JH, Krivit W. Acute parkinsonian syndrome with demyelinating leukoencephalopathy in bone marrow transplant recipients. *Pediatric Neurology*, 1991;7(6):457–463.

Lombardini L, Laszlo D, Rossi Ferrini P. Fatal herpesvirus 6 encephalitis after unrelated bone marrow transplant. *Bone Marrow Transplantation*, 1998;22(3):285–288.

Long SG, Leyland MJ, Milligan DW. Listeria meningitis after bone marrow transplantation. *Bone Marrow Transplantation*, 1993;12(5):537–539.

Lopez J, Ulibarrena C, Garcia-Larna J, Odriozola J, Perez de Oteyza J, Sastra JL, et al. Thalidomide as therapy for intestinal chronic GVHD. *Bone Marrow Transplantation*, 1993;11:251–252.

McGuire TR, Tallman MS, Yee GC, Nemunaitis JJ, Higano CS, McGuffin RW. Influence of infusion duration on the efficacy and toxicity of intravenous cyclosporine in bone marrow transplant patients. *Transplant Proceedings*, 1988;3(Suppl):501–504.

Mitchell RB, Wagner JE, Karp JE, Watson AJ, Brusilow SW, et al. Syndrome of idiopathic hyperammonemia after high-dose chemotherapy: review of nine cases. *American Journal of Medicine*, 1988;85:662–667.

Mohrmann R, Mah V, Vinters HV. Neuropathologic findings after bone marrow transplantation: an autopsy study. *Human Pathology*, 1990;21(6):630–639.

Montagna P. Acquired neuromyotonia after bone marrow transplantation. *Neurology*, 2000;54(6):1390–1391.

Mookerjee BP, Vogelsang G. Human herpes virus-6 encephalitis after bone marrow transplantation: successful treatment with ganciclovir. *Bone Marrow Transplantation*, 1997;20(10):905–906.

Moore D. Toxic leukoencephalopathy: a review and report of two chemotherapy-related cases. *Clinical Journal of Oncology Nursing*, 2003;7(4):413–417.

Moore IM, Espy KA, Kaufmann P, Kramer J, Kaemingk K, Miketova P, et al. Cognitive consequences and central nervous system injury following treatment for childhood leukemia. *Seminars in Oncology Nursing*, 2000;16(4):279–290; discussion 291–299.

Mulhearn R, Hancock J, Fairclough D. Neuropsychological status of children treated with brain tumors: a critical review and integrated analysis. *Medical Pediatric Oncology*, 1992;20:181–191.

Murphy P, Parker A, Hutchinson RM. High grade pyrexia following bone marrow transplantation: a neurotoxic complication of high-dose chemotherapy and radiotherapy in the UKALL XII Trial. *Bone Marrow Transplantation*, 1994;13:229–231.

Nagarajan R, Peteres C, Orchard P, Rydholm N. Report of severe neurotoxicity with cyclophosphamide. *Journal of Pediatric Hematology and Oncology*, 2000;22(6):544–546.

Nagashima T, Sato F, Chuma T, Mano Y, Sasaki I, Mori M, et al. Chronic demyelinating polyneuropathy in graft-versus-host disease following allogeneic bone marrow transplantation. *Neuropathology*, 2002;22(1):1–8.

Neitzert CS, Ritvo P, Dancey J, Weiser K, Murray C, Avery J. The psychosocial impact of bone marrow transplantation: a review of the literature. *Bone Marrow Transplantation*, 1998;22(5):409–422.

Nevo S, Vogelang GB. Acute bleeding complications in patients after bone marrow transplantation. *Current Opinions in Hematology*, 2001;8(5):319–325.

Norrell H, Wilson CB, Slagel DE. Leukoencephalopathy following the administration of methotrexate into the cerebrospinal fluid in the treatment of primary brain tumors. *Cancer*, 1974;33(4):923–932.

Onose M, Kawanishi C, Onishi H, Yamada T, Itoh M, Josaka K, et al. Neuroleptic malignant syndrome following BMT. *Bone Marrow Transplantation*, 2002; 29:803–804.

Openshaw H. Peripheral neuropathy after bone marrow transplantation. *Biology of Blood and Marrow Transplant*, 1997;3(4):202–209.

Owczarek J, Jasinska M, Orszulak-Michalak D. Drug-induced myopathies. An overview of the possible mechanisms. *Pharamcology Report*, 2005;57(1):23–34.

Ozon A, Topaloglu H, Cila A, Gunay M, Cetin M. Acute ascending myelitis and encephalopathy after intrathecal methotrexate in an adolescent boy with acute lymphoblastic leukemia. *Brain and Development*, 1994;16(3):246–248.

Packer RJ, Meadows AT, Roarke LB. Long-term sequelae of cancer treatment on the central nervous system in childhood. *Medical Pediatric Oncology*, 1987;15(5): 241–253.

Padovan CS, Sostak P, Reich P, Kolb HJ, Muller-Felber W, Straube A. Neuromuscular complications after allogeneic bone marrow transplantation. *Nervenarzt*, 2003;74(2):159–166. (Translated from German original article.)

Palmer B, Toto R. Severe neurologic toxicity induced by cyclosporine A in three renal transplant patients. *American Journal of Kidney Disease*, 1991;18(1):116–121.

Patchell RA, White CL, Clark AW, Beschorner WE, Santos GW. Neurologic complications of bone marrow transplantation. *Neurology*, 1985;35:300–306.

Pelgrims J, DeVos F, Van den Brande J, Schrijvers D, Prove A, Vermorken JB. Methylene blue in the treatment and prevention of ifosfamide-induced encephalopathy: report of 12 cases and a review of the literature. *British Journal of Cancer*, 2000;82(2):291–294.

Pomeranz S, Naparstek E, Ashkenazi E, Nagler A, Lossos A, Slavin S, et al. Intracranial haematomas following bone marrow transplantation. *Journal Neurology*, 1994; 241(4):252–256.

Prescott WA, Jr, Callahan BL, Park JM. Tacrolimus toxicity associated with concomitant metoclopromide therapy. *Pharmacotherapy*, 2004;24(4):532–537.

Price RA. Histopathology of CNS leukemia and complications of therapy. *American Journal of Pediatric Hematology Oncology*, 1979;1:21–30.

Rabinstein AA, Dispenzieri A, Micallef IN, Inwards DJ, Litzow MR, Wijdicks EF. Acute neuropathies after peripheral blood stem cell and bone marrow transplantation. *Muscle and Nerve*, 2003;28(6):733–736.

Rathi B, Azad RK, Vasudha N, Hissaria P, Sawlani V, Gupta RK. L-asparaginase-induced reversible posterior leukoencephalopathy syndrome in a child with acute lymphoblastic leukemia. *Pediatric Neurosurgery*, 2002;37:203–205.

Reddick WE, Glass JO, Langston JW, Helton KJ. Quantitative MRI assessment of leukoencephalopathy. *Magnetic Resonance Medicine*, 2002;47:912–920.

Reece DE, Frei-Lahr DA, Sheperd DE, Dorovini-Zis K, Gascoyne RD, Graeb DA, et al. Neurologic complications in allogeneic bone marrow transplant patients receiving cyclosporin. *Bone Marrow Transplantation*, 1991;8(5):393–401.

Reinohs S, Straube T, Baum P, Berrouschot J, Wagner A. Recurrent reversible cerebral edema after long term immunosuppression with tacrolimus. *Journal Neurology*, 2002;249(6):780–761.

Resar LM, Phillips PC, Kastran MB, Leventhal BG, Bowman PW, Civin CL. Acute neurotoxicity after intrathecal cytosine arabinoside in two adolescents with acute lymphoblastic leukemia of B-cell type. *Cancer*, 1993;71(1):117–123.

Richardson JK, Sandman D, Vela S. A focused exercise regimen improves clinical measures of balance in patients with peripheral neuropathy. *Archives of Physical Medicine and Rehabilitation*, 2001;82:205–209.

Roemer E, Blau IW, Basara N, Kiehl MG, Bischoff M, Gunzelmann S, et al. Toxoplasmosis, a severe complication in allogeneic hematopoietic stem cell transplantation: successful treatment strategies during a 5-year single-center experience. *Clinical Infectious Diseases*, 2001;32:e1–e8.

Roscrow MA, Kelsey SM, McCarthy M, Newland AC, Monson JC. Selective autonomic neuropathy as a novel complication of BMT. *Bone Marrow Transplantation*, 1992;10:469–470.

Sable CA, Donowitz GR. Infections in bone marrow transplant recipients. *Clinical Infectious Diseases*, 1994;18: 273–284.

Sakami H, Onozawa Y, Yano Y, Imai K, Sasaki T, Ibuka T, et al. Disseminated necrotizing leukoencephalopathy following irradiation and MTX therapy for central nervous system infiltration of leukemia and lymphoma. *Radiation Medicine*, 1993;11(4):146–153.

Sasaki T, Akaho R, Sakamaki H, Akiyama H, Yoshino M, Hagiya K, et al. Mental disturbances during isolation in bone marrow transplant patients with leukemia. *Bone Marrow Transplantation*, 2000;25(3):315–318.

Schagen SB, Muller MJ, Boogerd W, Van Dam FS. Cognitive dysfunction and chemotherapy: neuropsychological findings in perspective. *Clinical Breast Cancer*, 2002;3(Suppl 3):s100–s108.

Shah AK. Cyclosporine A neurotoxicity among bone marrow transplant recipients. *Clinical Neuropharmacology*, 1999;22(2):67–73.

Shimono T, Miki Y, Toyoda H, Egawaa H, Uemoto S, Tanaka K, et al. MR imaging with quantitative diffusion mapping of tacrolimus-induced neurotoxicity in organ transplant patients. *European Radiology*, 2003;13(5):986–993.

Singh N, Paterson DL. Encephalitis caused by human herpesvirus-6 in transplant recipients: relevance of a novel neurotropic virus. *Transplantation*, 2000;69(12): 2474–2479.

Slavney, P. *Psychiatric Dimensions of Medical Practice*. Baltimore, MD: Johns Hopkins University Press; 1998.

Smith EL, Whedon MB, Bookbinder M. Quality improvement of painful peripheral neuropathy. *Seminars in Oncology Nursing*, 2002,18:36–43.

Snider S, Bashir R, Bierman P. Neurologic complications after high-dose chemotherapy and autologous bone marrow transplantation for Hodgkin's disease. *Neurology*, 1994;44(4):681–684.

Solaro C, Murialdo A, Giunti D, Mancardi G, Uccelli A. Central and peripheral nervous system complications following allogeneic bone marrow transplantation. *European Journal of Neurology*, 2001;8(1):77–80.

Sommer, C. Painful neuropathies. *Current Opinion in Neurology*, 2003;16:623–628.

Sostak P, Padovan CS, Yousry TA, Ledderose G, Kolb HJ, Straube A. Prospective evaluation of neurological complications after allogeneic bone marrow transplantation. *Neurology*, 2003;60(5):842–848.

Srivastava A, Bradstock KF, Szer J, de Bortoli L, Gottlieb DL. Busulphan and melphalan prior to autologous bone marrow transplantation. *Bone Marrow Transplantation*, 1993;12:323–329.

Steg RE, Kessinger A, Wszolek ZK. Cortical blindness and seizures in a patient receiving FK506 after bone marrow transplantation. *Bone Marrow Transplantation*, 1999;23(9):959–962.

Syrjala K. Neurocognitive dysfunction after stem cell transplantation usually transient. *Blood*, 2004;104: 3386–3392.

Syrjala KL, Dikmen S, Langer SL, Roth-Roemer S, Abrams JR. Neuropsychiatric changes before transplantation to one year in patients receiving myeloablative allogeneic hematopoietic cell transplant. *Blood*, 2004: 104(100):3386–3392.

Tahsildar HI, Remler BF, Creger RJ, Cooper BW, Snodgrass SM, Tarr RW, et al. Delayed, transient encephalopathy after marrow transplantation: case reports and MRI findings in four patients. *Journal of Neuro-oncology*, 1996;27(3):241–250.

Tannock IF, Ahles TA, Ganz PA, van Dam FS. Cognitive impairment associated with chemotherapy for cancer: report of a workshop. *Journal of Clinical Oncology*, 2004;22(11):2233–2239

Teive HA, Brandi IV, Camargo CH, Bittencourt MA, Bonfirm CM, Friedrich ML, et al. Reversible posterior leucoencephalopathy syndrome associated with bone marrow transplantation. *Arquive Neuropsiquiatric*, 2001;59(3-B):784–789.

Thompson CB, Sanders JE, Fluornoy N, Buckner CD, Thomas ED. The risks of central nervous system relapse after bone marrow transplantation for acute myeloid leukemia. *Blood*, 1986;67:195–199.

Thompson CB, Sullivan KM, June CH, Thomas ED. Association between cyclosporin neurotoxicity and hypomagnesemia. *Lancet*, 1984;1116–1120.

Tichelli A, Gratwohl A, Egger T, Roth J, Prunte A, Nissen C, Speck B. Cataract formation after bone marrow transplantation. *Annals of Internal Medicine*, 1993;119(12):1175–1180.

Trullemans F, Grignard F, Van Camp B, Schots R. Clinical findings and magnetic resonance imaging in severe cyclosporine-related neurotoxicity after allogeneic bone marrow transplantation. *European Journal of Hematology*, 2001;67:94–99.

Tse N, Cederbaum S, Glaspy JA. Hyperammonemia following allogeneic bone marrow transplantation. *American Journal of Hematology*, 1991;38(2):140–141.

Turhal NS. Cyclosporin A and imipenem associated seizure activity in allogeneic bone marrow transplantation patients. *Journal of Chemotherapy*, 1999;11(5): 410–413.

van der Lelie J, Louwerse ES, Thomas LL, van Oers MH, von dem Borne AE. Acute ischaemic cerebrovascular accident after autologous bone marrow transplantation. *European Journal of Haematology*, 1996;56(1–2): 95–97.

Veroux P, Veroux M, Puliatti C, Morale W, Cappello D, Valvo M, et al. Tacrolimus-induced neurotoxicity in kidney transplant recipients. *Transplant Proceedings*, 2002;34:3188–3190.

Verstappen CC, Heimans JJ, Hockman K, Postma TJ. Neurotoxic complications of chemotherapy in patients with cancer: clinical signs and optimal management. *Drugs*, 2003;63(15):1549–1563.

Vidarsson B, Mosher DF, Salamat MS, Isaksson HJ, Onundarson PT. Progressive multifocal leukoencephalopathy after fludarabine therapy for low-grade lymphoproliferative disease. *American Journal of Hematology*, 2002;70:51–54.

Vogel H, Horoupian DS. Filamentous degeneration of neurons: a possible feature of cytosine arabinoside neurotoxicity. *Cancer*, 1993;71(4):1303–1308.

Vogelsang G, Morris L. Prevention and management of graft-vs-host disease: practical recommendations. 2003; *Drugs*, 45(5):668–676

Walker RW, Brochstein JA. Neurologic complications of immunosuppressive agents. *Neurology Clinics*, 1988; 6(2):261–278.

Wasserstein PH, Honig LS. Parkinsonism during cyclosporine treatment. *Bone Marrow Transplantation*, 1996;18(3):649–650.

Watanabe A. Portal-systemic encephalopathy in non-cirrhotic patients: classification of clinical types, diagnosis, and treatment. *Journal of Gastroenterology and Hepatology*, 2000;15:969–979.

Wen PY, Alyea EP, Simon D, Herbst RS, Soiffer RJ, Antin JH. Guillain-Barre syndrome following allogeneic bone marrow transplantation. *Neurology*, 1997;49(6): 1711–1714.

Wen PY, Blanchard KL, Block CC, Loeffler JF, Davis DG, Lacroix LA, et al. Development of Lhermitte's sign after bone marrow transplantation. *Cancer*, 1992;69: 2262–2266.

Whitley RJ, Lentnek A, McCracken GH. Evaluation of new anti-infective drugs for the treatment of viral encephalitis. *Clinical Infectious Diseases*, 1992;15(Suppl 1):S195–S199.

Wiznitzer M, Packer RJ, August CS, Burkey ED. Neurological complications of bone marrow transplantation in childhood. *Annals of Neurology*, 1984;16: 569–576.

Wong R, Beguelin GZ, de Lima M, Giralt SA, Hosing C, Ippoliti C, et al. Tacrolimus-associated posterior reversible encephalopathy syndrome after allogeneic hematopoietic stem cell transplantation. *British Journal of Haematology*, 2004;122:128–134.

Yalcin S, Nurlu G, Orhan B, Zeybek D, Muftuoglu S, Sarer B, et al. Protective effect of amifostine against cisplatin-induced motor neuropathy in rat. *Medical Oncology*, 2003;20(2):175–180.

Yoshikawa T. Human herpesvirus-6 and -7 infections in transplantation. *Pediatric Transplantation*, 2003;7:11–17.

Chapter 12

Late Effects of Bone Marrow Transplant

Kathy Ruble, RN, MSN, CPNP, AOCN®

The use of blood and marrow transplantation (BMT) as a therapeutic modality for the treatment of oncologic and nononcologic diseases continues to expand. It is estimated that there are 45,000 BMTs done yearly and currently 100,000 survivors of BMT after 5 or more years worldwide. Clearly, this aggressive form of therapy has led to increased survival for many patient populations. Although absence of disease is a paramount concern, so are the consequences of the therapy that afford this outcome. The intense therapies used prior to and during BMT can leave the survivor at risk for numerous medical late effects. A lifetime of surveillance and management is necessary to ensure that these patients continue to have optimal quantity, as well as quality of life. This chapter will address the potential late complications of bone marrow transplant and suggest screening and treatment where appropriate. For the purpose of clarity, *late effects* will be considered those conditions that the patient experiences 5 years or more after BMT. Although some of these effects may be seen prior to this time, we want to distinguish them from conditions that are acutely or subacutely associated with BMT.

Ophthalmologic Late Effects

Cataracts are a very common late effect after BMT and can be related to TBI or steroid use. One comprehensive study done by Kempen-Harteveld and colleagues (2002) examined the effects of TBI delivered in 1 or 2 fractions in 93 transplant survivors. The median age of the patients was 35, and the TBI was administered in 1 fraction of 8 Gy or 2 fractions of 5–6 Gy. Annual examinations were done over a 12-year period and found a 91% incidence of developing cataracts, with 44% of patients having cataracts significant enough to cause severe visual impairment (SVI). In this study, patients treated for GVHD with steroids were at greater risk of developing SVI, with a majority having SVI at 67 months post-BMT; the cataracts that developed later in follow-up were less likely to result in SVI. Other studies confirm that patients who receive TBI in multiple fractions are less likely to develop cataracts (Benyunes et al., 1995; Tichelli et al., 1996; Belkacemi et al., 1998), and in this study the cataracts that developed later in follow-up were less likely to result in SVI. Other studies have confirmed this high rate of cataract development and decreased risk with fractionation (Tichelli et al., 1996; Belkacemi et al., 1998).

Sicca syndrome, or dry eye, is another possible complication after BMT that results from scarring of the lacrimal duct. Dry eye has been reported in as many at 19% of BMT survivors and is usually related to scarring from radiation and/or GVHD (Tichelli et al., 1996). Patients with sicca syndrome may complain of dry or gritty-feeling eyes, which are easily irritated. Without appropriate treatment, sicca syndrome can lead to ulceration, scarring, or perforation. Sicca syndrome is diagnosed with a Schirmer's test and can frequently be treated with artificial tears. In severe cases, ligation of the lacrimal duct may be necessary (Jack and Hicks, 1981).

Pulmonary Late Effects

Pulmonary complications from BMT can be divided into two categories, infectious and noninfectious. With the exception of patients who do not have complete immunoreconstitution after transplant, there are few infectious pulmonary complications in the long-term follow-up period. The majority of noninfectious pulmonary effects from BMT will be experienced in the acute and early follow-up periods, (within 2 years of BMT). Bronchiolitis obliterans is one of the fatal late pulmonary complications after BMT and has rarely been diagnosed past 2 years post-BMT. Most pulmonary effects are static by the time the patient is seen in a late effects program, and maintenance is the primary objective. Some patients will persist with symptoms including cough, wheezing, and dyspnea, and other pa-

tients are asymptomatic but continue to display restrictive or obstructive changes on pulmonary function test (PFTs). Patients at risk for long-term restrictive or obstructive changes include those with significant infectious pulmonary complications during BMT, chronic GVHD, TBI, and/or chest irradiation for their primary disease, and chemotherapeutic agents known to cause pulmonary toxicity (busulfan, bleomycin, carmustine (BCNU), lonustine (CCNU)).

A large retrospective study in the pediatric population looked at pulmonary complications after BMT, and in 138 cases found 10 late/chronic severe pulmonary conditions. These conditions are listed in the **Table 12-1**.

In this study, five of the patients with chronic severe pulmonary conditions expired in the period of 1 to 8 years after BMT (Griese et al., 2000).

Routine pulmonary surveillance including history, physical exam, and PFTs are important for long-term BMT patients; particular care should be taken for patients with pretreatment risk factors including chest irradiation, surgery, or pulmonary toxic chemotherapeutic agents. Patient education should include good pulmonary hygiene, e.g., avoidance of smoking or environmental hazards.

Table 12-1 Chronic severe pulmonary condition.

Chronic bronchitis	1
Hepatopulmonary syndrome	1
Bronchiolitis obliterans	3
Pulmonary fibrosis	2
Idiopathic pneumonia syndrome	3

Cardiac Late Effects

Long-term cardiac dysfunction has been studied in many settings, including pediatric and adult survivors of BMT. The recurring difficulty with these studies is the inability to distinguish which deficits are due to the BMT therapies versus therapy the patients received prior to BMT. Known cardiotoxic cancer therapies include, primarily, anthracyclines and chest irradiation. Cardiac effects of these treatments include left ventricular dysfunction (LVD), decreased left ventricular mass, conduction abnormalities, valvular dysfunction, coronary artery disease, and complications from pericarditis (Steinherz et al., 1995; Lipshultz et al., 1991; Larsen, Jakacki et al., 1992b). Adding to the difficulty with attribution of cardiac abnormalities is the fact that they may be progressive over time and first appear in the late BMT period.

Eames and colleagues (1997) looked at 63 patients transplanted at < 18 years of age. Follow-up studies included chest radiograph (CXR), PFTs, ECG, echocardiogram (exercise and resting), treadmill testing, and cardiac symptoms. Findings indicated that 41.3% of patients had cardiac abnormalities found at a mean time of 3.3 years after BMT. The majority of these abnormalities were not identified pretransplant and two thirds were subclinical.

Other studies illustrate the importance of cardiac stress testing for BMT survivors. Larsen, Jakacki, and colleagues (1992) used a cross-sectional design to look at cardiac function after BMT during exercise and at rest. This study found that both adults and children had diminished cardiac function, including reduced exercise time, maximal oxygen consumption, anaerobic threshold, and cardiac output, although all had normal resting oxygen consumptions and cardiac indices at rest. Longitudinal assessments in a similar population revealed that these impaired cardiac findings are static and do not deteriorate over time (Hogarty et al., 2000).

Although the exact mechanisms for cardiac dysfunction in the BMT survivor population have not been fully defined, it is clear that they are at risk for diminished cardiac function. Those survivors whose pre-BMT treatment includes cardiotoxic therapies are at risk, independent of BMT, and need routine monitoring. Until there is a full understanding of the cardiac effects, the minimal follow-up should include periodic ECG, echocardiogram, history, and physical. Exercise and/or stress testing may also be considered for specific individuals. Patient education should include advisement on risks and healthy cardiovascular lifestyles.

Endocrine Late Effects

Endocrine dysfunction is a common late effect of BMT, and screening for endocrine abnormalities should be a standard of care for this population. Gonadal dysfunction is a frequently seen abnormality after BMT. Like other late effects, the risk of gonadal dysfunction is closely related to the sex, age at treatment, prior therapy, and preparative regimen. Ovarian failure is common in women who are transplanted after menarche, but normal pubertal development may progress in younger females (Tauchmanova et al., 2002; Shalet and Brennan, 2002). In general, females who undergo normal pubertal development and have spontaneous menstruation can be assumed to have sufficient ovary function. This may not guarantee the ability to successfully carry a pregnancy, since subtle changes in the uterus may impair its ability to respond appropriately to pregnancy-related changes (Bath et al., 1999). For women who do not resume menstruation after BMT, hormone replacement therapy (HRT) should be considered, especially for women well below the age for expected menopause. Depending on type of malignancy and other individual risk factors, HRT may not be appropriate, in which case monitoring for the effects of early menopause should be recommended. Even younger patients who develop spontaneous ovarian function after BMT may be at risk for early menopause and should be advised of this risk, which will allow them possible fertility options such as ova harvesting or other assisted reproductive technology.

The germinal epithelium of the male is much more sensitive to the toxic effects of BMT preparative regimens than the ovary is. In the male reproductive system, the germinal epithelium is responsible for spermatogenesis while the Leydig cells are responsible for testosterone production. With normal Leydig cell function, the majority of males can expect normal pubertal development and sexual function after BMT. Fertility for males after BMT is rare and can be predicted by measuring follicular stimulating hormone (FSH) levels. Elevated FSH indicates probable azoospermia, while semen analysis is the gold standard for diagnosing infertility (Shalet and Brennan, 2002). The literature does support the possibility of late recovery of spermatogenesis for the male BMT population and may be reflected by a normalization of the FSH (Sklar et al., 1984).

The thyroid is another endocrine gland that is vulnerable to late effects after BMT. The risk of thyroid dysfunction is greater after TBI, with decreasing incidence with increasing fractionation, although busulfan/cytoxan regimens have also been implicated in thyroid dysfunction

(Al-Fiar et al., 1997). Surveillance of thyroid function with serial thyroid stimulating hormone (TSH) and T4 measures can help to avoid clinical hypothyroidism and other complications from thyroid damage. Elevated TSH levels, even with normal T4/T3 levels, is reflective of thyroid impairment and may indicate the need for exogenous replacement. Animal studies have shown that giving exogenous hormone when TSH levels are elevated decreases the risk of developing a thyroid malignancy (Shalet and Brennan, 2002). After supplementation, some patients may recover normal thyroid function, but as yet there are no specific recommendations as to when, or if, it is appropriate to discontinue exogenous hormones in this population.

Growth hormone may also be impacted by BMT and is of particular concern to those who are transplanted in childhood. As with other late effects, the pretransplant therapies impact the risk of growth hormone deficiencies, as does TBI schedule, steroid use, and GVHD (Huma et al., 1995; Olshan et al., 1993). Growth charts, growth velocities, and growth hormone screening should be followed closely on all survivors of childhood BMT. If growth hormone deficiency is suspected, provocation tests, as well as bone age, should be evaluated.

Another important issue to consider in using growth hormone in the BMT population is the impact of radiation alone on growth. Any bone or soft tissue that is irradiated before it is fully developed will have a diminished growth capacity. Therefore, the radiation to the spine and epiphyseal areas will consequently impact the final height of the child, regardless of growth hormone status.

There is controversy over the use of growth hormone replacement in this population, because of the risks associated with second malignancies. As we will discuss in an upcoming section, second malignancies are a risk for BMT survivors. Growth hormone is known to cause cell proliferation in both benign and malignant cell lines. In animal models, cancers have been induced when supraphysiologic doses have been utilized. Studies looking at malignancies in humans treated with growth hormone have been inconclusive as to the exact risk (Ogilvy-Stuart and Gleeson, 2004). Until comprehensive studies and databases necessary to track these occurrences are established, it will be up to the health-care providers and families to weigh the risks versus benefits of growth hormone for an individual patient.

Renal Late Effects

The risk of renal dysfunction during BMT and in the time period immediately following BMT is significant. Although most patients have normal renal function going into transplant, the use of renal toxic preparative regimens (including TBI), the supportive care therapies (including cyclosporine, aminoglycosides, and antifungals), as well as complications (including sepsis and GVHD) make the likelihood of renal dysfunction high. Most studies looking at renal dysfunction after BMT have looked at the period of 1 to 2 years after BMT and describe an 11–25% probability of renal insufficiency (Cohen et al., 1993; Lawton et al., 1991; Kist-van Holthe et al., 2002). Fewer studies that look at longer term outcomes of renal function for this population are available. One long-term prospective study of autologous BMT in children found that patients were at risk for renal dysfunction in the 6 months following BMT; the authors attributed this long latency to the effects of radiation in combination with the slow turnover of endothe-

lium in the kidney. This study reported on the renal function of 26 patients with a median follow-up period of 10 years and found 7 patients with chronic renal impairment (defined as a GFR of < 70 m/min/1.73 m^2), all of whom had received TBI (Frisk et al., 2002).

Although there is still much to learn concerning renal function after BMT, a yearly screening with blood pressure, BUN, creatinine, and urinalysis for all patients at risk for renal insufficiency should be considered. Further evaluation with serum chemistries, creatinine clearance, or GFR is also important for those with any initial abnormal findings. Patients with established or new onset renal insufficiency should be followed in conjunction with nephrology to ensure the best possible outcome.

Gastrointestinal Late Effects

The majority of gastrointestinal complications of BMT are seen acutely or in the immediate post-transplant period. Graft-versus-host disease, gastritis/esophagitis, cytomegalovirus enteritis, bacterial enteritis, and toxic mucosal damage have been reported in the 16 months following BMT (Schulenburg et al., 2004), but fewer studies are available looking at longer periods after transplant. Baker and colleagues (2004) reported on late effects of survivors of chronic myelogenous leukemia (CML) who had undergone hematopoietic cell transplant and found that in self-report measures, survivors had 2.4 times higher risk of gallstones and 2.9 times higher risk of hepatitis when compared to siblings. Other complications, including oral health impairments and difficulty chewing or swallowing, were more frequently associated with chronic

GVHD, and dry mouth was more common in survivors regardless of cGVHD. Education for this population should include recommendations for good oral hygiene and routine dental care, as saliva plays an important role in maintaining the integrity of teeth and gums.

Screening of blood products and marrow has greatly reduced the number of BMT survivors contracting hepatitis and other blood-borne illnesses after transplant. Hepatitis risk is closely related to decade of transplant and the risks to the blood supply prior to screening. In the United States, blood product screening for hepatitis B began in 1972, and hepatitis C screening began in 1993. Patients who received blood products (packed red blood cells, whole blood, white cells, platelets, fresh frozen plasma, cryoprecipitate, immunoglobulin preparations, or clotting factors) prior to 1993 should be screened, as should any others who have abnormal liver function tests.

Musculoskeletal Late Effects

The primary musculoskeletal abnormalities seen after BMT include avascular necrosis, diminished bone mineral density, and osteochondromas. Avascular necrosis (AVN) is probably best characterized by a large French study looking at 4388 pediatric and adult allogeneic bone marrow transplant recipients (Socie et al., 1994, 1997). In this study, there were 77 cases of AVN reported, the majority of which occurred in patients > 20 years of age, with a median time to diagnosis of 22 months after transplant. The hip joint is the most common site for AVN in both children and adults (Matthes-Martin et al., 1999; Enright et al., 1990). The use of steroids

is the most important risk factor for the development of AVN (Enright et al., 1990; Fink et al., 1998; Socie et al., 1994). The most extreme cases of AVN may require joint replacement, and MRI scanning of the joints should be considered for any patient with persistent pain.

Diminished bone mineral density (BMD) in the form of osteopenia or osteoporosis is a common finding after BMT. Schimmer and colleagues (2001) found that over half of the 64 adult survivors of autologous transplant studied had evidence of diminished BMD, with older age being the only predictive variable of loss. Similar results were seen in a series of allogeneic bone marrow transplant survivors reported by Kauppila and colleagues (1999). Diminished BMD is a recognized complication of childhood cancer in general and may be associated with steroid use or can accompany other late effects such as hypogonadism or growth hormone deficiency. The study of BMD in childhood BMT survivors is complicated by the reduction in height for age seen in this population. Matthes-Martin and colleagues (1999) reported a 13% incidence of osteoporosis in allogeneic BMT survivors. Nysom and colleagues (2000) studied allogeneic survivors compared to healthy controls and survivors of conventionally treated acute lymphocytic leukemia (ALL). He found, when controlling for height and size-adjusted bone mass, that treated patients were very similar to controls in BMD and that whole-body mass was only marginally less after BMT as compared to conventionally treated ALL survivors.

Osteochondromas are present in 23–26% of survivors of BMT and may first appear > 5 years from transplant (Leung et al., 2000; Harper et al., 1998). These may appear as painless peripheral or central bony growths, or if nerves or blood vessels are involved they may become painful. Radiation has been closely associated with the development of osteochondromas and in rare circumstances these benign growths may develop into osteosarcoma or osteochrondrosarcoma (Poustchi-Amin et al., 1996; Jaffe et al., 1983).

Other related musculoskeletal abnormalities unique to the pediatric BMT survivor population have been reported and include slipped epiphysis, scoliosis, and metaphyseal growth abnormalities (Fletcher et al., 1994).

Immune Reconstitution and Late Effects

The time to immune reconstitution is primarily dependent on the type of transplant and chronic GVHD. In general, most immune function has returned to normal by 1 year posttransplant in patients who receive autologous product. Machatschek and colleagues (2003) found that in 58 children with autologous transplant, 75% had normal IgM levels by 6 months, and most infectious complications (77%) occurred in this period. In this study 90% of patients developed normal T cell function by 1 year posttransplant.

Survivors who have received an allogeneic product may have longer recovery periods and more late infectious morbidity. Delayed recovery of CD4+ T cells may be responsible for the infections occurring up to 1 year after allogeneic transplant (Storek et al., 1997). The delay in immune reconstitution is the rationale for delaying immunizations in the posttransplant period. Most experts would agree that immunizations should not be administered for a full year after transplant and/or discontinuance of immunosuppressive therapies. When immunizations are

instituted, a trial of diphtheria/tetanus (DT) vaccine should be used. A prevaccine DT level should be sent prior to immunization and a 6-week postimmunization level should be checked. If the patient is able to make an appropriate response to this vaccine, he may proceed to further immunizations safely.

By the time patients reach the long-term follow-up period of 5 years, a vast majority have normal immune function. The exception to this are patients who are functionally asplenic posttransplant. Hyposplenic or asplenic function is primarily found in patients with chronic GVHD and can be diagnosed by the presence of Howell-Jolly bodies in peripheral blood, reduced spleen size or blood flow, higher platelet counts, or higher indium-111-labeled autologous platelet recovery (Kalhs et al., 1988). More recently, sonography has been employed to diagnose this condition. The risk to patients who have diminished splenic function is infection with encapsulated organisms (Wollenberg et al., 2001). The use of triple vaccination for *Streptococcus* pneumonia, *Haemophilus* influenza type B, and meningococcus *Neisseria* may help provide protection, as does prophylaxis with penicillin; depending on the setting these interventions may be considered.

Second Malignancy after Bone Marrow Transplant

By far one of the most devastating consequences of bone marrow transplant is the development of a secondary malignant neoplasm (SMN). The SMN risk for the first decade after transplant consists primarily of posttransplant lymphoproliferative disorders (PTLD), myelodysplasia (MDS), and acute myeloid leukemia (AML).

PTLD is a condition associated primarily with Epstein-Barr virus and can be characterized as an uncontrolled proliferation of B lymphocytes in an environment of diminished cellular immunity. PTLD is seen primarily in the allogeneic transplant setting and occurs most often in the first 18 months after transplant. It has been reported that as many as half of SMNs after BMT may be due to PTLD, with an incidence of 1–1.6% (Curtis et al., 1999; Bhatia et al., 1996; Socie et al., 2000). While new therapies are under development, the mortality rate for PTLD is high.

Myelodysplasia and acute myeloid leukemia as SMNs are not limited to the BMT population and have long been recognized as late effects after therapy with alkylating agents and topoisomerase II inhibitors. Most studies have looked at MDS and AML in the autologous BMT population and report an actuarial risk ranging from 3–19.8% (Pedersen-Bjergaard et al., 2000). Studies that have looked at these conditions after autologous BMT and conventional therapies (without BMT) have found similar incidence between the two groups (Andre et al., 1998). These results may indicate that it is the prior or overall therapy that leads to this complication and not the BMT process itself.

The information on risks for solid tumors as SMNs continues to evolve as the population of survivors continues to age. One large study of autologous and allogeneic survivors reported by Baker and colleagues (2003) found a cumulative incidence of 3.8% at 20 years for the development of solid tumors after stem cell transplant. This incidence had not plateaued at 20 years, indicating that we have not yet seen the full effect of SMNs on the survivor population. Another large study published in 1997 looked at 19,229 survivors of allogeneic or syngeneic transplant and found a cumulative incidence of SMN of 6.7% at 15 years posttransplant. Malignant melanoma, oral cancers, central nervous system malignancies, and bone and connective tissue cancers were the most frequently seen in this study (Curtis et al., 1997). Other studies have confirmed these findings and additionally identified cervical, thyroid, and breast cancer as potential SMNs. Risk factors for SMNs, including TBI and chronic graft-versus-host disease, have been identified and should be kept in mind when evaluating patients with this history (Bhatia et al., 2001).

Clearly, SMNs will continue to be a real and frightening late effect in the transplant survivor population. While we continue to learn about the incidence of these diseases, we have very little data on the outcome of treatment for these SMNs. Clearly, in a population of aggressively treated patients, management of these SMNs will be a significant challenge.

Neurocognitive Late Effects

Pediatric practitioners have long recognized that the therapies employed for the treatment of cancer can have a negative impact on neurocognitive or neuropsychologic functioning. The first and most obvious therapy to be associated with this late effect was cranial irradiation. It is no surprise, then, that in the BMT population, this therapy is identified as a risk factor for this particular sequela. Studies that have looked at neuropsychologic functioning after BMT have found that the most detrimental effects occurred in patients receiving TBI and those with prior cranial irradiation, as well as those treated at a younger age, particularly those younger than 3 years of age (Cool et al., 1996). Conflicting data exist as to whether similar or less pronounced effects are seen in childhood BMT survivors who did not receive cranial irradiation or TBI, although there is some evidence in small studies that indicates impairment exists in this population (Kramer et al., 1997). The parameters examined in the majority of these studies include evaluation with standard neuropsychologic testing including IQ and find that especially for the irradiated group, there is a significant decline in IQ (Sanders et al., 1990; Christie et al., 1994).

Particular care should be taken when evaluating the survivor of pediatric BMT, including academic achievement and overall cognitive performance. Complete neuropsychologic evaluation should be recommended when any impairment is suspected or routinely recommended for those at greatest risk, namely young age at treatment or recipients of TBI or other cranial irradiation. Early identification of problems can lead to prompt intervention and a better academic outcome for the patient.

Although not as well documented, cognitive dysfunction is not exclusive to the pediatric population. Harder and colleagues (2002) reported on the cognitive functioning and quality of life in 40 adult survivors of bone marrow transplant. He found abnormal functioning in selective attention, executive function, information processing speed, verbal learning, and verbal and visual memory, when compared to population norms. Several factors may be involved in the adult neurocognitive experience and were identified in this study as fatigue, global health, and education level. Clearly, there is much more to be learned about the cognitive function of adult survivors of BMT, but it should be kept in mind when doing a comprehensive evaluation of this population.

Conclusion

In this chapter we have outlined some of the known late effects of BMT, but this is an evolving field of research and care, and much may yet be unknown. As this unique population of patients continues to age, and newer, more aggressive therapies are employed, we may find other unexplored areas.

Although exciting advances continue to evolve in the area of BMT therapies, it is equally important that parallel advances be achieved in the area of late effects. With a thorough understanding of late effects, we may be able to better design up-front therapies to minimize their long-term impact. Although cure of the underlying disease is critical, few would argue that the long-term outcomes are of utmost importance when evaluating any treatment. Patients who have endured and survived these aggressive therapies deserve our ongoing support and research.

References

Al-Fiar, F.Z., Colwill, R., Lipton, J., Fyles, G., Spaner, D., and Messner, H. 1997. Abnormal thyroid stimulating hormone (TSH) levels in adults following allogeneic bone marrow transplants. *Bone Marrow Transplantation, 19*, 1019–1022.

Andre, M., Henry-Amar, M., Blaise, D., Colombat, P., Fleury, J., Miliped, N., et al. 1998. Treatment-related deaths and second cancers risk after autologous stem cell transplantation for Hodgkin's disease. *Blood, 92*, 1933–1940.

Baker, K.S., DeFor, T.E., Burns, L.J., Ramsay, N.K., Neglia, J.P., and Robison, L.L. 2003. New malignancies after blood or marrow stem cell transplantation in children and adults: incidence and risk factors. *Journal of Clinical Oncology, 21*, 1352–1358.

Baker, K.S., Gurney, J.G., Ness, K.K., Bhatia, R., Forman, S.J., Francisco, L., et al. 2004. Late effects in survivors in chronic myeloid leukemia treated with hematopoietic cell transplant: results from the Bone Marrow Transplant Survivor Study. *Blood, 104*, 1898–1906.

Bath, L.E., Critchley, H.O., Chambers, S.E., Anderson, R.A., Kelnar, C.J., and Wallace, W.H. 1999. Ovarian and uterine characteristics after total body irradiation in childhood and adolescence: response to sex steroid replacement. *British Journal of Obstetrics and Gynaecology, 106*, 1265–1272.

Belkacemi, R., Sullivan, K.M., Deeg, H.J., Mori, M., Meyer, W., Fisher, L., et al. 1998. Cataracts after total body irradiation and bone marrow transplantation in patients with acute leukemia in complete remission: a study of the European Group for blood and marrow transplantation. *International Journal of Radiation Oncology, Biology, Physics, 41*, 659–668.

Benyunes, M.C., Sullivan, K.M., Deeg, H.J., Mori, M., Meyer, W., Fischer, L., et al. 1995. Cataracts after bone marrow transplantation: long term follow up of adults treated with fractionated total body irradiation. *International Journal of Radiation Oncology, Biology, Physics, 32*, 661–670.

Bhatia, S., Louie, A.D., Bhatia, R., O'Donnell, M.R., Fung, H., Kashyap, A., et al. 2001. Solid cancers after bone marrow transplantation. *Journal of Clinical Oncology, 19*, 464–471.

Bhatia, S., Ramsay, N.K., Steinbuch, M., Dusenbery, K.E., Shapiro, R.S., Weisdorf, D.J., et al. 1996. Malignant neoplasms following bone marrow transplantation. *Blood, 87*, 3633–3639.

Christie, D., Battin, M., Leiper, A.D., Chesells, J., Vargha-Khadem, F., and Neville, B.G. 1994. Neuropsychological and neurological outcome after relapse of lymphoblastic leukaemia. *Archives of Disease in Childhood, 70*, 275–280.

Cohen, E.P., Lawton, C.A., Moulder, T.E., Becker, C.G., and Ash, R.C. 1993. Clinical course of late-onset bone marrow transplant nephropathy. *Nephron, 64*, 626–635.

Cool, V.A. 1996. Long term neuropsychological risks in pediatric bone marrow transplant: what do we know? *Bone Marrow Transplantation, 18*, 45–49.

Curtis, R.E., Rowlings, P.A., Deeg, J., Shriner, D.A., Socie, G., Travis, L.B., et al. 1997. Solid cancers after bone marrow transplantation. *New England Journal of Medicine, 336*, 897–904.

Curtis, R.E., Travis, L.B., Rowlings, P.A., Socie, G., Kingma, D.W., Banks, P.M., et al. 1999. Risk of lymphoproliferative disorders after bone marrow transplantation: a multi-institutional study. *Blood, 94*, 2208–2216.

Eames, G.M., Crosson, J., Steinberger, J., Steinberger, J., Steinbuch, M., Krabill, K., et al. 1997. Cardiovascular function in children following bone marrow transplant: a cross-sectional study. *Bone Marrow Transplantation, 19*, 61–66.

Enright, H., Haake, R., and Weisdorf, D. 1990. Avascular necrosis of bone: a common serious complication of allogeneic bone marrow transplantation. *American Journal of Medicine, 90*, 733–738.

Fink, J.C., Leisenring, W.M., Sullivan, K.M., Sherrard, D.J., and Weiss, N.S. 1998. Avascular necrosis following bone marrow transplantation: a case-control study. *Bone, 22*, 67–71.

Fletcher, B.D., Crom, D.B., Krance, R.A., and Kun, L.E. 1994. Radiation-induced bone abnormalities after bone marrow transplantation for childhood leukemia. *Radiology, 191*, 231–235.

Frisk, P., Bratteby, L.E., Carlson, K., and Lonnerholm, G. 2002. Renal function after autologous bone marrow transplantation in children: a long-term prospective study. *Bone Marrow Transplantation, 29*, 129–136.

Griese, M., Rampf, U., Hofmann, D., Fuhrer, M., Reinhardt, D., and Bender-Gotze, C. 2000. Pulmonary complications after bone marrow transplantation in children: twenty-four years of experience in a single pediatric center. *Pediatric Pulmonology, 30*, 393–401.

Hard, G.C. 1998. Recent developments in the investigation of thyroid regulation and thyroid carcinogenesis. *Environmental Health Perspectives, 106*, 427–436.

Harder, H., Cornelissen, J.J., Van Gool, A.R., Duivenvoorden, H.J., Eijkenboom, W.H., and van den Bent, M.J. 2002. Cognitive functioning and quality of life in long term adult survivors of bone marrow transplantation. *Cancer, 95*, 183–192.

Harper, G.D., Dicks-Mireaux, C., and Leiper, A.D. 1998. Total body irradiation-induced osteochondromata. *Journal of Pediatric Orthopedics, 18*, 356–358.

Hogarty, A.N., Leahey, A., Zhao, H., Hogarty, M.D., Bunin, N., Cnaan, A., et al. 2000. Longitudinal evaluation of cardiopulmonary performance during exercise after bone marrow transplantation in children. *Journal of Pediatrics, 136*, 311–317.

Huma, Z., Boulad, F., Black, P., Heller, G., and Sklar, C. 1995. Growth in children after bone marrow transplantation for acute leukaemia. *Blood, 86*, 819–824.

Jack, M.K., and Hicks, J.D. 1981. Ocular complications in high-dose chemoradiotherapy and marrow transplantation. *Annals of Ophthalmology, 13*, 709–711.

Jaffe, N., Ried, H.L., Cohen, M., McNeese, M.D., and Sullivan, M.P. 1983. Radiation induced osteochondroma in long term survivors of childhood cancer. *International Journal of Radiation Oncology, Biology, Physics, 9*, 665–670.

Kalhs, P., Panzer, S., Kletter, K., Minar, E., Stain-Kos, M., Walter, R., et al. 1988. Functional asplenia after bone marrow transplantation. A late complication related to extensive chronic graft-versus-host disease. *Annals of Internal Medicine, 109*, 461–464.

Kauppila, M., Irjala, K., Koskinen, P., Pulkki, K., Sonninen, P., Viikari, J., et al. 1999. Bone mineral density after allogeneic bone marrow transplantation. *Bone Marrow Transplantation, 24*, 885–889.

Kempen-Harteveld, M.L., Struikmans, H., Kal, H.B., van der Tweel, I., Mourits, M.P., Verdonck, L.F., et al. 2002. Cataract after total body irradiation and bone marrow transplantation: degree of visual impairment. *International Journal of Radiation Oncology, Biology, Physics, 52*, 1375–1380.

Kist-van Holthe, J.E., Goedvolk, C.A., Brand, P., van Wheel, M.H., Bredius, R.G., van Oostayen, J.A., et al. 2002. Prospective study of renal insufficiency after bone marrow transplantation. *Pediatric Nephrology, 17*, 1032–1037.

Kramer, J.H., Crittenden, M.R., DeSantes, K., and Cowan, M.J. 1997. Cognitive and adaptive behavior 1 and 3 years following bone marrow transplantation. *Bone Marrow Transplantation, 19*, 607–613.

Larsen, R.L., Barber, G., Heise, C.T., and August, C.S. 1992. Exercise assessment of cardiac function in children and young adults before and after bone marrow transplantation. *Pediatrics, 89*, 722–729.

Larsen, R.L., Jakacki, R.I., Vetter, V.L., Meadow, A.T., Silber, J.H., and Barber, G. 1992. Electrocardiographic changes and arrhythmias after cancer therapy in children and young adults. *American Journal of Cardiology, 70*, 73–77.

Lawton, C.A., Cohen, E.P., Barber-Derus, S.W., Murray, K.J., Ash, R.C., Casper, J., et al. 1991. Late renal dysfunction in adult survivors of bone marrow transplant. *Cancer, 67*, 2795–2800.

Leung, W., Hudson, M.M., Strickland, D.K., Phipps, S., Srivastava, D.K., Ribeiro, R.C., et al. 2000. Late effects of treatment in survivors of childhood acute myeloid leukemia. *Journal of Clinical Oncology, 18*, 3273–3279.

Leung, W., Hudson, M., Zhu, Y., Rivera, G.K., Ribeiro, R.C., Sandlund, J.T., et al. 2000. Late effects in survivors of infant leukaemia. *Leukaemia, 14*, 1185–1190.

Lipshultz, S.E., Colan, S.D., Gelber, R.D., Perez-Acayde, A.R., Sallan, S.E., and Sanders, S.P. 1991. Late cardiac effects of doxorubicin therapy for acute lymphoblastic leukemia in childhood. *New England Journal of Medicine, 324*, 808–815.

Machatschek, J., Duda, J., Matthay, K., Cowan, M., and Horn, B. 2003. Immune reconstitution, infectious complications and post transplant supportive care measures after autologous blood and marrow transplantation in children. *Bone Marrow Transplantation, 32*, 687–693.

Matthes-Martin, S., Lamche, M., Ladenstein, R., Emminger, W., Felsberger, C., Topf, R., et al. 1999. Organ toxicity and quality of life after allogeneic bone marrow transplantation in pediatric patients: a single center retrospective analysis. *Bone Marrow Transplantation, 23*, 1049–1053.

Nysom, K., Holm, K., Michaelsen, K.F., Hertz, H., Jacobsen, N., Muller, J., et al. 2000. Bone mass after allogeneic BMT for childhood leukaemia or lymphoma. *Bone Marrow Transplantation, 25*, 191–196.

Ogilvy-Stuart, A.L., and Gleeson, H. 2004. Cancer risk following growth hormone use in childhood: implications for current practice. *Drug Safety, 27*, 369–382.

Olshan, J.S., Willi, S.M., Gruccio, D., and Moshang, T. 1993. Growth hormone function and treatment following bone marrow transplant for neuroblastoma. *Bone Marrow Transplantation, 12*, 381–385.

Pedersen-Bjergaard, J., Anderson, M.K., and Christiansen, D.H. 2000. Therapy-related acute myeloid leukemia and myelodysplasia after high dose chemotherapy and autologous stem cell transplantation. *Blood, 95*, 3273–3279.

Poustchi-Amin, M., Leonidas, J.C., and Elkowitz, S.S. 1996. Simultaneous occurrence of osteosarcoma and osteochondroma following treatment of neuroblastoma with chemotherapy, radiotherapy, and bone marrow transplantation. *Pediatric Radiology, 26*, 155–157.

Sanders, J.E. 1990. Late effects in children receiving total body irradiation for bone marrow transplantation. *Radiotherapy and Oncology, 18*, 82–87.

Schimmer, A.D., Mah, K., Bordeleau, L., Cheung, A., Ali, V., Falconer, M., et al. 2001. Decreased bone mineral density is common after autologous blood or marrow transplantation. *Bone Marrow Transplantation, 28,* 387–391.

Schulenburg, A., Turetschek, K., Wrba, F. Vogelsang, H., Greinix, H.T., Keil, F., et al. 2004. Early and late gastrointestinal complications after myeloablative and nonmyeloablative allogeneic stem cell transplantation. *Annals of Hematology, 83,* 101–106.

Shalet, S.M., and Brennan, B. 2002. Puberty in children with cancer. *Hormone Research, 57,* 39–42.

Sklar, C.A., Kim, T.H., and Ramsay, N.K. 1984. Testicular function following bone marrow transplantation performed during or after puberty. *Cancer, 53,* 1498–1501.

Socie, G., Cahn, J.Y., Carmelo, J., Vernant, J.P., Jouet, J.P., Ifrah, N., et al. 1997. Avascular necrosis of bone after allogeneic bone marrow transplantation: analysis of risk factors for 4388 patients by the Societé Francaise de Greffe de Moelle. *British Journal of Haematology, 97,* 865–870.

Socie, G., Curtis, R.E., Deeg, H.J., Sobocinski, K.A., Filipovich, A.H., Travis, L.B., et al. 2000. New malignant diseases after allogeneic marrow transplantation for childhood acute leukemia. *Journal of Clinical Oncology, 18,* 348–357.

Socie, G., Selmi, F., Seldel, L., Frija, T., Devergie, A., Esperou Bourdeau, H., et al. 1994. Avascular necrosis of bone after allogeneic bone marrow transplantation: clinical findings, incidence and risk factors. *British Journal of Haematology, 86,* 624–628.

Steinherz, L.J., Steinherz, P.G., and Tan, C. 1995. Cardiac failure and dysrhythmias 6–19 years after anthracycline therapy: a series of 15 patients. *Medical and Pediatric Oncology, 24,* 352–361.

Storek, J., Gooley, T., Witherspoon, R.P., Sullivan, K.M., and Storb, R. 1997. Infectious morbidity in long term survivors of allogeneic marrow transplantation is associated with low CD4 T cell counts. *American Journal of Hematology, 54,* 131–138.

Tauchmanova, L., Selleri, C., Rosa, G.D., Pagano, L., Orio, F., Lombardi, G., et al. 2002. High prevalence of endocrine dysfunction in long term survivors after allogeneic bone marrow transplantation for hematologic diseases. *Cancer, 95,* 1076–1084.

Tichelli, A., Duell,T., Weiss, M., Socie, G., Ljungman, P., Cohen, A., et al. 1996. Late-onset keratoconjunctivitis sicca syndrome after bone marrow transplantation: incidence and risk factors. European Group of Blood and Marrow Transplantation (EBMT) Working Party on Late Effects. *Bone Marrow Transplantation, 17,* 1105–1111.

Wollenberg, B., Riera-Knorrenschild, J., Neubauer, A., and Gorg, C. 2001. Functional hyposplenia after allogeneic bone marrow transplantation: a case report. *Ultraschall in der Medizin, 22,* 289–292.

Chapter 13

Family Issues and Perspectives

June Eilers, PhD, APRN, BC

Ann Breen, RN, MN, APRN, OCN®

Introduction

Blood and marrow stem cell transplantation (BMSCT) is a procedure with promise for the individuals involved, because it offers hope in the face of illness. But it is not without risk, and the reawakened hope offered through transplant may actually contribute to emotional stress (Patenaude et al., 1986). The stress of this risk is experienced not only by the transplant recipient, but also by family members, and thus, BMSCT has the potential to impact the family unit. Over time, clinicians and researchers have gained an increased understanding of the profound impact illness, disease, and treatment may have on the entire family unit involved with the transplant recipient. In fact, as early as 1979, Patenaude, Szymanski, and Rappeport reported on the intensity of the potential stress for the family of individuals undergoing transplantation and indicated that it can be one of the most stressful events for families to experience. Literature regarding psychosocial factors in BMSCT has continued to support that this early warning remains valid (Atkins and Patenaude, 1987; Patenaude, 1990; Tomlinson et al., 1993; Andrykowski, 1994a, 1994b; Lesko, 1994; Phipps and Mulhern, 1995; Stetz et al., 1996; Grimm et

al., 2000; Streisand et al., 2000). The challenge for the clinician attempting to prepare families for BMSCT is that the indications for and timing for transplant vary for different diagnoses. In addition, the extent of the impact varies related to extrinsic factors, such as the specific illness or disease and the treatment administered; to the severity of side effects and complications experienced; and to intrinsic factors regarding the family itself and the individuals that make up the family unit.

As BMSCT has become a more widely accepted treatment for many types of cancer and malignant and nonmalignant hematologic disorders as well as autoimmune diseases, the number of transplants continues to escalate (see Chapter 1 for further discssion). Consequently, the number of family members affected by BMSCT is also increasing exponentially. In order to provide optimum care to transplant recipients and their families, it is important to be aware of the potential stress associated with BMSCT and to view this stress and the related risks from the perspective of the family unit. Literature provides evidence for movement in this direction. Futterman and colleagues (1991) included family in their rating scale of emotional difficulties related to BMSCT. The importance of nursing attending to the family was indicated by Tomlinson and colleagues (1993), "the client is dependent on an environment organized to provide highly specific technological interventions, the acuity of illness is often of crisis proportions, and nursing care, though highly specialized, must incorporate family needs unique to this setting" (p. 246). This chapter will address factors related to BMSCT that contribute to the potential stress experienced, factors regarding the family that influence the impact of transplant on the family and their response, and implications for nursing.

Family Framework

"What is meant by family?" is a question that has been addressed over the years in the social sciences and psychology. Family can be understood as the social matrix within which we live and function. For some individuals, this family unit is very clearly delineated along traditional lines of formal marriage and offspring. In other situations, family units may not follow these definitions of family. The last several decades have seen multiple changes in what was formerly seen as the typical family. There are increasing numbers of single-parent families, second marriages, and blended families, as well as individuals who are cohabitants, but not married. All contribute to the wide diversity in family units today. This chapter will not attempt to identify and address each of the multiple options, but will address family generically as emotionally bonded individuals committed to the well-being of the BMSCT recipient. These individuals may or may not be related through bloodlines or by law, but function in such a way that they consider themselves to be family.

In addition, it is worthwhile to note that family is one of the few social organizations in

which membership is based strictly on who you are, rather than what you can do. This can provide comfort and security for the individual members who do not have to work to earn membership in a family, but simply become members by birth or marriage. However, it can add stress when individuals are not performing in the expected manner, but cannot be denied membership in the family. For the most part in this chapter, family will be presented as a single entity. Specific identities and relationships such as spouse/partner and parent/child will be addressed only as indicated to further enhance the content of the chapter.

Sociologists and psychologists have long attempted to gain an increased understanding of the family. Although we frequently hear about the impact of changing times on the family, and questions concerning whether the family can survive, the family unit has been in existence since the beginning of recorded history and is probably the longest standing social institution. As such, the family serves critical functions for society and the individuals involved in the family unit. The major functions of the family have evolved over time with societal changes and can be grouped into three categories: affection, economic cooperation, and socialization of children (Bahr, 1989).

If the family is to accomplish the identified functions efficiently and successfully, the individuals within the family unit must fulfill certain roles. Awareness of the roles of the family members in terms of essential tasks that must be completed for successful family life increases the clinician's ability to assess the impact of illness and treatment on the family. Nye (1976) identified the key roles as provider, housekeeper, child caregiver, child socialization provider, recreational assistant, kinship partner, sexual partner, and therapeutic provider. Families establish their own system for the roles based on the skills, talents, and abilities of the individuals. A family member may assume primary responsibility for a role, two or more individuals may share roles, or in some instances, family members may share the roles with others outside the unit. Once the family has established a system of functioning for the roles, normal interactions and function will be affected if individuals do not fulfill their respective roles. Illness and treatment can interfere with an individual's ability to perform the expected roles in the family. Adjustments must be made for the family to continue functioning in these situations. When a member of a family unit is ill and undergoes a potentially life-threatening procedure such as BMSCT, the rippling effect will be felt throughout the family.

Although nurses cannot be expected to be experts in the family, a basic understanding of family structure and functioning will enhance their ability to be supportive of the family unit. It also increases the likelihood that nurses will be attentive to both the needs of the family members and the critical role the family plays in successful long-term outcomes.

Family Units in BMSCT

Because the age of BMSCT recipients extends from infancy to adults, a wide range of family situations and relationships are represented in the transplant population. Therefore, it is difficult to describe the typical family in BMSCT. Family may be the parents of a child of any age, from infancy to adult; an adult child may be married or single, launched and independent, or remaining at home. Family may be the spouse or other partnered significant other. The partner relationship with the transplant recipient may have been in existence for years or for only a relatively short period of time. Children may be

the siblings of the transplant recipient, or they may be the children or grandchildren. They may be young and require significant direct care, nurturing, and supervision, or they may be older and function essentially independent.

The family units may be any of the multiple types (see **Table 13-1**). Two types of families should be added to this list presented by Schlesinger (1979), nonmarried couples with children and homosexual couples.

Family units in transplant present a varied picture, not only in terms of types and number of members, but also in terms of the ages of the members and duration of time as a family unit. *Family life cycle* is the term used to refer to a set of stages that a family unit typically passes through over the course of existence as a family (Glick, 1977).

As with the developmental stages for the life cycle of individuals, successful fulfillment of the tasks that commonly occur at each of the stages promotes satisfaction and facilitates the likelihood of smooth transition through the life cycle. The beginning of each stage is a time of critical transition that requires changes in roles and tasks

---

Table 13-1 **FAMILY TYPES.**

- Nuclear family: husband, wife, and children
- Childless couple: husband and wife only
- One-parent families: widowed, divorced, separated, and deserted spouses and never married mothers
- Adopted families: husband, wife, and adopted child(ren)
- Reconstituted families: second marriages and blended families
- Communal families: group of families living together with or without children

---

Source: Data from Schlesinger, 1979.

(Barnhill and Longo, 1978; Bahr, 1989). See **Table 13-2** for two examples of proposed stages and a listing of the tasks at the transition points.

The inclusion of the unattached young adult who is between families in Carter and McGoldrick's model (1980) is potentially im-

Table 13-2 STAGES OF FAMILY LIFE CYCLES AND TRANSITION TASKS.

Carter and McGoldrick*	Duvall**	Barnhill and Longo—Transitions***
Unattached young adult between families	Not addressed	Not addressed
New marriage	Married couple without children	Commitment of couple to each other
Family with young children	Childbearing family in which the oldest child is less than 30 months of age	Developing new parental roles, as husband and wife become mother and father
	Family with preschool children, in which the oldest child is from $2^{1}/_{2}$ to 6 years of age	Accepting the new personality as the child grows up
	Family with school children, with the oldest child between 6 and 13 years of age	Introducing the child to institutions outside the family, such as school, church, scouts, guides, sports groups, and so on
Family with adolescents	Family with teenagers, with oldest child between 13 and 20	Accepting adolescence, with the changed roles associated with this and the parents' need to come to terms with the rapid social and sexual changes occurring in their son or daughter
Launching the children and moving on	Family launching young adults, starting with the first child's departure from the home and ending when the last one goes	Allowing the child to experiment with independence in late adolescence and early adulthood; preparations to launch
	Middle-aged parents, from the "empty nest" to retirement	Come to accept their child's independent adult role, including starting his or her own family; letting go—facing each other again, husband and wife alone
Later life	Ageing family members, period from retirement to death	Accepting retirement and/or old age, with the changed lifestyle involved

Sources: *Carter and McGoldrick, 1980; **Duvall, 1977; ***Barnhill and Longo, 1978.

portant for BMSCT, since those involved in transplant frequently include these individuals, either as a recipient or as an adult child of an older BMSCT recipient. Duvall's (1977) delineation of family with children into more components based on age of the children allows clearer differentiation of families in these stages, because of the unique needs of children in the identified age groups. Therefore, in transplantation, it may be beneficial to utilize a combination of the two models. The transitions (Barnhill and Longo, 1978) can be seen as the changes the family must accomplish for smooth progression through the stages of the life cycle.

Numerous factors including illness, treatment, death, separation, divorce, and financial disaster can influence movement through the life cycle for families. Stress and strain from previous events in the life of the family unit can have a lasting effect and affect future coping ability. Thus, a family's current status may be influenced by previous events such as the initial diagnosis and treatment. Clinicians should also be aware of normative transitions that are occurring simultaneous to BMSCT and those that may have been affected by previous stressful events.

Diseases requiring transplant may have actually interfered with plans for marriage and/or children. Thus, individuals and couples may not be at the stage they had intended for themselves prior to the illness and treatment. Since a large portion of these models is based on the presence of children in the family, they may not always provide a direct fit for childless families or families with a wide span of age differences in their children. Although the diversity in families today and preexisting circumstances preclude stringent application of the stages and tasks as mandatory for all families to follow, the concept of family life cycles fosters increased understanding of family stressors that may occur at a given period in time for the family unit. Awareness of the family life cycle stage and accompanying responsibilities will increase clinicians' sensitivity to additional stressors the family unit may be experiencing during transplant.

Involvement of Family During the Transplant Trajectory

Although family involvement is not new to transplant, the focus has changed over time as advances in BMSCT and newer models of care delivery (see Chapter 1 for more information) allow and even expect increased family participation. The majority of the literature currently available regarding BMSCT, however, continues to focus on the transplant recipient. Articles make general references to families, but seldom address their unique needs. Research focusing on families in BMSCT is also limited and primarily pediatric and/or retrospective in nature (Eilers, 1993a, 1993b, 1996; Lee et al., 1994; Nelson, 1994; Sormanti et al., 1994; Phipps, 2002).

Family members have served as donors in allogeneic BMSCT since the time of the early transplants. After informed consent, these individuals were expected to be available for the transplant and potentially serve as a blood component donor if indicated. However, due to the isolation restrictions early in transplant history, direct family involvement with the transplant recipient was very limited. Family members were physically separated from their loved one, with limited, if any, direct contact or activity in the transplant recipient's room. At the same time, family units were frequently disrupted for an extended period of time by the expectation that the transplant recipient, frequently a young person, remain in the transplant city for 100 days posttransplant to allow for monitoring and treating graft-versus-host disease (GVHD).

Thus, at least a portion of the family unit would temporarily relocate to the transplant city. Since there were only a limited number of centers doing transplants, these family members frequently had to travel a great distance.

With gradual changes in transplant protocols and increased sensitivity to the potential benefit to family members and to the BMSCT recipient, more direct family involvement was allowed. Transplant isolation procedures have become less restrictive, and BMSCT has expanded to include autologous transplants. Autologous BMSCT extended the potential number of transplant candidates and the age range of transplant recipients. The expanded availability of pharmaceuticals for infections and the use of growth factors to decrease the length of neutropenia also facilitated this increased involvement by family members. With the shortened hospital stays, the availability of family members was essential so that the BMSCT recipient had a caregiver present as recovery continued in the outpatient setting. The ongoing changes in care delivery models seen in transplant today (see Chapter 1) have implications for families. Increasing numbers of centers are expanding into the practice of performing outpatient transplants (Cavanaugh, 1994). In some instances these programs have very abbreviated inpatient stays (Grimm et al., 2000); in others there is an attempt to provide all of the care outside the traditional acute care hospital setting (Schmit-Pokorny et al., 2003). Family members serve as the primary caregivers for the transplant recipient and are at risk for potential problems related to the roles they assume. As family involvement continues and even increases, there is a definite need for further study in this area.

Nurses are usually aware when family members are with the recipient during transplant and may indicate their presence in documentation. Larson's interviews with transplant recipients found that patients wanted their family members to be present to assist with nonmedical needs, assist with side-effect management, and provide emotional support (1995). The role the family plays in providing support and assistance and the impact of the transplant on the family present has received limited attention and requires further study, as does the impact of the family's emotional state on the transplant recipient (Lee et al., 1994; Winters et al., 1994; Phipps and Mulhern, 1995; Stetz et al., 1996; Grimm et al., 2000; Streisand et al., 2000; Manne, Duhamel, Ostroff, et al., 2003).

Clinicians have learned to value family involvement as a benefit for support and encouragement of BMSCT recipients. However, the ability of families to handle the situations encountered varies, as does the approach taken. At times, incorporation of the family unit may actually increase the time required to care for the transplant recipient. Lesko (1994) spoke to this issue in terms of family becoming second-order patients for nursing staff. BMSCT does not occur in isolation to the other activities and transitions in family life. Families come to transplant with varying prior experience and resources. Especially in the case of long-term illness, families are seldom dealing with only a single illness-induced stressor. An increased understanding of the interrelatedness of the multiple factors involved facilitates the clinician's ability to work effectively with the family unit.

Understanding Family Response to Stressful Situations

McCubbin and McCubbin (1993) use the concept of "pileup" to describe the accumulation of stressors, strains, and transitions over time that families bring with them into new situations. In their Resiliency Model of Family Stress, Adjustment, and Adaptation, the McCubbins have identified six broad categories of stressors and strains that impact how a family adapts to an illness-related situation (see **Table 13-3**).

The actual transplant is not the first major stressor for most of the families in BMSCT. Each has had to deal with the initial diagnosis and the potentially life-threatening aspect of the condition that brings them to transplant (Foster and McLellan, 2000). In addition, families frequently have encountered other nonillness-related stressful situations in their lives, such as natural disasters, job loss, accidents, and difficulties within the family unit. Sensitivity to the potential pileup of stressors and strains from any of the six categories identified is important for a more accurate picture of the family situation in transplant.

Since families respond to situations differently, merely having awareness of the family's previous experiences may not provide the clinician with an adequate view of what to expect from a family unit. Families may have had similar potentially stressful situations in

their lives, but have had differing responses and subsequently respond differently now also. According to the Resiliency Model by McCubbin and McCubbin (1993), family resources, strengths, and capabilities also vary and influence the impact of a given crisis situation. Capability for a family is the potential they have for meeting the demands of a given situation. Resources to aid in this process may be tangible or intangible and may come from the individual family members, the family unit as a whole, or from the community. The family's resources, strengths, and capabilities can actually moderate the impact of the potential crisis of BMSCT for the family (Phipps and Mulhern, 1995).

Therefore, just as it is important not to view only the transplant recipient and exclude family, the current episode in the family's life doesn't tell the whole story for the family unit. A family's previous experience with illness, treatment, and general crisis events in life can have two effects for the family unit. Families could have learned from their previous experience and can use it as stepping stone for future growth as they meet the challenges of BMSCT, or it could act as a

---

Table 13-3 CATEGORIES OF STRESSORS AND STRAINS THAT IMPACT FAMILY.

1. The illness and related hardships over time
2. Normative transitions in the life cycle of individuals and the family unit
3. Prior family strains accumulated over time
4. Situational demands and contextual difficulties
5. Consequences of family efforts to cope
6. Intrafamily and social ambiguity that leave the family and individuals with inadequate guidelines for how to act or cope

Source: McCubbin, M.A., and McCubbin, H.I. 1993. "Families coping with illness: The resiliency model of family stress, adjustment, and adaptation." In *Families, health, & illness,* ed. C.B. Danielson, B. Hamel-Bissell, and P. Winstead-Fry, pp. 21–63. St. Louis: Mosby.

stumbling block and interfere with the family's ability to cope with their current situation. As clinicians care for families in transplant, it is important to be aware of the effect of previous experience.

Family Assessment— Implications for Practice

Direct involvement of the family in BMSCT can increase the support available to the transplant recipient, allow family to have a better understanding of the transplant process, and potentially assist the family in coping with the stressor. However, since this involvement has the potential to actually increase the immediate stress experienced by family members, it is important for clinicians to provide family-focused care and attend to the needs of the family involved with the transplant recipient.

Conducting a family assessment is a critical component of caring for families in the transplant environment. The specific form or format is not as crucial as the information obtained.

This assessment may be performed by the nursing staff or may be provided by other professional psychosocial support services team members, such as psychology or social work specialists, depending on the availability of such services. As an initial step, knowing what type of family unit the transplant recipient's family represents (refer to Table 13-1) will facilitate the continued assessment and aid in the planning of care. Families come to transplant with varied histories and abilities to cope (Wolcott and Stuber, 1992) and cannot be regarded or treated as a homogenous group.

A theoretical model such as McCubbin's Resiliency Model of Family Stress and Coping (1993) can provide clinicians a framework for performing the necessary assessment and guide utilization of the information in planning care. See **Table 13-4** for the basic information that will provide an overview of the family to aid the clinician in developing a family-focused plan of care.

It is also important to be aware of how the BMSCT recipient's illness has affected the family to date. Since transplant is performed at

---

Table 13-4 BASIC FAMILY-FOCUSED ASSESSMENT INFORMATION.

1. Who is in the transplant recipient's family unit?
2. What stage of the family life cycle is the family in at this time?
3. If there are children in the family, what is their developmental stage?
4. Who is planning to be present during the transplant?
5. What is the relationship of these individuals to the transplant recipient?
6. Are there underlying reasons why some members of the family unit will not be present?
7. What other critical incidents has the family experienced? When did these occur?
8. How did the family cope with previous critical incidents?
9. Are there other preexisting or anticipated stressors in the family at the present time?

Source: McCubbin, M.A., and McCubbin, H.I. 1993. "Families coping with illness: The resiliency model of family stress, adjustment, and adaptation." In *Families, health, & illness*, ed. C.B. Danielson, B. Hamel-Bissell, and P. Winstead-Fry, pp. 21–63. St. Louis: Mosby.

various stages of disease trajectories, depending on the specific disease, families may be at different points in their adjustment to the diagnosis. If the diagnosis is fairly recent, families may still be in the crisis state of the initial shock of diagnosis. Other families may have thought they were free of worry of the disease because the individual had been in remission for an extended period of time, but then the disease came back. Such recurrence can be extremely stressful for these families who thought they had already dealt with all of the issues related to the disease. Still other families may have been living with the individual's diagnosis for an extended period of time, with little break from the stress involved.

Assessment of the capability of the family to meet the demands of their current situation involves the identification of the resources and strengths the family has and the coping behaviors and strategies used by the family (McCubbin and McCubbin, 1993). The resources may come from the individuals in the family, the family unit as a whole, or from the community around them. These resources may be tangible, such as financial assistance from the church in their local community, or may be intangible, such as a positive self-identity as a worthwhile individual. Families may see themselves as having a very large support system ready to provide support, or may see themselves as all alone in the process. Distance from home may also influence the perceived availability and importance of some resources for the family.

Although identification of this initial family-related information does not necessarily provide a complete picture of the family, it can aid the clinician in designing a family-focused approach to care. It can also help nurses to determine if more in-depth assessment is necessary and can provide the rationale for making referrals. Although we do not have sufficient research to predict family response to transplant, by collecting the previously identified information, clinicians can begin to identify families who may be at risk for high levels of stress during transplantation.

A word of caution: When multiple family members are present to provide the BMSCT recipient support during transplant, clinicians may obtain varying views regarding the family system from the different family members. Clinicians must be careful not to get caught up in the family struggles. Transplant is not a time to attempt to alter the normal functioning of the family system, unless their usual pattern of function will be detrimental to the well-being of the BMSCT recipient. If families require such extensive counseling, clinicians should refer them to an appropriately qualified therapist. In most situations, it is better to have the family seek such counseling after the current transplant crisis is past.

Potential Stress of BMSCT for Family Members

BMSCT-related factors also have the potential to cause transplantation to be a stressful experience for the transplant recipient and family. Uncertainty is a common theme in the literature regarding the psychological stress associated with transplantation (Atkins and Patenaude, 1987; Erse, 1992; Eilers, 1992, 1993a, 1993b; Lesko, 1994; Haberman, 1995). Mishel's (1988, 1990) theoretical work regarding uncertainty in illness provides a potential framework for increasing our understanding of this phenomenon. Within the context of this framework, it is important for clinicians to be aware that uncertainty is not inherently good nor bad. The impact of the uncertainty on the family is dependent on how the uncertainty is interpreted or framed. Another theme characteristic of BMSCT is the effect of the combination of the high-technology environment, the potential for life-threatening complications, and the hope for positive outcomes (McConville et al., 1990; Eilers, 1993a; Andrykowski, 1994a, 1994b; Lesko, 1994; Cooper and Powell, 1998). The interaction of these multiple factors associated with transplant contribute to the potential stress for the family. Literature review, clinical experience, and research in progress guide the following discussion of these factors and the family in transplant.

BMSCT Decision—Hope, Risk, and Program Selection

Prior to coming to transplant, the potential BMSCT recipients have usually been informed that based on current knowledge, their disease process will most likely lead to premature death unless a different, more aggressive treatment approach is utilized. Thus, family members have been confronted with the potential death of their loved one secondary to the disease process. BMSCT is offered as a treatment option, and at times, as the only hope to slow down the disease or to provide curative treatment (Eilers, 1992, 1993a; Stensland, 1993; Haberman, 1995). Families are also informed that BMSCT is not without significant risk, and if complications arise, they may actually result in the transplant recipient's death even sooner than would have been expected secondary to the disease otherwise. Thus, families must deal with considering an immediately life-threatening procedure at a time when they may or may not fully compre-

hend the life-threatening nature of the current condition. Parents of minor children struggle with the additional stress of having to make such life-and-death decisions for the child (Stevens and Pletsch, 2002). Transplant recipients and families have stated that they almost felt as though they had no choice; if they wanted a chance for longer life, BMSCT was the best option (Eilers, 1999). The uncertainty triggered at the time of the initial discussion about BMSCT continues throughout the transplant process, and can be perceived as stressful, or as presenting hope and promise for the future.

Once the family has connected emotionally with the potential for hope with BMSCT, issues related to insurance coverage, financial eligibility, and program acceptance may become stressors. Insurance coverage for transplantation is not automatic in this era of cost containment in health care. Families without adequate insurance coverage may shift their focus from the stress related to the potential risks of transplantation to a fight with the insurance company or a massive fund-raising campaign. In some instances, families struggle with the uncertainty of not knowing if their loved one will be eligible for BMSCT based on disease-related factors. Families who have experienced stressors in these areas prior to transplant may come into BMSCT with their resistance partially worn down, or they may have been energized by the success of overcoming barriers. The needs of the families who do not make it into transplant programs for reasons related to insurance coverage, financial eligibility, and programs' acceptance criteria have received limited attention in the literature and are beyond the scope of this chapter, but deserve future study.

Although at times transplant recipients/families are offered a choice of transplant programs, in some instances they may not find themselves in the anticipated location. Preferred provider contracts, program experience/specialty, and physician referral patterns influence transplant program selection. This may mean utilizing a transplant center other than the one closest to home and in an unfamiliar community. When transplant recipients/families are offered a choice of programs, they may struggle with uncertainty regarding how to select the right program. Some families conduct extensive information-gathering missions; others select the one that is most convenient. If the transplant recipient develops complications later, the program selection process issue may resurface for those involved in the decision.

Being Away from Home

Since the majority of transplants are performed at large cancer treatment facilities, transplant recipients and families frequently have to travel considerable distances for BMSCT. Thus, they find themselves far removed from usual supports, in an unfamiliar environment, encountering what may be one of the most stressful events in their lives. This may become particularly important for staff to remember if the transplant recipient becomes critically ill, and the spouse or significant other is then left to make major decisions under stress, without the aid or support of their loved one. For some, this may be the first time they have to make critical decisions alone.

The impact of the distance from home has been noted to actually have a varied effect on family members (Eilers and Stensland, 1990; Eilers, 1993a). The greater distance may or may not be an additional stressor. When the transplant center is close to home, family members are often tempted to try to maintain their usual schedule, plus visit and support the transplant

recipient. If the center is too far away to allow frequent short trips back and forth, family members are more likely to have to actually separate from the daily responsibilities of the home environment. These family members have had to do more extensive preparation prior to leaving home and at the time of the BMSCT have commented that once at the transplant site they had to let go of those home maintenance concerns.

The fact that other aspects of the family's life go on while the transplant recipient is having the transplant can cause additional stress for families. The normal functional responsibilities of the family presented earlier in this chapter continue even if the family is separated due to the transplant. Responsibility for practical tasks such as mail, bills, lawn care, and home maintenance may need to be delegated. The ability to accomplish this will depend on the availability of family and community support. The ease with which families are able to do this varies. Family members also struggle with child care responsibilities and their inability to maintain involvement in other family activities, e.g., children's sports games, birthdays, and special events at school.

If there are dependent children in the family, decisions regarding their care must be made prior to the transplant. This includes the range of responsibilities from nurturing and affection to planning for transportation to various activities. Children left at home in the care of others may experience stress related to adjusting to the parent substitutes. In addition, they will experience normal development transitional struggles and may want to know when their parents are returning home. Family members have to strive to find the right balance of time at the transplant center and time at home. They often struggle with the need and desire to be two places at once. Attempts to do so will add to the stress experienced and may lead to exhaustion from making frequent trips between home and the transplant center.

Although there may be adequate insurance coverage for the transplant, this may not include financial coverage for transportation, housing, food, and living expenses for the family member(s) spending time with the BMSCT recipient. Maintaining regular phone contact with other family members not at the transplant center can also add to the expenses. Families experience the stress of these additional out-of-pocket expenses that occur at a time when their income is most likely decreased.

Being at the Transplant Center

Transplant centers usually recommend (and often require) that families consider having someone accompany the transplant recipient to the transplant city and remain available for BMSCT recipient support. This has become particularly true as transplant centers have moved to transitioning more of the transplant services to the outpatient setting and require the presence of a caregiver during the outpatient care. Decisions regarding which family members accompany the BMSCT recipient to the transplant facility are made by family members on an individual basis, on a variety of criteria, and may be a source of contention within the family.

Financial demands on the family, work-related regulations, individual coping abilities, and personal commitments may influence which family members are able to be present at the transplant site. Because membership in families is automatic based on who one is and not on satisfactoriness of relationships and role performance, clinicians should be aware that indi-

vidual family members present may not be accustomed to being together, and may not find the relationship mutually supportive. In addition, the stress of BMSCT may contribute strain to previously stressed relationships and may also impact supportive relationships.

As discussed previously, families in transplant span a wide spectrum in terms of age, relationships, and stage of family life. In some instances, multiple family members who make up an extended family for the BMSCT recipient may share responsibility for being present and supporting the transplant recipient. These family members may take turns being present, or may alternate and attempt to "pass the baton" from one to another.

Parents of adult children who previously have been independent potentially face unique challenges as they accompany their children to transplant settings (Eilers and Stensland, 1989). Although the transplant recipients are adults, able to and required to make their own informed decisions and sign consent forms, to the parents, the adult BMSCT recipient is still their child. These parents struggle with concerns regarding their child's well-being. Since their child has been independent and in some instances already married, the closeness of their relationship varies. In addition, the parent may or may not have been present during the information sharing and informed consent process pretransplant. Thus, they may not be adequately informed regarding the indications for transplant and the potential side effects.

Knowing What to Expect

Preparing families for what to expect in transplant is not a straightforward process (Lesko, 1994). As discussed previously and in other chapters, there are many different BMSCT scenarios,

Families must be adequately prepared for the possible complications, yet be able to maintain a positive attitude and provide support for the BMSCT recipient. A common approach from family members interviewed prior to the transplant of a loved one was a process identified as preparing for the worst and hoping for the best (Eilers, 1993a).

Since the normal expected course for BMSCT varies widely, it is difficult to adequately prepare family members for precisely what to expect. Among the factors that influence the course are the type of transplant, the preparatory regimen, and the overall condition of the transplant recipient prior to transplant. Some transplant recipients have relatively simple courses of short duration and return to a normal level of function fairly soon. Others experience multiple life-threatening complications and repeated setbacks, have extended stays in the hospital, and require an extremely long recovery period. Unfortunately, others experience multiple life-threatening complications and do not survive. Since clinicians cannot predict the precise BMSCT course for a given individual, family members must deal with an inherent amount of uncertainty.

The need for isolation precautions and the risk of life-threatening infections contribute further to the potential stress of BMSCT. Families struggle with the fear of causing a serious infection and frequently assume the role of guard to watch others around their loved one. At the same time, transplant recipients and family members alike often experience the need for closeness, touch, and affection. Thus they struggle as they may not be certain what is allowed or what is too risky.

Although technically under isolation precautions of varying intensity, patients and family members often feel bombarded with excess stimuli. Transplant routines and the involvement of multiple team members limit the amount of private, uninterrupted time. In addition, BMSCT recipients and family members often struggle with the fact that due to the necessary sharing of information among transplant team members, they may feel that everyone knows them, but they don't even know the names of many of the team members. This can especially be problematic in large transplant units and teaching centers.

Making plans and recommendations for visitors while the transplant recipient is at the transplant center may be problematic. Visitors to the transplant center may be allowed as a source of support for the family member who is staying with the transplant recipient. However, family members often experience guilt over their own need for emotional support (Andrykowski, 1994a, 1994b). Families may allow visitors in an attempt to provide additional support to the BMSCT recipient, or to allow the visitor to remain connected with the transplant recipient (especially for children of an adult BMSCT recipient). When transplant recipients experience complications and are at risk of dying, allowing children to visit may be especially important to prepare them emotionally. These same children may require the presence of additional adults to care for them between brief visits to the recipient's room.

Family members who are staying with the transplant recipient may struggle with mixed feelings regarding visitors (Eilers, 1993a). They need to determine if they will assume the role of entertaining the visitors or separate from that responsibility. The condition of the transplant recipient and the willingness of the family member to leave the transplant recipient influence this decision. Some family members want breaks from the facility, and others are not comfortable leaving.

Monitoring visitors to be certain they don't place the transplant recipient at risk for life-threatening infections places additional responsibility on the family members. Some families decide not to allow visitors in an attempt to decrease the risk of exposure to infections. Allowing young children to visit, while beneficial for parents and children, stimulates concerns regarding exposure to contagions and the ability of the child to report symptoms.

Being Family During Transplant

Once the actual transplant process begins and the recipient starts the preparatory treatment, family members' concerns focus on the preparative regimen (Eilers, 1993a, 1993b). Depending on the transplant recipient's diagnosis, stage of disease, and their own prior involvement with the transplant recipient's previous treatment, family members have varying levels of knowledge regarding chemotherapy and radiation therapy. Based on pretransplant information, they often regard the current doses as super high and very dangerous. In fact, they sometimes use the term *supra-lethal* to describe the chemotherapy. At times, family members will make reference to how many times higher the current dose is compared to normal chemotherapy. Although appropriate use of medications can control the majority of the nausea and vomiting for the BMSCT recipient, family member anxiety and recall of this portion of the transplant is intense. They struggle with knowing that high doses are essential to overcome the disease process and not wanting to see their loved one suffer. The conditioning phase of transplant is a very structured time period with specific times for the treatments. Due to the intensity of the treatment and the high expectations for effectiveness, family members are often extremely tense during the

conditioning time period. The medications for treatment and prevention of side effects may alter the cognitive function of the transplant recipients and limit their connectedness with family members, thus the family members may have a sense of being alone.

Family member response to transplant day is varied (Eilers, 1993a, 1993b). For some transplant recipients the day is seen as anticlimactic after the intensity of the preparatory regimen. This same sense is seen in a portion of family members who see it as the transplant team just giving an infusion of blood cells. For others, it is a highly charged, highly emotional day. Since this day signifies the beginning of a new start—hope for the future—they are very concerned that everything goes well. These individuals become concerned if staff portray an attitude that may not indicate adequate attention to detail. Some have indicated that transplant day takes on an almost religious connotation of rebirth. Some family members actually find it physically and emotionally difficult to be present in the room during the transplant. They want to be kept informed regarding progress, and then to know as soon as it is over—that all has gone well. Once the day of the infusion is over, family members become anxious for engraftment and recovery. The uncertainty of the length of time for this to occur contributes to the impact transplant has for them.

When the treatments that are an integral part of transplant cause disfigurement and pain, family members struggle emotionally and in an almost helpless state with the physical impact of the treatment on their loved one (Eilers, 1993a; Lesko, 1994). These changes can include severe mucositis, jaundice, fluid retention, and skin alterations including rashes, blisters, and peeling. Due to the dose intensity in transplant, these physical changes are often much more pronounced than families have seen previously. Not only do family members experience the stress related to these problems occurring in their loved one, but also, due to the intensity of the environment and close identification with family members of other BMSCT patients, just knowing that other transplant recipients are experiencing difficulty can add to the stress (Wolcott and Stuber, 1992). Although their loved one may have experienced side effects with previous chemotherapy treatments, the extremely high doses utilized in BMSCT cause heightened concern. Often these side effects alter the transplant recipient's ability to interact with family members in a pleasant, meaningful manner. Thus the family members may feel all alone and at times rejected by their loved one. Since most family members have not experienced transplant previously, they are uncertain if the side effects they are witnessing are normal or an indication of the potentially severe complications that can lead to death.

Decision making when the transplant recipient becomes critically ill is an area of particular concern for family members. For the spouse of the transplant recipient, it may be the first time in their relationship that a major decision is made without discussing the situation as a couple. When the family members responsible for making the decisions for the adult transplant recipient are the parents of that transplant recipient, they may struggle with feeling they didn't realize just how critical the situation was for their child. If the adult transplant recipient's spouse and parents are both present at the transplant facility, it often requires careful discussions with all members present. Parents of young children also struggle with making decisions for their child, and they may question

their earlier decision for a transplant. Families with multiple adult children sharing the responsibility of being with their parent during transplant often find it difficult to have everyone adequately informed. In each of the family member combinations, family members struggle with not wanting to see their loved one suffer, yet not wanting to give up hope if there is a chance for recovery. Although the transplant recipient must make the decision regarding the transplant initially, if severe complications occur, family members are left with the burden of critical decisions regarding specific aspects of life-support measures. For some families, this is the first time they have had to make such critical decisions regarding another individual's life.

Knowing that the BMSCT recipient's condition can change very quickly has been identified as being even worse than the roller coaster existence discussed with cancer in general. Family members have said it is "more like a yo-yo, it can change so quickly" (Eilers, 1993a). They never quite know what to expect from morning to afternoon and are uncertain when they leave the transplant recipient's hospital room at night what it will be like when they return in the morning. Although family members have been informed regarding potential side effects and complications, it is difficult for them to ascertain if what they are seeing is normal for transplant. Family members usually find it easier to cope with what the transplant recipient is experiencing if the particular changes are within the normal range of what happens in transplantation. Not only are rapid changes stressful for family members who are present, but such changes make it difficult to keep those who are not at the transplant center informed. In addition, BMSCT remains a poorly understood process by those who have not been directly involved. Families are asked by others back home, "Is the surgery is over yet?" "Now that he has had his transplant, is he better?" and so on. Dealing with these individuals can add to family member stress at a time they have little reserve.

Since the length of time of the wait for engraftment varies greatly, family members again face the uncertainty of not knowing (Eilers, 1992, 1993a, 1993b). After the preparatory regimen is completed, the time frame becomes much less predictable. For those involved in coaching the transplant recipient's active participation in care to prevent complications, the inability to impact the return of white cells may be difficult. Growth factors have decreased the length of aplasia in transplantation in general; however, not all cell lines or individuals respond in a predictable manner to the growth factors. The transplant recipient may experience flulike symptoms and other side effects secondary to the growth factors; thus, although the growth factors are seen as potentially beneficial, once again family members struggle with knowing that the transplant recipients have to tolerate bad to get better. In addition, not knowing how long engraftment will take makes it difficult for family members to plan their length of stay at the transplant center. This then makes it difficult for them to plan and make arrangements for their own lives posttransplantation.

Beyond the Acute Phase

Two changes in BMSCT have resulted in decreased number of inpatient days for transplant: earlier dismissals and transitioning of portions of transplant care to the outpatient setting. Whereas families used to be informed they should prepare for a 6- to 8-week hospitalization, stays for most BMSCT recipients are now considerably shorter. This move towards shorter length of inpatient stay and increased care in the outpatient setting has had a mixed impact for families. Transplant recipients and families alike are frequently anxious to be released from the hospital. This gives them the opportunity to be in a more homelike atmosphere in outpatient housing and to gain some sense of control and independence. However, it can also be frightening for family members as caregivers. In the hospital they knew highly skilled staff were always readily available to assist if anything changed. Confidence in the staff helped to decrease concern regarding potential side effects. Family members may find themselves being taught to administer treatments and cares that were formerly provided by staff. They are often uncertain if they will know what to do if something changes, or if they will detect important changes (Eilers, 1992, 1993a, 1993b). Thus, family members question their ability to assume the responsibility being placed on them by the transplant center. For some, the dismissal to outpatient care has been equated to a cutting of the umbilical cord.

Expectations that families will continue care in the outpatient setting can have a mixed effect. Transplant recipients enjoy knowing they no longer require hospitalization and they like being away from the constant reminders of the transplant that are present in the hospital room. Family members appreciate knowing that the BMSCT recipient is well enough to leave the hospital. They are often concerned about the caregiver responsibilities and potential risks that remain. They are insecure regarding their own skill level as care providers and monitors of symptoms. Long hours in the outpatient treatment setting for continued care can also contribute to family member stress during this phase of transplant. When immediate side effects decrease with time and engraftment continues, thus decreasing the risk of infections, family members become more at ease and anticipate a return to normal. As BMSCT continues to change and increasing numbers of transplant recipients have outpatient transplants, its impact on transplant recipients and families will require close monitoring.

Families of transplant recipients who develop graft-versus-host disease (GVHD) and other long-term complications such as renal failure experience new uncertainties. When GVHD persists, the situation encountered by the family is not unlike that reported by cardiac transplant families (Mishel and Murdaugh, 1987). They find they may have traded one disease process for another. They had hoped for the best and anticipated a return to good health. When GVHD or other problems change the reality of the outcome of BMSCT, they need to redesign their dream. Fear and uncertainty persist as they realize the GVHD may become life-threatening. Family response in these situations requires further study.

Intervening for the Family in BMSCT

As the discipline with the largest number of members on the team and the most direct contact time with the transplant recipient and family, nurses play a key role in both promoting and providing family-focused care in transplant programs. In addition to their responsibility for the traditional direct physical care of the BMSCT recipient, nurses serve as educators, advocates, comforters, and care directors. Throughout these responsibilities, nurses role model many aspects of the care needed.

Emotional, educational, and social support need to be integrated into all aspects of the transplant program. The different phases of transplantation require focused nursing interventions that are designed to promote adjustment along the transplant trajectory. (See **Figure 13-1** for an illustration of the phases of transplant and recipient-related problems that may occur during the different time periods.) Nurses should meet formally with the transplant recipients and family members to provide them with information at each major transition throughout the transplant trajectory. Vital transitions include discharge from the hospital and departure from the transplant center to home. Recipients and caregivers need extensive counseling, education, and support at each of these transitions. Remaining accessible by asking recipients and caregivers/family members if they have any unanswered questions or unmet needs throughout the process promotes trust in the nurse and facilitates individualization of nursing interventions based on the family's experience.

Group classes are another effective form of intervention and education. Recommended class topics include overview of the transplant process, transplant definitions, team member roles, patient and caregiver roles, infection control, symptom management, common situations, and medications. Providing a quick reference guide regarding potential side effects and situations helps family members to determine when a symptom or concern requires emergent care or when consultation at the next scheduled appointment is soon enough.

Classes that review scenarios and typical clinical examples facilitate anticipatory guidance and educational and psychological preparation. The scenarios promote discussion within the family and the opportunity to rehearse potential prob-

---

Figure 13-1 TIME FRAME FOR RECOVERY PROCESS: STEPS ALONG THE ROAD.

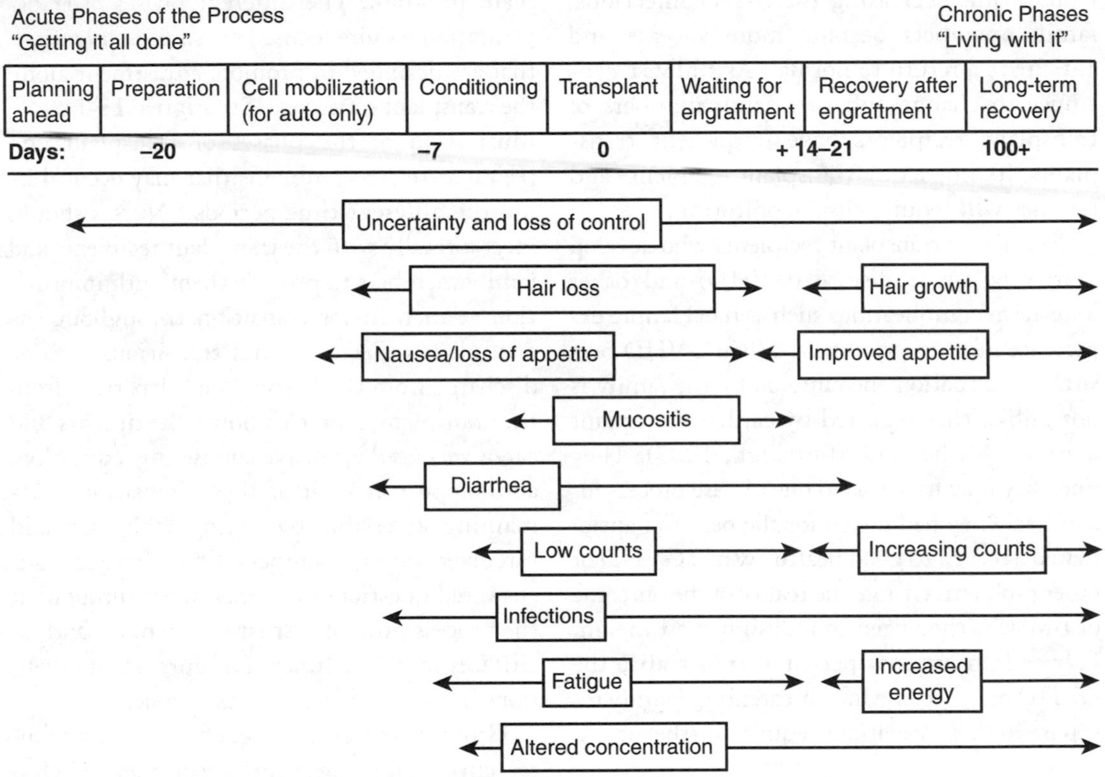

Acute Phases of the Process   Chronic Phases
"Getting it all done"   "Living with it"

Planning ahead	Preparation	Cell mobilization (for auto only)	Conditioning	Transplant	Waiting for engraftment	Recovery after engraftment	Long-term recovery
Days:	−20		−7	0	+14–21		100+

Uncertainty and loss of control

Hair loss   Hair growth

Nausea/loss of appetite   Improved appetite

Mucositis

Diarrhea

Low counts   Increasing counts

Infections

Fatigue   Increased energy

Altered concentration

Source: Adapted from Seattle Cancer Care Alliance. (2001). *Preparing for Transplants.* Seattle, WA:

---

lems. Recipients and family caregivers can "try on" some situations and consider how they would handle the common outpatient transplant situations. Role-playing typical clinical examples allows the BMSCT recipient and family to develop confidence in handling the myriad problems that may develop throughout the treatment process. It also provides a dose of stress inoculation, which creates self-confidence before there is a need to act in an urgent or emergent situation.

The emotional and educational needs in all phases of treatment can be overwhelming from both the caregiver/family member and BMSCT recipient's perspective. Therefore, information should be tailored to suit the treatment phase as well as the learning and emotional styles of the family members and BMSCT recipients. One guiding principle for individualizing care is assessing the ability and desire of the learner to hear or receive the information. The level of involvement and need or desire for information also varies from person to person. The educational and support processes must provide many opportunities for teaching, assessment, repetition, and reinforcement. The nurse must acknowledge and assess level of uncertainty, depression, stress, role strain, and anxiety at every phase of the transplant process.

Since it is possible that not all family members have received the pretransplant information shared with the transplant recipient, the nurse should determine what family members already know about transplant. Providing a resource manual that outlines the transplant process is beneficial upon arrival at the transplant center. A suggested outline is as follows: the transplant program, navigating the clinic, navigating the inpatient departments, steps through the transplant process, managing care at home, managing central lines, medications, and long-term recovery (Seattle Cancer Care Alliance, 2001). The manual is then available as a reference to guide families not only in the acute phases of transplantation, but also through long-term follow-up after the BMSCT recipient leaves the center. The manual can be used by all of the team members as a method to introduce and reinforce information throughout the transplant trajectory. Use of the manual also helps to create consistency among treatment providers and families, thereby enhancing confidence in the treatment team and system.

Throughout the transplant process nurses should ensure that caregivers/family members and recipients are able to meet their safety needs. The focus should be on essential knowledge first and enrichment if time and emotional energy allow them to appreciate the additional information. Safety needs include line care, infection control guidelines, and understanding access to medical and nursing assistance 24 hours a day. Detailed discussions regarding side effects and possible complications need to occur when the caregiver and recipients are able to process the information. Information needs to be repeated in multiple formats and methods with an awareness of when they are going to need the information for self-care and increased understanding of signs and symptoms (see Figure 13-1).

The high-tech environment that is so common to transplant center staff is often foreign and therefore possibly threatening to family members. Nurses play a critical role in fostering a sense of familiarity with the technology in the environment and an adequate level of understanding regarding what is expected (Cooper and Powell, 1998). Bridging this gap between the medical environment and the family is critical throughout the transplant trajectory as family members strive to ascertain if the current problem or concern is cause for panic. Staff can aid family members in determining what side effects and problems are common to transplant versus those that are cause for major concern for the life of the recipient by reviewing the expected side effects and potential life-threatening complications for each phase of the trajectory.

Advocating for Family Members

It is important for nurses to advocate for family-focused care in BMSCT. Transplantation actually places family members in a paradoxical situation. They have been informed of the negative of the underlying disease process and the hope that transplantation offers, but that transplantation is not without significant risk. Thus, they come to transplant prepared for the worst and hoping for the best (Eilers, 1999). Their behaviors must be understood from this perspective. BMSCT recipients and family members may require additional help when no one is listening or they are responding in a manner that is not typical for them. Nurses can assist family members to articulate their concerns and can serve as interpreters of information they may not have understood. In a similar manner, nurses serve as care directors, helping families identify the need to involve team members from other disciplines. Scheduling appointments and confirming the availability of family members as caregivers often also falls within the realm of nursing in the outpatient setting.

Facilitating Coping

The emotional support provided by a nurse with a listening ear can facilitate coping during the stressful times of transplant. Support becomes especially important when the transplant recipient is critically ill and the family members need to make difficult decisions. This may become even more important if the transplant recipient dies and the family members feel responsible based on the decisions they made.

Different coping strategies can be effective depending upon personality and lifetime patterns of stress management (Folkman et al., 1996). Some individuals require more information and factually based strategies that promote understanding. These people tend to respond well when information provides them with the ability to make informed choices concerning treatment needs and strategies. Others want only the information that they need to know at any given point in time. At times the need to know may shift from minimal to maximal detail and back again. Careful listening and assessment allows for accommodations at the appropriate times to enhance coping and learning.

Self-efficacy training or other interventions that facilitate the participant's confidence in their own self-control can help the participant feel as if they have more instrumental control. This is especially important when the partici-pants perceive the illness and treatment process as an external influence leaving them powerless and ineffective. Objective, structured clinical examinations (OSCEs) have been tested as an approach for validating family members' competency as caregivers (Heermann et al., 2001).

Needs of Family as Caregivers

Family members in the role of caregiver can benefit from a clear understanding of their responsibilities. This can be in the form of a job description and information regarding methods of coping with the role that has been thrust upon them (see **Figure 13-2**). Family members need to understand the rationale for self-care. They often struggle with the concept of self-care for themselves because they are so concerned about the BMSCT recipient's well-being (see **Figures 13-3** and **13-4**). The transplant team should explain to family members that if they do not take care of themselves they will find themselves frustrated and irritable, lose perspective, and possibly become physically ill. This explanation assists them to see the rationale for self-care and hopefully makes them feel as if they have permission to take care of themselves. Self-care in the form of exercise, eating right, and taking time for self are examples that have been beneficial. Keeping a diary or journal and accepting help from volunteers should also be encouraged as potential options.

Acknowledge the role confusion and strain that affect normal family relations and responsibilities as the transplant recipient necessarily becomes more dependent through the transplant process. When people arrive at the transplant center, their anxiety level is very high until they build trust with the transplant team. Transplant staff should promote normal family functioning whenever possible (e.g., school attendance for school-aged

---

Figure 13-2 Outline of typical caregiver responsibilities.

Making Arrangements
  Transportation
  Financial
  Tracking appointments

Giving Emotional Support
  Being physically present
  Giving encouragement

Providing Physical Care
  Identifying changes in patient's condition
  Reporting patient's symptoms to health-care staff
  Obtaining medical care if needed
  Monitoring patient compliance in self-administration of oral medications
  Recording medications taken/administered
  Acquiring and maintaining medical supplies
  Performing tasks such as central line care
  Administering fluids and medications using an intravenous pump

Maintaining the Home Environment
  Cleaning
  Food preparation
  Shopping

Patient Advocacy
  Gathering information and assuring that pertinent information is given to medical staff
  Helping with decision making

Providing Assistance/Support to Others
  Serving as a communication link with other family members or friends
  Imparting information to children
  Providing child care

Source: Adapted from Seattle Cancer Care Alliance, 2001.

children) and work with the child-life specialists to promote age-appropriate information. Younger children often appreciate a specially designed coloring book that provides a simple overview about the process, such as *My Journey: Through a Bone Marrow/Stem Cell Transplant* (Beasley et al., 1999). Family should be encouraged to celebrate birthdays, anniversaries, and other significant dates whenever possible.

Distance from their home community and the availability of significant others influence the social support perceived by individuals during transplant (Amato et al., 1998). Enhancing

family participation in transplantation increases the support available for the transplant recipient, but may add stress for the family member who feels isolated. Support groups and peer-to-peer linkups contribute support during the transplant trajectory. Internet access permits the creation of virtual communities and serves as a new method to facilitate social coping. Caregivers may want to consider a group e-mail, voice mail, or make special arrangements for phone message updates to be passed on to multiple individuals so they have an efficient method of keeping other friends and family

---

Figure 13-3 Taking care of the caregiver.

Caregivers are encouraged to take care of themselves through exercise, proper diet, and adequate sleep. The caregivers can benefit from breaks.
   Here are some helpful tips from Rosalynn Carter's book, *Helping Yourself Help Others*:

1. Listen to your friends. Be open to others' observations.
2. Let go. Know your limits.
3. Focus on your loved ones' strengths.
4. Learn relaxation techniques.
5. Take care of your health.
6. Maintain a life outside your caregiving role.
7. Keep a daily "burnout log."
8. Insist on private time.
9. Build a caregiving team.
10. Rely on your sense of humor.
11. Appreciate the benefits of leisure time.
12. Help your loved one find a support group.
13. Seek professional help.
14. Appreciate your own efforts.
15. Seek spiritual renewal.

Source: Adapted from Seattle Cancer Care Alliance, 2001.

---

members informed as they go through this long experience. These methods allow the caregivers to conserve time and emotional energy through the acute and demanding phase of transplant and yet sense the support of others. Families may also want to have friends videotape activities in the local community so they can remain connected. This may be especially beneficial if children at home are involved in sports activities and other events the parent would normally attend in person. Perceived social support has been identified as contributing to transplant related quality of life (Molassiotis et al., 1997).

Complementary therapies can be beneficial for family members experiencing stress during transplantation. Family members should be encouraged to continue stress reduction measures such as relaxation and music therapy that they have practiced previously. Creating context with humor and perspective at every stage of the transplant process can also help the recipient cope with the challenges of illness and treatment. Humor has been associated with a reduction in maternal depressive symptoms during the transplant process (Phipps, 2002; Manne et al., 2003).

Transplant Phase— Guided Care

A family's educational and psychological needs can be divided into two major time periods (see Figure 13-1). During the initial acute needs time period, care recipients tend to focus first on the need to know and second on getting it all done. This first phase can be broken down into steps including planning ahead, preparation, conditioning, transplant, waiting for engraftment, and recovery after engraftment. Most of these steps occur during the recipient's time at the transplant center.

The second major phase, long-term recovery, begins as the individuals recognize the fact that the recovery process is actually a chronic one. The transplant recipient and family members need to learn about living with it. In addition, it is important to remember that family members may not move through the phases simultaneously or in concert with the recipient. Awareness of where the family members are in the adjustment process will aid nurses as they provide care. The transition between the major phases is gradual. The steps may not always occur at a specific point in time or in the same sequence. However, a common psychological shift occurs when recipients depart from the transplant center.

Figure 13-4 Recommendations for caregiver support during the transplant process.

We hope these recommendations will assist families in anticipating the need for caregiver support. **Patients' needs change throughout the transplant process.** Patients benefit from different levels of caregiver support during the different phases.

Inpatient Phase: Patients do not require caregivers, but do appreciate and benefit from emotional support from family and friends.

Ambulatory Phases and Support Levels: Caregivers are very important in providing care when the patient is ambulatory.

A. **Consistent Support:** *Definition*—Caregiver is present the majority of the time; breaks should be less than 3 to 4 hours. **Patients left alone should have access to the phone, the ability to contact emergency services, the ability to operate ambulatory pumps, the ability to get to the restroom, and access to food and fluids.**
   Criteria for recommending a consistent caregiver for the patient are:
   1. During conditioning (including phenytoin administration), chemotherapy, and radiation therapy
   2. First 1 to 2 weeks in the clinic after initial discharge after transplant
   3. Three different IV infusions such as hydration, medications, or hyperalimentation over a 24-hour period
   4. Neutropenia (absolute neutrophil count [ANC < 500])
   5. Altered mental status—drowsy, confused, impaired judgment, poor memory
   6. Weakness/limited mobility (cannot walk without assistance)
   7. Sliding scale insulin (when starting therapy)
B. **Intermittent Support:** *Definition*—Does not need a caregiver majority of hours within a 24-hour period. A caregiver is available 2 to 3 times per day to provide assistance with dressing changes, medications, transportation, and processing information provided during conferences or clinic visits.
C. **Minimal Support:** *Definition*—Patients do not require a caregiver, but do benefit from emotional support during a clinic visit and conferences.

Source: Adapted from Seattle Cancer Care Alliance, 2001.

The detailed information traditionally associated with the acute phase of the transplant trajectory as depicted in Figure 13-1 provides for more targeted interventions. This helps families learn to anticipate how to cope with the specific problems such as mucositis, nausea, loss of appetite, and diarrhea that commonly occur during specific time periods, as included in the figure. If the caregiver knows when to make saline rinses in an outpatient or home setting and when to call for help, the caregiver and transplant recipient feel more confident in the outpatient home setting. Enhancing the awareness of the overall time frame from pretransplant through the recovery phase provides families a positive perspective during the very serious acute phases of transplantation. The care recipients need to understand what the expected side effects are, what interventions are indicated, and what possible complications may occur during the acute phase of the process. Family members engage in watchful waiting during the acute phase and need the opportunity to ask questions frequently each day.

Prior to Arrival

Although seldom addressed in the literature, potential transplant recipients and family members often are initially informed of the need to consider a transplant long before their first contact with an actual transplant center. It is at this time that they may seek information from health-care providers who are not adequately informed about transplantation. These individuals may inadvertently provide answers that will misguide the information seeker. For this reason it is important for transplant programs to strive to inform non-BMSCT health-care providers and the public about transplantation. Professional organizations such as the Oncology Nursing Society and the National Bone Marrow Donor Program can also play a role in facilitating networking among health-care providers.

Programs need to have an organized process in place to provide information and education before the transplant recipient and family arrive at the transplant center. Efforts should focus on being certain that from the initial point of contact with the transplant center, all information provided to families is accurate and consistent. All personnel must be adequately informed to be able to connect families with the team members responsible for providing the initial information. It is beneficial when informed individuals answer questions over the phone and provide an overview of the transplant process. Following this with written and video information that outlines the transplant process can facilitate anticipatory coping to help the family prepare for its forthcoming experience. Suggested content includes overview of the clinical program, basics of transplant biology, role of the donor, fertility, steps of the transplant process, role of the caregiver, and definition of terms. Nurses should encourage questions and provide a list of phone numbers so people can ask questions before they arrive for transplantation. The potential BMSCT recipient should be encouraged to share the information they receive with family members and other individuals who will be involved with them during the transplant process.

Upon Arrival and Prior to Transplant

During the pretransplant period, nurses have a responsibility to work closely with the transplant team to be certain that the transplant recipient and family are adequately informed regarding transplant in order to make the best decision at the time. An extended meeting with the physician and other team members provides the transplant recipient and family an opportunity to hear information that is specific for their own situation as compared to the generalized information in the mass communication options. Although it is essential to be sure the transplant recipient and family have made an informed decision regarding transplantation, once the decision has been made clinicians must be careful not to cause continued second-guessing regarding the wisdom of the decision. Families need to conserve their coping energy to proceed through the process, instead of questioning prior decisions and events.

The transplant team should assess the family communication and stress management style, particularly noting the coping strategies that have worked for them in the past. The assessment ideally should be done by the social worker, psychologist, or nurse on the family's arrival to the center. The information obtained from this assessment should form the entire transplant team's approach towards working with the family (Saleh and Brockopp, 2001).

The assessment can be a guide initially to provide tailored and individualized intervention. The team should inform transplant recipients and families of the psychosocial services available, including one-to-one counseling and support groups, and of the spiritual services offered inpatient, outpatient, and in the community.

During Conditioning and on the Day of Transplant

As the transplant recipient starts on the conditioning regimen, reinforce the information offered during the initial time period. Offer to answer questions and review the expected side effects and complications related to this time period. Nurses should remain aware that the perception of family members and the transplant recipients are likely to differ during this time since the recipients may be medicated to prevent nausea and vomiting. If so, this lack of connectedness with the recipient and/or the desire to not cause additional stress for her or him may cause family members to feel alone. Therefore, it is important to provide consistent psychological support during this highly stressful time for the family. The transplant team should reinforce the availability of psychological and spiritual resources.

Posttransplant Recovery

Ongoing care after the day of transplant involves reviewing what to expect in the immediate posttransplant period. Care recipients in the hospital posttransplant and their family members need preparation for discharge so that they are aware of their care responsibilities. Nursing staff should review infection control, how to access help 24 hours per day, a typical outpatient time frame, common posttransplant problems, medications, coping with the recovery process,

home infusion, and schedules. The length of time at the transplant center for this phase depends on the type of transplant and the transplant recipient's complications. Staff shold use relevant metaphors to help everyone maintain a realistic and productive perspective of the experience during what can be an extended time period (e.g., this is like a triathlon and you are in the swimming phase with more phases to go).

Long-Term Recovery— Living with It

Transplant-related problems are not always emergent or acute, nor do they end when the transplant recipient is dismissed to return home. As families are getting ready to leave the center and return to their home environment, they need assistance preparing to cope with long-term problems. Dismissal teaching prior to the BMSCT recipient's departure from the center can assist with this transition. The needs of the allogeneic and autologous recipient are quite different at this stage of the process. Depending on the type of transplant and the conditioning regimen, instruction should include such topics as monitoring for and preventing infection, human sexuality, early menopause, infertility, cataracts, fatigue, joint changes, and steroid-induced diabetes. Posttransplant recipients are often tired and sick of being tired. Since a leading complaint after 1 year posttransplant is fatigue (Baker, Zabora, et al., 1999), and 50% of patients who have had an allogeneic transplant are at risk of developing chronic graft-versus-host disease, which can affect many body systems (Flowers et al., 2002), these topics are especially crucial.

Chronic physical and neuropsychological problems take a toll on the recipient and family members. Many patients report depression posttransplant. Loss of memory and ability to focus is one of the most frustrating aspects of the long-term recovery process.

In addition, transplant recipients and family members have to live with the lingering concern of recurrence and may need additional support as they address this issue. These are large burdens to cope with, and they often surface after the families have left the transplant center (White, 1994). Thus they need to know who to turn to for the necessary ongoing support and information. Emotional adjustment and reintegration into the community, work, and school settings are also important.

Some families describe the reintegration process as smooth, and others describe a more challenging process. Individuals describe delayed stress disorders after transplant (Manne et al., 2002); others describe feeling as though they are apart from other people after the transplant experience. Recovery takes more than a year for many allogeneic transplant patients. Some patients are not themselves for 3 to 5 years (Syrjala et al., 2004). Role adjustments are necessary when the transplant recipient reclaims roles in the family as he or she gradually experiences increased strength and concentration.

Transplant recipients are glad to be alive, but frustrated with physical and emotional problems they are left to live with as a result of the treatment. Refer to Chapter 12 for information on long-term late effects that challenge transplant recipients and their family members. Parents of young children often face additional problems. Sormanti, Dungan, and Rieker (1994) found that although most parents cope well posttransplant, financial strains and fears of relapse remain. In general, families express a new appreciation for life and a realignment of priorities. Further study will be necessary to

better understand the long-term impact of BMSCT on families.

Implications for Future Research

More research is needed to advance the science of nursing care of the family in BMSCT. At this time, limited research has been conducted in the arena. Challenges to family-focused research in BMSCT stem from the diversity of the individuals involved, the wide spectrum of transplant trajectories, and the multiple interactions possible. The potential for future family-focused research in BMSCT is great because we lack the necessary replication to advance the science of our care. As clinicians, we are dependent on other sources of evidence to guide our practice and establish standards for care.

Conducting psychosocial research in BMSCT requires the use of valid and reliable measures. This includes measures of the independent variables that can be used for individuals and for families. Unfortunately, few instruments have been tested in this population. In addition, we still lack consensus regarding the outcome measures that best reflect the desired dependent variables. Measurement of the dose of nursing interventions such as teaching and support are also lacking.

Research of families in BMSCT should not be limited to the families during and after transplantation. The individuals/families who decide against transplant or are not eligible for transplantation also deserve careful attention. In addition, families of individuals who died during transplantation require careful study. Does the grief process for these individuals differ significantly from that of families who experience the death of individuals who decided not to attempt BMSCT or were regarded as not eligible for the procedure?

Summary

Family involvement in BMSCT has changed greatly since the early transplants when the recipients were in strict isolation for extended periods of time and family members were not allowed in the rooms. Today a concern at the other end of the continuum may well be the burden on the family of serving in a primary caregiver role during a potentially life-threatening procedure. Family members are extremely important in BMSCT. They provide the recipient with essential emotional support, serve as a connection with the past and future in terms of motivation for having the transplant, provide health-care practitioners with knowledge regarding the recipient, assist with care, and oversee daily routines. Family members' abilities and resources to fulfill these roles varies greatly. Since we lack solid research data regarding proven interventions for supporting families in transplant, we must base our care on the currently available information, the experience of individuals with expertise in transplant, and information that can be extrapolated from other clinical areas. Nurses play a key role in supporting families and enabling them to cope with the stressors associated with transplantation.

References

Amato, J.J., Williams, M., Greenberg, C., Bar, M., Lo, S., and Tepler, I. 1998. Psychological support to an autologous bone marrow transplant unit in a community hospital: A pilot experience. *Psycho-Oncology* 7: 121–125.

Andrykowski, M.A. 1994a. Psychiatric and psychosocial aspects of bone marrow transplantation. *Psychosomatics* 35(1):13–24.

Andrykowski, M.A. 1994b. Psychosocial factors in bone marrow transplantation: A review and recommendations for research. *Bone Marrow Transplantation* 13: 357–375.

Atkins, D.M. and Patenaude, A.F. 1987. Psychosocial preparation and follow-up for pediatric bone marrow transplant patients. *American Journal of Orthopsychiatry* 57(2):246–252.

Bahr, S.J. 1989. *Family Interaction.* New York: Macmillian.

Baker, F., Marcellus, D., Zabora, J., Polland, A.S., Jodrey, B.A., and Jodrey, D. 1997. Psychological distress among adult patients being evaluated for bone marrow transplantation. *Psychosomatics* 38(1):10–19.

Baker, F., Zabora, J., Polland, A., and Wingard, J. 1999. Reintegration after bone marrow transplantation. *Cancer Practice* 7(4):190–197.

Barnhill, L.H., and Longo, D. 1978. Fixation and regression in the family life cycle. *Family Process* 17:469–478.

Beasley, B., Charuhas, P., Chouinard, M., Lange, L., Sever, S., Springer, B., et al., 1999. *My journey: Through a bone marrow/stem cell transplant.* Seattle, WA: Fred Hutchinson Cancer Research Center.

Carter, G.A., and McGoldrick, M. 1980. *The family life cycle: A framework for family therapy.* New York: Gardner Press.

Carter, R. and Golant, S.K. 1995. *Helping yourself help others: A book for caregivers.* New York: Random House.

Cavanaugh, C.A. 1994. Outpatient autologous bone marrow transplantation: A new frontier. *Quality of Life— A Nursing Challenge* 3(2):25–29.

Cooper, M.C., and Powell, E. 1998. Technology and care in a bone marrow transplant unit: Creating and assuaging vulnerability. *Holistic Nursing Practice* 12(4): 57–68.

Duvall, E.M. 1977. *Marriage and family development.* 5th ed. Philadelphia: J.B. Lippincott.

Eilers, J. 1992. Qualitative research: An approach to increase our understanding of the impact of BMT on family members. *Oncology Nursing Forum* 19(2):311.

Eilers, J. 1993a. The experience of family members of bone marrow transplant patients. Presentation at International Bone Marrow Transplant Symposium. Seattle, WA.

Eilers, J. 1993b. Measurement of uncertainty in family members of bone marrow transplant patients. *Oncology Nursing Forum* 20(2):334.

Eilers, J. 1996. Factors that influence the impact of bone marrow transplantation for family caregivers of adult transplant recipients. Diss. for PhD at University of Nebraska Medical Center College of Nursing.

Eilers, J. 1999. The care partner's perspective: Is the glass half empty or half full? Paper presented at Blood and Marrow Stem Cell Transplantation: Mobilizing Our Potential for the Next Millennium conference. Sept. 30–Oct. 2, Omaha, NE.

Eilers, J., and Stensland, S. 1989. *Parents of adults with cancer: An initial look at the experience.* Unpublished paper.

Eilers, J., and Stensland, S. 1990. Survey of patients' and family members' perceptions of bone marrow transplantation. *Oncology Nursing Forum* 17(2 Suppl.):211.

Ersek, M. 1992. The process of maintaining hope in adults undergoing bone marrow transplantation for leukemia. *Oncology Nursing Forum* 19(6):883–889.

Flowers, M.E., Parker, P.M., Johnston, L.J., Matos, A.V., Storer, B., Bensinger, W.I., et al. 2002. Comparison of chronic graft-versus-host disease after transplantation of peripheral blood stem cells versus bone marrow in allogeneic recipients: Long-term follow-up of a randomized trial. *Blood* 100(2):415–419.

Folkman, S., Lazarus, R.S., Dunkel-Schetter, C., DeLongis, A., and Gruen, R. 1996. Dynamics of a stressful encounter: Cognitive appraisal, coping, and encounter outcomes. *Journal of Personality and Social Psychology* 50(5):992–1003.

Foster, L., and McLellan, L., 2000. Cognition and the cancer experience. *Cancer Practice* 8(1):25–31

Futterman, A.D., Wellisch, D.K., Bond, G., and Carr, C.R. 1991. The psychosocial levels system: A new rating scale to identify and assess emotional difficulties during bone marrow transplantation. *Psychosomatics* 32(2):177–186.

Glick, P.C. 1977. Updating the life cycle of the family. *Journal of Marriage and the Family* 39:5–13.

Grimm, P.M., Zawacki, K.L., Mock, V., Krumm, S., and Frink, B.B. 2000. Caregiver responses and needs: An ambulatory bone marrow transplant model. *Cancer Practice* 8(3):120–128.

Haberman, M. 1995. The meaning of cancer therapy: Bone marrow transplantation as an exemplar of therapy. *Seminars in Oncology Nursing* 11(1):23–31.

Heermann, J.A., Eilers, J., and Carney, P. 2001. Use of modified OSCEs to verify technical skill performance and competency of lay caregivers. *Journal of Cancer Education* 16:93–98.

Larson, P.J. 1995. Perceptions of the needs of hospitalized patients undergoing bone marrow transplant. *Cancer Practice* 3(3):173–179

Lee, M.L., Cohen, S.E., Stuber, M.L., and Nader K. 1994. Parent-child interactions with pediatric bone marrow transplant patients. *Journal of Psychosocial Oncology* 12(4):43–60.

Lesko, L.M. 1994. Bone marrow transplantation: Support of the patient and his/her family. *Supportive Care in Cancer* 2:35–49.

Manne, S., Duhamel, K., Nereo, N., Ostroff, J., Parsons, S., Martini, R., et al. 2002. Predictors of PTSD in mothers of children undergoing bone marrow transplantation: The role of cognitive and social processes. *Journal of Pediatric Psychology* 27(7):607–617.

Manne, S., Duhamel, K., Ostroff, J., Parsons, S., Martini, R., Williams, S., et al. 2003. Coping and the course of mother's depressive symptoms during and after pediatric bone marrow transplantation. *Journal of the American Academy of Child & Adolescent Psychiatry* 42(9):1055–1068.

McConville, B.J., Steichen-Asch, P., Harris, R., Neudorf, S., Sambrona, J., Lampkin, B., et al. 1990. Pediatric bone marrow transplants: Psychological aspects. *Canadian Journal of Psychiatry* 35:769–775.

McCubbin, M.A., and McCubbin, H.I. 1993. Families coping with illness: The resiliency model of family stress, adjustment, and adaptation. In *Families, health, & illness*, eds. C.B. Danielson, B. Hamel-Bissell, and P. Winstead-Fry (21–63). St. Louis: Mosby.

Mishel, M.H. 1988. Uncertainty in illness. *Image: Journal of Nursing Scholarship* 20(4):225–232.

Mishel, M.H. 1990. Reconceptualization of the uncertainty in illness theory. *Image: Journal of Nursing Scholarship* 22(4):256–262.

Mishel, M.H., and Murdaugh, C.L. 1987. Family adjustment to heart transplantation: Redesigning the dream. *Nursing Research* 36:332–338.

Molassiotis, A., Akker, V.D., and Boughton, B.J. 1997. Perceived social support, family environment and psychosocial recovery in bone marrow transplant long-term survivors. *Social Science & Medicine* 44(3): 317–325.

National Cancer Institute. Take time: Support for people with cancer and the people who care about them. Retrieved December 27, 2005, from www.nci.nih.gov/cancertopics/takingtime

National Cancer Institute. When someone in your family has cancer. Retrieved December 27, 2005, from www.cancer.gov/cancertopics/when-someone-in-your-family

Nelson, A. 1994. Parents' responses when their child has a bone marrow transplant. *Oncology Nursing Forum* 21(2):371.

Nye, F.I. 1976. *Role structure and analysis of the family.* Beverly Hills, CA: Sage.

Patenaude, A.F. 1990. Psychological impact of bone marrow transplantation: Current perspectives. *The Yale Journal of Biology and Medicine* 63:515–519.

Patenaude, A.F., Levinger, L., and Baker, K. 1986. Group meetings for parents and spouses of bone marrow transplant patients. *Social Work in Health Care* 12(1): 51–65.

Patenaude, A.F., Szymanski, L., and Rappeport, J. 1979. Psychological costs of bone marrow transplantation. *American Journal of Orthopsychiatry* 49(3):409–422.

Phipps, S. 2002. Reduction of distress associated with pediatric bone marrow transplant: Complementary health promotion interventions. *Pediatric Rehabilitation* 5(4):223–234.

Phipps, S., and Mulhern, R.K. 1995. Family cohesion and expressiveness promote resilience to the stress of pediatric bone marrow transplant: A preliminary report. *Developmental and Behavioral Pediatrics* 16(4):257–263.

Saleh, U.S., and Brockopp, D.Y. 2001. Quality of life over one year following bone marrow transplantation: Psychometric evaluation of the quality of life in bone marrow transplant survivors tool. *Oncology Nursing Forum* 28(9):1457–64.

Schlesinger, B. 1979. *Families: Canada.* Montreal: McGraw-Hill Ryerson: 8.

Schmit-Pokorny, K., Franco, T., Frappier, B., and Vyhlidal, R.C. 2003. The cooperative care model: An innovative approach to deliver blood and marrow stem cell transplant care. *Clinical Journal of Oncology Nursing,* 7(5):1–7.

Seattle Cancer Care Alliance. 2001. *Preparing for transplant.* Seattle, WA.

Sormanti, M., Dungan, S., and Rieker, P.P. 1994. Pediatric bone marrow transplantation: Psychosocial issues for parents after a child's hospitalization. *Journal of Psychosocial Oncology* 12(4):23–42.

Stensland, S. 1993. Bone marrow transplant patient responses to admission interview questions: A descriptive study. Paper presented at the National Association of Oncology Social Work Annual Conference, New York.

Stetz, K.M., McDonald, J.C., and Compton, K. 1996. Needs and experiences of family caregivers during marrow transplantation. *Oncology Nursing Forum* 23(9):1422–1427.

Stevens, P.E., and Pletsch, P.K. 2002. Ethical issues of informed consent: Mothers' experiences enrolling their children in bone marrow transplantation research. *Cancer Nursing* 25(2):81–87.

Streisand, R., Rodrigue, J.R., Houck, C., Graham-Pole, J., and Berlant, N. 2000. Brief report: Parents of children undergoing bone marrow transplantation: Documenting stress and piloting a psychological intervention program. *Journal of Pediatric Psychology* 25(5): 331–337.

Syrjala, K.L., Langer, S.L., Abrams, J.R., Storer, B., Sanders, J.E., Flowers, M.E.D., et al. (2004). Recovery and long-term function after hematopoietic cell transplantation for leukemia or lymphoma. *Journal of the American Medical Association* 29(19):2335–2343.

Tomlinson, P.S., Kirschbaum, M., Tomczyk, B., and Peterson, J. 1993. The relationship of child acuity, maternal responses, nurse attitudes and contextual factors in the bone marrow transplant unit. *American Journal of Critical Care* 2(3):246–252.

White, A. (1994). Parental concerns following a child's discharge from a bone marrow transplant unit. *Journal of Pediatric Oncology Nursing* 11(3):93–101.

Winters, G., Miller, C., Maracich, L., Compton, K., and Haberman, M.R. 1994. Provisional practice: The nature of psychosocial bone marrow transplant nursing. *Oncology Nursing Forum* 21(7):1147–1154.

Wolcott, D., and Stuber, M. 1992. Bone marrow transplantation. In *Psychiatric Aspects of Organ Transplantation*, eds. J. Craven and G.M. Rodin (189–204). Oxford: Oxford University Press.

Chapter 14

Ethical Issues Inherent to Blood and Marrow Transplantation

Joyce L. Neumann,
RN, MS, AOCN®

Introduction

Ethical dilemmas are inherent in treatment options such as blood and marrow transplantation (BMT). Due to the aggressive nature of the treatment, with high risk for complications and the fact that many patients offered this treatment may be facing their only chance at cure or significant control of their disease, clinicians and patients/ family members may face difficult and sometimes desperate situations. Although overall survival post-BMT has improved throughout the last decades, some of the previously recognized barriers such as age, limited source for stem cells, disease status at the time of BMT, and complications such as graft-versus-host disease (GVHD) have been challenged and present new ethical consideration.

With the recent development of nonmyeloablative transplantation, older patients, even those in the seventh decade of life and who have preexisting comorbid conditions, are being offered this treatment option, which is adding questions as to the appropriateness of this therapy (Little and Storb, 2002). One of the technological barriers, namely the lack of appropriate donors, has been challenged by the use of multiple or expanded cord blood transplantation in adults and haploidentical donors. These new therapies, however, are associated with prolonged neutropenia (cord blood) and increased risk for GVHD (haploidentical BMT). Although GVHD has been associated with fewer patients experiencing relapse of disease, certain characteristics of GVHD are predictive of poorer overall survival. These were identified by Lee and colleagues (2002) as higher Karnofsky performance scale, diarrhea, weight loss, and cutaneous and oral involvement of GVHD.

Oncology nursing practice is guided by the standards of the professional nursing organizations. In 1996, the Oncology Nursing Society and the American Nurses Association published the "Statement on the Scope and Standards of Oncology Nursing Practice" (Brant et al., 1996). Included in this document is the standard on ethics, which calls for decisions and actions by oncology nurses on behalf of clients to be determined in an ethical manner. It also encourages oncology nurses to examine their own philosophy; discuss ethical issues with other colleagues; address advance directives with patients and families; act as patient advocates; maintain sensitivity to patients' cultural diversity; protect patient autonomy, dignity, and rights; and seek resources to examine issues and formulate ethical decisions (Brant et al., 1996). Because of the research aspect of this treatment option, members of the nursing staff may have difficulty accepting the aggressive nature of the therapy. Nurses new to transplantation practice or research settings may have difficulty understanding the goals of the research program and acknowledging that the patient has accepted the experimental nature of the treatment. Nurses may have the perception of being caught in the middle of competing goals of the medical team and the patient and family (Hamric, 2001). It may take skill and diplomacy on the nurse's part to make sure that mutual goals are understood.

The following is a list of the ethical principles and considerations relevant to the care of the BMT patient, which will be discussed in this chapter. Case studies at the beginning of each section are used to focus the discussion and are similar to actual cases from the author's experience.

Bioethical Principles

1. **Beneficence:** to benefit or help persons.
2. **Nonmaleficence:** to prevent or avoid harm to persons, to "do no harm."
3. **Sanctity of Life:** Human life is held in high regard and respect.
4. **Justice:** Professionals have a duty to act with fairness, giving every individual what is owed them.
5. **Personal Autonomy:** Competent individuals or their surrogates have a right to decide for or against treatment.
6. **Benefit–Burden:** Only medical treatments that provide more benefit than burden are ethically mandated (Beauchamp and Childress, 2001).

Case Study 14-1

Peter was a 23-year-old patient with primary refractory Hodgkin's disease who was referred by a physician in a city 150 miles away from the cancer center. Despite aggressive treatment, he achieved only a partial response. He was single; his mother lived close to him and worked full-time. Peter had a history of substance abuse, but stated he had not used any illegal drugs recently. He did require frequent narcotic analgesia for abdominal pain relief. He also had periods of extreme anxiety, including almost hysterical behavior if in pain. He always came to his clinic appointment alone and was frequently late. His BMT physician recommended an allogeneic transplantation as the only method to cure Peter, but he did not have a sibling match, so a matched, unrelated donor search was started. The physician decided to treat with an autologous procedure until the donor was found.

Ethical Considerations in Clinical Situations

1. **Norms of Family Life:** Familial relationships give rise to moral responsibility. Nurses expect families to act in the best interest of the patient.
2. **Relationship between Clinician and Patient:** Clinicians have a fiduciary responsibility to care for patients. There needs to be mutual trust, and the patient must be treated as a whole person.
3. **Professional Integrity of Clinicians:** Clinicians have no responsibility to offer treatment that is not medically indicated.
4. **Cost-Effectiveness and Justice:** In a system with limited resources, allocation needs to be prioritized for the most appropriate use. Medical personnel need to be stewards of their resources.
5. **Cultural and/or Religious Variations:** Differences in beliefs or cultural norms may create disparity in values and principles (Fletcher, 1993).

When to Offer BMT as a Treatment Option

In Case Study 14-1, Peter met the medical eligibility criteria, but due to the refractory nature of his disease, the physician gave him only a 20% chance of cure with the matched unrelated donor (MUD) BMT; the plan of the autologous procedure was to provide time to secure a donor. Included in the eligibility criteria are those physiological parameters (cardiac and lung function) that are considered minimum to safely use the treatment option. The staff had concerns about offering treatments to patients when there is little or no chance for cure or control of disease and felt conflicted between the ethical principles of beneficence and nonmaleficence. Clinicians may feel that as long as the patient knows the survival outcome data, all treatment options should be offered and administered if the patient so chooses. This stance may conflict with what may be considered the best medical practice, perhaps less aggressive therapy could be administered if cure is not possible. Additionally, consideration must be given to resource allocation. The financial burden, as well as the shortage of beds and personnel that many busy transplant centers are experiencing, can make the implications profound.

The landmark case of Coby Howard of Oregon in the late-1980s has heightened the debate related to resource allocation (Fox and Leichter, 1991). Coby was a 7-year-old boy with leukemia who needed a bone marrow transplant. Initially, Oregon Medicaid had agreed to fund the procedure to be performed in the neighboring state of Washington. Before the transplant process was started, however, the Oregon legislature voted to discontinue funding of solid organ and bone marrow transplantation, which was expected to benefit only 34 people over a 2-year period. The $2.8 million in savings were to be used to fund 1,500 low-income mothers and children needing prenatal and pediatric care. Coby died waiting for the funds needed for the transplant (Pentz, 1999). The competing ethical principles facing lawmakers was in deciding justice (Coby was entitled to what was promised) and benefit versus burden (the greater good for the most people).

More recently, the efficiency of transplantation for women with breast cancer was negatively affected by the unethical reporting of research results by a group of Bezwoda researchers in South

Africa. When the promising Bezwoda results were reported at the 1999 American Society of Clinical Oncologists and were later found to be fraudulent, the efficiency of offering this treatment was put into question and the number of women receiving BMT declined. The study protocol used several unethical research practices (i.e., the protocol, written in 1990, cited a 1997 paper in its bibliography; the control group was given an inferior regimen; and ineligible patients were enrolled and their informed consent was not documented). There were also justice issues related to this underserved population (Pentz, 2004).

Post-BMT care factors also need to be examined prior to offering this treatment. The aftercare of the patient requires compliance with sometimes complex medication schedules, clinic visits to monitor blood counts and physical exams, and compliance with guidelines for self-care activities. A requirement of many programs is an available caregiver at all times. Many centers have developed a pathway or process for evaluating special needs or situations, which may put the patient at risk for harm (*nonmaleficence*) with the therapy (Neumann, 2001). Ideally, these issues should be addressed and resolved before the patient begins therapy, whether inpatient or outpatient. In Peter's case, a psychosocial assessment was performed by the social worker on the third attempt (Peter had missed his two previous appointments). The need for a full-time caregiver was discussed and Peter indicated he would have one available, but was unable to list names. The assessment also prompted a referral to psychiatry for anxiety management.

It is important that there is a consensus among all team members that certain ethical considerations will be upheld; some of these are as follows: Team members have an obligation to provide potential life-saving treatment (*beneficence*) independent of socioeconomic status; other factors, in addition to medical eligibility, will impact outcomes and patient safety (*nonmaleficence*); and success is dependent on a team of professionals who are empowered to make decisions. There are also certain behavioral factors that affect success for the patient, the health-care team, and the program; these include:

- Patient's verbal commitment, which is be demonstrated with actions (compliance with appointments, tests, treatments).
- The fact that individuals (patients) do not change coping styles during a life event such as BMT, and maladaptive coping skills (e.g., drug and alcohol abuse, violent or threatening behavior, morbid obesity) need to be addressed prior to the start of therapy.
- Refusal of psychosocial assessment and intervention can be just as serious as refusal of cardiac medications to a patient with congestive heart failure or insulin to a diabetic (Neumann, 2004).

Molassiotis and colleagues (1997) and Neitzert and colleagues (1998) have studied the importance of a social support system for the patient's success and quality of life after transplantation. In studies by Prieto and colleagues (2002) and Akaho and colleagues (2003), psychological factors of the BMT recipients were examined. Gender and mood status pre-BMT were suggested to be factors associated with prognosis post-BMT in the Japanese study (Akaho et al., 2003). Issues related to religious or cultural beliefs also need to be addressed prior to BMT. For patients who espouse the religious beliefs of Jehovah's Witnesses (JW), the nonacceptance of blood products may make BMT an unacceptable treatment option for both the patient and the care team. There have been few anecdotal reports of successful autologous BMT in JW patients (Kerridge et al., 1997; Mazzi et al., 2000). The responsibility of BMT programs to provide consistent assessment and support for the patient and caregiver can be paramount to the success of the treatment.

Other variables that may influence the clinician's decisions related to offering this treatment include the patient's age, toxicities, and cost. Elderly patients frequently receive less aggressive therapy because of regimen-related toxicity or a clinician's biases (Hutchins et al., 1999; Clarke, 2001). In the past, HSCT has been a treatment modality for young patients, but with the advent of nonmyeloablative stem cell transplantation therapy, it can include all age groups. Although the toxicity of nonmyeloablative transplantation is less than myeloablative transplantation, complications related to comorbid conditions of the older patient can make management equally as complex. Comorbidity

has recently been examined by Shahjahan and colleagues (2004). Using the Charlson comorbidity index (CCI), the retrospective study of 78 patients with acute myelogenous leukemia (AML) or myelodysplastic syndome (MDS) in first remission indicated that a lower comorbid score and an age younger than 40 years were strong predictors of better overall survival, event-free survival, and nonrelapse mortality.

In a study by Barker and colleagues (2002) in MUD, risk factors for nonsurvival for patients with chronic myelogenous leukemia (CML) (54%) and other leukemia and lymphoma diagnoses were non-CML diagnosis, age over 35 years, diagnosis to transplant time of greater than 18 months, and Grade 3–4 acute GVHD. The best overall survival rate (77%) was identified in patients younger than 35 years with early CML-chronic phase 2 year. The feasibility of offering treatment like BMT when known risks factors (disease status, comorbid conditions, age or psychosocial issues) for nonsurvival are high, needs to be considered prior to offering the treatment. Finally, putting a healthy donor at risk during collection of allogeneic stem cells for a therapy that is questionable in

Case Study 14-2

Francisco is an 18-year-old from Spain who traveled to the United States with his parents for treatment of his ALL, which had not responded to any other therapy. His parents searched the Internet and found that haploidentical BMTs were being performed at a Midwest cancer center. Since Francisco had no siblings or donor in the registry, his parents felt this was his only treatment option. During the initial clinic visit, his parents asked the clinic staff not to tell Francisco about all the risks and complications involved because this would make their son more anxious.

terms of chance for success is also an ethical responsibility that needs to considered before treatment.

Informed Consent

A great deal has been written about shared decision making as an ethical imperative (Charles et al., 1999; Whitney, 2003). Typically, models for decision making have been characterized as being paternalistic (common 3 to 4 decades ago, in which the physician assumed the dominant role); informed (involves providing patient education), in which case the patient makes the decision with little guidance from the medical team except to give information; and shared, in which information and decisions are made jointly (Charles et al., 1999). The purpose of informed consent is to give the recipient of care information related to the treatment plan, medications to be given, side effects, complications, risks, cost, benefits, and rights (Jacoby et al., 1999). The recipient can then make the appropriate decision for himself or his family member. It is important that the patient is aware of the major and frequently occurring minor effects of treatment. Clinicians vary concerning telling patients about side effects that occur infrequently. Some clinicians believe that patients only should be aware of side effects or complications that have a higher chance of occurring.

In the case of research protocols, a written informed consent document is used as a tool to provide information and obtain the patient's permission to receive treatment, with a signed copy supplied to the patient. It also serves the purpose of documentation and registration of the patient on the protocol. Providing and having patients sign an informed consent for standard of care therapies is a suggested practice but is not uniformly practiced. By signing consent, even for what would be considered standard of care treatment, the patient assumes an increased sense of responsibility by both the practitioner and herself to understand the treatment planned (Jacoby et al., 1999).

Veracity or truth-telling regarding the treatment and prognosis can pose the greatest concerns in the process of informed consent. Veracity is defined by Beauchamp and Childress (2001, p. 284) in the health-care setting as "comprehensive, accurate, and objective transmission of information, as well as to the way the professional fosters the patient's understanding." Frequently, families, in an attempt to protect the patient, will request altering of truth, so that their loved ones will not give up hope or decide to stop treatment. If the patient is very young or old or from a different ethnic background, there may be a surrogate or proxy who will be the decision-maker or spokesperson. The clinician, either nurse or physician, is faced with the challenge of ensuring the patient's wishes or interests are met and protected (Crawley et al., 2002).

The communication skills of clinicians are of great importance when presenting the information to patients and families. There is increasing study and training in how to give bad news. It is very apparent that better communication skills with compassionate and clear messages lead to decreased conflict and fewer ethical dilemmas. Informed consent involves both social and individual values recognition (Holmes-Rovner and Wills, 2002). In a study by Brown and colleagues (2004), consultations between medical oncologists and their patients were taped and analyzed using qualitative methodology. Strategies were identified for physicians to encourage collaborative decision making; these include the following:

1. Introduce joint decision-making process;
2. Use language that relays and reflects patient autonomy;
3. Check preferred decision-making style (involved or not);
4. Check information preferences of patient; invite questions and comments;
5. Check patient's medical knowledge and understanding;
6. Explicitly offer choice of treatment;
7. Acknowledge uncertainty of treatment benefits;
8. Declare professional recommendation;
9. Provide opportunity for amplification of patient voice;
10. Provide time and opportunity to discuss concerns in detail;
11. Offer decision delay, and offer ongoing decision support/answer to future questions.

Patient care discussion related to treatment options and informed consent should include alternative treatment options. There may be concerns about a conflict of interest when the patient's physician is also the research protocol principle investigator (Wendler, 2000). Information about alternative therapies and potential conflict of interest has been added to most informed consent documents currently being used. As discussed earlier, the risk for BMT may vary depending on the type of BMT performed and the patient risk factors. Communicating risks while trying to maintain a sense of hope can be difficult (Back et al., 2003); this is especially difficult when the risk is unknown. Calman (2002) identifies three factors relevant to communication of risk: the certainty of the risk (the evidence base), the level of risk (high or low), and the ef-

fect of the risk on the individual. The concept of uncertainty has been studied by Mishel (1988) and others. Assisting the patient to cope with uncertainty by providing information about what is known or BMT program outcomes would be helpful to most patients in the decision-making process. Patients' coping styles may be another variable in communicating information about treatment and risks. Coping styles are different, and patients' need or desire for information about procedures and risks, including uncertain outcomes, may vary. Whereas some patients want much detail, others may want little or no information and may practice risk-aversion behaviors or relegate family members or caregivers to be the receivers of this information (the bad news). Andrykowski (1994) suggests that research should focus on pretreatment decision making as it related to after-treatment outcomes, including the examination of patients' expectations for a range of treatment outcomes.

When the patient is a child or adolescent there are additional issues related to consent, especially when treatment is involving research, usually the case in BMT. There is continuing debate related to the age at which consent can or should be obtained; this may also have cultural variation. Based upon the Nuremberg Code (1947), persons from whom consent is being sought should be provided with information about the nature, duration, and purpose of the procedure; its methods and means; all reasonably expected inconveniences and hazards; and any effects on the person from involvement in the process (Lind et al., 2003). It is important to be aware of the common law and legislation, which may vary within countries. In Canada, the law is province-based and may vary from ages 14 to 16 years (Lind et al., 2003). Children younger than this age are not considered to have decision-making capacity, and decisions are made by proxy, usually by the parents. In this circumstance, most would use the process of assent instead of consent, which is considered between autonomous consent and no involvement in the consent process. This, however, may not be considered as pertinent when the child takes a position of dissention to participation in research, as pointed out by the authors. In a recently published study by Stevens and Pletsch (2002), 12 mothers whose children had undergone bone marrow transplantation were interviewed about their experiences giving informed consent. Their stories reveal complex ethical issues of informed consent, including the life and death circumstances and the urgency to begin treatment, which may have affected decision making and the voluntary nature of the research. Mothers in this study (Stevens and Pletsch, 2002) also shared later feelings of regret and self-recrimination about the decision to consent. The authors recommended including the emotional aspects of the decision during the informed consent procedure and relationship building to ensure informed consent over the duration of the clinical trial.

Patient Education

Many refer to the informed consent procedure as a process that continues after the official document is signed and includes a continuum of patient education (Holmes-Rovner and Wills, 2002). Frequently, the oncology nurse *validates the patient's understanding* of the plan and goal of care. The nurse may assist the patient to formulate questions and give additional information concerning the long-term consequences of the planned therapy. Expectations regarding return to work and the emotional and physical recov-ery after BMT should be discussed when the patient is making a decision concerning treatment. Full physical and emotional recovery, including return to work, may take as long as 3 to 5 years as identified by Syrjala and colleagues (2004). Ideally, these questions and concerns should be addressed before treatment begins. Patient information should be provided in order to give a more detailed explanation of what the patient might expect and the care requirements during the therapy. Some BMT centers also provide a care contract or agreement document that specifically outlines what is expected of the patient or caregiver and what they can expect of the health-care facility and providers of care (Neumann, 2004). This is especially helpful if there is concern about the patient's and care-giver's understanding or level of commitment. Letting patients also know that there are care requirements that are nonnegotiable may help to avert difficult care situations and ethical issues (e.g., noncompliance or nonadherence to the plan of care) in the future.

An assessment of patients' information needs and expectations pre-BMT and post-BMT that included measurement of their perception of uncertainty and coping style would help to individualize their learning and care planning. It is perceived that knowledge of the behavioral style of these individuals will be important in helping to determine the amount and perhaps timing of information sharing that will have an impact on decision making. Frequently when discussing the treatment plan, forgotten questions or concerns may relate to fertility issues, plans to return to work or normal life, the plan if complications occur, and end-of-life care (Andrykowski, 1994). Ideally, these questions and concerns should be addressed before treatment begins.

It is important when conducting Phase I clinical trials that the patient understands that there may be little or no benefit to them and that the goal of the trial is to define the maximum tolerated dose (Daugherty, 2004). Studies suggest that even after being instructed that the study they have been enrolled in is a Phase I study, patients believe they will personally gain a clinical benefit from their participation (Daugherty, 2004). With the advent of the Internet, perceptive consumers have many opportunities to explore options—both standard therapy and unproven therapies—and many make their decisions about participation in a particular trial before the first clinic visit (Daugherty, 2004).

Donor Issues

There is an ethical responsibility to inform the normal donor of the risks associated with the donation of stem cells through bone marrow harvest or collection through apheresis procedure. The risks to a normal healthy donor are minimal, with life-threatening complications occurring in 0.4% of donors (Buckner et al., 1994) for either procedure. When the donor is older (even in her seventies), as with the sibling of a patient receiving nonmyeloablative therapy, the risk may be greater (Anderlini et al., 1997). There have been few recent studies examining issues related to donors. In a small ($n = 18$) study by Wolcott and colleagues (1986), donors reported little

---

Case Study 14-3

A patient from the Middle East (a country that did not participate in the international bone marrow registry) with chronic myelogenous leukemia was treated with chemotherapy in the United States and returned home in remission. BMT was recommended in the event that he should experience a relapse. Within 4 months, the patient relapsed and requested a BMT, having found a donor in his country. The physicians at the transplant center assumed this was a related donor and began planning for peripheral blood stem cell collection, which was the norm for related BMT. After the patient and donor arrived in the United States,

it was discovered that the patient found the donor by an unauthorized search of hospital records and that the donor was typed several years earlier when her daughter had leukemia. The donor was a poor woman from a rural village who was convinced to travel to the United States to perform this donation. As she was worked up, it was decided that a bone marrow harvest would be more suitable. This necessitated her staying in the United States for a week longer than she had planned. The patient was living with the donor and his family, which also created a very strained situation for the donor. There were concerns about coercion of the donor.

emotional distress, high self-esteem, current life satisfaction, and little change in their relationship with donors. There seems to be a relationship between the recipient's condition and the donor's psychosocial status (Wolcott et al., 1986).

Special consideration is required when the donor is a child or minor. If the treatment has a low chance of success, the risks to the normal donor may be a factor in the decision not to proceed, although this was not the case in a study examining the use of pediatric donors as reported by Chan and colleagues (1996). Patients and families may become desperate to find treatment options. Normal donors' rights must be protected through program and/or institutional policies that provide a mechanism to assure voluntary, confidential, and safe practices when harvesting stem cells, whether through apheresis or bone marrow procurement (Pentz et al., 2004).

When the donor is a minor, extensive psychosocial and developmental assessment by experts in child psychology is recommended. The emotional impact may be profound due to the age of both the patient and donor or, in the case of a haploidentical donor (i.e., child-to-parent or parent-to-child), the urgency for decision making. Most centers would recommend a separate health-care team for the donor to eliminate the possibility of competing interests. With regard to informed consent for a minor donor, most centers will obtain consents from the donor, as well as the parent(s), if possible (Massimo, 1996). In the case of a very young or incompetent minor donor, a formal ethics consult may be standard practice during the consenting process. In the extreme case, the legal system may need to resolve the infrequent issue of dissension between the minor donor's joint-custody parents. If there are any concerns about

donor rights or interests, regardless of age, a formal ethics consult should be initiated by any member of the health-care team.

In the case of an unrelated donor, the national and international bone marrow registries (ABMTR and IBMTR) have set strict guidelines to protect the normal donor's and patient's rights and confidentiality. Assessment of the donor for possible increased risk factors related to general anesthesia in the case of bone marrow harvest or increased fluid and electrolyte shifts during an apheresis procedure is completed. Concerns about potential withdrawal of consent by the donor after the patient's conditioning regimen is started are dealt with by evaluation of level of commitment and obtaining the donor's signature on a letter of intent. Selection of date may be somewhat complicated and is sometimes inflexible once set. Specific information (e.g., donor's name and address) is provided to the patient and/or donor after a year only if both parties agree.

With the development of umbilical cord blood (UCB) technology, ethical issues related to procurement, equitable use and distribution, marketing practices, and timing of informed consent have been identified and discussed (Sugarman et al., 1997). The efficiency of UCB use in adults has been explored with some programs developing multiple cords or ex vivo expansion of UCB product to meet the minimum cell dose requirements. Occasionally there has been some confusion by patients or others as to the difference between UCB and embryonic stem cells. In the current climate embryonic research is considered an ethical, social, and political issue, so clarification of the differences becomes extremely important (Sandel, 2004).

Caring for international patients coming from countries where ethics considerations are different poses other challenges, as in Case Study 14-3. The institutional ethics committee and administrative review board were both involved in the resolution of this case. The institutional minor donor policy was applied to provide additional protective measures for the donor (i.e., separate housing was provided). The ethicist met the donor and offered the options of returning home or donating bone marrow before returning home. For situations similar to this in the future, a policy was created to ensure donors would be directly contacted and interviewed prior to traveling to the transplant center.

Case Study 14-4

John was a patient with lymphoma who was in a third relapse of his disease. He had previously had an autologous transplant and was being offered an allogeneic transplantation from his sister donor, who was a one-antigen mismatch. Since his last BMT, he has had fungal pneumonia, which has cleared from his last CT scan, and he has lost 20 kilograms. His physician in consult with other BMT physicians and the BMT team determined that an allogeneic BMT was reasonable to offer John at that time, but that he needed to understand the increased risk. Since he did not meet the eligibility criteria for the protocol, a compassionate investigational new drug (CIND) was written. During the work-up process, John was asked by the social worker if he had an advance directive (AD); he replied that he did not. He was given the forms for living will and durable power of attorney. In the follow-up meeting, the clinic nurse asked John about his AD; he had not filled out the paperwork and was not interested in doing so. The clinic nurse shared this with the physician. During the consenting procedure, the physician again informed John that he was a high-risk patient and asked if he thought about what he would want done if he needed mechanical ventilation or had severe refractory GVHD. He was also asked about whom he would want to make decisions for him, if he was not able to. John's physician informed him that mechanical ventilation could be a temporary procedure, and if his condition did not improve, that his family would be consulted, the ventilator would be turned off, and he would be allowed to die. John became very upset and said because of religious beliefs he did not want his sister (next of kin) to be asked to help make this decision because she would suffer in the afterlife if she took part in the decision to end his life. John asked that he be kept alive until he recovered or his heart stopped.

Advance Care Planning/Advance Directives

Independence and self-reliance have been virtues sought after and cultivated in traditionally Protestant, Western societies throughout history (Hanssen, 2004). This autonomous sense of self may present a profound contrast to members of Middle Eastern or Eastern societies, in which collectivism or interdependence is valued and utilized in decision making related to advance care planning (Matsumura et al., 2002). With the advent of the civil rights and women's rights movements in the 1960s, the principle of *personal autonomy or self-determination* has gained even greater importance in the American culture (Rajput and Bekes, 2002). In 1976, the same year the Karen Quinlan case was argued in the judicial system to allow substituted judgment or surrogate decision making at the end of life, California became the first state to recognize living wills in the Natural Death Act. In 1990, the U.S. Congress enacted the Patient Self-Determination Act, which mandates that at the time of admission to a federally funded hospital, patients must be asked if they have advance directives. If they do, they are asked to submit a copy, and if not, they are provided with the necessary forms for completion. This act was created in response to the U.S. Supreme Court statement the same year, which identified that a person has a constitutionally protected right in the interest of liberty to refuse unwanted treatment that is upheld even in the case of mental capacity loss (Jonsen et al., 2002). In lieu of the living will document, the surrogate decision maker of an incompetent person or person lacking capacity is asked to consider not what they would want or what they want for their loved one, but what the patient would want for themselves (Quill, 2005). This has never been so widely debated or contested as with the recent case of Terri Schiavo (Annas, 2005).

The term advance directive (AD) usually refers to three separate documents: the living will, the medical power of attorney, and in many states the out-of-hospital do-not-resuscitate order. Decision making about continued treatment for patients with poor prognostic indicators for survival (see next section) may be more traumatic unless the patient and family members/caregivers are prepared for that possibility (Tilden et al., 2001). It is assumed that satisfaction with the decision-making process can be better achieved when patients' and family members'/caregivers' coping style and degree of perceived decisional uncertainty are taken into consideration (Parascandola et al., 2002).

When first developed, the living will was written by persons who did not wish to be kept alive by artificial means if they were in conditions considered irreversible. Irreversible condition is defined by each state's judicial system. In the state of Texas it is defined as "a condition, injury or illness: that may be treated, but is never cured or eliminated; that leaves a person unable to care for or make decisions for the person's own self; and that, without life-sustaining treatment provided in accordance with the prevailing standard of medical care is fatal" (Advance Directive Act, 1999). Recently, an additional statement has been added to the living will (initiated by the Right to Life coalition) in some states so that the individual can indicate they want everything done regardless of the nature of the condition. The additional statement reads, "I request that I be kept alive in this *terminal* condition using available life-sustaining treatment, and I request that I be kept alive in this *irreversible* condition using available life-sustaining treatment. This does not apply to hospice care" (Directive to Physicians and Family or Surrogates, 2000). Although this is thought to give more choices to the individual, it has the potential to create a barrier to clinicians exercising what they would view as sound medical practice or actions in the patient's best interest, for example if CPR is not indicated for a patient who is in the final stages of terminal illness. Many believe this reflects the principle of self or autonomy taken to the extreme (Meier and Morrison, 2002). Finally, if the AD documents are truly to reflect patient autonomy, one might question why they do not include the additional choices of physician-assisted suicide or active and passive euthanasia for those people whose wishes may include ending or shortening their lives if their condition is intolerable to them (Snelling, 2004).

These documents need to reviewed and ideally become a forum for preemptive discussions, especially when the patient is about to undergo treatment regimens that have a high risk for complications that may necessitate intensive care or intubation (Quill and Brody, 1996). The time and quality of patient–physician discussions regarding advance directives has been studied. A qualitative study by Tulsky and colleagues (1998) reported that in conversations between 56 physicians and patients (age 65 years or older or with serious medical diagnosis) the average time spent discussing advance directives was less than 6 minutes; physicians spoke for two thirds of the time and frequently used vague language. Physicians, of course, are not the only health-care professionals who have a responsibility to discuss advance directives with patients; social workers and nurses share

this responsibility (Douglas and Brown, 2002; Jezewski et al., 2003). Current nursing literature and research support the fact that there appears to be a deficit in nurses' understanding and comfort level with advance directives and the Patient Self-Determination Act (Shapiro and Bowles, 2002).

One of the most widely published, ambitious, and well-funded (through a multi-million-dollar donation from the Robert Wood Johnson Foundation) studies examining patient preferences was the Study to Understand Prognosis and Preferences for Outcomes and Risks of Treatment (SUPPORT). This prospective study involving 6800 hospitalized patients at five teaching hospitals in the United States that evaluated ways to improve end-of-life decision making and reduce the frequency of a mechanically supported, painful, and prolonged process of dying (Weeks et al., 1998; Prendergast, 2001). Although the study introduced several interventions to encourage and support discussion between physicians and patients, none of these had an impact on increasing the communication between practitioner and patient or on diminishing the fear surrounding the process of dying in this country (Teno et al., 2002). Another activity of the foundation that funded the SUPPORT project was the formation of the Last Acts Partnership, a coalition of more than 100 prominent organizations working to improve the quality of care for dying people. The Last Acts Partnership supports bills like the one currently before the U.S. Senate (S. 2545) that would cover the cost of a physician consultation visit for Medicare beneficiaries to discuss advance directives and make these documents portable across state lines (Advance Directives Improvement and Education Act, 2004). This allows the work of improving the quality of care for dying people to continue.

Although durable power of attorney continues to be recommended, the use of living wills has recently come under criticism as a costly exercise to try to predict how the patient will decide about care in the abstract at some point in the future should they become incompetent (Fagerlin and Schneider, 2004; Loewy, 1998; Kessler and McClellan, 2004; Dresser, 2003; Meier and Morrison, 2002). The Joint Commission on Accreditation of Healthcare Organizations (JCAHO) has mandated that hospitals requesting accreditation demonstrate that patients are asked if they have advance directives at the time of admission and provided information if they do not have the documents. Despite these measures and other attempts by hospitals and community groups aimed at encouraging patients to complete living wills, the number of patients completing the documents remains dismal at less than 30% (Baer, 2001). The use of a living will (and certainly the durable power of attorney), however, is supported before planned treatment options or situations where high risks for undesirable outcomes may occur, such as BMT.

Some religious and social groups (the Center for Bioethics and Human Dignity at Trinity International University, Americans United for Life, Christian Medical and Dental Associations) are interested in combining the two documents with the inclusion of a statement specifically disallowing any form of assisted suicide or euthanasia. There also has been support for advance care planning to provide more information about patients' values instead of using treatment-based directives that may be left open for interpretation when applied later to actual clinical situations (Kolarik et al., 2002).

Finally, expectations of treatment become important in both the informed consent process and in advance care planning. In a study by Lee and colleagues (2001), discrepancies between patients' and physicians' estimates for the success of stem cell transplantation were examined. Results of the study indicated that of the 313 patient participants, those with intermediate and advanced disease receiving an allogeneic BMT tended to be more optimistic than their physicians, and they failed to recognize the higher risks associated with their situations (Lee et al., 2001).

In Case Study 14-4, an ethics consult was requested by the patient's clinic physician. This was attended by the patient, his sister, three members of the ethics committee (a physician, nurse, and social worker), a chair of the ethics committee, the physician's clinic nurse, and the BMT program director. The patient started the discussion with a compelling argument asserting that he could not sanction withdrawal of life-sustaining treatment on religious grounds, nor could he allow his sister to be part of this decision. He requested to be allowed to be kept alive until his heart stopped and could not be restarted. The ethics committee recommendation in this case was to uphold what was considered to be standard practice, which was identified as stopping mechanical ventilation and allowing the patient to die if he experienced multiorgan failure or relapse disease, or required maximum ventilator or vasoactive support with little or no chance of reversal. After this recommendation, the patient decided to seek care elsewhere, and the BMT team helped facilitate transfer of information to another BMT center of the patient's choice.

Unfortunately, most ethics consults are performed once this aggressive supportive care has been rendered, at which time families are having to deal with the impending loss of their loved ones, as well as participation in the decision-making process (Foxall and Gaston-

Johansson, 1996). This has the potential to increase ICU days, ventilator days, and the unnecessary use of artificial nutrition and hydration (Schneiderman et al., 2000).

Few studies have examined the cultural differences concerning advance directives. Perkins and colleagues (2002) performed one such study; it structured open-ended interviews that were conducted with Mexican-American, Euro-American, and African-American patients on two general medicine units. Fifty-eight patients were interviewed, with the highest number of participants (26) being Mexican-Americans. Interestingly, the study indicated that Mexican-Americans and African-Americans believed that the health-care system controlled the treatment; the Euro-Americans held this belief infrequently. The Euro-Americans and Mexican-Americans expressed trust in the system, whereas most African-Americans did not. In addition, both the Euro-Americans and the Mexican-Americans believed the AD helped the staff to know and implement the patient's wishes, whereas most African-American participants believed they should wait to until they were very sick to express their wishes. The Euro-American participants had particular wishes about life support, other care, and acceptable outcomes, and the Mexican-Americans expressed the desire to be allowed to die if treatment was futile (Perkins et al., 2002).

Disproportionate Care (When Burden Outweighs Benefit of Care)

The do-not-resuscitate order is a medical decision made by the patient's physician that usually prohibits the use of extraordinary measures (e.g., CPR, defibrillation, emergency medications, intubations) in conditions that are considered-irreversible. Furthermore, the use of such measures will not change the outcome for the patient, nor is there reasonable hope for recovery. Terms used in current literature that are replacing the terms *extraordinary* and *ordinary* are *proportionate* (more benefit than burden) and *disproportionate* (increased burden without clear benefit for the patient) care. The principle of proportionality examines the obligation to recommend or provide medical interventions as an estimated ratio of promised benefit over its attendant burden (Jonsen et al., 2002). The physician will want to discuss continued care with the patient (if possible), family, and/or the person with the authority for substituted judgment (surrogate decision-maker). It is never recommended to do this unilaterally, nor should the physician put the burden of the DNR decision on the patient or family exclusively. It is clear that there frequently is disparity in definitions and the meaning of DNR among patients, providers, and families, which can lead to conflict in the process (Olver et al., 2002). Focusing on care or no care versus prolongation of life, quality of life, or the full range of end-of-life decisions is a common pitfall in developing a plan of care for patients who lack decision-making capacity (Lang and Quill, 2004). Acceptance of the fact that there is little or nothing left to offer in terms of treatments for cure is a process for BMT patients and families that may take some time to reach. The condition of the patient may warrant continuation of aggressive therapy up until the point of needing intubation or CPR because of the uncertainty related to prognosis. Patients and families may assume that they are required to sign the DNR order, which is the case in some institutions or states. In New York, there is a state statute that mandates that the adult patient's (or designees) verbal or written consent be obtained before a physician writes an order to withhold resuscitation. In a comparative study of inpatient do-not-resuscitate forms used at 30 National Cancer Institute–designated cancer centers, 25% required patient and/or surrogate signatures (Zhukovsky et al., 2004). There is still the perception by some that the quality of nursing care will be less if they authorize a DNR order, or that it is like a death sentence, or that the patient will lose all hope and just give up if they write a DNR.

There is a wide variety of practice patterns involving the DNR order even within National Cancer Institute–designated cancer centers (NCICC). Some institutions have created a preprinted order sheet, on which the physician has a menu of measures to choose from (including cardiac defibrillation, vasoactive drugs, antiarrythmic drugs, cardiac pacemaker, tracheotomy, chemotherapy, antibiotics, dialysis, blood products, hyperalimentation, tube feeding, intravenous fluids, oxygen, and tests) and specifies that patient comfort always takes priority. Only 13 of 30 NCICCs use forms that allow for identification of additional levels of treatment limitations other than resuscitation efforts (Zhukovsky et al., 2004). Establishing the specific goal of care is paramount in deciding which of these measures to withhold.

Evaluating what our experience has demonstrated with certain complications is critical in making sound judgments about which conditions may be considered irreversible in BMT patients. Studies published by Hinds and colleagues (2001) and Groeger and colleagues (1998) identified variables that impact the mortality of cancer patients admitted to the intensive care unit. They included CPR within 24 hours prior to admission, intubations, intracranial mass, allogeneic BMT, recurrence of disease, poor baseline performance status, prothrombin time longer than 15 seconds, albumin less than 2.5 gm/dl, bilirubin greater than 2.0 mg/dl, BUN greater than 50 mg/dl, and number of hospital days prior to ICU admission. Allogeneic BMT patients who are intubated and have an infection or have a gastrointestinal bleed have decreased (4%) chance of survival (Price et al., 1998). In a study by Huaringa and colleagues (2000) of 60 BMT patients who required mechanical ventilation for pneumonia or diffuse alveolar hemorrhage, only 5% were alive at 6 months, including the 18% who were extubated and discharged from ICU. Poor prognostic indicators were graft-versus-host disease, prolonged ventilation (more than 14 days), and late development of respiratory failure (greater than 30 days after BMT). Patients with breast cancer and pulmonary edema had a favorable predictive factor in this study. In another study reported by Hennessy, White, and Crotty (1997), all 15% of their total of 141 BMT patients who required ventilation died. Preemptive conversation about decision making with the patient and family decreased the number of patients transferred to the ICU to less than 15% versus 25–40% as reported in other studies. The appropriateness of ICU transfers in the BMT patient population has been controversial because of the historical perception of generally poor outcomes (Shemie, 2003), although overall survival seems to be improving (Rubenfeld and Crawford, 1996). In the pediatric BMT population, there is evidence to support the presumption that this treatment modality (BMT) is not a factor-influencing outcome of ICU admission. Jacobe and colleagues (2003) reported that underlying diagnosis, age, time of admission post-BMT, type of transplantation, conditioning regimen, and GVHD did not influence outcome in their pediatric BMT patients admitted to ICU, and multiorgan failure was the most important predictor of survival.

Discontinuation of Medically Inappropriate Care (Futility)

At times, measures are instituted when it is not clear if the patient's condition is reversible. When it becomes apparent that there is little or no chance of recovery, the decision may be made to discontinue those measures that are life-sustaining with the goal of a peaceful death with dignity. This is extremely difficult for families, and they may liken it to euthanasia. The concept of futility, as examined by Bailey (2003), presents many value-laden judgments of care and assumptions about the quality and quantity of life that may be ethically unjustifiable. Many factors need to be considered when having this discussion, such as individual preferences, religious beliefs, and cultural traditions. For example, individuals of the Muslim faith may believe removing ventilator support would be totally unacceptable under any circumstances. Institutions and hospitals, especially those with religious affiliations, may hold the ethical principle of the sanctity of life in highest regard. This may lead to conflict with what practitioners might consider appropriate medical care regarding termination of care. With the exception of aggressive relapsed disease, the transplant medical team frequently has difficulty discontinuing aggressive therapy for complications of transplantation. In an article by Perry, Rivlin, and Goldstone (1999), a review of literature of decision making and practices related to stopping treatment for BMT patients with life-threatening organ failure was presented. The authors stressed the importance of these discussions during pretransplant counseling, including the identification of treatment limits. Tools to predict outcomes have been developed using severity measures (Iezzoni et al.,1995; Cook et al., 2003) although studies indicate physicians' perception of patient preference, physicians' prediction of survival, the likelihood of poor cognitive function, and the use of inotopes or vasopressors were equally important to specific measurements.

When families and clinicians disagree on medical care, an ethics consult may be called, and the institutional medical futility (inappropriate medical care) policy may need to be enacted. In 1999, Texas was the first state to adopt a law regulating end-of-life decisions, providing a legislatively sanctioned, extrajudicial, due-process mechanism for resolving medical futility disputes and other end-of-life ethical disagreements (Fine and Mayo, 2003). This usually involves a review process that includes clinical experts not directly involved in the case, members of the ethics committee, the patient's family, the medical team, and a representative from the hospital administration. If the decision is made to terminate life support, a designated waiting period will be established in order for the patient/family to find another care facility that will continue to provide the level of care requested. During this process, there are usually provisions to maintain the same level of life-sustaining care as well as an agreement (within the institution's physician group) that no other physician will take over the case, thereby changing the goal and plan of care as decided by the committee. If the family does not choose to move the patient, life-sustaining measures will be discontinued, and comfort measures will be continued until the patient dies (Fine and Mayo, 2003).

Summary

Blood and marrow transplantation nurses experience many ethical issues in their roles as caregivers and patient advocates. Kelly and colleagues (2000) do well in describing the emotional labor faced by BMT nurses in providing care that may not benefit the patient (moral schizophrenia, a term used by an earlier author) and its impact on staff morale. Initial studies are being done to try to quantify the issues nurses face in their practice (Fry and Duffy, 2001). Nurses working in research centers where Phase I trials are being performed may have additional issues because of the unknown results of these studies and the possibility of severe side effects and complications as new therapies are being developed.

The ethical obligations inherent during interchange between the nurse and patient must occur within the boundaries of professional interdependence and complex organizational structures, and in a matter that is unique for the culture (Penticuff, 1997). Nurses' demand for patients to be autonomous, especially when caring for patients from different cultures, may in some cases conflict with the concepts of respect, integrity, and human worth that the principle of autonomy is meant to protect (Hanssen, 2004).

Nurses are encouraged to become involved in institutional ethics committees and writing policies that can help define practice and lessen potential conflicts. Dodd and colleagues (2004) describe ethical activism (where nurses try to make hospitals be more receptive to nurses' participation in deliberation on ethical issues) and ethical assertiveness (nurses participate in deliberation without a formal invitation) as two important activities nurses may want to take on. Measures to support the nurse in the role of caregiver and patient advocate should also be examined (Neumann, 2004; Davis et al., 2003). At MD Anderson Cancer Center, monthly ethics rounds on the inpatient BMT unit were initiated. Results of a staff survey after 1 year of ethics rounds indicate that the nurses have an increased knowledge of ethical principles, and the nursing staff feels more comfortable discussing ethical issues with physician colleagues (Neumann et al., 2001). Other strategies to empower nurses to delve into ethical activities need to be examined and incorporated into programs of nursing education and management (Peter et al., 2004).

Nurses, like physicians, have the responsibility to be good stewards of limited resources and create criteria with guidelines for judicious use of therapies, especially new therapies with high risk and those that tend to be extremely costly. Nurses also have a responsibility to know their states' current regulations, as well as the policies of their institutions, related to the issues presented here. Finally, in order to truly advocate for patients, it is imperative to know the goal of care and challenge inconsistencies if they arise between the patient's understanding of that goal and the medical plan of care.

References

Advance Directive Act of 1999, Texas Health and Safety Code, Chapter 166.046. 1999.

Advance Directives Improvement and Education Act of 2004 (S. 2545). U.S. Senate Bill.

Akaho, R., Sasaki, T., Mori, S., Akiyama, H., Yoshino, M., Hagiya, K., et al. (2003). Psychological factors and survival after bone marrow transplantation in patients with leukemia. *Psychiatry and Clinical Neurosciences, 57*, 91–96.

Anderlini, P., Przepiorka, D., Lauppe, J. Seong, D., Giralt, S., Champlin, R., et al. (1997). Collection of peripheral blood stem cells from normal donors 60 years of age or older. *British Journal Haematology, 97*(2), 485–487.

Andrykowski, M.A. (1994). Psychosocial factors in bone marrow transplantation: a review and recommendations for research. *Bone Marrow Transplantation, 13*, 357–375.

Annas, G. (2005). "Culture of Life" politics at the bedside—the case of Terri Shiavo. *New England Journal of Medicine, 352*(16), 1717–1715.

Back, A., Arnold, R., & Quill, T. (2003). Hope for the best, and prepare for the worst, *Annals of Internal Medicine, 138*(5), 439–442.

Baer, C.L. (2001). Good news, bad news! *Critical Care Medicine, 29*(12), 2391–2392.

Bailey, S. (2003). The concept of futility in health care decision-making. *Nursing Ethics, 11*(1), 77–83.

Barker, J.N., Davies, S.M., DeFor, T.E., Burns, L.J., McGlave, P.B., Miller, J.S., et al. (2002). Determinants of survival after human leucocyte antigen-matched unrelated donor bone marrow transplantation in adults. *British Journal Haematology, 118*(1), 101–107.

Beauchamp, T., & Childress, J. (2001). *Principles of Biomedical Ethics* (5th ed.). New York: Oxford University Press.

Brant, J., Iwamoto, R., Rumsey, K., & Summers, B. (1996). Statement on the scope and standards of oncology nursing practice. In J. Brant (Ed.), *American Nurses Association, Oncology Nursing Society* (pp. 28–29). Washington, DC: American Nurses Publishing.

Brown, R., Butow, P., Butt, D., Moore, A., & Tatersall, M. (2004). Developing ethical strategies to assist oncologists in seeking informed consent to cancer clinical trials. *Social Science and Medicine, 58*(2), 379–390.

Buckner, C.D., Peterson, F.B., & Bolonesi, B.A. (1994). Bone marrow donors. In S.J. Forman, K.G. Blume, & E.D. Thomas, (Eds.), *Bone Marrow Transplantation* (pp. 259–269). Boston: Blackwell Scientific Publications.

Calman, K.C. (2002). Communication of risk: choice, consent and trust. *Lancet, 360*(9327), 166–168.

Chan, K.W., Gajewski, J., Supkis, D., Pentz, R., Champlin, R., Bleyer, W. (1996). Use of minors as bone marrow donors: current attitude and management. A survey of 56 pediatric transplantation centers. *Journal of Pediatrics, 128*(5), 644–648.

Charles, C., Gafni, A., & Whelan, T. (1999). What do we mean by partnership in making decisions about treatment? *British Medical Journal, 319*, 780–782.

Clarke, C.M. (2001). Rationing scarce life-sustaining resources on the basis of age. *Journal of Advanced Nursing, 35*(5), 799–804.

Cook, D., Rocker, G., Marshall, J., Sjokvist, P., Dodek, P., Griffith, L., et al. (2003). Withdrawal of mechanical ventilation in anticipation of death in the intensive care unit. *New England Journal of Medicine, 349*(12), 1123–1132.

Crawley, L., Marshall, P., Lo, B., & Koenig, B. (2002). Strategies for culturally effective end-of-life care. *Annals of Internal Medicine, 136*(9), 673–679.

Daugherty, C. (2004). Ethical issues in phase 1 clinical trials. *Clinical Advances in Hematology & Oncology, 2*(6), 358–360.

Daugherty, C., Ratain, M., & Grochowski, E. (1995). Perceptions of cancer patients and their physicians involved in phase I trials. *Journal of Clinical Oncology, 13*(9), 1062–1072.

Davis, S., Kristjanson, L., & Blight, J. (2003). Communicating with families of patients in an acute hospital with advanced cancer. *Cancer Nursing, 26*(5), 337–345.

Directive to Physicians and Family or Surrogates (Living Will), State of Texas, 2000. Advance Directive Act (see 166.033, Health and Safety Code).

Dodd, S., Jansson, B., Brown-Saltzman, K., Shirk, M., & Wunch, K. (2004). Expanding nurses' participation in ethics: an empirical examination of ethical activism and ethical assertiveness. *Nursing Ethics, 11*(1), 15–27.

Douglas, R., & Brown, H.N. (2002). Patients' attitudes toward advance directives. *Journal of Nursing Scholarship, 34*(1), 61–65.

Dresser, R. (2003). Precommitment: a misguided strategy for securing death with dignity. *Texas Law Review, 1823*, 1–23.

Fagerlin, A., & Schneider, C. (2004). Enough: the failure of the living will. *Hastings Center Report, 34*(2), 30–42.

Fine, R.L., & Mayo, T. (2003). Resolution of futility by due process: early experience with the Texas Advance Directives Act. *Annals of Internal Medicine, 138*(9), 743–746.

Fletcher, J. (Ed.). *Introduction to Clinical Ethics*. University of Virginia, Center for Biomedical Ethics, 1993, pp. 15–17.

Fox, D.M., & Leichter, H.M. (1991). Rationing care in Oregon: the new accountability. *Health Affairs, 10*(2), 7–27.

Foxall, M.J., & Gaston-Johansson, F. (1996). Burden and health outcomes of family caregivers of hospitalized bone marrow transplant patients. *Journal of Advanced Nursing, 24*, 915–923.

Fry, S.T., & Duffy, M.E. (2001). The development and psychometric evaluation of the Ethical Issues scale. *Journal of Nursing Scholarship, 33*(3), 272–277.

Groeger, J., Lemshow, S., Price, K., Nierman, D., White, P., Klar, J., et al (1998). Multicenter outcome study of cancer patients admitted to the intensive care unit: a probability of mortality model. *Journal of Clinical Oncology, 16*(2), 761–770.

Hamric, A.B. (2001). Reflections on being in the middle. *Nursing Outlook, 49*(6), 254–257.

Hanssen, I. (2004). An intercultural nursing perspective on autonomy. *Nursing Ethics, 11*(1), 28–41.

Hennessy, B.J., White M., & Crotty, G.M. (1997). Predicting death in mechanically ventilated recipients of bone marrow transplants. *Annals of Internal Medicine, 127*(1), 88.

Hinds, P.S., Oakes, L., Furman, W., Quargnenti, A., Olson, M.S., Foppiano, P., et al. (2001). End-of-life decision making by adolescents, parents, and healthcare providers in pediatric oncology. *Cancer Nursing, 24*(2), 122–136.

Holmes-Rovner, M., & Wills, C.E. (2002). Improving informed consent—insights from behavioral decision research. *Medical Care, 40*(9), 30–38.

Huaringa, A.J., Leyva, F.J., Giralt, S.A., Blanco, J., Signes-Costa, J., Velarde, H., et al. (2000). Outcome of bone marrow transplantation patients requiring mechanical ventilation. *Critical Care Medicine, 28*(4), 1232–1234.

Hutchins, L., Unger, J., Crowley, J., Coltman, C., & Albain, K. (1999). Underrepresentation of patients 65 years of age or older in cancer-treatment trials. *New England Journal of Medicine, 341*(27), 2061–2067.

Iezzoni, L.I., Ash, A.S., Shwartz, M., Daley, J. Hughes, J.S., & Mackiernan, Y.D. (1995). Predicting who dies depends on how severity is measured: implications for evaluating patient outcomes. *Annals of Internal Medicine, 123*(10), 763–770.

Jacobe, S., Hassan, A., Veys, P., & Mok, Q. (2003). Outcomes of children requiring admission to an intensive care unit after bone marrow transplantation. *Critical Care Medicine, 31*(5), 1299–1305.

Jacoby, L.H., Maloy, B., Cirenza, E., Shelton, W., Goggins, T., & Balient, J. (1999). The basis of informed consent for BMT patients. *Bone Marrow Transplantation, 23*, 711–717.

Jezewski, M.A., Meeker, M.A., & Shrader, M. (2003). Voices of oncology nurses: what is needed to assist patients with advance directives. *Cancer Nursing, 26*(2), 105–112.

Jonsen, A., Siegler, M., & Winslade, W. (2002). *Clnical Ethics* (5th ed.). New York: McGraw-Hill.

Kelly, D., Ross, S., Gray, B., & Smith, P. (2000). Death, dying and emotional labour: problematic dimensions of the bone marrow transplant nursing role? *Journal of Advanced Nursing, 32*(4), 952–960.

Kerridge, I., Lowe, M., Seldon, M., Enno, A., & Deveridge, S. (1997). Clinical and ethical issues in the treatment of a Jehovah's Witness with acute myeloblastic leukemia. *Archives of Internal Medicine, 25*(157), 1753–1757.

Kessler, D., & McClellan, M. (2004). Advance directives and medical treatment at the end of life. *Journal of Health Economics, 23*, 111–127.

Kolarik, R.C., Arnold, R.M., Fischer, G.S., & Hanusa, B. (2002). Advance care planning: a comparison of values statements and treatment preferences. *Journal of General Internal Medicine, 17*, 618–624.

Lang, F., & Quill, T. (2004). Making decisions with families at the end of life. *American Family Physician, 70*, 719–723, 725–726.

Lee, S., Fairclough, D., Antin, J., & Weeks, J. (2001). Discrepancies between patient and physician estimates for the success of stem cell transplantation. *Journal of the American Medical Association, 285*(8), 1034–1038.

Lee, S.J., Klein, J.P., Barrett, A.J., Rinden, O., Antin, J.H., Cahn, J.Y., et al. (2002). Severity of chronic graft-versus-host disease: association with treatment-related mortality and relapse. *Blood, 15*, 406–414.

Lind, C., Anderson, B., & Oberle, K. (2003). Ethical issues in adolescent consent for research. *Nursing Ethics, 10*(5), 504–511.

Little, M.T., & Storb, R. (2002). History of haematopoietic stem-cell transplantation. *Nature Reviews Cancer, 2*, 231–237.

Loewy, E.H. (1998). Ethical considerations in executing and implementing advance directives. *Archives of Internal Medicine, 158*, 321–324.

Massimo, L. (1996). Ethical problems in bone marrow transplantation in children. *Bone Marrow Transplantation, 18*(2), 8–12.

Matsumura, S., Bito, S., Liu, H., Kahn, K., Fukuhara, S., Kagawa-Singer, M., et al. (2002). Acculturation of attitudes toward end-of-life care: a cross-cultural survey of Japanese Americans and Japanese. *Journal of General Internal Medicine, 17*, 531–539.

Mazzi, P., Palazzo, G., Amurri, B., Cervellera, M., Rizzo, C., & Mazzi, A. (2000). Acute leukemia in Jehovah's Witnesses: a challenge for hematologists. *Haematologica, 85*(11), 1221–1222.

Meier, D., & Morrison, R.S. (2002). Autonomy reconsidered. *New England Journal of Medicine, 346*, 1087–1089.

Mishel, M. (1988). Uncertainty in illness. *State of the Science, 20*(4), 225.

Molassiotis, A., van den Akker, O., & Boughton, B. (1997). Perceived social support, family environment and psychosocial recovery in bone marrow transplant long-term survivors. *Social Science and Medicine, 44*(3), 317–325.

Neitzert, C.S., Ritvo, P., Dancey, J., Weiser, K., Murray, C., & Avery, J. (1998). The psychosocial impact of bone marrow transplantation: a review of the literature. *Bone Marrow Transplantation, 22*, 409–422.

Neumann, J., Pentz, R., & Flamm, A. (2001). Evaluating the impact of ethics rounds on nurses' roles as caregiver and patient advocate [abstract]. *Oncology Nursing Society Congress*, San Diego. Abstract 206.

Neumann, J.L. (2001). Ethical issues confronting oncology nurses. *Nursing Clinics of North America, 36*, 827–841.

Neumann, J.L. (2004). Ethical consideration in the hematopoietic stem cell transplantation nursing. In S. Ezzone (Ed.), *Hematopoietic Stem Cell Transplantation: A Manual for Nursing Practice* (pp. 221–235). Pittsburgh, PA: Oncology Nursing Society.

The Nuremburg Code, 1947. (1949). In A. Mitscherlich & F. Mielke (Eds.), *Doctors of Infamy: The Story of the*

Nazi Medical Crimes (pp. xxiii–xxv). New York: Schuman.

Olver, I., Eliott, J., & Blake-Mortimer, J. (2002). Cancer patients' perception of do not resuscitate orders. *Psycho-Oncology, 11*, 181–187.

Parascandola, M., Hawkins, J., & Danis, M. (2002). Patient autonomy and the challenge of clinical uncertainty. *Kennedy Institute of Ethics Journal, 12*(3), 245–264.

Penticuff, J.H. (1997). Nursing perspectives in bioethics. In K. Hoshino (Ed.), *Japanese and Western Bioethics* (pp. 49–60). Boston: Kluwer Academic Publishers.

Pentz R. (1999). Case presentation—core curriculum. Fellows ethics course. MD Anderson Cancer Center, Houston, TX.

Pentz, R.D. (2004). *Ethics: are we making progress?* Paper presented at the IBMTR/ASBMT Tandem meeting, Orlando, FL.

Pentz, R.D., Chan, K.W., Neumann, J.L., Champlin, R.E., & Korbling, M. (2004). Designing an ethical policy for bone marrow donation by minors and others lacking capacity. *Cambridge Quarterly of Healthcare Ethics, 13*(2), 149–155.

Perkins, H.S., Geppert, C.M.A., Gonzales, A., Cortez, J.D., & Hazuda, H.P. (2002). Cross-cultural similarities and differences in attitudes about advance care planning. *Journal of General Internal Medicine, 17*(1), 48–57.

Perry, A.R., Rivlin, M.M., & Goldstone, A.H. (1999). Bone marrow transplant patients with life-threatening organ failure: when should treatment stop? *Journal of Clinical Oncology, 17*(1), 298–310.

Peter, E., Lunardi, V., & Macfarlane, A. (2004). Nursing resistance as ethical action: literature review. *Journal of Advanced Nursing, 46*(4), 403–416.

Prendergast, T.J. (2001). Advance care planning: pitfalls, progress, promise. *Critical Care Medicine, 29*(2), 34–39.

Price, K.J., Thall, P.F., Kish, S.K., Shannon, V.R., & Andersson, B.S. (1998). Prognostic indicators for blood and marrow transplant patients admitted to an intensive care unit. *American Journal of Respiratory Critical Care Medicine, 158*(3), 876–884.

Prieto, J.M., Blanch, J., Atala, J., Carreras, E., Montserrat, R., Cirera, E., et al. (2002). Psychiatric morbidity and impact on hospital length of stay among hematologic cancer patients receiving stem-cell transplantation. *Journal of Clinical Oncology, 20*(7), 1907–1917.

Quill, T. (2005). Terri Shiavo—a tragedy compounded. *New England Journal of Medicine, 352*(16), 1630–1633.

Quill, T.E., & Brody, H. (1996). Physician recommendations and patient autonomy: finding a balance between physician power and patient choice. *Annals of Internal Medicine, 125*(9), 763–769.

Rajput, V., & Bekes, C.E. (2002). Ethical issues in hospital medicine. *Medical Clinics of North America, 86*(4), 869–870.

Rubenfeld, G.D., & Crawford, S.W. (1996). Withdrawing life support from mechanically ventilated recipients of bone marrow transplants: a case for evidence-based guidelines. *Annals of Internal Medicine, 125*(8), 625–633.

Sandel, M. (2004). Embryo ethics—the moral logic of stem-cell research. *New England Journal of Medicine, 351*(3), 207–209.

Scanlon, C. (2003). Ethical concerns in end-of-life care: When questions about advance directives and the withdrawal of life-sustaining interventions arise, how should decisions be made? *American Journal of Nursing, 103*(1), 48–55.

Schneiderman, L., Gilmer, T., & Teetzel, H.D. (2000). Impact of ethics consultations in the intensive care setting: a randomized, controlled trial. *Critical Care Medicine, 28*, 3920–3924.

Schneiderman, L.J., Jecker, N.S., & Jonsen, A.R. (2001). Abuse of futility. *Archives of Internal Medicine, 161*(1), 128–130.

Shahjahan, M., Alamo, J., deLima, M., Khouri, I., Gajewski, J., Andersson, B., et al. (2004). Effect of comorbidities on allogeneic hematopoietic stem cell transplant outcomes in AML/MDS patients in first complete remission [abstract]. Presented at Tandem BMT Meetings, Orlando, FL. Abstract 150143.

Shapiro, J., & Bowles, K. (2002). Nurses' and consumers' understanding of and comfort with the Patient Self-Determination Act. *Journal of Nursing Administration, 32*(10), 503–508.

Shemie, S. (2003). Bone marrow transplantation and intensive care unit admission: what really matters? *Critical Care Medicine, 31*(5), 1579.

Snelling, P. (2004). Consequences count: against absolutism at the end of life. *Journal of Advanced Nursing, 46*(4), 350–357.

Stevens, P., & Pletsch, P. (2002). Ethical issues of informed consent: mothers' experiences enrolling their children in bone marrow transplantation research. *Cancer Nursing, 25*(2), 81–87.

Sugarman, J., Kaalund, V., Kodish, E., Mashall, M., Reisner, E., Wilfond, B., et al. (1997). Ethical issues in umbilical cord blood banking. *Journal of the American Medical Association, 278*(11), 938–943.

Syrjala, K., Langer, S., Abrams, J., Storer, B., Sander, J., Flowers, M., et al. (2004). Recovery and long-term function after haemapoietic cell transplantation for leukemia or lymphoma. *Journal of the American Medical Association, 291*(19), 2335–2343.

Teno, J., Fisher, E., Hamel, M., Coppola, K., & Dawson, N. (2002). Medical care inconsistent with patients' treatment goals: association with 1-year Medicare resource use and survival. *Journal of American Geriatrics Society, 50*, 496–500.

Tilden, V., Tolle, S., Nelson, C., & Fields, C. (2001). Family decision-making to withdraw life-sustaining treatments from hospitalized patients. *Nursing Research, 50*(2), 105–115.

Tulsky, J., Fischer, G., Rose, M., & Arnold, R. (1998). Opening the black box: how do physicians communicate about advance directives. *Annals of Internal Medicine, 129*(6), 441–449.

Weeks, J., Cook, F., O'Day, S., Peterson, L., Wenger, N., Reding, D., et al. (1998). Relationship between cancer patients' predictions of prognosis and their treatment preferences. *Journal of the American Medical Asssociation, 279*, 1709–1714.

Wendler, D. (2000). Informed consent, exploitation and whether it is possible to conduct human subjects research without either one. *Bioethics, 14*(4), 310–339.

Whitney, S.N. (2003). A new model of medical decisions: exploring the limits of shared decision making. *Medical Decision Making, 23*, 275–280.

Wolcott, D.L., Wellisch, D.K., Fawzy, F.I., & Landsverk, J. (1986). Psychological adjustment of adult bone marrow transplant donors whose recipient survives. *Transplant, 41*(4), 484–488.

Zhukovsky, D., Hwang, J., Palmer, J., Smith, M., Flamm, A., & Wiley, J. (2004). A comparative analysis of inpatient do not resuscitate (DNR) forms used at National Cancer Institute–designated cancer centers (NCICC). *Journal of Clinical Oncology, 22*(145), 8222.

Chapter 15

Hematopoietic Cell Transplantation: The Trajectory of Quality of Life

Liz Cooke, RN, MN, ANP, AOCN®

Marcia Grant, RN, DNSc, FAAN

Deborah Eldredge, PhD, RN

History and Changes in Transplant

There were an estimated 33,440 new cases of leukemia and 62,250 new cases of lymphoma for the year 2004, and many of these patients experienced a hematopoetic cell transplant (HCT) (American Cancer Society [ACS], 2004). Thousands of HCTs are performed each year, with the number of transplants increasing for treatment of malignant diseases (King, 1996; Andrykowski et al., 1999). Along with the increase in the number of transplants and the refinement of medical treatment, survival rates after HCT have steadily improved since the late 1960s. Mortality rates at 100 days posttransplant vary from 5% to 42%, depending on diagnosis and stage of disease at the time of transplant (Loberiza, 2003). This increase in survival is due to improvements in human leukocyte antigen (HLA) matching, transfusion medicine, antibiotic coverage, graft-versus-host prophylaxis and treatment, gene therapy, stem cell collection with early engraftment, growth factors, and changes in transplant conditioning with reduced intensity and nonmyeloablative

transplants that have led to a revolution in theoretical treatment of transplants (Whedon and Fliedner, 1999).

During the 1960s and 1970s, cure was the goal of transplant science, as well as the outcome desired. However, beginning in the late 1980s and into the 1990s, with the increase in survival, psychosocial aspects of the cancer survivor became more of an essential component of care (Zebrack, 2000). Aaronson and colleagues (1991), in their review article of quality of life (QOL) research, discussed the fact that QOL should be an integral part of medical care. Zebrack (2000), in his article, discusses that QOL became a major outcome measure in the mid-1990s, replacing the terms "adaptation" and "psychosocial adjustment." Subsequently, QOL became the psychosocial outcome desired. With increases in survival rate, physical and psychosocial issues have been better identified. Several studies have described major QOL issues after transplant. These issues include physical symptoms such as fatigue, pain, dyspnea, insomnia, poor concentration, appearance, concern about body image, and physical restrictions; psychological symptoms such as fear of the future, loss of control, anxiety, and depression;

social issues such as reintegration into the family, workforce, social roles, sexuality, and dealing with financial issues; and existential/religious issues (Altmaier et al., 1991, Kopp et al., 1998, Baker et al., 1999, Baker, 1994, Molassiotis, 1996, Vickberg et al., 2001, Wettergren et al., 1997). Thus, transplant continues to be associated with a substantial risk of mortality and morbidity, increasing the burden on patients, families, and health-care providers (Blume and Amylon, 1999). The purpose of this chapter is to define QOL as used in HCT patient assessment, to summarize major QOL findings divided by time since transplant and by the four dimensions of the QOL model, to summarize QOL studies on pediatric patients and for caregivers, and to discuss intervention studies to date. Case studies are used to demonstrate typical problems faced by patients after transplant.

QOL History/Construct

QOL History

Quality of life (QOL) assessment is an important aspect of the current care provided to the cancer patient, and it has been successfully used as an outcome in describing HCT patients. Whereas traditional outcomes in response to cancer treatment have included disease-free survival, tumor response, and overall survival, assessment of quality of life adds an outcome of significant importance to the clinician, the patient, and the family. Information on QOL outcomes provides valuable information when requesting consent from patients, planning education interventions to assist patients in adaptation, and evaluating alternative treatment approaches.

The increasing interest in and importance of QOL as an outcome is illustrated by the grow-

ing number of studies that include this concept. QOL measurements are used in all new anticancer clinical trials, in health services research, in acute care, and in chronic illness (Eiser and Morse, 2001; Mandelblatt and Eisenberg, 1995). Quality of life publications have increased dramatically over the last 30 years. The first listing of the citation *quality of life* appeared in Index Medicus in 1972 with 15 citations. By 2003 more than 15,000 citations had accumulated with *quality of life* as the major topic or subtopic.

QOL Definition

A challenge to the use of QOL assessments in the clinical area is the lack of a common definition of QOL. Most definitions used today are derived from the World Health Organization's definition of health as not only the absence of disease and infirmity, but also a positive state of physical, mental, and social well-being (WHO, 1993). This definition includes six broad domains: physical health, psychological state, levels of independence, social relationships, environmental features, and spiritual concerns. Some definitions may also include a measure of the patient's satisfaction with their level of function in the various domains (Gotay et al., 1992; Ferrans, 1996; Moinpour et al., 1989). For example, the level of functioning may be assessed, as well as the satisfaction the patient has with that level of functioning. One important aspect of the multiple domain definition is that more than one domain needs to be measured. That is, if only one dimension is measured, for example, psychological well-being, then that is a study of psychological well-being, and not quality of life. An example of a measure that does not assess QOL is the Karnofsky score, which measures only functional status.

To limit the broad definition of QOL, researchers interested in disease and treatment-related QOL have used health-related quality of life (HRQOL) as a way to keep the focus on health and disease. This approach provides the rationale for excluding such aspects as housing and education in the definition of HRQOL. This results in some limits to the construct being measured; however, the multiple dimensions that still remain are frequently composed of many items each. Multiple questionnaires or instruments have been developed to measure QOL, and the science for establishing the reliability and validity of these measures has evolved with some clear recommendations and procedures for establishing a new instrument (Scientific Advisory Committee of the Medical Outcomes Trust, 2002).

Definitions of QOL within the nursing literature have paralleled other disciplines' definitions with a focus on the multidimensional nature of the concept. Ferrans (1990) reviewed the QOL literature in relation to definitions and conceptual issues included, and identified five broad categories into which QOL definitions could be grouped. These categories focus on the patient's 1) ability to lead a normal life, 2) happiness/satisfaction, 3) achievement of personal goals, 4) ability to lead a socially useful life, and 5) physical and/or mental capabilities (actual or potential).

Research by Grant, Padilla, and Ferrell has emphasized the need for a multidimensional definition of QOL, including an existential/spiritual dimension (Grant, Ferrell, and Sakurai, 1994). These investigators have identified QOL as consisting of four dimensions or domains: physical well-being, psychological well-being, social well-being, and spiritual well-being. Each dimension consists of generic items of concern to all cancer populations, as well as items specific to a type of cancer or treatment. The model has been validated across studies in a number of

cancer patient populations (Ferrell et al., 1992b; Ferrell et al., 1997; Ferrell et al., 1998a, 1998b; Grant, 1999a, 1999b; Greimel et al., 1997; Padilla et al., 1990). Work has also included development of an instrument specific to measuring QOL in HCT patients (Ferrell et al., 1992a, 1992b; Grant et al., 1992). **Figure 15-1** identifies the QOL model as it applies to HCT patients. This model was identified through qualitative analysis of HCT survivor data describing positive and negative aspects of QOL. The resulting instrument has been used in a number of other QOL studies of HCT patients (Saleh and Brockopp, 2001; Whedon et al., 1995; King et al., 1995).

QOL Assessment

QOL assessment can include several levels of measurement. A global assessment of QOL can be obtained with a single item asking patients to rate their QOL on a given scale. The next level of assessment includes the broad domains or aspects of QOL. For example, physical well-being, functional status, psychological well-being, social well-being, spiritual well-being, and economic well-being. A single score can also be used to assess each of these domains. The third level is the individual item level, wherein specific aspects of each domain are measured. For example, under the physical well-being domain, one could measure fatigue levels, nausea, and mouth sores; under the psychological well-being domain, one could measure typical QOL concerns, such as anxiety, depression, and control; under the social well-being domain, one could measure family distress, roles and relationships, and work; under the spiritual domain, one could measure the meaning of the illness, and hope. When an assessment instrument contains many items, summary scores for subscales can be calculated. Such

Figure 15-1 QOL-BMT model.

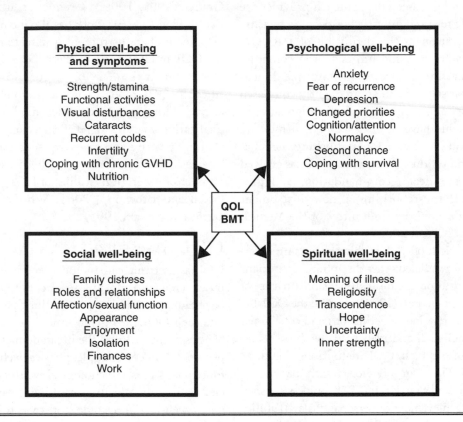

calculations generally involve adding up the items in a specific domain and dividing by the number of items to obtain a mean score. All three levels of measurement can provide important information in caring for cancer patients and survivors—the overall assessment of QOL, the domain scores, and specific item scores. Overall scores provide a score that may or may not change much over time, whereas subscale or domain scores may identify what concerns the patient faces at specific time periods. Item scores provide specific aspects that could be used to test

interventions; for example, fatigue may be an item that impacts the physical well-being domain. Developing approaches to relieving fatigue could impact not only fatigue, but also the physical well-being domain and overall QOL.

Many questionnaires and surveys have been developed to measure QOL, with some of them specific to the HCT population. Hacker, in her review article (2003), created an exceptional table reviewing QOL tools and studies. She discusses sample size, patient population, design, measurement points, instruments used, and major finding with each study. Selection of an instrument should be based on the purpose of the assessment—is it a research endeavor? A clinical endeavor? What will the investigator do with the results of the assessment? Examining a number of questionnaires and selecting one that is reliable, valid, and fits the purpose is an important step in obtaining the right data for the questions posed. **Table 15-1** lists some of the more common instruments used to measure QOL in the HCT population and dimensions measured. Some of these are general instruments and others have been developed specifically for the HCT population. All have been used in research on QOL in HCT patients.

QOL Score

QOL is an important outcome assessment in HCT patients, and can be used before, immediately after, and for years following the transplant discharge. Studies have included multiple dimension measurements of functional status, physical well-being, psychological well-being, social well-being, and spiritual well-being (Ferrell et al., 1992a, 1992b; Grant et al., 1992; Baker et al., 1999; Bush et al., 1995; Andrykowski, Greiner, et al., 1995; Syrjala et al., 1993; McQuellon et al., 1998; Molassiotis and Morris, 1999). These studies have contributed valuable data in understanding

Table 15-1 EXAMPLES OF INSTRUMENTS FOR ASSESSING QOL DIMENSIONS IN HCT PATIENTS.

Name of Instrument	Generic	HCT Specific	Dimensions
City of Hope Quality of Life for Hematologic Cell Transplant		X	Physical, psychological, social, spiritual
POMS (Profile of Mood State)	X		Psychological
FLIC (Functional Living Index—Cancer)	X		Physical, psychological, family interaction, social ability, somatic sensation
PAIS (Psychosocial Adjustment to Illness Scale)	X		Health, sex role, social support, interpsychic functioning
QLI-Ferrans (Quality of Life Index—Ferrans)	X		Health and functioning, socio-economic functioning, psychological functioning, family functioning
FACT-BMT (Functional Assessment of Cancer Therapy—Bone Marrow Transplant)		X	Physical, role, emotional, social, cognitive functioning

the impact of HCT on patients' and families' lives, and they provide a valuable foundation for designing studies to improve survivors' QOL.

QOL in HCT Patients First Year Posttransplant

Physical Quality of Life

Physical well-being impacts QOL significantly in HCT survivors up to 3 years post-HCT, and evidence indicates that the time since transplant greatly impacts how QOL is rated (Baker, 1994; Prieto et al., 1996; Sutherland et al., 1997; Vose et al., 1992). Broers et al. (2000) noted that a large portion of patients experience functional limitations and somatic symptoms within the first year. Heinonen and colleagues (2001) studied allogeneic patients during the first 3 years after transplant and found that patients perceived their physical well-being as worst in the first year. Generally, after 1 year, most patients carry on with daily activities, with 68% actively participating in work, school, or household activities. Another study validated this information, indicating that most patients returned to full-time employment (76%); however, patients with extremely physical positions such as manual workers were less likely to return to work compared to office workers (Vose et al., 1992). The most common clinical factors affecting physical well-being that have been reported to affect QOL include fatigue, gastrointestinal symptoms, infection potential, GVHD, and sexual issues. Other physical symptoms listed within the first 5 years included headaches, dizziness, loss of hair, shivering, and shortness of breath (van Agthoven et al., 2001; Molassiotis et al., 1995).

FATIGUE

Fatigue is the most common distressing significant symptom posttransplant, and it is higher the first year than in subsequent years (Andrykowski, Brady et al., 1995; Baker et al., 1999; Kopp et al., 1998; Molassiotis et al., 1996a). Although allogeneic transplant patients experience significant fatigue, even autologous transplant patients report a significant amount (van Agthoven et al., 2001). Along with fatigue, related symptoms have been identified such as insomnia and energy level. Chao and colleagues (1992) reported that 90 days post-HCT, 34% of autologous patients reported difficulty sleeping, and Andrykowski and colleagues (1997) reported that 51% of survivors mentioned the presence of sleep difficulty over the first 5 years. McQuellon et al. (1998) measured psychosocial recovery over the first year after HCT— at baseline, hospital discharge, 100 days, and 1 year post-HCT. Effect over time on fatigue or energy ratings was significant. The percentage of patients reporting 75% or greater of normal energy at each time point was: discharge, 10.5%; 100 days, 33.3%; 1 year, 51%. Fatigue, insomnia, and energy level are all significant symptoms in the first year, with one study indicating that these symptoms may even impact the patients' psychological status (Andrykowski et al., 1997).

ADDITIONAL SYMPTOMS

Gastrointestinal (GI) difficulties are very common the first year, with poor appetite being probably the most common GI symptom cited (Chao et al., 1992; Molassiotis et al., 1996a; Vose et al., 1992). Most studies indicate that eating difficulties subside the first year (Baker et al., 1999). Other related symptoms include changes in taste, oral mucositis, sore mouth when swallowing, dry mouth, nausea, vomiting, and changes in bowel patterns (Bellm et al., 2000; Hengeveld et al.,

1988; Kopp et al., 1998; Molassiotis et al., 1995; Molassiotis et al., 1996a). Infections are listed by patients as a continued health concern the first year. One study reported that 34% of patients experienced frequent colds (Baker et al., 1999; Chao et al., 1992). The presence of graft-versus-host disease (GVHD) is a factor that predicts lower QOL (Chiodi et al., 2000). Also, patients 1 year posttransplant list GVHD as a major concern (Baker et al., 1999). Some of these physical aspects may become permanent and impact QOL (McQuellen and Andrykowski, 2004).

SEXUAL ISSUES

Sexual issues can become a QOL issue within the first 6 to 12 months. The literature indicates that issues such as fertility and a decrease in sexual interest or libido are common. (Vose et al., 1992; Molassiotis et al., 1995; Baker et al., 1999). Both men and women experience sexual issues. Spinelli et al. (1994) noted that women who received total body irradiation as part of the conditioning regimen before allogeneic transplant had decreased estrogen, and increased follicle stimulating hormone (FSH) and luteinizing hormone (LH) post-HCT. At the 6-month follow-up, 78% reported vasomotor symptoms and 94% reported sexual difficulties. Syjrala et al. (1998) reported that men's arousal problems doubled after transplant, then returned to normal at 3 years. Testosterone levels also decreased initially and then increased for most men.

Psychological Quality of Life

Psychological issues within the first year are numerous. Initially, most of the patients focus on the physical aspects of transplant, and then are surprised to find that the psychological distress may become quite overwhelming and is slow to decrease (Keogh et al., 1998). Level of psychosocial distress has been explored by Twillman and colleagues (1993). A three-point level of risk was proposed, with level 1 including patients at low risk for developing psychosocial complications, level 2 representing moderate, and level 3 representing high risk. Although most patients within the first year report good QOL and also report that distress improves slowly throughout the first year, a significant number report severe psychological distress after transplant (Baker et al., 1999; Wettergren et al., 1997). Many studies have looked at vulnerable time points surrounding the transplant experience. The following time points of distress have been identified: before admission, during admission, directly before the transplant, discharge from the inpatient setting, and for the allogeneic patients, between 3 to 5 months and 6 to 9 months posttransplant (McQuellon et al., 1998; Fife et al., 2000; Gaston-Johansson and Foxall, 1996; Leigh et al., 1995). In contrast, other studies show decreases in anxiety and depression 1 week after transplant, and the periods of least emotional distress were at 3 months and 1 year (Fife et al., 2000; Leigh et al., 1995). By 1 year after transplant, feelings of loss of control, difficulty with dependence, anxiety, depression, and being more cautious all decreased.

Factors that relate to psychological distress and health are numerous and may relate to HCT morbidity and mortality (Andrykowski, 1994; Andrykowski et al., 1994; Broers et al., 2000; Colon et al., 1991). For example, one study noted a significant negative relationship between depressive symptoms and improved survival for patients at 31 days posttransplant (Colon et al., 1991). Identified factors that relate to psychological health and distress are the following: pre-HCT emotional and psychological status, anxious preoccupation, poorer functional QOL, disease recurrence, negative mood, type of transplant, locus of control, degree of social support, and relatives' distress (Andrykowski, 1994; Andrykowski et al., 1999; Curbow et al., 1993; Meyers et al., 1994; Keogh et al., 1998). Fears identified by HCT patients during the first year are low energy level, difficulty returning to normal, and fear of the future (Baker et al., 1999). Pretransplant family conflict, marital status, and presence of GVHD predicted emotional distress at 1 year.

Some studies have identified coping styles or themes that patients have used within the first year. Shuster and colleagues (1996) identified five themes of coping within the first 4 weeks: psychologic functioning, alertness, attitude, social relationships, and spirituality. Coping methods during the first year were the following: hope, directing attention, maintaining control over the situation, and acceptance. Effective coping mechanisms were used by patients who demonstrated less mood disturbance, whereas patients experiencing psychological maladjustment during isolation used ineffective coping styles (Molassiotis et al., 1996a).

Social Quality of Life

Social support for the transplant patient within the first year is life-sustaining; in fact, Colon and colleagues (1991) found that on the median day 31 there was a significant positive relationship between perceived support and improved survival. The first year is a time when patients can feel quite powerless about their social world and negotiating a new social role for themselves (Steeves, 1992). Common social concerns within the first year involve the following: social/role function, separation from home and loved ones, problems with family and children, stigmatization, difficulties with hospital bills, financial difficulties, job or work difficulties, discrimination in the workplace, health or life insurance,

difficulty making future plans, and difficulties with personal or intimate physical relations (Hjermstad et al., 1999; McQuellon et al., 1998; Baker et al., 1999). Hjermstad and colleagues (1999) did an interesting study titled "Do patients who are treated with stem cell transplantation have a health-related quality of life comparable to the general population?" The outcomes of this prospective study 1 year after transplant revealed that stem cell patients had significantly lower social and role function, with financial difficulties being a significant issue.

Spiritual Quality of Life

Very few studies specifically examine the spiritual aspect of transplant patients within the first year. Shuster and others (1996) identified five themes of coping for patients posttransplant within the first 4 weeks; spirituality was one of them. In Steeves's (1992) hermeneutic study, patients within the first 100 days were interviewed about the meaning of their lives during and following the transplant. In finding meaning, patients renegotiated their social position when faced with a new situation and they tried to reach a personal understanding about the transplant experience as a whole. These findings revealed the personal spiritual challenges that faced the transplant patient, whose life dramatically changed from pre- to posttransplant.

QOL in HCT Patients 1 to 5 Years Posttransplant

Physical Quality of Life

Andrykowski, Greiner, and colleagues (1995) evaluated patients 12 to 124 months after transplant and found that slightly fewer than half of the patients considered themselves back to normal; 48% considered themselves back to normal with the problem areas being sexuality, physical activity, and work outside the home. Reports of less than normal cognitive, physical, occupational, and sexual and/or interpersonal functioning were common. Physical well-being was a significant predictor of satisfaction with QOL in patients 1 to 3 years after transplant (Heinonen et al., 2001). Factors that predicted a poorer QOL in transplant patients 1 to 5 years posttransplant were age, long-term sequelae, chronic GVHD (cGVHD), and short follow-up. A large portion of patients experienced functional limitations and somatic symptoms up to 3 years after transplant (Broers et al., 2000). Discordance between pre-HCT expectations for returning to normal and current functional status was associated with greater current psychological distress. Another study seemed to suggest that patients beyond 3 years posttransplant were indistinguishable from the normal population in most domains, although some still experienced troublesome symptoms (Sutherland et al., 1997).

FATIGUE

Fatigue, lack of energy, and sleep issues continue to be factors 1 to 5 years after transplant, with Andrykowski and colleagues (1997) noting that 65% of transplant survivors within 5 years reported problems with energy and 51% reported the presence of sleep difficulty. Also, Molassiotis and Morris (1999) found that fatigue had significant associations with other variables such as depression, general pain, infections, overall psychosocial adjustment, weight loss, anxiety, cognitive impairment, mouth/throat problems, insomnia, and loss of appetite.

COGNITIVE CHANGES

As early as the 1980s, the QOL literature began to indicate the existence of cognitive issues in adult patients. Andrykowski and colleagues (1989) studied 16 patients over three points in time. Patients exhibited long-term issues with difficulties in concentration and thinking, forgetfulness, slowed reaction time, and clumsiness. These neurological symptoms increased within the second and third time points, with the last two points in time being mostly less than 5 years apart. Another Andrykowski and colleagues (1990) study in patients 12 to 96 months from transplant reported that the increased dose of TBI was associated with increased cognitive dysfunction involving symptoms such as slowed reaction time, reduced attention and concentration, and difficulties in reasoning and problem solving (Andrykowski et al., 1990). These findings were confirmed in a study comparing HCT patients with nontransplanted adults (Wenz et al., 2000). Results showed a rapid decline of cognition ability after transplant. Harder and colleagues (2002) reported that the central neuropsychological difficulty reported by HCT patients was that of the speed with which information is processed. Predications of these deficits have not yet been reported.

OTHER

Bush and colleagues (1995) identified other issues such as skin and eye problems posttransplant in patients. Marks and colleagues (1999) found that unrelated transplant patients 1 to 5 years posttransplant were dissatisfied with physical strength and appearance. Molassiotis and Morris (1999) surveyed 28 unrelated patients 13 to 92 months after transplant and found that difficulty doing strenuous activity was reported by 53.6% of patients; 50% had difficulty taking a long walk. Incidence rates of symptoms were as follows: fatigue (55.9%), mouth and throat problems (25.3%), skin problems (26.9%), eye problems (48.9%), cognitive impairment (38.9%), general pain (41%), insomnia (42.7%), diarrhea (24.2%), and constipation (26.6%).

Psychological Quality of Life

Andrykowski, Brady, and others (1995) tested 172 allogeneic/autologous transplant patients 12 to 124 months after transplant and found that only a minority of patients considered themselves back to normal. Reports of less than normal cognitive, physical, occupational, and sexual or interpersonal functioning were common. Discordance between pre-HCT expectations for returning to normal and current functional status was associated with greater psychological distress. One study reported on patients 3 months to 5 years posttransplant and identified three trajectories and the related psychosocial concerns: 1) post-SCT recovery (disease recurrence, energy level, returning to normal); 2) during recovery (quality medical care and overprotectiveness of others); and 3) later in the course of recovery (feeling tense/anxious, sexual life, sleep relationship with spouse or partner, ability to be affectionate) (Andrykowski et al., 1999).

Certain factors have been associated with favorable psychological outcomes: higher external locus of control, more satisfaction with quality of life, and less psychological distress 3 years after HCT (Broers et al., 2000). In contrast, certain factors have been associated with unfavorable outcomes: A higher systemic symptomatology score, a shorter time post-HCT, a higher number of major infections, and lower educational level were predictive factors of a higher psychosocial distress (Prieto et al., 1996). Problem areas identified by patients during this time were the following: emotional dysfunction, skin and eye problems, cGVHD, sleep disturbances, and sexual dysfunction (Bush et al., 1995).

Molassiotis and colleagues (1995) compared autologous patients to allogeneic patients. Autologous patients mainly reported problems such as decreased sexual interest (35%), worrying thoughts (30%), anxiety (28.5%), lack of energy (23.8%), desperate feelings about the future (23.8%), tiredness (19%), depressed mood (19%), nervousness (14.3%), and difficulty concentrating (14.3%). Allogeneic patients mainly reported more physical problems such as dry mouth (38.5%), tiredness (38.5%), lack of energy (34.6%), tension (24%), headaches (26.2%), decreased sexual interest (20%), irritability (16%), worrying thoughts (15.4%), low back pain (15.4%), sore mouth/pain when swallowing (15.4%), and shortness of breath (15.3%). Eighty-six percent of the autologous patients described QOL as good, and 73% of the allogeneic patients described their QOL as good. When specifically looking at unrelated allogeneic patients, the incidence of emotional dysfunction was 63.3%. Areas of psychosocial dysfunction were found to be vocational environment, sexual relationships, social environment, and psychological distress, with high individual variability. Women showed significantly higher dysfunction compared with men in relation to overall psychosocial adjustment, vocational adjustment, social adjustment, and psychological distress. In a later study, correlations showed that younger age at diagnosis and younger age at HCT were both associated with better overall psychosocial adjustment, better sexual relationships, better adjustment with domestic environment, and better adjustment with vocational environment (Molassiotis and Morris, 1999).

Social Quality of Life

Posttransplant expectations of returning to family roles or back to work and resuming a normal life may be unrealistic. Molassiotis and Morris (1999) did a qualitative study to assess perceptions about QOL 13 to 98 months after HCT. Quality of life was described in terms of "normality," enjoyment, and fulfillment in life: being psychologically and physically healthy, being independent, having family and relationships, having work, experiencing happiness, and having material support. Social factors identified by survivors included frustration caused by the inability to function in life, family life, returning to work, and infertility. Main concerns about the future were related to health status, the long-term effects of the transplant, financial concerns, infertility, the normalization process, and the family.

The importance of family support is clear even years after transplant. Molassiotis et al. (1997) examined perceptions of social support and family dynamics in 91 HCT long-term survivors 6 to 122 months after HCT. Results indicated that the HCT group received more social support than a maintenance chemotherapy group and that the main sources of support were immediate family members. Strong family relationships were associated in both groups with significantly better adjustment with respect to their domestic, extended family or social environment, and psychological distress. Fromm and colleagues (1996) surveyed 90 HCT survivors (autologous/allogeneic), 1 to 10 years posttransplant. Negative sequelae included increased uncertainty about the future (59%), emotional taxing of family (52%), depression (43%), and family's increased uncertainty about the future (40%).

Role retention following transplant is significantly related to higher quality of life (Baker et al., 1991; McQuellen and Andrykowski, 2004). Role changes and caregiver burden continue several years after transplant (Boyle et al., 2000). After the transplant, importance is placed on the following roles: family member, caregiver, worker,

and friend. Declines in the roles of worker, caregiver, home maintainer, friend, and hobbyist occur while increases in student, volunteer, family member, religious participant, and participant in organizations occur (Baker et al., 1991). Patients have expressed concern over the role of the worker, or provider. Many studies indicate that 25–35% of patients do not return to full-time work within 1 to 2 years (Molassiotis et al., 1995; Marks et al., 1999; Syrjala et al., 1993; Baker et al., 1991). Issues in the workplace include being unable to work due to physical condition, being hindered in new jobs by medical history, delaying finishing school, job discrimination problems, and problems obtaining insurance (Belec, 1992).

Sexual issues after transplant are well documented in the literature, and they are also linked to greater psychological distress (Mumma et al., 1992). Issues include a decrease in sexual desire, inability to achieve an erection at least 50% of the time, inability to ejaculate, decrease in sexual satisfaction or pleasure, decrease in sexual activity, or even a complete cessation of sexual activity (Vose et al., 1992; Molassiotis and Morris, 1999; Zittoun et al., 1997). For men, difficulties with erection or ejaculation were associated with inability to attain sexual satisfaction. For women, loss of menses was associated with inability to attain sexual satisfaction. In a multivariate analysis, factors associated with sexual satisfaction were younger age at the time of HCT, the diagnosis of aplastic anemia rather than malignancy, satisfaction with appearance, overall life satisfaction, and a satisfying relationship with a significant other (Wingard et al., 1992).

Spiritual Quality of Life

Roles in religious or spiritual organizations, priorities and values, and beliefs all may change after transplant. Baker and others (1991) interviewed 135 allogeneic/autologous HCT patients 6 to 149 months post-HCT and showed that increases in volunteerism, religious participation, and participation in organizations occurred. Belec (1992) looked at quality of life issues in 24 autologous/allogeneic patients 1 to 3 years posttransplant. Results indicated that for 90% of the subjects, the transplant experience led to a reassessment of their priorities and values: leading fuller, more meaningful lives, greater appreciation of life, spending more time with family, reducing time at work, and making a concerted effort to enjoy life more, strive for new goals, and become better people. Curbow and colleagues (1993) sent out surveys to 135 allogeneic/autologous patients 6 to 149 months post-HCT, and 67.5% reported a positive change in beliefs about what is important in life. Fromm and others (1996) looked at 90 HCT survivors (autologous/allogeneic), 1 to 10 years post-HCT. Positive sequelae reported were new philosophy of life (59%), change in personal attributes (74%), improved family relationships (52%), more supportive family (51%), and greater appreciation of life (47%).

QOL in HCT Patients More Than 5 Years Posttransplant

Physical

Duell and colleagues (1997) evaluated the health and functional status of 798 long-term survivors of allogeneic transplants at 5, 10, and 15 years. Mortality at 10 years was 8% and at 15 years was 14%. The most common cause of death more than 5 years posttransplant was

relapse, followed by cGVHD. Prieto and colleagues (1996) found that a higher symptomatology score, a lower educational level, an older age at transplant, a shorter time posttransplant, female gender, and impotence were significant predictors of an impaired overall quality of life in patients 6 months to 154 months after HCT.

Patients 6 to 18 years posttransplant experienced persistent colds, influenza, memory problems, fatigue, shingles, and pain. The physical complications that were listed as difficult to cope with were the following: diabetes, eye problems, shingles, eating habits, GVHD, lack of stamina, no regrowth of hair, headaches, lung problems, sexual difficulties, memory loss, loss of mobility, weight gain, weaning from prednisone, skin problems, colds, flu, visual impairment, cavities, gingivitis, and joint and muscle pain (Haberman et al., 1993). Bush and others (1995) did a descriptive study on 125 adults surviving 6 to 18 years after transplant. In regard to general quality of life, 74% of the patients reported their QOL was the same or better than before the transplant, 80% related current health status and QOL as good to excellent, and 88% said the benefits of HCT outweighed the side effects. Side effects and complications listed were the following: fatigue, eye problems, sleep disturbances, general pain, and cognitive dysfunction.

CHRONIC GVHD

Most patients who are > 5 years posttransplant report good QOL scores; however, there is a subgroup of patients for which this is not true (Molassiotis and Morris, 1999; Wingard, 1994; Prieto et al., 1996; Duell et al., 1997; Deeg et al., 1998; Chiodi et al., 2000). The symptoms listed identifying this subgroup of patients suggest cGVHD. In fact, findings from a small randomized study suggest that the presence of cGVHD may cause a lower quality of life (De Souza et al., 2002). Physically, cGVHD has been linked to suboptimal levels of physical capability and reduced performance, poor health, inadequate rehabilitation, and increased fatigue, and it remained the dominant risk factor for complications such as avascular necrosis due to treatment with steroids, cataracts, musculoskeletal diseases, pulmonary problems, and possibly posttreatment malignancy (Molassiotis and Morris, 1999; Kiss, 2002; Prieto et al., 1996; Duell et al., 1997; Deeg et al., 1998; Chiodi et al., 2000).

Psychologically, cGVHD causes symptoms and more infections, and both factors are linked to increased psychological distress. Socially, patients with cGVHD have greater loss of employment, difficulty with reentry into societal roles, and impairment of social activity.

PSYCHOLOGICAL QUALITY OF LIFE

Fromm and colleagues (1996) looked at HCT survivors 5 to 10 years after HCT and found that positive psychosocial sequelae were frequently reported often conjunctively with negative psychosocial sequelae. Some positive sequelae were: new philosophy of life (59%), greater appreciation of life (47%), making changes in personal characteristics (71%), finding support within the family (51%), improving relationships with family (52%), and finding help and support from friends (39%). Some negative sequelae were: increased uncertainty with the future (59%), emotional tax on family (52%), and depression (43%). Patients who had a poorer prognosis going into HCT had more psychosocial benefits.

Social Quality of Life

Haberman and others (1993) interviewed 125 adult survivors 6 to 18 years after HCT and found that for some patients, the adjustment by family, friends, and peers is a dominant theme (18%). Dealing with family, friends, and peers was also listed as one of the three things that were the most difficult. These dealings included divorce, marriage, losing a twin, unexpressed emotions in the family, disrupting a parent's life, keeping children in school, being dependent on others, being angry at people who would send their sick kids over to play, people deciding to either be guarded or stay away entirely because of the cancer, people constantly saying "Are you sure you should be doing that?", and wanting to be near their children but being afraid of their germs. Heinonen and colleagues (2001) found that after 5 years, satisfaction with social support and education proved to be significant predictors of contentment with life.

Pediatric Population

There is a wealth of information about childhood survivors of cancer and long-term quality of life issues; however, few pediatric studies examine the quality of life of children within the first year of transplant. Two recent articles based on one study with the pediatric population during the first 6 months is worth mentioning (Phipps, Dunavant, Garvie, et al., 2002; Phipps, Dunavant, Lensing, et al., 2002). Phipps, Dunavant, and colleagues (2002) prospectively examined descriptive, medical, and demographic outcomes at various phases during the first 6 months among 153 children undergoing transplant. Results indicated that children undergoing transplantation enter the hospital with an already heightened level of distress that increases dramatically following the conditioning regimen and peaks at approximately one week after transplant. These levels return to basal levels by 4 to 6 months posttransplant. Results indicated that the children undergoing unrelated donor transplants experienced the highest level of distress whereas those undergoing autologous transplants experienced the lowest level of distress. Younger patients experienced lower levels of distress and better quality of life than older children or adolescents. Those patients with lower socioeconomic status had greater quality of life disturbance and distress.

Caregiver

Although the HCT patient and family caregiving unit survives the HCT experience in tandem, there are few studies that look specifically at the quality of life of family caregivers. The focus instead is on the responsibilities of the caregivers and the emotional impact that results. The concept of family-based cancer care (Schumacher, 1996) is a multifaceted, dynamic endeavor elicited by the occurrence of an illness. Dimensions of family-based illness care in cancer proposed by Schumacher are managing symptoms and side effects; providing optimal nutrition; promoting emotional well-being; maintaining the sense of self; maintaining social activities; communicating with extended family members; communicating with health professionals; carrying on the medical regimen; negotiating the health-care system; seeking out holistic, complementary, or supplemental therapies; reallocating household responsibilities; and preparing for an uncertain future. Caregiving for HCT patients incorporates all of these responsibilities, but it may be more involved because of the intensity of

the conditioning therapy and variation in the recovery trajectory. Families must manage a complex and variable medication routine based on symptoms and side effects of treatment, support patients through a higher level of uncertainty regarding outcome of the transplant than with chronic progressive illnesses, communicate with a large number of health-care professionals, and often relocate to the transplant center, leaving their usual systems of support.

In the clinical literature, nurses are instructed to teach caregivers how to manage central lines, facilitate adherence to a sophisticated medication regimen, anticipate and manage patient symptoms, and provide emotional support to patients (Lonergan et al., 1996; Whedon and Wujcik, 1997). In the 3 months following hospitalization, researchers reported that caregiving involved providing physical care, protecting patients from harm and misinformation, maintaining patients' connections with their social worlds, and serving as advocates (Stetz et al., 1996). Although caregivers are taught about what to expect before and after HCT, most report the experience was not what they anticipated (Stetz et al., 1996). Younger patients or caregivers often have younger family responsibilities (Rolland, 2005), such as working outside the home and raising young children. Caregivers tend to be spouses or adult children, but may include siblings, in-law relations, and friends. Caregivers also accept responsibility for young children, relocate to the geographic region for the transplant, and manage the daily functions of the household (Eilers, 1997). Patients can become quite dependent quickly, leaving caregivers little time to prepare for caregiving. Importantly, patients recovering from HCT are likely to experience fluctuations in functional and cognitive abilities, making it necessary for caregivers to negotiate care tasks with patients and for caregivers to be flexible with caregiving patterns.

The bulk of research with caregivers of HCT patients has focused on identifying stressors and describing emotional outcomes. Most of the studies have collected data during clinical time frames, with several assessments during hospitalization and again at 6 to 12 months. Caregivers are highly emotionally distressed in the days before the HCT and continue to have elevated levels of anxiety and fatigue as patients prepare to leave the hospital (Foxall and Gaston-Johansson, 1996; Keogh et al., 1998). In addition to managing complex medical care, caregivers report uncertainty about patients' surviving the HCT procedure, recurrence of the primary illnesses, and the development of life-threatening complications (Eilers, 1997; Haberman, 1995). Often patients and caregivers temporarily relocate to live near the transplant center, introducing additional stresses of social isolation and financial burdens associated with running separate households (Eilers, 1997). Caregivers report additional anxiety as they transition from hospital to home, leaving the safe haven of the hospital (Wochna, 1997).

For caregivers, the time of hospital discharge represents the beginning of significantly more responsibility for responding to patients' needs. At 6 months following transplant, HCT caregivers reported emotional and physical exhaustion related to patients' ongoing problems with fatigue and continued need for supervision (Zabora et al., 1992). Most caregivers expected patients would have resumed their former roles and responsibilities within the family but this did not occur. In addition, as patients' health improves, caregivers often report that reintegrating patients back into the family system is a difficult transition (Eilers, 1997). The most

common theme among HCT caregivers interviewed between 1 and 6 years is that some sense of normalcy had returned to the family unit, but there were continued caregiving demands and fluctuation in role responsibilities (Boyle et al., 2000). As expected, patients reported significantly more problems with physical functioning, role limitations, energy/fatigue, social functioning, pain, and general health than caregivers; however, patients and caregivers report similar disruption in emotional well-being and emotional role limitations (Boyle et al., 2000). Less attention has been paid to functional outcomes for HCT care partners. Higher amounts of caregiving were related to lower reports of physical health in HCT caregivers, less attention to personal health concerns (Foxall and Gaston-Johansson, 1996), exhaustion, and limited social interactions (Rivera, 1997). A clear need exists for additional QOL-specific research in this area.

Interventions

Unfortunately there are very few quality of life intervention studies in the transplant population. We will, however, list the few available studies, offer some case examples and suggestions, and provide a comprehensive table of possible interventions based on the problems identified in the literature (see **Table 15-2**). Table 15-2 divides up the suggested interventions by the trajectory of quality of life. Many of these interventions are not research-based since the literature is scarce in this area, but they are drawn from clinical expertise and suggestions from the literature. Some of these suggestions come from the expanding body of literature focused on long-term follow-up for which there are few evidence-based practice guidelines. This section will touch on general

Table 15-2 INTERVENTIONS.

Time Period	Primary Issues/Needs	Interventions
1st year	Physical, fatigue	Consistent close hematologic ambulatory follow-up care with laboratory monitoring, screening for complications such as organ toxicity or GVHD, and medication management
		Assurance that time affects physical recovery
		Suggest less physically demanding work, or working fewer hours per day
		Inpatient or outpatient exercise program
		Physical/occupational therapy referral for all patients with exercises tailored to individual needs
		Regular progressive exercise
		Guarding energy and balancing activities
		Frequent rest periods
		Restorative activities such as exposure to beauty and pleasurable experiences
		Drug treatment for anemia if needed; consider keeping the hemoglobin over 10–12 g/dL
		Sleep interventions if needed, such as sleep hygiene training
	GI	Consider IV hydration overnight in the home/outpatient setting
		Nutrition consultation with a dietitian
		Mucositis management—such as management of pain and mouth care
		Infection assessment and patient teaching to discern differences in GI infection vs. GVHD vs. slow healing
		Treatment of nausea/vomiting with adequate antiemetics
		Assessment of GI GVHD: mouth and upper and lower GI

	Issue	Intervention
	Infection	CDC guideline education for HCT patients regarding neutropenic precautions
	GVHD	Prompt treatment of GVHD with patient education to assess early symptoms
	Sexual issues	Fertility counseling pretransplant/sperm banking or fertility preservation
		Posttransplant sexual counseling
		Assess possibility of hormone replacement treatment for both men and women, and consider treating even if hormone levels are borderline normal
		Gynecologic referral for women
		Urologic referral for men
Psychological	Distress	Pretransplant psychological assessment
	Anxiety	Assurance of common feelings
	Depression	Patient education of possible delayed response
	Loss of control	Psychological support throughout the transplant process
		Support group for transplant patients
	Difficulty with dependence	Psychological support and counseling
		Encourage coping styles such as hope, maintaining control, use of social support, spirituality, acceptance
		Focus on common stressful time points—before admission, during admission directly before transplant, discharge
Social	Powerlessness	Exploring new possible roles such as a change in jobs or expectations of role chores
	Change in role	Consistent and present social support
	Separation from home	Job counseling/retraining
	Problems with family/children	Family therapy
	Stigmatization/discrimination	Caregiver support group and/or caregiver resources from ACS, NIH, Leukemia and Lymphoma Society, or other transplant organizations
	Financial difficulties	
	Job issues	
	Sexuality	

(continues)

Table 15-2 INTERVENTIONS *continued.*

Time Period	Primary Issues/Needs	Interventions
	Spirituality	Exploration of spiritual issues such as search for meaning, change in life priorities
	Search for meaning	
1–5 years	Physical (see previous intervention)	Long-term follow-up recommendations such as organ function analysis (PFTs, thyroid, ophthalmic), antibiotic prophylaxis, regular yearly oncologic and hematologic screening, osteoporosis prevention, immunization follow-up, chronic GVHD assessment and management
	Medical management	
	Fatigue	Examine possible symptom clusters with fatigue, such as depression, pain, infections, psychological adjustment, weight loss, anxiety, cognitive impairment, mouth/throat issues, insomnia, loss of appetite, GVHD
	Cognitive issues	Regular assessment of cognitive issues
		Memory tools
		Decrease multitasking
		Patient education on symptoms—forgetfulness, slowed reaction, and expectations
	Psychological	Support group
	Discordance with pre-BMT expectations	Counseling
		Encourage contact with other patients if not interested in support group
		Increase patient control
		Monitor patients with risk factors such as lack of social support, history of depression, and increased morbidity
	Social	See previous recommendations
	Role distress	Financial counseling
	Sexual issues	Psychological support for role adjustment/changes
	Vocational adjustment	Education re: caregiver burden and self-care
	Discordance with pre-BMT expectations	Continued family support/therapy

	Spirituality	Change in spiritual/religious roles	See previous recommendations
			Volunteerism
			Journaling
			Serving as a partner to a new patient
			Religious participation
More than 5 years	Physical	Persistent physical symptoms with GVHD	See previous recommendations
			Teaching on long-term side effect management to encourage partnership with patient for recommendations
			Aggressive treatment for chronic GVHD
			Referrals for psychological ongoing support
			Sexual counseling
			Vocational training
			Fatigue management
			Encourage support group attendance
			Health maintenance and lifestyle changes for complications
			Vigilant monitoring for infection if chronic GVHD present
	Psychological	Positive/negative feelings	See previous recommendations
	Social	Continued family adjustment	Encourage coping with any permanent long-term disability
			See previous recommendations

Interventions are based either on evidence (when available) or clinical expertise.

concepts from this body of literature, while other chapters within this textbook devote more detail to this critical area of long-term follow-up recommendations.

In regard to interventions that affect physical quality of life, Courtneya and others (2000) did an exercise intervention study during the transplant process and showed that those patients who did exercise throughout the transplant experience had higher QOL scores. Another exercise program by Dimeo and colleagues (1996) showed a significant improvement in maximal walking distance and a significant lowering of the heart rate with equivalent workloads. Their conclusion was that fatigue and loss of physical performance in patients undergoing transplant can be corrected with adequate rehabilitative measures. The benefits of exercise for other populations cannot be understated. These two studies provide valuable data to consider incorporating a regular exercise program for all uncomplicated transplant patients in the inpatient and clinic setting. Suggested goals would be to maintain strength and mobility, decrease fatigue, maintain organ function such as respiratory and cardiac function, provide an outlet for the patients to socialize and obtain support, and improve mood and a sense of well-being.

Another intervention that affects physical and social quality of life for these patients focuses on sexuality. Since the early 1990s, hormone replacement therapy has been reported as reducing women's sexual difficulties, improving frequency and enjoyment of sex, and improving the amount of sexual activity (Spinelli et al., 1994). Syrjala and colleagues (1998) suggest hormone replacement therapy to be in place for women by the first year. Failure may result in increased sexual dissatisfaction at 3 years post-

transplant. Hormone replacement therapy following transplantation is a complex decision involving evaluation of risk factors such as cardiac dysfunction and osteoporosis, while at the same time balancing the research of transplant patients' sexual satisfaction following transplantation. It would be reasonable to obtain a gynecologic referral for all women at 100 days after transplant to discuss hormone replacement therapy with a gynecologist knowledgeable about posttransplant care.

In regard to psychological quality of life, various forms of therapy are indicated. McQuellon and others (1998) measured psychosocial recovery over the first year after transplant. Those who did not receive some form of counseling had decreased mean scores on the emotional well-being scale. Hypnosis has been reported to be effective in reducing oral pain (Syrjala et al., 1992). During the first year, professional psychologic support was related to lower anger/hostility, depression, anxiety, confusion, and mood disturbance (Molassiotis et al., 1996b). Psychologic support is essential for patients who are dealing with a myriad of stressors including a life-threatening illness, crisis, potential for prolonged hospitalization and isolation, pain, intense treatment, family adjustment, and financial issues. Psychologic support should be initiated at consultation stage and maintained throughout the first year with regular sessions during the inpatient or intensive outpatient stage. Participation within a support group for transplant patients is often extremely helpful for patients through the shared experience and as a forum for expressing emotions and obtaining information from other patients and facilitators. An added benefit would be to have a concurrent family support group at the same time to assist family members with coping, caregiver fatigue, and recovery from the intense crisis affecting the family.

In order to illustrate quality of life interventions, three case studies will be presented with follow-up recommendations to illustrate the suggestions listed within the literature and Table 15-2. Each case study will present a patient in the various trajectory periods after transplantation, within the first year, within 1 to 5 years and more than 5 years.

Case Study 15-1　Within the First Year

Stan is a 45-year-old man with a diagnosis of AML in first remission who had an allogeneic transplant from an HLA-compatible brother 6 months ago. He is married to a supportive wife, and they have three small children ages 1, 3, and 5. He owns his own computer consulting business and has tried to manage his business from home for the last few months. His immediate posttransplant inpatient course was complicated by neutropenic fever, azotemia, nausea, vomiting, diarrhea, skin rash and blistering, and mucositis, all resolved at discharge. Stan was discharged on day 30 and has been home for 5 months with no readmissions. The patient developed acute GVHD of the skin on day 40, which resolved with the addition of steroids to the normal regimen of cyclosporine.

At 6 months, physically, he manifests some evidence of cGVHD of the mouth with lichenoid patches on the mucosa, palate, and gums. He complains of a burning sensation and tenderness when eating acidic or spicy foods, and finds that he has some taste alterations. Otherwise he feels good; he has had two colds, but no other infections since discharge. He continues on tapering doses of cyclosporine and prednisone.

Psychologically he describes himself as a "driver" and copes by meeting crises head-on, gathering information, and taking control. He has not had any issues with depression and anxiety, but is concerned about his exposure to possible infections while being on immunosuppressive medications and also having small children. His wife continues to be supportive, although at times she feels overwhelmed with the care of three small children and her husband. They both have supportive families and friends. Socially, he has felt frustrated with his decrease in work hours, feels the pressure of being a provider for his family, and would like to start work again full-time. Spiritually, they attend a church, but the patient does not list religion or spirituality as a significant part

(continues)

Case Study 15-1   *(continued)*

of his life. The wife, however, does find that her religion and belief in God has given her strength to cope with the challenges of the past year.

Physical Recommendations

- Continued medical follow-up for issues of cGVHD and medication management
- Teaching regarding foods to avoid with cGVHD of the mouth with nutritional consult
- Dental referral
- Teaching regarding infection risk, especially viruses such as colds, zoster reactivation
- Discuss strategies of dealing with sick children and decreasing exposure such as avoidance, sleeping arrangements, importance of hand-washing, and temporary use of masks
- Reinforce simple needed behaviors such as hand-washing
- Teach energy conservation
- Explore issues of sexuality with the patient and refer for counseling; also assess testosterone level and replace if needed, and refer to a urologist for issues of impotence

Psychological Recommendations

- Address anxiety about infection with information regarding infection prevention

Social Recommendations

- Support the caregiver with referral to social worker and support group for caregivers
- Teach about crisis intervention and emphasize the essential need for social support
- Encourage spouse to utilize social supports in a structured manner by offering suggestions on definite tasks

Spiritual Recommendations

- Open the dialogue regarding spirituality to establish availability for the future
- Encourage wife to continue with her religious/spiritual activities

Case Study 15-2   Within 1 to 5 Years

Sarah is a 38-year-old married Native American woman with a diagnosis of NHL 19 months after allogeneic transplant. She has two small children, ages 1 and 4. Her occupation is a special education teacher, and she has not worked since her transplantation. Her immediate inpatient posttransplant course was complicated by neutropenic fever, *Clostridium difficile* infection, acute gut GVHD, mucositis, and pulmonary infiltrate, all resolved at discharge by day 35. Within the first 6 months after transplantation, she developed CMV viremia, was admitted and treated with antiviral therapy, and has had negative evidence of subsequent CMV infection. At 9 months posttransplant, she was admitted for headaches and seizure and diagnosed with encephalitis, unknown organism. She experienced severe disability after the encephalitis and needed intensive rehabilitation with speech and occupational and physical therapy. At 19 months after transplantation she no longer uses an assistive device with walking; her speech is hesitant, but understandable; she has not had any seizures; and she continues to have difficulty holding utensils and with coordination of her upper extremities. She describes her fatigue as an 8 on a scale of 1 to 10 and has difficulty caring for her children. She is also experiencing sleep abnormalities, with frequent wakening and difficulty falling back to sleep. During the day she feels drained, and she finds herself frequently yelling at her children. She describes her husband as unsupportive. According to her, he does not understand why she is unable to return to the household roles she was able to do before transplant. She has no family members living close by; most of her family lives in Mexico. She has experienced feelings of depression and is currently being seen by a psychiatrist to manage her antidepressant therapy. She does not feel that religion or spirituality is important in her life.

Physical Recommendations

Continued medical follow-up for issues of cGVHD and medication management

Continued PT/OT

Fatigue management: teaching on energy conservation, need for exercise, creativity outlets, restorative concepts

Referral for sleep evaluation and teaching on sleep hygiene tips such as: sleep just long enough, wake up and go to bed at the same time every day, exercise regularly, get light exposure every day, reduce or

(continues)

Case Study 15-2   *(continued)*

eradicate noise, regulate room temperature, eat a bedtime snack, avoid daytime naps or limit to 30 minutes at a time, avoid stimulants, limit alcohol consumption, get out of bed if not asleep within 20 minutes, do not use tobacco

Psychological Recommendations

Referral to a psychologist for individual therapy and family therapy to strengthen the dyad relationship

Explore the issue of child abuse and inform Child Protective Services if suspect

Encourage parenting classes at a local college

Encourage attendance at a support group

Continue with antidepressant therapy as indicated

Social Recommendations

Referral to a social worker for assisting the patient in getting state disability to pay for issues such as house cleaning, child care, and laundry, and assistance with any eligible programs with governmental or community programs

Job retraining

Spiritual Recommendations

None

Case Study 15-3   More Than 5 Years

Tom is a 55-year-old single male with CML who is 10 years post-sibling allogeneic transplant. His inpatient transplant course was typical and uncomplicated except for developing acute graft-versus-host disease of the gut and liver, which resolved. Subsequently, one year after getting a transplant, he developed chronic graft-versus-host disease of the skin, eyes,

and oral mucosa, which has continued to the present. He also notes a decrease in his muscle strength and overall stamina. With treatment on steroids, he developed anxiety, agitation, and an aggressive personality, which limited higher doses of steroids. Approximately 5 years after transplantation, he developed memory difficulties and changes in speech. Neurological exam at the time found no abnormality, and he continues with the neurological symptoms. He was, however, placed on antidepressant therapy for treatment of anxiety and depression by his primary care physician. He verbalizes issues with body image from the cGVHD feeling that he looks different and is uncomfortable going out in public. He has not had a significant dating relationship in 8 years. He has not been able to work since transplantation, and he is living on disability. Spiritually, he verbalized that initially he was angry at God about his state of health and feeling useless; however, he has come to some peace about it and started attending a Presbyterian church in the last year.

Physical Recommendations

Referral to a transplant center and a cGVHD clinic for aggressive management of his skin, eyes, and oral mucosal symptoms, including skin care, infection prevention, and ophthalmology referral

Follow general long-term follow-up guidelines such as yearly hematologic screening, yearly oncologic screening, osteoporosis management, antibiotic prophylaxis, regular pulmonary function screening, thyroid function exam, and immunization follow-up

Refer for follow-up neurological exam and diagnostic studies for persistent neurological deficits with follow-up on a yearly basis

Referral to a neuropsychologist to teach memory enhancement techniques

Psychological Recommendations

Referral to a psychologist to help him deal with body image and sexuality issues

Continue antidepressant therapy

Encourage participation and attendance in a support group

Social Recommendations

Encourage volunteer work, which would encourage socialization and be less stressful and demanding than a paid position, and could be a position that would take his infection issues into account

Spiritual Recommendations

Consider pastoral counseling and support

Consider finding a volunteer opportunity through the Presbyterian church

Summary

Quality of life after transplantation is a major area of importance to our patients and their families. Now that survival is improving, often patients are living with long-term complications, disability, and physical and psychological concerns after transplantation. Sadly, often the supporting resources are not available to cope with these long-term concerns that both patients and caregivers live with daily. QOL assessment from the first year following transplant to many years posttransplant can provide valuable clues as to what persistent problems plague the HCT survivors, as well as offer suggested interventions. Much research in the past decades has focused on assessing the issues these patients encounter. Hopefully in the decades ahead, there will be more studies focused on testing interventions to assist these patients and their families in coping with issues and disabilities.

References

Aaronson, N.K., Meyerowitz, B.E., Bard, M., Bloom, J.R., Fawzy, F.I., Feldstein, M., et al. (1991). Quality of life research in oncology: Past achievements and future priorities. *Cancer, 67*(3 Suppl), 839–843.

Altmaier, E.M., Gingrich, R.D., & Fyfe, M.A. (1991). Two-year adjustment of bone marrow transplant survivors. *Bone Marrow Transplantation, 7*(4), 311–316.

American Cancer Society. (2004). *Facts and Figures.* Atlanta, GA: ACS.

Andrykowski, M.A. (1994). Psychosocial factors in bone marrow transplantation: A review and recommendations for research. *Bone Marrow Transplantation, 13,* 357–375.

Andrykowski, M.A., Altmaier, E.M., Barnett, R.L., Otis, M.L., Gingrich, R., & Henslee-Downey, P.J. (1990). The quality of life in adult survivors of allogeneic bone marrow transplantation. *Transplantation, 50*(3), 399–406.

Andrykowski, M.A., Brady, M.J., Greiner, C.B., Altmaier, E.M., Burish, T.G., Antin, J.H., et al. (1995). Returning to normal following bone marrow transplantation: Outcomes, expectations and informed consent. *Bone Marrow Transplantation, 15*(4), 573–581.

Andrykowski, M.A., Brady, M.J., & Hanslee-Downey, P.J. (1994). Psychosocial factors predictive of survival after allogeneic bone marrow transplantation for leukemia. *Psychosomatic Medicine, 56,* 432–439.

Andrykowski, M.A., Carpenter, J.S., Greiner, C.B., Altmaier, E.M., Burish, T.G., Antin, J.H., et al. (1997). Energy level and sleep quality following bone marrow transplantation. *Bone Marrow Transplantation, 20,* 669–679.

Andrykowski, M.A., Cordova, M.J., Hann, D.M., Jacobsen, P.B., Fields, K.K., & Phillips, G. (1999). Patients' psychosocial concerns following stem cell transplantation. *Bone Marrow Transplantation, 24*(10), 1121–1129.

Andrykowski, M.A., Greiner, C.B., Altmaier, E.M., Burish, T.G., Antin, J.H., Gingrich, R., et al. (1995). Quality of life following bone marrow transplantation: Findings from a multicentre study. *British Journal of Cancer, 71,* 1322–1329.

Andrykowski, M.A., Henslee, P.J., & Barnett, R.L. (1989). Longitudinal assessment of psychosocial functioning of adult survivors of allogeneic bone marrow transplantation. *Bone Marrow Transplantation, 4,* 505–509.

Baker, F. (1994). Psychosocial sequelae of bone marrow transplantation. *Oncology (Huntington), 8*(10), 87–92, 97; discussion 87–101.

Baker, F., Curbow, B., & Wingard, J.R. (1991). Role retention and quality of life of bone marrow transplant survivors. *Social Science in Medicine, 32*(6), 697–704.

Baker, F., Wingard, J.R., Curbow, B., Zabora, J., Jodrey, D., Fogarty, L., et al. (1994). Quality of life of bone marrow transplant long-term survivors. *Bone Marrow Transplantation, 13,* 589–596.

Baker, F., Zabora, J., Polland, A., & Wingard, J. (1999). Reintegration after bone marrow transplantation. *Cancer Practice, 7*(4), 190–197.

Belec, R.H. (1992). Quality of life: Perceptions of long-term survivors of bone marrow transplantation. *Oncology Nursing Forum, 19*(1), 31–37.

Bellm, L.A., Epstein, J.B., Rose-Ped, A., Martin, P., & Fuchs, H.J. (2000). Patient reports of complications of bone marrow transplantation. *Support Care Cancer, 8,* 33–39.

Blume, K.G. & Amylon, M.D. (1999). The evaluation and counseling of candidates for hematopoietic cell transplantation. In E. Thomas, K. Blume, & S. Forman (Eds.), *Hematopoietic cell transplantation.* (2nd ed., pp. 371–380). Malden, MA: Blackwell Science, Inc.

Boyle, D., Blodgett, L., Gnesdiloff, S., White, J., Bamford, A.M., Sheridan, M., et al. (2000). Caregiver quality of life after autologous bone marrow transplantation. *Cancer Nursing, 23*, 193–203.

Broers, S., Kaptein, A.A., Le Cessie, S., Fibbe, W., & Hengeveld, M.W. (2000). Psychosocial functioning and quality of life following bone marrow transplantation: A 3-year follow-up study. *Journal of Psychosomatic Research, 48*, 11–21.

Bush, N.E., Haberman, M., Donaldson, G., & Sullivan, K.M. (1995). Quality of life of 125 adults surviving 6–18 years after bone marrow transplantation. *Social Science in Medicine, 40*(4), 479–90.

Chao, N.J., Tierney, D.K., Bloom, J.R., Long, G.D., Barr, T.A., Stallbaum, B.A., et al. (1992). Dynamic assessment of quality of life after autologous bone marrow transplantation. *Blood, 80*(3), 825–830.

Chiodi, S., Cpinelli, S., Ravera, G., Petti, A.R., van Lint, M.T., Lamparelli, T., et al. (2000). Quality of life in 244 recipients of allogeneic bone marrow transplantation. *British Journal of Haematology, 110*(3), 614.

Claisse, J.P., Hirsch, I., & Gluckman, E. (1994). Quality of life after allogeneic bone marrow transplantation: The patient's point of view. *Nouvelle Revue Francaise d'Hematologie, 36*(Suppl. 1), S83–S84.

Colon, E.A., Callies, A.L., Popkin, M.K., & McGlave, P.B. (1991). Depressed mood and other variables related to bone marrow transplantation survival in acute leukemia. *Psychosomatics, 32*(4), 420–425.

Courneya, K.S., Keats, M.R. & Turner, A.R. (2000). Physical exercise and quality of life in cancer patients following high dose chemotherapy and autologous bone marrow transplantation. *Psycho-Oncology, 9*, 127–136.

Curbow, B., Somerfield, M.R., Baker, F., Wingard, J.R., & Legro, M.W. (1993). Personal changes, dispositional optimism, and psychological adjustment to bone marrow transplantation. *Journal of Behavioral Medicine, 16*(5), 423–443.

De Souza, C.A., Duraes, M.I., Vigorito, A.C., Penteado, Aranha, F.J., Oliveira, G.B., et al. (2002). Quality of life in patients randomized to receive a bone marrow or a peripheral blood allograft. *Haematologica, 87*(12), 1281–1285.

Deeg, J.H., Leisenring, W., Storb, R., Nims, J., Flowers, M.E.D., Witherspoon, R.P., et al. (1998). Long-term outcome after marrow transplantation for severe aplastic anemia. *Blood, 91*(10), 3637–3645.

Dimeo, F., Bertz, H., Finke, J., Fetscher, S., Mertelsmann, R., & Keul, J. (1996). An aerobic exercise program for patients with haematological malignancies after bone marrow transplantation. *Bone Marrow Transplantation, 18*(6), 1157–1160.

Duell, T., van Lint, M.T., Ljungman, P., Tichelli, A., Socie, G., Apperley, J.F., et al. (1997). Health and functional status of long-term survivors of bone marrow transplantation. *Annals of Internal Medicine, 126*(3), 184–192.

Eilers, J.G. (1997). Family issues and perspectives. In M.B. Whedon & D. Wujcik (Eds.), *Blood and marrow stem cell transplantation: Principles, practice, and nursing insights* (2nd ed., pp. 442–456). Sudbury, MA: Jones and Bartlett Publishers.

Eiser, C., & Morse, R. (2001). A review of measures of quality of life for children with chronic illness. *Archives of Disease in Childhood, 84*(3), 205–211.

Ferrans, C. (1990). Development of a quality of life index for patients with cancer. *Oncology Nursing Forum, 17*, 15–21.

Ferrans, C.E. (1996). Development of a conceptual model of quality of life. *Scholarly Inquiry for Nursing Practice, 10*(3), 293–304.

Ferrell, B., Grant, M., Schmidt, G., Rhiner, M., Whitehead, C., Fonbuena, P., et al. (1992a). The meaning of quality of life for bone marrow transplant survivors, Part I: The impact of bone marrow transplant on quality of life. *Cancer Nursing, 15*(3), 153–160.

Ferrell, B., Grant, M., Schmidt, G., Rhiner, M., Whitehead, C., Fonbuena, P, et al. (1992b). The meaning of quality of life for bone marrow transplant survivors; Part II: Improving the quality of life for bone marrow transplant survivors. *Cancer Nursing, 15*(4), 247–253.

Ferrell, B.R., Grant, M., Funk, B., Otis-Green, S., & Garcia, N. (1997). Quality of life in breast cancer, Part I: Physical and social well being. *Cancer Nursing, 20*(6), 398–408.

Ferrell, B.R., Grant, M.M., Funk, B., Otis-Green, S.A., & Garcia, N.J. (1998a). Quality of life in breast cancer survivors: implications for developing support services. *Oncology Nursing Forum, 25*(5), 887–895.

Ferrell, B.R., Grant, M., Funk, B., Otis-Green, S., & Garcia, N. (1998b). Quality of life in breast cancer, Part II: Psychological and spiritual well being. *Cancer Nursing, 21*(1), 1–9.

Fife, B.L., Huster, G.A., Cornetta, K.G., Kennedy, V.N., Akard, L.P., & Broun, E.R. (2000). Longitudinal study of adaptation to the stress of bone marrow transplantation. *Journal of Clinical Oncology, 18*(7), 1539–1549.

Foxall, M.J., & Gaston-Johansson, F. (1996). Burden and health outcomes of family caregivers of hospitalized bone marrow transplant patients. *Journal of Advanced Nursing, 24*, 915–923.

Fromm, K., Andrykowski, M.A., & Hunt, J. (1996). Positive and negative psychosocial sequelae of bone marrow transplantation: Implications for quality of life assessment. *Journal of Behavioral Medicine 19*(3), 221–240.

Gaston-Johansson, F., & Foxall, M. (1996). Psychological correlates of quality of life across the autologous bone marrow transplant experience. *Cancer Nursing 19*(3), 170–176.

Gotay, C.C., Korn, E.L., McCabe, M.S., Moore, D.T., & Cheson, B.D. (1992). Quality-of-life assessment in cancer treatment protocols: Research issues in protocol development. *Journal of the National Cancer Institute, 84*(8), 575–579.

Grant, M. (1999a). Assessment of quality of life following hematopoietic cell transplantation. In E. Thomas, K. Blume, & S. Forman (Eds.), *Hematopoietic cell transplantation* (2nd ed., pp. 407–413). Malden, MA: Blackwell Science, Inc.

Grant, M. (1999b). Quality of life issues in colorectal cancer. *Developments in Supportive Cancer Care, 3*(1), 4–9.

Grant, M., Ferrell, B., & Sakurai, C. (1994). *Defining the spiritual dimension of quality of life assessment in bone marrow transplant survivors.* Poster session presented at the 8th International Cancer Nursing Conference, Vancouver, BC, Canada.

Grant, M., Ferrell, B., Schmidt, G.M., Fonbuena, P., Niland, J.C., & Forman, S.J. (1992). Measurement of quality of life in bone marrow transplantation survivors. *Quality of Life Research, 1*(6), 375–384.

Greimel, E.R., Padilla, G.V., & Grant, M.M. (1997). Self care responses to illness of patients with various cancer diagnoses. *Acta Oncologica, 36*(3), 141–150.

Haberman, M. (1995). The meaning of cancer therapy: Bone marrow transplantation as an exemplar of therapy. *Seminars in Oncology Nursing, i*(1), 23–31.

Haberman, M., Bush, N., Young, K., & Sullivan, K.M. (1993). Quality of life of adult long-term survivors of bone marrow transplantation: A qualitative analysis of narrative data. *Oncology Nursing Forum, 20*(10), 1545–1553.

Hacker, E.D. (2003). Quantitative measurement of quality of life in adult patients undergoing bone marrow transplant or peripheral blood stem cell transplant: A

decade in review. *Oncology Nursing Forum, 30*(4), 613–629.

Hann, D.M., Garovoy, N., Finkelstien, B., Jaconsen, P.B., Azzarello, L.M., & Fields, K.K. (1999). Fatigue and quality of life in breast cancer patients undergoing autologous stem cell transplantation: A longitudinal comparative study. *Journal of Pain and Symptom Management, 17*, 311–319.

Hann, D.M., Jaconsen, P.B., Martin, S.C., Kronish, L.E., Azzarello, L.M., & Fields, K.K. (1997). Quality of life following bone marrow transplantation for breast cancer: A comparative study. *Bone Marrow Transplantation, 19*, 257–264.

Harder, H., Cornelissen, J.J., Van Gool, A.R., Duivenvoorden, H.J., Eijkenboom, W.M., & van den Bent, M.J. (2002). Cognitive functioning and quality of life in long-term survivors of bone marrow transplantation. *Cancer, 95*, 183–192.

Heinonen, H., Volin, L., Uutela, A., Zevon, M., Barrick, C., & Ruutu, T. (2001). Quality of life and factors related to perceived satisfaction with quality of life after allogeneic bone marrow transplantation. *Annals of Hematology, 80*(3), 137–143.

Hengeveld, M.W., Houtman, R.B., & Zwaan, F.E. (1988). Psychological aspects of bone marrow transplantation: A retrospective study of 17 long-term survivors. *Bone Marrow Transplantation, 3*(1), 69–75.

Hjermstad, M.J., Evensen, S.A., Kvaloy, S.O., Fayers, P.M., & Kaasa, S. (1999). Health-related quality of life 1 year after allogeneic or autologous stem-cell transplantation: A prospective study. *Journal of Clinical Oncology, 17*(2), 706–718.

Keogh, F., O'Riordan, J., McNamara, C., Duggan, C., & McCann, S.R. (1998). Psychosocial adaptation of patients and families following bone marrow transplantation: A prospective, longitudinal study. *Bone Marrow Transplantation, 22*, 905–911.

King, C., Ferrell, B.R., Grant, M., & Sakurai, C. (1995). Nurses' perception of the meaning of quality of life for bone marrow transplant survivors. *Cancer Nursing, 18*(2), 118–129.

King, C.R. (1996). Latent effects and quality of life one year after marrow and stem cell transplantation. *Quality of Life—A Nursing Challenge, 4*(2), 40–45.

Kiss, T.L., Abdolell, M., Jamal, N., Minden, M.D., Lipton, J.H., & Messner, H.A. (2002). Long-term medical outcomes and quality-of-life assessment of patients with chronic myeloid leukemia followed at least 10 years after allogeneic bone marrow transplantation. *Journal of Clinical Oncology, 20*(9), 2334–2343.

Kopp, M., Schweigkofler, H., Holzner, B., Nachbaur, D., Niederwieser, D., Fleischhacker, W.W., et al. (1998). Time after bone marrow transplantation as an important variable for quality of life: Results of a cross-sectional investigation using two different instruments for quality-of-life assessment. *Ann Hematol*, 77(1-2), 27–32.

Larsen, J., Gardulf, A., Nordstrom, G., Bjorkstrand, B., & Ljungman, P. (1996). Health-related quality of life in women with breast cancer undergoing autologous stem-cell transplantation. *Cancer Nursing*, 19, 368–375.

Leigh, S., Wilson, K.C., Burns, R., & Clark, R.E. (1995). Psychosocial morbidity in bone marrow transplant recipients: A prospective study. *Bone Marrow Transplantation*, 16(5), 635–40.

Litwins, N.M., Rodrigue, J.R., & Weiner, R.S. (1994). Quality of life in adult recipients of bone marrow transplantation. *Psychological Reports*, 75(1 Pt. 1), 323–328.

Loberiza, F. (2003). Report on state of the art in blood and marrow transplantation. *IBMTR/ABMTR Newsletter*, 10(1), 7–10.

Lonergan, J.N., Kelley, C.H., McBride, L.H., & Randolph, S.R. (1996). Homecare management of the bone marrow transplant patient (2nd ed.). Sudbury, MA: Jones and Bartlett Publishers.

Mandelblatt, J.S., & Eisenberg, J.M. (1995). Historical and methodological perspectives on cancer outcomes research. *Oncology (Huntington)*, 9(11 Suppl), 23–32.

Marks, D.I., Gale, D.J., Vedhara, K., & Bird, J.M. (1999). A quality of life study in 20 adult long-term survivors of unrelated donor bone marrow transplantation. *Bone Marrow Transplantation*, 24, 191–195.

McQuellon, R.P., & Andrykowski, M.A. (2004). Psychosocial complications. In K. Atkinson, R. Champlin, J. Ritz, W.E. Fibbe, P. Ljungman, & M.K. Brenner (Eds.), *Clinical bone marrow and blood stem cell transplantation* (3rd ed., pp. 1591–1604). Cambridge, UK: Cambridge University Press.

McQuellon, R.P., Craven, B., Russell, G.B., Hoffman, S., Cruz, J.M., Perry, J.J., et al. (1996). Quality of life in breast cancer patients before and after autologous bone marrow transplantation. *Bone Marrow Transplantation*, 18, 579–584.

McQuellon, R.P., Russell, G.B., Cella, D.F., Craven, B.L., Brady, M., Bonomi, A., et al. (1997). Quality of life measurement in bone marrow transplantation: Development of the Functional Assessment of Cancer Therapy-Bone Marrow Transplant (FACT-BMT) scale. *Bone Marrow Transplantation*, 19, 357–368.

McQuellon, R.P., Russell, G.B., Rambo, T.D., Craven, B.L., Radford, J., Perry, J.J., et al. (1998). Quality of life and psychological distress of bone marrow transplant recipients: The "time trajectory" to recovery over the first year. *Bone Marrow Transplantation*, 21(5), 477–486.

Meyers, C.A., Weitzner, M., Byrne, K., Valentine, A., Champlin, R.E., & Przepiorka, D. (1994). Evaluation of the neurobehavioral functioning of patients before, during, and after bone marrow transplantation. *Journal of Clinical Oncology*, 12(4), 820–826.

Moinpour, C.M., Feigl, P., Metch, B., Hayden, K.A., Meyskens, F.L., Jr., & Crowley, J. (1989). Quality of life endpoints in cancer clinical trials: Review and recommendations. *Journal of the National Cancer Institute*, 81, 485–495.

Molassiotis, A. (1996). Late psychosocial effects of conditioning for BMT. *British Journal of Nursing*, 21, 1296–1302.

Molassiotis, A., Boughton, B.J., Burgoyne, T., & van den Akker, O.B. (1995). Comparison of the overall quality of life in 50 long-term survivors of autologous and allogeneic bone marrow transplantation. *Journal of Advanced Nursing*, 22(3), 509–516.

Molassiotis, A., & Morris, P. J. (1999). Quality of life in patients with chronic myeloid leukemia after unrelated donor bone marrow transplantation. *Cancer Nursing*, 22(5), 340–349.

Molassiotis, A., van den Akker, O.B.A., & Boughton, B.J. (1997). Perceived social support, family environment and psychosocial recovery in bone marrow transplant long-term survivors. *Social Science & Medicine*, 44(3), 317–325.

Molassiotis, A., van den Akker, O.B.A., Milligan, D.W., Goldman, J.M., & Boughton, B.J. (1996a). Psychological adaptation and symptom distress in bone marrow transplant recipients. *Psycho-Oncology*, 5, 9–22.

Molassiotis, A., van den Akker, O.B., Milligan, D.W., Goldman, J.M., Boughton, B.J., Homes, J.A., et al. (1996b). Quality of life in long-term survivors of marrow transplantation: Comparison with a matched group receiving maintenance chemotherapy. *Bone Marrow Transplantation*, 17, 249–258.

Mumma, G.H., Mashberg, D., & Lesko, L.M. (1992). Long-term psychosexual adjustment of acute leukemia survivors: Impact of marrow transplantation versus conventional chemotherapy. *General Hospital Psychiatry*, 14(1), 43–55.

Padilla, G.V., Ferrell, B., & Grant, M.M. (1990). Defining the content domain of quality of life for cancer patients with pain. *Cancer Nursing, 13*(2), 108–115.

Phipps, S., Dunavant, M., Garvie, P.A., Lensing, S., & Rai, S.N. (2002). Acute health-related quality of life in children undergoing stem cell transplant, Part I: Descriptive outcomes. *Bone Marrow Transplantation, 29*(5), 425–434.

Phipps, S., Dunavant, M., Lensing, S., & Rai, S.N. (2002). Acute health-related quality of life in children undergoing stem cell transplant, Part II: Medical and demographic determinants. *Bone Marrow Transplantation, 29*(5), 435–442.

Prieto, J.M., Saez, R., Carreras, E., Atala, J., Sierra, J., Rovira, M., et al. (1996). Physical and psychosocial functioning of 117 survivors of bone marrow transplantation. *Bone Marrow Transplantation, 17*, 1133–1142.

Rivera, L.M. (1997). Blood cell transplantation: Its impact on one family. *Seminars in Oncology Nursing, 13*, 194–199.

Rolland, J.S. (2005). Chronic illness and the family life cycle. In B. Carter & M. McGoldrick (Eds.), *The expanded family life cycle: Individual, family and social perspective* (3rd ed., pp. 492–511). Boston: Allyn and Bacon.

Saleh, U.S., & Brockopp, D.Y. (2001). Quality of life one year following bone marrow transplantation: Psychometric evaluation of the quality of life in bone marrow transplant survivors tool. *Oncology Nursing Forum, 28*, 1457–1464.

Schumacher, K.L. (1996). Reconceptualizing family caregiving: Family-based illness care during chemotherapy. *Research in Nursing & Health, 19*, 261–271.

Scientific Advisory Committee of the Medical Outcomes Trust. (2002). Assessing health status and quality-of-life instruments: Attributes and review criteria. *Quality of Life Research, 11*, 193–205

Shuster, G.F., Steeves, R.H., Onega, L., & Richardson, B. (1996). Coping patterns among bone marrow transplant patients: A hermeneutical inquiry. *Cancer Nursing, 19*(4), 290–297.

Spinelli, S., Chiodo, S., Bacigalupo, A., Brasca, A., Menada, M.V., Petti, A.R., et al. (1994). Ovarian recovery after total body irradiation and allogeneic bone marrow transplantation: Long-term follow up of 79 females. *Bone Marrow Transplantation, 14*(3), 373–380.

Steeves, R.H. (1992). Patients who have undergone bone marrow transplantation: Their quest for meaning. *Oncology Nursing Forum, 19*(6), 899–905.

Stetz, K.M., McDonald, J.C., & Compton, K. (1996). Needs and experiences of family caregivers during marrow transplantation. *Oncology Nursing Forum, 23*, 1422–1439.

Sutherland, H.J., Fyles, G.M., Adams, G., Hao, Y., Lipton, J.H., Minden, M.D., et al. (1997). Quality of life following bone marrow transplantation: A comparison of patient reports with population norms. *Bone Marrow Transplantation, 19*, 1129–1136.

Syrjala, K.L., Chapko, M.K., Vitaliano, P.P., Cummings, C., & Sullivan, K.M. (1993). Recovery after allogeneic marrow transplantation: Prospective study of predictors of long-term physical and psychosocial functioning. *Bone Marrow Transplantation, 11*(4), 319–27.

Syrjala, K.L., Cummings, C., & Donaldson, G.W. (1992). Hypnosis or cognitive behavioral training for the reduction of pain and nausea during cancer treatment: A controlled clinical trial. *Pain, 48*(2), 137–146.

Syrjala, K.L., Roth-Roemer, S.L., Abrams, J.R., Scanlan, J.M., Chapko, M.K., Visser, S., et al. (1998). Prevalence and predictors of sexual dysfunction in long-term survivors of marrow transplantation. *Journal of Clinical Oncology 16*(9), 3148–3157.

Twillman, R.K., Manetto, C., Wellish, D.K., & Wolcott, D.L. (1993). The transplant evaluation rating scale. A revision of the psychosocial level system for evaluating organ transplant candidates. *Psychosomatics, 34*, 144–153.

van Agthoven, M., Vellenga, E., Fibbe, W.E., Kingma, T., & Uyl-de Groot, C.A. (2001). Cost analysis and quality of life assessment comparing patients undergoing autologous peripheral blood stem cell transplantation or autologous bone marrow transplantation for refractory or relapse non-Hodgkin's lymphoma or Hodgkin's disease. A prospective randomized trial. *European Journal of Cancer, 37*(4), 1781–1789.

Vickberg, S., Duhamel, K., & Smith, M. (2001). Global meaning and psychological adjustment among survivors of bone marrow transplant. *Psycho-Oncology, 10*, 29–39.

Vose, J.M., Kennedy, B.C., Bierman, P.J., Kessinger, A., & Armitage, J.O. (1992). Long-term sequelae of autologous bone marrow or peripheral cell transplantation for lymphoid malignancies. *Cancer, 69*(3), 784–789.

Watson, M., Zittoun, R., Hall, E., Solbu, G., & Wheatley, K. (1996). A modular questionnaire for the assessment of longterm quality of life in leukemia patients: The MCR/EORTC QLQ-LEU. *Quality of Life Research, 5*(1), 15–19.

Wellisch, D.K., Centeno, J., Guzman, J., Belin, T., & Schiller, G.J. (1996). Bone marrow transplantation vs. high-does cytorabine-based consolidation chemotherapy for acute myelogenous leukemia: A long-term follow-up study of quality-of-life measures of survivors. *Psychosomatics, 37,* 144–154.

Wenz, F., Strinvorth, S., Lohr, F., Fruehauf, S., Wildermuth, S., Van Kampen, M., et al. (2002). Prospective evaluation of delayed central nervous system (CNS) toxicity of hypertractionated total body irradiation (TBI). *International Journal of Radiation, Oncology, Biology, Physics, 48,* 1497–1501.

Wettergren, L., Langius, A., Bjorkholm, M., & Bjorvell, H. (1997). Physical and psychosocial functioning in patients undergoing autologous bone marrow transplantation—a prospective study. *Bone Marrow Transplantation, 20*(6), 497–502.

Whedon, M.B., & Fliedner, M.C. (1999). Nursing issues in hematopoietic cell transplantation. In E. Thomas, K. Blume, & S. Forman (Eds.), *Hematopoietic cell transplantation* (2nd ed., pp. 381–385). Malden, MA: Blackwell Science, Inc.

Whedon, M., Stearns, D., & Mills, L. E. (1995). Quality of life of long-term adult survivors of autologous bone marrow transplantation. *Oncology Nursing Forum, 22,* 1527–1535.

Whedon, M.B., & Wujcik, D. (1997). *Blood and marrow stem cell transplantation: Principles, practice, and nursing insights* (2nd ed.). Sudbury, MA: Jones & Bartlett Publishers.

Winer, E.P., Lindley, C., Hardee, M., Sawyer, W.T., Brunatti, C., Borstelmann, N.A., et al. (1999). Quality of life in patients surviving at least 12 months following high dose chemotherapy with autologous bone marrow support. *Psycho-Oncology, 8,* 167–176.

Wingard, J.R. (1994). Functional ability and quality of life of patients after allogeneic bone marrow transplantation. *Bone Marrow Transplantion, 14* (Suppl. 4), S29–S33.

Wingard, J.R., Curbow, B., Baker, F., Zabora, J., & Piantadosi, S. (1992). Sexual satisfaction in survivors of bone marrow transplantation. *Bone Marrow Transplantation, 9,* 185–190.

Wochna, V. (1997). Anxiety, needs, and coping in family members of the bone marrow transplant patient. *Cancer Nursing, 20,* 244–250.

World Health Organization, Division of Mental Health. (1993). *WHO-QOL study protocol: The development of the World Health Organization quality of life assessment instrument (MNG/PSF/93.9).* Geneva, Switzerland: WHO.

Zabora, J.R., Smith, E.D., Baker, F., Wingard, J.R., & Curbow, B. (1992). The family: The other side of bone marrow transplantation. *Journal of Psychosocial Oncology, 10,* 35–46.

Zebrack, B. (2000). Cancer survivors and quality of life: A critical review of the literature. *Oncology Nursing Forum, 27*(9), 1395–1401.

Zittoun, R., Achrard, S., & Ruszniewski, M. (1999). Assessment of quality of life during intensive chemotherapy or bone marrow transplantation. *Psycho-Oncology, 8,* 64–73.

Zittoun, R., Suciu, S., Watson, M., Solbu, G., Muus, P., Mandelli, F., et al. (1997). Quality of life in patients with acute myelogenous leukemia in prolonged first complete remission after bone marrow transplantation (allogeneic or autologous) or chemotherapy: A cross-sectional study of the EORTC-GIMEMA AML 8A trial. *Bone Marrow Transplantation, 20,* 307–315.

Chapter 16

Models of Care Delivery for Hematopoietic Stem Cell Transplant Patients

Theresa Franco,
RN, MSN

Rosemary C. Ford,
RN, BSN, OCN®

Blood and bone marrow transplantation has undergone many changes in the past decade. Expanding the use of transplant in a variety of disease states, increasing the age of candidates who qualify for therapy, and advancing the technology to enhance safety and efficiency have shaped the current transplant environment. In the 1990s, the use of mobilized peripheral blood progenitor cells and hematopoietic colony stimulating factors led to more rapid engraftment. The continued development of pharmaceutical agents to improve high-dose regimens and more effectively manage symptoms such as nausea and vomiting also played a critical role (Dix and Gellar, 2000). These clinical components, combined with the increasing competition for transplant dollars through contracting arrangements, forced transplant programs to evaluate existing clinical environments in which transplant and the associated care was performed. Blood and bone marrow transplant, which had been primarily an inpatient-driven service model, needed to be overhauled.

More questions than answers surfaced. What changes needed to occur in program goals? What pieces of the infrastructure required modification? Can critical services be delivered in a safe and timely manner in a different setting? What new care delivery models should be designed? What revisions must take place in the transplant team? What will happen to program outcomes and reputation? Most importantly, how and where do the patient and family fit into a new model?

The traditional care delivery models with significant inpatient lengths of stay, the need for sterile environments, the degree of resource utilization, and the role of the transplant team were reexamined (Peters et al., 1994). This analysis of the entire transplant trajectory led many programs to redesign or revise care strategies, shift service allocation, explore other venues for care, and realign team members. Transitioning a portion, or perhaps all transplant care, to the outpatient area no longer seemed unreasonable or unrealistic. This outpatient movement, which had the potential to be quality driven, cost efficient, and patient empowered, would significantly change care delivery models of transplant care.

Changing Models of Care

A spectrum of innovative care delivery models has evolved in response to the changes in transplant. The shift to a greater ambulatory focus has produced hybrids of traditional patient care models and outpatient resource utilization. Hospital inpatient admissions are based on the patients' clinical needs, not simply on the initiation of transplant therapy. Yet, every transplant program still needs an inpatient care model to support intensive assessment and care delivery.

Inpatient Care Delivery

The traditional inpatient care delivery model remains for those transplant therapies with significant toxicity potential and for clinical complications that must be managed in an inpatient area with transplant expertise. Inpatient accommodations range from a dedicated, 2-bed area on a general oncology floor to a dedicated transplant unit with 20 or more beds. These environments may be HEPA-filtered to provide the most optimal environment for performing high-risk transplant (Dykewicz et al., 2000). The inpatient staff must be well educated in all types of transplants to effectively manage transplant therapies and associated complications.

Intensive Care

Complications of transplant affect every system and can become life-threatening. Intensive care strategies may be required to manage complications such as septic shock, pneumonia, disseminated intravascular coagulation (DIC), and Grade 3 or 4 graft-versus-host disease (GVHD).

Severe mucositis threatening the airway, respiratory distress syndrome, and cardiopulmonary toxicity necessitate intensive treatments. Ventilator support and Swan-Ganz monitoring may be initiated. Renal failure from drug therapy or systems failure may be treated by dialysis performed on the transplant unit or may be severe enough to require intensive care monitoring (Shapiro, 1995).

Transplant patients who need intensive measures may be kept on the inpatient transplant unit or be transferred to an intensive care unit. Of the 66 transplant centers listed on the Oncology Nursing Society's Blood and Marrow Stem Cell Transplant (BMSCT) Special Interest Group's Web site, 19 do not transfer their critical patients to an intensive care unit (Special Interest Group BMSCT Oncology Nursing Society Directory, 2004). A poll by the American Society of Bone Marrow Transplants in December 2003 suggests that the number of transplant patients who require critical interventions, the degree of comfort of the transplant team to provide intensive care, and facility/equipment needs impact the integration of this level of care into an inpatient transplant unit. Keeping patients who need critical care modalities in the inpatient transplant unit requires that all or a portion of the nursing staff be trained in therapies such as ventilator care and cardiac monitoring (ASBMT, n.d.). Achieving competence in these skills is related to the frequency with which these measures occur in each program's patient population. An educational program coupled with periodic practice scenarios or a skills lab is crucial to maintaining the staff's expertise (Ford et al., 2004). Some transplant units make arrangements with the intensive care area to provide support in critical situations by moving an intensive care nurse to the transplant unit. Others send a transplant nurse with the patient to the intensive care unit to provide the continuum of transplant expertise. Little evidence supports that one care methodology results in better patient outcomes. Transplant programs must weigh all factors and individually decide which care model is optimal for their patient population

Outpatient Models

One of the earliest outpatient models in transplant was developed by Peters and colleagues (1994) at Duke University. Women with primary metastatic breast cancer who received high-dose chemotherapy and autologous bone marrow and peripheral blood progenitor cells were discharged to an outpatient clinic after these therapies were completed. The patients' follow-up care continued daily in the ambulatory setting with readmission to the inpatient unit only for complications such as febrile neutropenia, viral pneumonia, and dehydration that could not be managed safely in the outpatient environment. This pioneering effort using the outpatient setting for transplant care resulted in impressive outcomes with a reported length of stay reduction from 37 to 24.5 days initially and from 24.5 to 7 days subsequently, and a decrease in charges of 50% over time (Peters et al., 1994).

The belief that an outpatient care model had a place in transplant was reinforced by Weaver and colleagues in their treatment of lymphoma patients in 21 community medical centers across the United States (Weaver et al., 1997). The sequencing of events was different in this outpatient model. The high-dose chemotherapy regimens and the peripheral blood stem cell (PBSC) infusions were administered in the out-

patient facility, and patients were admitted posttransplant for care and surveillance. Most of the patients (96%) were hospitalized for a median of 14 days, while three patients were treated entirely as outpatients. It was evident from the data that a well-tested, high-dose chemotherapy regimen with a PBSC infusion could be administered safely in a community cancer center's outpatient arena (Weaver et al., 1997). These successes prompted other centers to pilot models for transplant care in the outpatient setting.

An approach that allowed for the entire transplant process to be delivered in the ambulatory area was developed. Comprehensive management of the transplant patient could be done successfully as an outpatient if there was a firm commitment to resources, ongoing coordination, and communication with the transplant team. This approach requires the patient and family to demonstrate a willingness to be actively engaged in every step of the process. In the complete outpatient model, the transplant patient receives the high-dose regimen, actual transplant, and posttransplant care all on an outpatient basis. An admission to the inpatient sector occurs only if complications become too difficult or severe to treat as an outpatient (Meisenberg et al., 1998; Ruiz-Argüelles et al., 1998; Dix and Gellar, 2000). This entire outpatient strategy has the advantage of shorter lengths of stay coupled with cost containment. It does, however, have significant impact on the outpatient setting, requiring realignment of resources to ensure quality patient management and safety (Jagannath et al., 1997).

Going beyond the outpatient setting to deliver care is another alternative that has been explored. Westerman and colleagues (1999) advanced transplant care into the home. Encouraged by the successful management of patients in the outpatient clinic, a cohort of patients were discharged to home following stem cell infusion, and all subsequent supportive care was done by specialized home-care professionals. Readmissions to the hospital did occur in this subset as well as in a subset of patients who were managed entirely as outpatients. Most of these individuals, however, were discharged quickly after a brief observation period and appropriate interventions for fever, indwelling catheter malfunctioning, or chemotherapy-related toxicity (Westerman et al., 1999).

With the cooperation of astute home-care professionals, this shift to home was possible. Patients were safe, they reported a positive experience that enhanced their quality of life, and there was increased availability of beds in the inpatient setting for the higher acuity patient (Westerman et al., 1999). Unfortunately, the logistics of providing such services at home and the cost compared to delivering services in a centralized outpatient locale may make this care model undesirable to many transplant programs that treat patients from distant areas (Reed and Armitage, 1999).

All of this hard work paved the way for many centers to seriously entertain the possibility of performing all or a portion of transplant care in the outpatient arena. Success in this endeavor calls for reconsideration of many facets of the transplant program. The first step is to review the goals and philosophy of the program.

Philosophy/Goal

The goals and philosophy of the transplant program must be evaluated whenever significant changes in transplant occur. This ensures that ongoing transplant discoveries are leveraged to the program's advantage and contribute to the highest level of care for the transplant patient. The advances of the past have driven every program to alter its care delivery systems and utilization of services. This reexamination is necessary as nonmyeloblative conditioning regimens, new applications for stem cell transplantation, novel drug agents, and ongoing competition for payers demand change.

Any assessment of a transplant program should focus on the vision and mission of the program, existing limitations in care delivery, multidisciplinary support systems, desired outcomes, and future directions (Corcoran Buchsel and Kapustay, 1997). A program whose foundation is research will need to incorporate investigational protocols and research initiatives into resource allocation and care delivery decisions. For example, a Phase I clinical trial often dictates inpatient assessment for safety considerations.

The number and type of transplants that a facility forecasts is a strong consideration. If a program is primarily focused on autologous transplant, the ability to move patients into other care environments will be less cumbersome than a program that has a significant allogeneic patient base. The rigorous nature of the conditioning regimens, management of side effects, and timely response to potential complications for the allogeneic transplant patient will require more attention and resources when planning a shift to outpatient care.

Age is another factor to consider when evaluating an outpatient program. Adult transplant patients are typically viewed as appropriate outpatient candidates. Their ability to comply with the expectations placed on them in the outpatient setting provides a higher comfort level. In contrast, pediatric patients are more often treated as inpatients, although most parents are capable of assisting with care in the outpatient setting with appropriate support. Additional issues that deserve consideration in shaping the program are current and future technology pursuits, the degree of competition with other centers, and existing payer relationships.

Model of Care Change Implications for the Transplant Team

New care delivery models have significant impact on transplant team members. Physicians are required to reevaluate their entire approach to treatment and selection of candidates in the transplant program. The population of patients eligible for transplant, information requirements, and engaging support from significant others takes on a different perspective. Nurses are challenged to practice complex, comprehensive care in creative ways in new settings. Pharmacists are expected to expand their role and revise administration practices. Many other critical disciplines are faced with assessing their current workload to support shifting care initiatives. Table 16-1 outlines key team member and departmental responsibilities in the transplant program.

At the center of this transition are the patient and their significant others. It is apparent that success in an ambulatory setting hinges on the ability of the patient and his or her family to accept greater responsibilities in care (Dix and Gellar, 2000). Greater educational and care demands are placed on both the patient and his or her caregivers or care partners, who become more intimately involved in transplant care. The primary caregiver in this evolution, which traditionally has been the nurse at the inpatient bedside, now is a family member or friend who

agrees to become a member of the health-care team. Determining the scope of these newly acquired responsibilities by the entire transplant team and evaluating one's ability to fulfill them become a significant challenge for all.

Facility Resources

Facility resources have a major impact on the ease and ability to implement and sustain an outpatient transplant model of care. Most transplant programs have designated inpatient space to manage inpatient treatment. In the outpatient model, functional activities need to be identified and space reconfigured to accommodate the level and types of outpatient activities.

Ideally, the outpatient environment should be adjacent or in close proximity to the inpatient unit. Clinic activities, which include physician visits and treatment episodes, may be performed next to the acute care setting or, in some instances, within a portion of the inpatient unit. This assists in creating a full continuum of care for the transplant patient. An inpatient/outpatient adjacency can result in greater efficiencies in care delivery by sharing personnel, equipment, and transplant expertise. Unfortunately, competing space priorities of other service providers, physical design limitations, and different practice patterns may make this ideal location impossible to achieve.

Outpatient Clinic

The outpatient clinic must be large enough to serve the needs of the outpatient transplant population. On a daily basis, exam rooms and the consultation area must be available for physicians or midlevel providers to evaluate the outpatient, modify the plan of care, and assess the ability of the patient and family to comply with

Table 16-1 CLINICAL SERVICES REQUIRED FOR TRANSPLANT PROGRAMS.

Service	Interface with Transplant (special considerations in italics)
Medical staff	Determine goals of transplant program in terms of population, types of transplant. Establish research initiatives. *Hours of availability in clinic may determine possibility of transferring therapies to outpatient setting.*
Transplant coordinator	Coordinates plan of care and research interface between physicians and patients. Interfaces with the National Marrow Donor Program. *These roles vary between transplant centers.*
Registered nurses	Integral to coordinating care on inpatient and outpatient settings. Primary responsibility for assessment, patient teaching, discharge planning, medication administration and home infusion. Provide 24-hour patient triage in outpatient setting. Assess learning readiness of patients and caregivers. Coordinate materials and classes for patients and caregivers specific to the transplant process.
Nutrition services	Conducts initial assessment. Coordinates nutrition, fluid therapy, and related patient education.
Social work	Conducts initial assessment. Coordinates ongoing psychosocial assessment, intervention, and support. Provides referral to pastoral care as appropriate.
Pastoral care	Addresses spiritual needs.
Pharmacy	Conducts initial assessment. Teaches patients regarding medications and administration.
Home infusion	Most patients will require intravenous infusions at home. During the transplant process, medications and hydration must be supplied and families taught how to administer to the patient. Insurance companies often have preferred provider contracts with specific home infusion agencies. *The acuity of transplant patients and the resulting frequency of changes in infusion therapies is often challenging for home infusion therapies to support.*
Clinic infusion	Administers infusions and transfusion therapies, including high-dose chemotherapy and stem cell infusions. Monitors patients throughout these therapies. *Hours of operation need to include evening and weekend options for successful outpatient programs.*
Procedure suite	Provides procedures with or without sedation, including bone marrow aspirations and lumbar punctures.
Clinical labs	Provide laboratory testing required for patient assessment in a timely manner. *Note increased outpatient acuity often requires same-day lab results for patient safety.*
Research and specialty labs	*Labs such as cryogenetics and pharmacokinetics will need to coordinate the specifics of their operations with various care delivery models in terms of timing and logistics.*
Health information management	Obtain medical records from referring physicians. Coordinate patients' medical records in inpatient and outpatient departments.

Table 16-1 CLINICAL SERVICES REQUIRED FOR TRANSPLANT PROGRAMS *continued.*

Service	Interface with Transplant (special considerations in italics)
Materiel management	Coordinates supplies and equipment needed to perform required patient care.
Patient financial	Coordinates approval of services with the patients' insurance.
Housing	Assists patients and families in finding housing close to transplant center.
Services and payers	Provide documentation regarding justification and rationale for services provided. *Interface with payers must be coordinated with nurses communicating with payers' case managers.*
Medical subspecialists: Infectious disease Pulmonary Renal Gastrointestinal Psychiatry Neurology Dermatology Ophthalmology	Provide expert consultation on request of the transplant medical team. *Must be available on short notice for both inpatient and outpatient requests due to the potentially rapid-changing clinical needs of transplant patients.*
Oral medicine	Conducts initial assessment. Collaborates to assess patients' oral health status before and after transplant.
Pulmonary function	Conducts initial assessment. Collaborates to assess patients' pulmonary status before and after transplant.
Radiation oncology	Coordinates total body irradiation treatment. *Availability of linear accelerator may dictate timing of conditioning therapies.*
Radiology	Provides diagnostic procedures as needed. Coordinates insertion and removal of central venous catheters. *Need to consider on-demand requirements for increased acuity of outpatients.*
Blood bank	Coordinates blood product requirements. Coordinates response to blood product transfusions. *Type of blood products ordered can be very complicated in an ABO mismatched allogenic transplant.* *Blood product required for transplant programs can be a large percentage of a geographic area's total service requirement.*
Patient transport	*The move to outpatient care requires transplant programs to consider shuttles or other means of transportation to the clinic.*
Ambulance	*The move to outpatient care requires transplant programs to develop relationships with ambulance companies for both urgent and emergent transport.*
Long-term follow-up support	Assesses and suggests treatment for patients who have returned to their referring physicians after transplant. *With the increasing number of patients surviving posttransplant, the need for expertise in the unique problems of these patients is expanding.*

care expectations. This space can be multipurpose, shared with other service providers, or utilized to accommodate other aspects of the transplant process, such as evaluating candidates for transplant. However, there should be some type of designated flow pattern to facilitate smooth and timely delivery of care.

In addition, consideration should be paid to the layout of the waiting area for this population. Patients' immunosuppressive condition warrants careful attention. Infection control policies must be in place to minimize risk and ensure patient safety. Potential manifestations of side effects such as nausea and vomiting, hair loss, skin rashes, and other issues related to body image challenge one to create private niches within public spaces to demonstrate sensitivity to the patient's experience.

Infusion/Treatment Center

The outpatient model adopted by the transplant program and the number of patients will drive the type and hours of operation of the treatment or infusion center. Identifying the interventions that will be performed is crucial in determining space, equipment, and staffing. If the preparative regimen will be administered in the infusion center, accommodations and protocols for safe administration and disposal of the agents must be in place. Drugs requiring special handling or monitoring, along with a host of other intravenous medications, must be factored into the setting. Pharmaceutical service is a key element in the provision of care. Agreements can range from securing existing pharmaceutical support within the hospital to an actual satellite pharmacy within or next to the infusion area. Aside from drug support, spatial consideration should be given for blood products administration, central line and peripheral lab draws, and procedures such as bone marrow biopsies or aspirates, and discontinuance of central lines.

The milieu in which treatment will be provided is of utmost importance. An open concept with treatment chairs or a combination of private/semiprivate rooms is another decision in design planning. Some patients desire to have a private setting for their care, whereas others benefit from interacting with patients who are undergoing a similar experience.

Furniture in the treatment center should be functional and sturdy. Comfortable recliners for patients who may spend up to 16 hours in the area are critical. Many infusion centers have hospital beds for patients to use during stem cell infusions or other treatments that are tiresome or very complex. Due to the common side effects such as nausea, vomiting, and diarrhea, bathrooms within the area or close to the infusion area are essential. Space for supplies and equipment storage must be identified, and a small nutritional area for patients and families is a desired amenity.

The entire ambulatory area should be under the diligent surveillance of both infection control and housekeeping to minimize infectious transmission and maintain cleanliness. Policies and procedures that address regimens for cleaning and culturing are of utmost importance.

Apheresis Area

The blood stem cell collection procedure can be done in a variety of ways, but space should be allocated within a reasonable distance to the inpatient or outpatient area. Approximately 40 square feet per patient is needed to accommodate the machinery and to deliver services (Corcoran Buchsel and Kapustay, 1997). The actual amount of space will be determined by the number of patients who require apheresis at any given time, allowing 2 to 4 hours per typical episode. Many different staffing models are feasible. Inpatient or outpatient staff may be trained to do the apheresis procedure or a partnership with a blood service organization such as the American Red Cross may exist. Proximity to the cryopreservation laboratory to process the product must also be considered.

Educational Areas/ Conference Space

Orientation and ongoing education of the patient and caregiver is of primary importance in outpatient transplant. Space must be designated to allow for participation in one-on-one coaching, group teaching, and counseling sessions. A place for classes to deliver comprehensive information related to all phases of transplant, labs to practice skills, and a location to house support meetings and diversional activities need to be identified. This space can be flexible in nature and can also satisfy the educational and conferencing needs of the transplant staff with appropriate scheduling.

Other Considerations

A day surgical suite for catheter placement and other procedures, a lounge area to escape from the entire transplant experience, and a resource center to house information and provide online access are ideal additions. Unfortunately, space is a precious commodity in most programs. Therefore, much creativity must be invoked to provide a satisfying environment for all those participating in aspects of care.

Housing

The success of outpatient models for transplant is dependent on the degree of participation of the patient and family who accept the responsibilities of care. To ensure timely access to services, the patient and care partner should be housed close to the facility. For safety, many centers require the patient who wants to commute from home to live within a certain distance—typically within 30 minutes or 30 miles—from the center.

For the patient who is not local, housing may range from being within the actual transplant center to a few miles away in a hotel or apartment. The housing may be owned by the transplant facility or a hotel corporation, or a partnership may exist between the two entities to provide lodging for transplant patients. Transportation may be provided by the hotel or the transplant facility by means of a shuttle service or prepaid taxi services. Reimbursement for housing and accompanying expenses may or may not be part of the financial transplant package.

One of the main concerns that must be addressed is the cleaning of the residential space. Policies and procedures endorsed by the infection control department or infectious disease specialists should be established to decrease risks to the patient. Random walk-throughs should be done to determine adherence to policies. In-service meetings should be held with the appropriate staff to improve understanding of the correct procedures.

Caregiver Issues

The shift in transplant care delivery models radically changed the role of the patient's significant other from one of primarily psychosocial support to one who is essential to the patient's acceptance into some transplant programs. Many centers may not accept or have difficulty accepting a patient for transplant if the patient does not have a competent adult caregiver available. Although this may seem harsh, third-party payers will not pay for inpatient days not clinically required, and neither the patient nor the transplant center can absorb this cost. One possibility for the patient without a caregiver is to be admitted to a skilled nursing facility (SNF) during periods when the patient is too clinically labile to live alone. This option is not widely entertained, however, because most SNFs do not meet transplant standards regarding private rooms, private baths, specific infection control practices, or staff able to administer infusions.

Some centers have defined periods of time during the transplant process when caregivers are mandatory and other times when they are encouraged to be present. (See Figure 13-4 in Chapter 13.) Mandatory periods include episodes in the ambulatory setting during conditioning, preengraftment, infusion therapy, or impaired mobility. The workup phase, inpatient days, and a clinically stable postengraftment period may not mandate caregiver presence. Some patients plan for a series of caregivers to come at various intervals during the transplant process. It is important that the transplant nurses educate each of these caregivers directly to ensure correct information is transmitted instead of one caregiver educating the next one.

Caregiver Responsibilities

Typical caregiver responsibilities are discussed below and summarized in Figure 13-2 in Chapter 13.

MONITORING OF PATIENT

Assessment and monitoring of the patient's temperature, level of consciousness, skin condition, fluid intake, food intake, sleep patterns, pain, fatigue, and signs of upper respiratory infection can all be done by the caregiver. The caregiver is asked to keep written records of such things as medication administration, food intake, and temperatures to assist the transplant team in planning appropriate interventions. The caregiver attends all clinic activities to relay his or her assessment of the patient to the staff.

MEDICATION ADMINISTRATION

Administration of oral medications and selected intravenous medications and hydration can also be a part of the caregiver's activities. Medications include antivirals, antibiotics, and cyclosporine. The first dose of many of these medications is usually given in the clinic to ensure immediate availability of expertise if a reaction occurs.

ADHERENCE TO PATIENT SCHEDULE

The caregiver provides transportation to and from the clinic and coordinates the patient's medication and infusion schedule with clinic visits.

INFECTION CONTROL

One of the major concerns with transferring care of neutropenic patients to the ambulatory setting is infection control. Studies have shown that neutropenic patients can be in the ambulatory setting with prophylactic antibiotic therapy (Wingard and Leather, 2004). It is important to teach patients and caregivers to use common sense in avoiding infections, while at the same time not instilling in them an unwarranted degree of fear. Simple measures such as frequent hand-washing, avoiding crowds, washing fruits and vegetables, other food safety practices, and daily personal hygiene should be the focus of their efforts. Caregivers should know the initial signs of infection, especially the importance of taking the patient's temperature at least twice a day.

CENTRAL VENOUS CATHETER CARE

Every model of care delivery must include teaching the patient or caregiver the basic care of the central venous catheter. This includes removing the exit site dressing, inspection of the exit site for signs of infection or dislodgement, cleansing the site according to program policy, and reapplying the dressing. In addition, the catheters need to be flushed periodically according to policy, and this is usually done by the patient or caregiver between clinic appointments. It is also essential that basic safety measures be taught to the patient and caregiver, including what to do if the line falls out, becomes dislodged, breaks, or the cap is lost.

The stress of these responsibilities cannot be underestimated. It is crucial that the transplant staff acknowledge this stress and include assessment of the caregiver's ability to cope during the patient's clinic visits. It is important that the caregiver plan respite time for him- or herself and be cognizant of his or her own health needs during this time.

Outpatient Flow of Services

One of the most challenging aspects of ambulatory models is the logistics of how and when the patient will get needed services. Inpatient models have the advantage of the constant availability of the patient, with many services either delivered at the bedside or within the hospital. In the ambulatory setting, the patient's primary location may be his or her own home or a housing facility. There must be a plan for every service that the patient may need to access. Each center must evaluate its own staffing and facility resources and determine how outpatients will interface with these resources on a routine as well as emergent basis (see Table 16-1 for services to be considered). There should be recognition that the transplant patient is often fatigued, and grouping visits when possible can conserve precious energy. It is essential for the transplant staff to determine standards for the frequency of clinic visits. During conditioning, the patient will warrant daily visits, including weekends. A decision for clinic support during neutropenia must be finalized. There may be times when it is appropriate for a transplant nurse to assess the patient independently between the required physician visits.

Hours of Operation/ Emergency Plan

Hours of clinic operation must be discussed when planning an outpatient model. Key staff and services such as physicians, triage nurses, infusions, lab, and radiology must be available seven days a week for a program to be successful. Unless these services are always available, after-hours accommodations must be in place.

An emergency plan should be developed and well articulated to the patient and caregiver. There should be a transplant triage nurse available by phone at all times to assist with immediate problem solving. The emergency department may not be the ideal location for these complex patients to be assessed or treated. Lack of timeliness in being seen in a busy emergency room with other individuals who may potentially harbor dangerous infectious agents can put the transplant patient at risk. Many centers utilize the inpatient transplant unit for after-hours calls and emergencies or maintain 24-hour coverage in their outpatient setting.

Patient and Caregiver Teaching

Teaching is the critical intervention for successful transition of care to the ambulatory setting. The caregiver becomes the conduit for the basic nursing assessments performed in traditional care models and must be instructed on key aspects to monitor.

It is a challenge for the patient and caregiver to understand everything that they must in a relatively short period of time, so resources must be available. Ambulatory nurses must develop excellent teaching skills as well as possess the ability to evaluate the learners' comprehension. Many centers assign nurse case managers to patients so that the patient has a primary source for continuity of approach, information, and reinforcement. Most centers have a transplant manual that outlines the entire transplant process for the patient. Some have videotapes for such topics as the transplant process, insertion and care of the central venous catheter, use of an ambulatory pump for infusions, and coping strategies. Large centers have found that some common topics such as hands-on ambulatory pump function, introduction to the responsibilities of the caregiver, food safety, and departure preparation can be successfully taught to groups of patients and caregivers in a classroom setting. The final responsibility for individualized patient teaching, however, rests with the ambulatory nurse, who must assess and intervene in all areas of care within the time constraints of a clinic visit.

Teaching begins as soon as the patient makes initial contact with the transplant center. Information is mailed to the patient and donor, if applicable, and a specific staff member is assigned to be available for questions by phone. Many patients come to the center for a consult with the medical staff before deciding to pursue transplant. This is an ideal time for nurses to offer an overview of the program and to answer questions. Once the patient is accepted for transplant, workup usually takes about 1 to 2 weeks to complete. This is the pivotal opportunity to educate the patient and caregiver about the transplant process as well as clinic operations. Patient teaching is a multidisciplinary effort, and it should be clear what each discipline will cover. Research centers must ensure that the patient has all the information required to give informed consent for the protocols being offered. The nurse can provide a great deal of information regarding the specifics of various clinical trials and can assist the patient in formulating questions for the physician before consent is obtained. It is helpful for patients to receive consent forms in advance so they can be prepared to address their issues prior to consenting.

The nurse must plan ahead and ensure that caregivers are competent when therapies are initiated. It may seem awkward to teach about therapies for which the patient has not yet consented or been financially approved, but time becomes limited. Once the workup is completed, consents signed, and financial approval secured, there is often an urgency to start conditioning to meet deadlines for unrelated donor harvesting or to accommodate linear accelerator schedules. Teaching at this stage centers on what to expect with the conditioning therapies and management of supportive interventions such as antiemetics and infusions. The patient will have a central venous catheter inserted, which necessitates preoperative teaching and instruction about the dressing change and flushing. If the patient will require home infusion, this is the time to ensure the caregiver is competent in managing the infusion pump.

Patient and caregiver teaching is a significant part of every clinic visit throughout the transplant process. As new therapies, side effects, or complications arise, the patient and caregiver must be educated on how this will affect them and what responsibilities they can expect.

It is not unusual for patients to be admitted during some phase of the transplant process. During these times the nursing staff assumes the primary responsibility from the caregiver for assessment and therapies. Patient teaching is focused on understanding the immediate therapies being delivered and how they affect the clinical condition of the patient. When the patient approaches discharge, it is again time to plan for continued, expected outpatient therapies and reassess the caregiver's competence.

The importance of a discharge plan cannot be underestimated. Every center should have a comprehensive discharge teaching plan and identify an individual or group to be responsible for its implementation with the patient and caregiver.

At the end of the patient's transplant course, instruction specific to resuming the patient's previous life activities must be given. The timing of these recommendations is individual and takes into account the patient's clinical condition at the time of departure from the transplant center. It is important that the physician assuming care for the patient be informed about the plan of care and resources to access should consultation with the transplant team be necessary. When the patient returns for the long-term follow-up assessment, teaching should be based on the results of the assessment and questions from the patient.

Interface with Third-Party Payers

A major focus in transplant care has been to reduce cost while maintaining quality. Moving care to the outpatient setting has proven to be cost effective (Rizzo et al., 1999).

The intensive specialized care required to support a patient through the process costs on average $145,000 for autologous, $232,000 for related, and $295,000 for unrelated allogeneic transplant (Hauboldt & Ortner, 2002). Sophisticated, dedicated patient financial services are a vital part of every transplant program (Adams and Johns, 2004). Financial counselors must work with the patients from the time of initial contact with the transplant medical staff. Patients are informed of the costs of transplant and assisted in evaluating their financial status and insurance benefits. The financial services staff also is responsible for maintaining a strong communication link with each patient's insurance carrier, representing both the patient's and the medical center's interests.

Many transplant centers have contracts with individual insurance carriers likely to cover patients referred to that center. These contracts benefit the payers by offering discounts in cost and benefit the transplant centers by assuring patient referrals. Some insurance companies have established "centers of excellence" ratings where they critique centers for specific quality outcomes and subsequently refer patients preferably to these centers.

Other insurance companies contract with companies that specialize in coverage for catastrophic illnesses and treatments. One example is United Resource Network (www.urnweb.com), which has contracts with transplant centers negotiating discounted reimbursement for the various types of transplants. Contracts often designate a specific sum or case rate for an identified period of time during treatment. Examples of case rate definitions are from the first day of conditioning to day 35 posttransplant for autologous patients and to day 50 posttransplant for allogeneic patients. Transplant centers are guaranteed that case rate regardless of actual cost.

Some patients will begin the workup for transplant with approval for coverage confirmed by their insurance company. Others will have the cost of the workup approved, but the transplant approval will be pending the insurance company's review of workup data. Still others may arrive with approval denied but pending appeal by the transplant center's medical staff. The increasing influence of third-party payers on patient care affects every transplant program today. It is not unusual for approval for transplant to come from the insurance provider within days or even hours of the plan to start conditioning. This can be anxiety-provoking for the patient and staff. It is critical for a member of the clinical staff to know the specifics of each patient's coverage, especially for outpatient pharmacy, home infusion, skilled nursing facility, and physical therapy benefits, as well as whether preapproval is needed for procedures such as central line insertion or radiology scans. Insurance contracts may impact a patient in the ambulatory setting by allowing the patient to receive medications and home infusion from the transplant center during the case rate period, but then requiring the patient to obtain services outside of the case rate from payer-contracted retail pharmacies or home infusion companies.

Communication with third-party payers should be consistent throughout the transplant process. Most insurance companies have nurse case managers assigned to a transplant patient caseload to ensure questions and concerns are addressed. Likewise, transplant centers should have a designated individual, usually a nurse or social worker, who is responsible for communication with these case managers. This individual is skilled at describing transplant therapy as well as the changing clinical status of the patient as he or she progresses through transplant. This can often assist in obtaining specific approval for additional services that the patient needs.

Innovative Care Delivery Models

The dramatic changes in transplant have motivated some transplant centers to develop innovative care models that place the patient and family member(s) clearly at the center of care. In the mid 1990s, the Johns Hopkins Oncology Center developed a unique model of care delivery for its blood and bone marrow transplant patients and families. This model, called IPOP, inpatient/outpatient care continuum, permits patients to remain in a homelike atmosphere with their selected caregivers during some phases of care. The caregivers, after receiving appropriate education, assist the patient with many care activities. This allows the patients to more fully access the ambulatory setting, while reducing the length of time spent in the inpatient setting (Grimm et al., 2000). IPOP is a patient-focused care delivery model that maximizes the resources of the outpatient environment, yet provides 24-hour access to care. This results in the provision of continuity of care by the transplant team across different locations. Selected patients visit the IPOP clinic each day but spend their nights in a residential living facility with a caregiver. A critical pathway that includes the same components as inpatient care is followed in the outpatient arena. Significant complications such as organ dysfunction, febrile episodes, and graft-versus-host disease may result in an inpatient admission, but once resolved, the patient is quickly transitioned back to the ambulatory side of care. This design has resulted in IPOP patients spending less than 10 days in an inpatient area (Johns Hopkins, 2004).

The benefits of this ambulatory transplant model extend beyond the patient to the caregiver. Grimm and colleagues (2000) conducted a study comparing the emotional responses and needs of caregivers of transplant patients in the IPOP setting with those in inpatient settings. The findings reveal that IPOP caregivers had significantly less mood disturbance at several points in the care continuum before discharge than their inpatient counterparts. They reported greater satisfaction in the meeting of their psychological needs and reported less feelings of isolation. It was determined that caregiver education and the assessment and interventions to meet caregiver psychological needs is of extreme importance when designing different care models.

Cooperative Care

Another creative approach in transplantation has been established at the University of Nebraska Medical Center with the development of a cooperative care model. In an effort to meet the ongoing challenges of transplant, the medical center adapted a cooperative care model that was designed by Dr. Anthony Grieco and his team at New York University Medical Center. This care delivery model centers on the belief that with appropriate education and training, the patient and a selected lay person, usually a family member, can actively participate in many cares required in an acute health-care setting (Grieco et al., 1994). At Nebraska, this individual becomes the primary caregiver to the patient during the acute phase of transplant. The caregiver, through classroom instruction, skills labs, and one-on-one reinforcement with the health-care team, becomes comfortable in participating in a variety of functions. These include such things as assisting with activities of daily living, taking vital signs, administering medications, and recording relevant data. Because the caregiver becomes a vital member of the team and is given much accountability, an assessment of his or her readiness to accept this role is completed by a nurse prior to the patient's admission into cooperative care.

The cooperative care model includes amenities and accommodations that are very different than the typical hospital or outpatient setting. The patient and care partner are housed in suites that combine care functions with comfort and privacy. Each one-bedroom suite has defined living and bedroom space, a kitchenette, and a bathroom. Adjustable lighting, space for supplies and personal belongings, an entertainment center, and computer access help establish a homelike atmosphere. This assists the patient and care partner in promoting recovery while enhancing autonomy and diversion during their transplant stay.

Outcomes of the cooperative care model include reduction in medication errors, patient falls, and length of stay. Patient satisfaction with transplant care is higher than the inpatient satisfaction rates and cost efficiencies have been experienced (Schmit-Pokorny et al., 2003). As a result, this exciting care model is being expanded to other patient populations.

Summary

There are many models of care delivery for blood and marrow stem cell transplant programs that safely provide patients with the comprehensive services required throughout the transplant continuum. Each transplant center must determine its own care model based on unique goals, strategic direction, and operational and staff resources. Outside influences such as cooperative research protocols, accreditation requirements, and National Marrow Donor Program (NMDP) criteria will drive some aspects of care planning within a program. Models of care will continue to evolve as transplant therapies change and new discoveries emerge. Innovative options, alternative approaches, and exciting opportunities will shape the care models of the future.

References

Adams, L.L., & Johns, A.A. (2004). Nursing issues in hematopoietic cell transplantation. In Blume, K.G., Forman, S.J., & Appelbaum, F.R. (Eds.), *Thomas' hematopoietic cell transplantation* (3rd ed., pp. 463–468). Malden, MA: Blackwell.

ASBMT. (n.d.) ASBMT survey. Retrieved February 15, 2004, from http://www.ASBMT.org

Corcoran Buchsel, P., & Kapustay, P. (1997). Models of ambulatory care for blood cell and bone marrow transplantation. In Bakitas Whedon, M., & Wujcik, D. (Eds.), *Blood and marrow stem cell transplantation* (2nd ed., pp. 525–561). Sudbury, MA: Jones & Bartlett.

Dix, S.P., & Gellar, R.B. (2000). High-dose chemotherapy with autologous stem cell rescue in the outpatient setting. *Oncology, 14*(2), 171–185.

Dykewicz, C.A., Jaffe, H.W., & Kaplan J.E. in collaboration with the Guidelines Working Group Members from the CDC, the Infectious Diseases Society of America, and the American Society of Blood and Marrow Transplantation. (2000). Guidelines for preventing opportunistic infections among hematopoietic stem cell transplant recipients. *Biology of Blood Marrow Transplantation, 6*, 659–737.

Ford, R.C., Campbell, J., & Madison, J. (2004). Nursing issues in hematopoietic cell transplantation. In Blume, K.G., Forman, S.J., & Appelbaum, F.R. (Eds.), *Thomas' hematopoietic cell transplantation* (3rd ed., pp. 469–482). Malden, MA: Blackwell.

Grieco, A.J., Glassman, K.S., & Garnett, S.A. (1994). Origins of cooperative care. In Grieco, A.J., McClure, J.L., Komiske, B.K., & Menard, R.F. (Eds.), *Family partnership in hospital care: The cooperative care concept* (pp. 3–14). New York: Springer.

Grimm, P.M., Zawacki, K.L., Mock, V., Krumm, S., & Frink, B.B. (2000). Caregiver responses and needs: An ambulatory bone marrow transplant model. *Cancer Practice, 8*(3), 120–128.

Hauboldt, R., & Ortner, N. (2002). 2002 organ and tissue transplant costs and discussion. Retrieved December 29, 2005, from http://www.milliman.com/pubs/HRR_07-2002.pdf

Jagannath, S., Vesole, D.H., Zhang, M., Desikan, K.R., Copeland, N., Jagannath, M., et al. (1997). Feasibility and cost-effectiveness of outpatient autotransplants in multiple myeloma. *Bone Marrow Transplantation, 20*, 445–450.

Johns Hopkins. (2004). JHH Comprehensive Transplant Center bone marrow transplantation. Retrieved February 15, 2004, from http://www.hopkinsmedicine.org/Transplant/programs/bonemarrow/index.html

Meisenberg, B.R., Ferran, K., Hollenbach, K., Brehm, T., Jollon, J., & Piro, L.D. (1998). Reduced charges and costs associated with outpatient autologous stem cell transplant. *Bone Marrow Transplantation, 21*, 927–932.

Peters, W.P., Ross, M., Vredenburgh, J.J., Hussein, A., Rubin, P., Dukelow, K., et al. 1994. The use of intensive clinic support to permit outpatient autologous bone marrow transplantation for breast cancer. *Seminars in Oncology, 21*(4 Suppl 7), 25–31.

Reed, E., & Armitage, J.O. (1999). Stem cell transplant at home: Glimpse of the future. *Annals of Oncology, 10*, 493–494.

Rizzo, D., Vogelsang, G.B., Krumm, S., Frink, B., Mock, V., & Bass, E.B. (1999). Outpatient-based bone marrow transplantation for hematologic malignancies: Cost saving or cost shifting? *Journal of Clinical Oncology, 9,* 2811.

Ruiz-Argüelles, G.J., Ruiz-Argüelles, A., Pérez-Romano, B., Marín-López, A., & Delgado-Lamas, J.L. (1998). Non-cryopreserved peripheral blood stem cells autotransplants for hematological malignancies can be performed entirely on an outpatient basis. *American Journal of Hematology, 58,* 161–164.

Schmit-Pokorny, K., Franco, T., Frappier, B., & Vyhlidal, R. (2003). The cooperative care model: An innovative approach to deliver blood and marrow stem cell transplant care. *Clinical Journal of Oncology Nursing, 7,* 509–514.

Shapiro, T.W. (1995). Intensive care management of the BMT patient: Administrative and clinical issues. In Buchsel, P., & Wheedon, M.P. (Eds), *Bone marrow transplantation: Administrative strategies and clinical concerns* (pp. 69–96). Boston: Jones & Bartlett Publishers.

Special Interest Group BMT Oncology Nursing Society. (2004). Directory. Retrieved December 27, 2005, from http://www.ons.org/clinical/treatment/directory.shtml

Weaver, C.H., Schwartzberg, L., Zhen, B., Mangum, M., Leff, R., Tauer, K., et al. (1997). High-dose chemotherapy and peripheral blood stem cell infusion in patients with non-Hodgkins lymphoma: Results of outpatient treatment in community cancer centers. *Bone Marrow Transplantation, 20,* 753–760.

Westerman, A.M., Holtkamp, M.M.J., Linthorst, G.A.M., van Leeuwen, L., Willemse, E.J.M., van Dijk, W.C., et al. (1999). At home management of aplastic phase following high-dose chemotherapy with stem-cell rescue for hematological and non-hematological malignancies. *Annals of Oncology, 10,* 511–517.

Wingard, J.R., & Leather, H.L. (2004). Bacterial infections. In Blume, K.G., Forman, S.J., & Appelbaum, F.R. (Eds.), *Thomas' hematopoietic cell transplantation* (3rd ed., pp. 665–682). Malden, MA: Blackwell.

Chapter 17

Transplant Networks and Standards of Care: International Perspectives

Susan Ezzone, MS, RN, CNP

Monica Fliedner, MSN

Jan Sirilla, MSN, RN, OCN®

During the later part of the 20th century, blood and marrow stem cell transplant (BMT) has evolved into a conventional treatment modality for a variety of malignant and nonmalignant diseases, and its use continues to evolve. The use of autologous transplantation following high-dose chemotherapy for aggressive treatment of solid tumors was a major focus in the 1990s. During the late 1990s and early 21st century, interest has grown in the use of nonmyeloablative preparative regimens and donor lymphocyte infusions. Rapid changes occurring in the specialty have made it difficult for healthcare professionals to remain up to date on current practice and trends in transplantation. Several organizations have published standards of care or recommendations for practice for BMT. This chapter will review the known networks and standards of care established in blood and marrow stem cell transplantation.

International Nursing Networks

For many years, nurses working in blood and marrow stem cell transplantation have exchanged ideas and knowledge related to the specialty through participation in conferences offered in the United States, Canada, and European and other countries. The following is a review of the known networks established, but it is not meant to be an exhaustive description.

Nursing Networks within the United States

The Oncology Nursing Society (ONS) is an internationally recognized organization of more than 28,000 members whose mission is to promote excellence in oncology nursing. In the early years of marrow transplantation, the ONS provided a forum for networking among transplant nurses through attendance at the ONS Annual Congress. Many of the initial educational offerings focusing on bone marrow transplant nursing were provided through the ONS Annual Congress and in later years through the Fall Institute conference. Since ONS member needs are very broad and reach all aspects of oncology nursing, transplant nurses searched for ways to meet their needs related to education, practice, administration, and research issues in transplantation.

In 1989, ONS approved the development of several special interest groups (SIGs) to provide a forum for nurses working in oncology specialty areas to network and collaborate in education, practice, administration, and research. The Bone Marrow Transplant (BMT) SIG was formed in 1989, and the first strategic plan was developed in 1992. The plan provides direction for SIG activities towards accomplishing the mission statement and strategic goals. The SIG recently changed its name to Blood and Marrow Stem Cell Transplant (BMSCT) SIG. The BMSCT SIG, as an organization of more than 600 members within ONS, collaborates with other ONS committees or SIGs to promote an expanded transplantation knowledge base to oncology nurses. Some of the activities of the BMSCT SIG include offering educational programs at ONS congress and institutes of learning (formerly known as Fall Institute), publishing a newsletter, disseminating new information, distributing a BMT nursing resource directory, publishing a manual of recommendations for education and practice, conducting nursing research, and offering regional workshops. Information about the BMSCT SIG, the latest newsletter, and the resource directory are now available on the ONS SIG Web site (http://www.ons.org/clinical/treatment/directory.shtml). The BMSCT SIG meets yearly at the ONS Annual Congress to discuss and plan activities and communicates throughout the year via the newsletter, mailings, and phone contact.

In recent years, transplant nursing educational sessions have been offered at the annual tandem meeting of the International Bone Marrow Transplant Registry (IBMTR) and Autologous Blood and Marrow Transplant Registry (ABMTR). This conference provides an opportunity for networking among nurses, physicians, pharmacists, data managers, and administrators. Conference education and research topics provide an up-to-date review of current practices in the specialty of blood and marrow transplantation.

Nursing Networks within Europe and Canada

The European Blood and Marrow Transplant-Nurses Group (EBMT-NG) was formed in January 1985 with the encouragement and support of physicians working in transplantation. Since most European countries have small transplant centers, the need to share information grew rapidly. The first meeting of the EBMT-NG was held in Bad Hofgastein, Austria, as a 1-day conference, which later expanded to a 2-day conference. Now, a 3-day nursing conference is held in conjunction with the physician conference and offers many concurrent abstract and instructional sessions. The joint conference provides a forum for nurses, physicians, allied health professionals, and data managers to network and share information about new developments in treatment modalities. The conference has been lengthened to allow nurses opportunities to share expertise and clinical knowledge among European countries. Over the years, learning needs of conference attendees have changed and currently reflect an increased need for sessions on symptom control, care for the caregiver, and family nursing. Interactive sessions, such as workshops, roundtable sessions, and debates on current hot topics, were introduced.

Every year, the board of the EBMT-NG, which consists of the president, president-elect, secretary, treasurer, and delegates from the hosting country where the conference takes place, invites internationally well-known speakers. In the past, speakers included not only physicians who gave updates on new developments in transplantation, but also nurses who have performed important work related to nursing care of the transplant patient.

Since there are approximately 26 countries participating in the EBMT-NG who speak many different languages, there are difficulties in communication among countries. Many nurses speak only their native language and have difficulty communicating in other languages. Therefore, it is not always possible to translate protocols or research studies into the primary language of the host country. Each country has its own culture, meaning of nursing care, status of nurses, educational preparation of nurses, and health-care system. Especially with new treatment modalities like transplantation, it is difficult to translate and transcribe nursing care strategies to another language. With these challenges, nurses need an effective communication network to be able to exchange new ideas. Nurses and other health-care professionals committed to developing care for the patient undergoing a transplant can become individual or group members of the EBMT-NG. In recognition of the importance of teamwork, the EBMT-NG organization opened its membership to nurses and data managers in 2003. This will facilitate and promote more involvement of nurses in the work of EBMT-NG.

To facilitate networking within Europe, the EBMT-NG established a group of contact persons from every country. These contact persons receive announcements for the next conference and distribute them within their country. Also, the contact persons meet at the conference to receive an update on the work of the board and

then report important information to their countrymen in their primary language. Many transplant centers within the same country may be located so far apart that nurses don't communicate regularly throughout the year. These countries organize meetings of their fellow nurses during the conference to exchange information. The EBMT-NG holds a national nursing group meeting during the conference to facilitate networking. Nurses in some countries, like Switzerland, Germany, Great Britain, and the Netherlands, are organized in national BMT/blood cell transplant (BCT) working parties. Many topics have been discussed during the past 15 EBMT-NG meetings. Abstracts of the presentations are published together with the medical abstracts in the *Journal of Bone Marrow Transplantation*.

In the beginning of the EBMT nurses group, the presentations at the conferences were published in the proceedings and sent to all attendees of the conference, which allowed distribution of the information to only a limited number of nurses. Since 1992, the EBMT-NG develops and distributes an EBMT-NG journal in which most presentations of the conferences are published along with other articles and important information on transplant nursing. The journal is published twice a year and is received by all attendees of the conference and all nurses who are members of the EBMT nurses group. Publication of the journal provides the information presented at the conference to nurses who did not attend. Other information throughout the year is published in the interdisciplinary *EBMT News*. This enhances the communication between the medical and nursing group. Over the past few years, a mission statement and strategic goals have been developed. The strategy includes five areas on which the EBMT-NG will focus over the next 4 years: profile and public relations; communication; research; education and training; and clinical nursing practice. For each area an action plan is developed. It will be very interesting for centers from many different countries to work together on several specific topics.

The Joint Accreditation Committee-EBMT ISCT (International Society for Cellular Therapy) Europe (JACIE) was established in 1999. This accreditation program aims to create a standardized system of accreditation across Europe. So far, 12 countries participate in this centralized program, which maintains the same strictness, criteria, and standards in different European countries. These standards are based on the standards of the Foundation for the Accreditation of Cellular Therapy (FACT), which were developed initially by the ISCT and a subcommittee of the American Society for Blood and Marrow Transplantation (ASBMT). Nursing aspects will be included in the accreditation process of the EBMT-NG in the future.

In Canada, the Canadian Association of Nurses in Oncology (CANO) is an organization that promotes excellence in oncology nursing practice and education. In recent years, marrow/stem cell nurses who attended the annual CANO conference met to network and share ideas related to transplant nursing. For 3 consecutive years, a transplant workshop was offered during the CANO conference in an effort to meet the educational needs of transplant nurses. Since transplant centers in Canada are separated by hundreds of miles, networking is difficult. The formation of special interest groups within CANO is under consideration and may provide a more effective networking opportunity among Canadian transplant nurses.

International Medical Networks

Medical Networks within the United States

For many years, physicians within the United States and other countries have participated in specialty organizations such as the American Society of Clinical Oncology (ASCO), the American Society of Hematology (ASH), and regional cooperative oncology groups. These organizations provide physicians the opportunity to share information related to the treatment of persons with cancer and/or hematologic diseases and to collaborate on developing and conducting research. Advancements in technology and knowledge as well as research findings are presented at annual conferences. In the past, ASCO's annual conference has been held immediately following the ONS Annual Congress, which facilitates a forum for collaboration among physicians and nurses, and offers a joint session coordinated by ASCO and ONS members. Presentations on marrow/BSC transplantation are given during the annual conferences.

Cooperative oncology groups were formed in 1955 by the National Cancer Institute (NCI) for the purpose of developing and coordinating controlled clinical trials jointly among researchers to expand the science and treatment of cancer (Cheson, 1991). The clinical trials are funded through the NCI through cooperative agreements, and clinical trials are conducted at several centers in an effort to expedite patient accrual and development of new knowledge and treatments for cancer. Investigative studies evaluating the effectiveness of bone marrow and/or BSC transplant are being conducted by many of the cooperative groups for a variety of diseases.

The International Bone Marrow Transplant Registry (IBMTR) was formed in the 1970s for the purpose of collecting, organizing, and analyzing all data on allogeneic and syngeneic bone marrow transplantation. Transplant centers are encouraged to participate in the IBMTR by submitting data to the registry on every transplant performed. The international data collated through the IBMTR provides a large database for analyzing trends or changes in practice and outcomes of transplantation. The results of the IBMTR data are published in medical journals and presented at international scientific meetings. In 1990, the Autologous Blood and Marrow Transplant Registry (ABMTR) was formed to facilitate efforts in international data collection on autologous transplant, similar to the IBMTR. The first meeting of the ABMTR was held in January 1995 prior to the American Society for Blood and Marrow Transplantation conference in Keystone, Colorado. The IBMTR and ABMTR are coordinated through the Medical College of Wisconsin at Milwaukee. Uniform data reporting forms are provided by the IBMTR/ABMTR to transplant centers that submit data. Data reporting forms are available in handwritten and/or computerized format.

The American Society for Blood and Marrow Transplantation (ASBMT) was formed to advance the research and clinical practice of stem cell transplantation. According to the ASBMT Web site (ASBMT, 2005), the organization focuses on seven broad areas: research, representation, clinical standards, regulation, communications, accreditation, and reimbursement. There are four levels of membership:

1. *Member*—MDs or PhDs with expertise in stem cell transplantation (either publication of 2 papers or 2 years clinical experience in SCT)
2. *Associate*—other MDs or PhDs
3. *Affiliate*—other allied professionals with an interest in transplantation
4. *In Training*—fellows-in-training in transplantation

All members receive the monthly journal, *Biology of Blood and Marrow Transplantation* as well as the ASBMT's bulletin, *Marrow Transplantation Reviews*.

In 1999, a special interest group was formed for BMT administrative directors. Membership in this group is available for no additional cost to affiliate members of ASBMT. The goal of this group is to address administrative and operational issues of BMT programs. The special interest group has been instrumental in developing a standard RFI (request for information) to be used as the annual reporting mechanism to payers and in developing new current procedural terminology (CPT) codes for stem cell transplantation procedures. They also provide an educational track for BMT administrators at the annual BMT tandem conference.

In Ohio, a unique network called the Ohio Bone Marrow Transplantation Consortium (OBMTC) has been established. This consortium was founded in 1992 to ensure excellence in patient care, enhance and support timely patient access, promote fiscal responsibility, and develop a spirit of cooperation and collaboration among transplant centers in Ohio (Ohio BMT Consortium, 1992). The OBMTC has developed membership standards, conducts annual reviews of transplant program progress, and maintains a statewide patient registry to track patient outcomes. The consortium is available to assist third-party payers in determining selection criteria for transplantation, providing expert reviews, and developing funding strategies to assist in providing indigent care. Efforts are made to avoid duplication of services and to support reasonable use of health-care dollars through appropriate patient selection. An annual scientific meeting is offered to promote collaborative research among Ohio transplant centers.

Medical Networks within Europe and Canada

In 1975, the first European meeting was held in St. Moritz, Switzerland, when 10 physicians from Switzerland, France, and the Netherlands met to exchange experiences and knowledge on clinical aspects of BMT. In 1977, three other countries (United Kingdom, Germany, and Italy) joined the working party and together formed the EBMT, with their first president Professor B. Speck, MD, from Basel, Switzerland. Over the years, the physicians formed 10 working parties to discuss acute leukemia, chronic leukemia, lymphoma, solid tumors, aplastic anemia, immunobiology, autoimmune diseases, infectious diseases, late effects, and pediatric diseases. The EBMT working parties publish regular reports on their collaborative activities in their official *Journal of Bone Marrow Transplantation*. The number of transplant centers that participate in the EBMT increases every year. In 2005 more than 2500 individual members from about 500 centers in almost 60 countries were members of the EBMT.

The Canadian Bone Marrow Transplantation medical organization is composed primarily of physicians but may also include transplant coordinators and transplant laboratory personnel.

Traditionally, the organization's biannual conference has been targeted to physicians, transplant coordinators, and research laboratory personnel. Recently, the organization has expanded its offer of membership to nurses, and a nurses group meets during the biannual conferences.

Development of Standards of Care

Nursing Standards in Transplantation

Bone marrow transplant nursing has been recognized as a subspecialty of oncology nursing for many years. Initially, transplant nurses derived guidelines for practice from other nursing specialty areas such as hematology, oncology, critical care, burn care, infectious disease, transfusion therapy, and ambulatory care. Although similarities in practice between transplant nursing and these specialties exist, it was evident that marrow/blood stem cell transplantation was a unique practice area. Many of the initial publications on marrow transplantation originated from nurses in the Seattle, Washington, area and focused on describing the process of transplantation, complications, and specific practice issues (Hutchinson and Itoh, 1982; Stream et al., 1980). In 1981, de la Monataigne and colleagues from Memorial Sloan Kettering Cancer Center published standards of care for the patient with graft-versus-host disease, which still provides the basis for nursing management for this unique complication. Over the next 10 years, marrow transplant nursing practice was integrated into oncology nursing textbooks such as *Guidelines for Oncology Nursing Practice* (Davis, 1991), *Core Curriculum for Oncology Nurses* (Wikle, 1992), and *Cancer Nurs-*

ing: Principles and Practice (Buchsel, 1993). In addition, professional journals have dedicated an issue or part of an issue to marrow transplantion. These include *Seminars in Oncology Nursing* (Buchsel and Ford, 1988; Wujcik, 1994), *Nursing Clinics of North America* (Hutchinson, 1983; Buchsel and Kelleher, 1989; Ford and Eisenberg, 1990), and the American Association of Blood Banks (1990). In recent years, papers on nursing research, practice, quality of life, and patient education have appeared frequently in professional journals. In addition, several nursing textbooks and manuals have been developed to provide essential content for transplant nursing and to describe the standard of care among transplant centers. A summary of these textbooks is included in **Table 17-1**. All of these and other publications assist to define the standards of practice of marrow/blood stem cell transplantation.

A resource developed by the BMT SIG is the *BMT Nursing Resource Directory*, which is published by ONS every 2 years and is now available on the ONS SIG Web site (http://bloodmarrow.ons.wego.net). The directory provides a comprehensive overview of transplant centers in the United States and Canada and has become a valuable and demanded reference by transplant nurses, other health-care providers, and patients. Demographic information for each center includes contact name and phone numbers for nurses, number of beds, number of transplants per year, identification as adult and/or pediatric facility, type of transplant, type of room, patient acuity, verification of orientation and policy/procedure manual available, description of nursing research conducted, and patient education contact and materials available. The information provided in the directory is not available through any other resource and allows easy access to contact persons for networking, collaboration, and

biannual updates on the standard of care in transplantation.

The use of transplantation as a treatment modality was traditionally offered at academic and/or research institutions, but currently, aspects of care are provided through home-care agencies, ambulatory clinics, physician offices, and community settings. Many home health-care/infusion agencies have recruited transplant nurses as experts in the specialty to provide clinical leadership in developing transplant home-care programs and training staff. Comprehensive resources for staff education for care of the transplant patient have been developed by several of the home-care agencies (Lonergan et al., 1994). These resources are a valuable contribution to developing the standard of care in nontraditional settings in marrow/blood stem cell transplant. Collaboration between the transplant center and the home-care agency should occur to provide continuity of care throughout the transplant continuum.

The challenge of providing patient education to patients and families undergoing marrow/stem cell transplantation is complicated by the complexity and variation of the treatment modality as well as the availability of materials. Most transplant programs have developed materials that discuss transplantation specific to the center. Numerous patient/family educational resources are available through institutions or the pharmaceutical industry for purchase, and with permission, may be adapted to meet the needs of individual transplant centers. The development of these and other patient education materials has created a standard for providing patient education materials. One of the most used patient education materials available is a book titled, *Bone Marrow Transplant: A Book of Basics for Patients*, which was written by a former transplant patient (Stewart,

Table 17-1 Examples of nursing textbooks in blood and marrow transplantation.

Textbook	Description
Ezzone, S., & Camp-Sorrell, D. (Eds.). (1994). *The Manual for Bone Marrow Transplant Nursing: Recommendations for Education and Practice*. Pittsburgh, PA: ONS Press.	The purpose of the manual is to present an overview of BMT nursing practice and provide a framework for developing orientation courses or educational programs for transplant nursing. A scope of practice provides a definition of the specialty of transplant nursing and a basis for the nursing practice across the continuum of care through the transplant process.
Buchsel, P.C., & Whedon, M.B. (Eds.). (1995). *Bone Marrow Transplantation: Administrative and Clinical Strategies*. Sudbury, MA: Jones & Bartlett.	This textbook provides a valuable focus on administrative and management issues of transplant programs as well as new clinical issues. An attempt is made to provide basic critical pathways for the medical care of the transplant recipient through the continuum of care.
Ezzone, S. (Ed.). (1997). *Manual for Blood Stem Cell Transplantation: Recommendations for Nursing Education and Practice*. Pittsburgh, PA: ONS Press.	Provides the first guidelines for nursing care of the patient undergoing peripheral blood stem cell transplant.
Buchsel, P., & Kaputstay, P.M. (2000). *Stem Cell Transplantation: A Clinical Textbook*. Pittsburgh, PA: ONS Press.	Provides a notebook format text that allows chapters to be added over time to update current practice in transplantation.
Shapiro, T.W., Davison D.B., & Rust, D.M. (1997). *A Clinical Guide to Stem Cell and Bone Marrow Transplantation*. Sudbury, MA: Jones and Bartlett.	A pocket guide to stem cell transplant. Provides a comprehensive overview of the transplant process, including pretransplant evaluation, conditioning regimens, procurement and infusion of stem cells, management of transplant complications, diagnostic tests, pharmacologic management, transfusion therapy, and long-term follow-up care.
Ezzone, S. (Ed.). (2004). *Hematopoietic Stem Cell Transplant: A Manual for Nursing Practice*. Pittsburgh, PA: ONS Press.	This book was developed to replace the previously mentioned ONS Press publications and to combine them into one reference.
Oncology Nursing Society. (2004, October 5). *BMT Nursing Resource Directory*. Pittsburgh, PA: Author.	Provides a comprehensive overview of transplant centers in the United States and Canada. Available on the ONS SIG Web site (http://bloodmarrow.ons.wego.net).

1992). In addition, Stewart publishes a bi-monthly newsletter on pertinent topics related to bone marrow and blood stem cell transplant; the newsletter may be ordered by patients, families, and health-care providers. Each issue of the newsletter provides valuable information on a variety of topics, such as types of transplant, treatment of specific diseases, complications of transplant, and available resources, as well as articles highlighting individual experiences through the transplant process.

Several networks that provide patient education or information are available through international computer networks, such as the Internet and America Online (AOL). These networks offer online, interactive chat rooms that allow users to access information from universities, the National Cancer Institute (NCI), and government agencies. The BMT newsletter described earlier is available through the Internet, as is other useful patient education material. Users communicate with others on a variety of topics through online messages and responses that all users have access to read. A few of the available interactive computer online forums include Living with Cancer, BMT Talk, NCI's CancerNET, Cancer-List, Hematology/Oncology List, Breast Cancer List, Ovarian List, and NCI Physical Data Query (PDQ) (Flatau, 1995; Frankel, 1995). Access to communication through the Internet has provided many transplant recipients the ability to share and receive information about personal experiences through the treatment process.

Medical Standards in Transplantation

Over the past 40 years, the specialty of bone marrow transplantation has evolved rapidly and is now considered conventional treatment for leukemia, lymphoma, aplastic anemia, and other diseases. As advances in scientific knowledge and technology have expanded, the use of blood stem cells for transplantation has become a treatment option for many persons who otherwise would be ineligible for transplant. Standards for the use of transplantation as treatment for malignant and nonmalignant disease can be derived from the numerous scientific studies and reports in the medical literature. Several publications that provide information on the basic and advanced concepts of transplantation, guidelines for the use and practice of transplantation, and scientific investigations performed are available.

Medical textbooks that comprehensively discuss the evolution, current approaches, and future directions of transplantation have been published (Atkinson, 1994; Deeg et al., 1992; Forman et al., 1994). In addition, symposium proceedings have been published through the BMT journal and independent publications and serve to distribute up-to-date information to transplant centers.

IBMTR/ABMTR Standards

The IBMTR/ABMTR publishes reports on the clinical investigations conducted at transplant centers throughout the world in an effort to determine factors that affect the success and failure of transplantation. Collecting, analyzing, and reporting data from the international registry assists in describing the standard of care and use of transplantation as a therapeutic treatment option.

In 1986, the first issue of the journal *Bone Marrow Transplantation* was published through the efforts of the EBMT medical group, under the leadership of the editor, John Goldman,

MD, of London. The journal has become a widely recognized international publication that provides information on all aspects of the basic and clinical science of transplantation. In recent years, a very informative newsletter titled *Marrow Transplantation Reviews* has been published by the ASBMT, providing information on numerous topics in the field of transplantation. In the fall of 1995, the ASBMT published the first issue of a journal titled *Biology of Blood and Marrow Transplantation*. The newsletter and journal are included in the membership of ASBMT. An IBMTR newsletter distributed to participating centers summarizes the activities of the IBMTR/ ABMTR and data on the use and outcomes of transplantation (IBMTR, 2003, 2004). The IBMTR conducts periodic assessments through survey data to determine the pattern and frequency of transplantation.

The IBMTR/ABMTR and the ASBMT hold a combined meeting early every year. During odd years, the meeting is held in Keystone, Colorado, and during the even years, the meeting is held in an alternate site with a warm climate.

The meeting includes 5 days of scientific sessions and workshops on blood and marrow transplantation. The registration fee also includes access to several related conferences that are held at the same time and location. These include BMT Pharmacists Conference, Clinical Research Associate Data Management Workshops, BMT Medical Directors Conference, BMT Center Administrators Conference, and Transplant Nursing Conference. FACT (Foundation for the Accreditation of Cellular Therapy) training courses for inspection and inspectors are also available at an additional cost.

The ASBMT has developed and approved guidelines for clinical centers and training in bone marrow transplantation, which were published in the first issue of the journal *Biology of Blood and Marrow Transplantation* (Appelbaum et al., 1995; Phillips et al., 1995). The guidelines discuss requirements that must be present to ensure the highest quality of medical practice. Guidelines for clinical centers describe recommendations for program size; type of staff including physicians, consulting physicians, nurses, transplant coordinators, pharmacy staff, dietary staff, social service staff, physical therapy staff, and data management staff; data assessment and quality assurance; and inpatient, outpatient, and other facilities. Specific guidelines for training of medical staff are recommended; they include cognitive and procedural skills, method of training, board certification, and training in the care of transplant patients.

ASBMT Guidelines

The American Society for Blood and Marrow Transplantation (ASBMT) was formed to develop standards of practice and guidelines for autologous and allogeneic stem cell transplant. Evidence-based reviews have been developed for the use of transplantation for the treatment of multiple myeloma and diffuse large B-cell lymphoma (Hahn et al., 2003; Hahn et al., 2001). Guidelines have been developed for clinical centers for use in training and in preventing infections among transplant recipients. A joint public policy on legislative and regulatory affairs has also been written (ASBMT, 2003).

ASCO and ASH Guidelines

In 1990, the American Society of Clinical Oncology (ASCO) and the American Society of Hematology (ASH) published a special report in two peer review journals that described the minimum criteria necessary to provide a safe and successful environment in which to perform transplantation (ASCO/ASH, 1990a, 1990b). This document was endorsed by the board of directors of both organizations and was recognized by new transplant centers as the standard for program development. Adherence to these guidelines assisted transplant centers with the special preparation and commitment for providing transplant as a treatment modality. Topics in this document included patient volume, facilities, personnel, treatment outcome, and data reporting. In addition, ASCO published recommendations for the use of hematopoietic colony stimulating factors (CSFs) (ASCO, 1994; ASCO, 2003a). Among other uses of CSFs, recommendations are given for the use of CSFs in patients undergoing high-dose chemotherapy and autologous transplantation and in mobilizing BSCs for transplantation. In addition, ASCO published a special report of clinical practice guidelines for platelet transfusions (ASCO, 2003b).

Cooperative Group Guidelines

NCI-organized cooperative oncology groups are involved in conducting clinical trials involving allogeneic and autologous bone marrow and BSC transplantation, which allows large patient samples to be accrued in short time intervals. The Eastern Cooperative Oncology Group (ECOG) published a position paper that provides recommended guidelines for the management of autologous and allogeneic bone marrow transplantation (Rowe et al., 1994). Since cooperative group clinical trials require uniformity in care and assurance of quality, ECOG developed basic guidelines for the acceptance of centers into the cooperative group trials. In addition, the ECOG guidelines may be useful to new

transplant centers during program development. The ECOG guidelines include recommendations for GVHD prophylaxis and treatment, treatment of infections, management of hepatic venoocclusive disease, use of hematopoietic growth factors, reconstitution of the hematopoiesis, peripheral blood progenitor cell transplants, use of intravenous immunoglobulins, and blood bank support.

NMDP Standards

The National Marrow Donor Program (NMDP) was established in 1987 to expand the availability of volunteer, unrelated, HLA-matched marrow donors for transplantation (Welte, 1994). The NMDP has the expectation that each program that participates with the NMDP will comply with its standards. The NMDP has standards for facility characteristics, medical director, personnel, support services, policies and procedures, and applicant center for each of the following: donor centers, donor recruitment groups, cord blood banks, marrow collection centers, apheresis collection centers, and transplant centers. In addition, there are standards for the recruitment of donors; donor selection and screening; the collection, transportation, processing, and labeling of hematopoietic progenitor cells (HPC); and record retention. The latest standards, the 19th edition, became effective September 13, 2004 (NMDP, 2004).

State Regulations

Some states have regulations for certain healthcare services. In Ohio, those services include stem cell transplant. Health-care services are expected to comply with these rules, which have been effective since March 1, 1997. These rules were reviewed in March 2003 (Ohio Department of Health, 2003).

There are rules governing all selected health-care services, as well as specific rules for each particular service. General rules cover inspections and audits, patient care policies, service standards, medical record requirements, complaints, variances, and waivers. In addition, there are general and specific rules for personnel and staffing, facilities and safety, quality assessment, and data collection. For stem cell transplant, there are also rules for patient selection. The patient selection criteria include pulmonary, cardiac, renal, and hepatic function and performance status; criteria for exclusion; and disease indications for autologous, allogeneic, and repeat transplants, donor lymphocyte infusions (DLI), and storage of cells.

In June 2003, the Ohio Department of Health notified all health-care organizations in Ohio that inspections of selected health-care services would begin in July 2003. Sites would be randomly selected with the goal of inspecting all sites every 3 years. The purpose of the inspections is to ensure compliance with the rules.

Each state defines its own rules. Some states do not regulate stem cell transplant centers at all, whereas other states have specific criteria. For instance, Missouri has no guidelines, West Virginia only regulates the number of transplant beds, and Massachusetts requires all hematopoietic stem cell services to have FACT accreditation. It is important to be knowledgeable about your state's rules.

European Standards

The number of transplant centers and the number of transplants done using blood stem cells (BSCs) is increasing rapidly. In Europe, in 1973, only 16 allogeneic transplants and no autologous marrow transplants were performed. Thirty years later, in 2003, this number had increased to more than 21,000 hematopoietic stem cell transplants (HSCTs) performed, reported from 597 centers in 42 European countries (Gratwohl et al., 2003).

The density of transplant teams and transplants performed for hematologic malignancies and nonhematologic disease varies among European countries. According to data from the EBMT, it is obvious that the use of reduced-intensity conditioning regimens in allogeneic transplant has steadily increased since 1999, although up to that time no study had yet proven that these regimens are superior to the standard approach of myeloablative transplant. This implies a challenge for the nursing care as the patients face different problems like a change in the pattern of graft-versus-host disease.

One of the most controversial and emotional areas of transplantation is the treatment of metastatic breast cancer with high-dose chemotherapy (HDC) and autologous bone marrow and/or BSC transplant. The effectiveness of HDC with transplant versus conventional treatment in improving survival rates has been debated by oncologists, hospital administrators, and insurers, with varying agreement or resolution of this issue. Although the lack of data from controlled studies makes it difficult to form conclusions about appropriate treatment for metastatic breast cancer, data are promising that longer disease-free survival (DFS) may occur with the use of HDC with transplantation (Eddy, 1992). As this debate continues, it would be anticipated that standards for use of HDC with transplantation for the treatment of metastatic breast cancer will be established through the input of health-care providers, administrators, insurers, and patients.

Due to the current focus on cost reduction in health care, it would be remiss not to discuss, at least briefly, issues related to cost versus benefits of transplantation. Controversies of the medical, social, ethical, and financial consequences of transplantation are debated by hospitals, insurers, governmental agencies, health-care providers, patients, and families. Difficult questions remain unanswered regarding the appropriateness of transplantation for the treatment of certain diseases and considerations for end-of-life decisions when complications occur. At times, cost considerations influence insurers and health-care providers in determining these life-and-death decisions. Numerous journal articles in the United States, Europe, and other countries have been published in an attempt to concretely define the cost versus benefits of transplantation (Dufoir et al., 1992; Griffiths et al., 1993; Mitchell et al., 1993). Caution should be used in utilizing the research findings published in clinical practice, since great variation exists among centers in use of techniques of transplantation, preparative regimens, supportive and therapeutic pharmaceutical agents, laboratory, radiology, protective environment, and administrative costs. A survey mailed to pharmacists at 92 U.S. BMT programs described that inpatient BMT drug costs accounted for 12% of the total inpatient drug budget as well as a significant component of the cost of transplant (King et al., 1994). Transplant centers should consider cost versus benefits of medications used in transplantation based on documented scientific and clinical experience. For example, the reduced cost of autologous transplantation with the use of hematopoietic growth factors is reflected in the decreased use of resources such as drug therapy, laboratory testing, transfusion requirements, and hospital days (Petros and Peters, 1993). Controversy regarding the benefits of autologous transplant for the treatment of metastatic breast cancer raises important questions regarding the use of health-care dollars.

FACT Standards

The FACHT (Foundation for the Accreditation of Hematopoietic Cell Therapy) was cofounded in 1996 by the ASBMT and the ISCT (International Society for Cellular Therapy). According to Warkentin and colleagues (2000), "The major objective of FACHT is to promote quality medical and laboratory practice, through its program of voluntary standards, inspection and accreditation" (p. 213). The first edition of the standards was published in 1996 and the inspection program began in June 1997.

In December 2001 FACHT became FACT (Foundation for the Accreditation of Cellular Therapy) to allow for the inclusion of other types of cellular therapies. The second edition of the standards became available in March 2002 (FACT, 2002). The standards are divided into four parts: Part A, Terminology, Abbreviations and Definitions; Part B, Clinical Program Standards; Part C, Hematopoietic Progenitor Cell Collection Standards (applicable to both harvest and apheresis collections); and Part D, Hematopoietic Progenitor Cell Processing Standards (see **Table 17-2** for further breakdown of the description of the standards). An organization may seek accreditation for the entire program or just the portion that applies to it. For example, an organization may only provide stem cell processing, and it would then seek accreditation according to Part D.

Once an organization makes the decision to seek FACT accreditation, the organization

Table 17-2 FACT STANDARDS.

Clinical Program Standards		Hematopoietic Progenitor Cell Collection Standards		Hematopoietic Progenitor Cell Processing Standards	
B1.000	General	C1.000	General	D1.000	General
B2.000	Clinical Unit	C2.000	Hematopoietic Progenitor Cell Collection Facility	D2.000	Laboratory Facilities
B3.000	Personnel	C3.000	Personnel	D3.000	Personnel
B4.000	Quality Management	C4.000	Quality Management	D4.000	Quality Management
B5.000	Policies and Procedures	C5.000	Policies and Procedures	D5.000	Policies and Procedures
B6.000	Donor Evaluation, Selection and Management	C6.000	Donor Evaluation and Management	D6.000	Hematopoietic Progenitor Cell Collection Processing
B7.000	Therapy Administration	C7.000	Hematopoietic Progenitor Cell Collection	D7.000	Cryopreservation
B8.000	Clinical Research	C8.000	Labels	D8.000	Labels
B9.000	Data Management	C9.000	Records	D9.000	Issue of Product for Infusion
B10.000	Records			D10.000	Conditions for Storage
				D11.000	Transportation
				D12.000	Disposal
				D13.000	Records

Source: Adapted from FACT, Hematopoietic Progenitor Cell Collection, Processing, and Transplantation: Accreditation Manual, Second Edition. FACT. Omaha, Nebraska, 2002.

submits a three-page registration form and fee to the FACT office. With this registration, the clock starts ticking. FACT allows the organization up to 12 months to complete the next step, which is the submission of a checklist of documentation (see Table 17-3) and additional fees. The FACT staff will review the submissions and offer feedback to the organization. The organization then has an opportunity to provide additional documentation. The inspection, which is the next step, is scheduled within 3 months of the submission of the checklist.

The inspection team will include a physician team leader who is also responsible for the clinical facility inspection as well as inspectors for the collection and/or processing facilities if those are included in the organization's program. The on-site inspection includes an initial interview, site visits, chart and document review, and an exit conference. During the exit interview, the inspectors will review their key findings. The on-site team does not make the accreditation decision but submits its findings to the FACT board for its review.

The FACT office informs the organization of the results of the inspection within 3 months (see Table 17-4). The organization then has 2 to 4 months to formulate a response and make required changes. Necessary reinspections are scheduled within 2 months.

The accreditation period is 3 years. Approximately 6 months prior to the end of the accreditation period, FACT sends a renewal packet to the organization. The facility has 1 month to complete the documentation and return it to the FACT office with the appropriate fees. Inspections are scheduled within 2 months and FACT informs the facility of the outcome within 3 months. Currently, there are approximately 132 organizations accredited and 227 registered. For more information, go to the FACT Web site, http://www.factwebsite.org.

U.S. Food and Drug Administration (FDA)

Although the U.S. Food and Drug Administration (FDA) does not regulate BMT programs, it has published a rule (Code of Fedeal Regulations, 2001) requiring all facilities that process cellular and tissue-based products to register with the FDA. Since cellular products include stem cells, the collection facilities and processing laboratories associated with each transplant program are required to register. In May 2004, the FDA finalized a rule called, "Suitability Determination for Donors of Human Cellular and Tissue-Based Products." The third rule applicable to HSCT programs, "Current Good Tissue Practices for Manufacturers of Human Cellular and Tissue-Based Products; Inspection and Enforcement," was finalized in November 2004. HSCT programs were expected to demonstrate compliance with these rules by May 25, 2005.

The "Suitability Determination for Donors of Human Cellular and Tissue-Based Products" rule regulates the testing and screening of donors for possible infectious diseases. The goal is to prevent the transmission of communicable diseases to the recipients of cells and/or tissue (Code of Federal Regulations, 2004b). The rule has both general and specific guidelines about testing, quarantine, and labeling (see Table 17-5 for a listing of the individual sections). Transplant programs, apheresis facilities, and stem cell processing laboratories will need to work collaboratively to meet these requirements.

The "Current Good Tissue Practices for Manufacturers of Human Cellular and Tissue-Based Products; Inspection and Enforcement"

Table 17-3 FACT ACCREDITATION PROGRAM DOCUMENTATION TO ACCOMPANY CHECKLIST.

Clinical Program	Collection Facility	Processing Laboratory
• List of patients for a 12-month period	• Medical director	• Physical map
• Copy of JCAHO certificate	• License	• Facility organizational chart
• Program organizational chart	• Curriculum vitae	• Laboratory director curriculum vitae
• Physical map	• Examples of completed labels	• Laboratory medical director
• Copy of American Society of	• Physical map	• License
Histocompatibility and Immunogenetics	• Facility organizational chart if not	• Curriculum vitae
(ASHI) certificate for HLA laboratory	included with clinical program	• Quality management plan
• Program director	• Quality management plan	• Table of contents for policy and
• License	• Table of contents for policy and	procedure manual
• Board certifications	procedure manual	• Examples of completed labels
• Curriculum vitae	• Blank consent forms	• Biohazard label
• Documentation of training/experience		• Copy of instructions for infusion
• Educational activities		• Example of completed infusion form
• Competencies		
• Other attending physicians		
• Same as program director		
• Midlevel practitioners		
• National certification and/or license		
• Training		
• Competencies		
• Educational activities		
• Consulting physicians—board		
certification for at least one physician		
in each category		
• Quality management plan		
• Table of contents for policy and		
procedure manual		
• Blank consent forms		

Source: Adapted from FACT, Hematopoietic Progenitor Cell Collection, Processing, and Transplantation: Accreditation Manual, Second Edition. FACT. Omaha, Nebraska, 2002.

Table 17-4 POTENTIAL OUTCOMES OF ON-SITE INSPECTION.

1. No deficiencies; full accreditation for 3 years.
2. Few minor deficiencies or variances; written response, chairman and staff review before accreditation.
3. Significant deficiencies; written response, board review before accreditation.
4. Significant deficiencies in specific area(s); written response followed by focused reinspection, full board review.
5. Significant deficiencies in all areas; written response followed by focused reinspection, full board review.
6. Nonaccreditation requiring reapplication.

Source: Adapted from Warkentin, P.I., Nick L., and Shpall, E.J. (2000). FACHT accreditation: common deficiencies during on-site visits. *Cytotherapy, 2*(3), 213–220.

rule requires "all human cellular and tissue-based products to be manufactured in compliance with current good tissue practice (CGTP)" (Code of Federal Regulations, 2004a). These rules have specific requirements for facilities where cells and tissue are processed. For BMT purposes, this will be the stem cell processing laboratory. (See **Table 17-6** for a listing of the sections.) Although these rules apply only to the processing laboratory, each BMT program will need to evaluate the impact on the rest of the program whether in cost or processes that overlap departments.

Summary

Marrow and BSC transplantation continues to be a rapidly growing and changing specialty that requires collaboration and sharing of knowledge and ideas among health-care disciplines and transplant centers. As trends in this dynamic treatment modality continue to evolve, it will be imperative for health-care professionals to develop standards of care for all aspects of transplantation. New approaches used in transplantation have been introduced in this book, including preparative regimens, GVHD prophylaxis and treatment, biologic agents, gene therapy, outpatient transplant, consecutive transplants, alternative stem cell sources, and the management of transplant complications. In

Table 17-5 RULES AND REGULATIONS, DONOR SUITABILITY.

1271.50	Determination of donor suitability
1271.55	Records of donor suitability determination
1271.60	Quarantine pending determination of donor suitability
1271.65	Quarantine and disposition of human cellular or tissue-based product from a donor determined to be unsuitable
1271.75	Donor screening
1271.80	Donor testing; general requirements
1271.85	Donor testing; specific requirements
1271.90	Exceptions from the requirement of donor suitability determination; labeling requirements

Source: Code of Federal Regulations. Suitability Determination for Donors of Human Cellular and Tissue-Based Products. 21 C.F.R. §1271 (2004b). Department of Health and Human Services: Food and Drug Administration.

Table 17-6 Rules and regulations, current good tissue practices for manufacturers of human cellular and tissue-based products.

1271.150	Current good tissue practice: general
1271.155	Exemptions and alternatives
1271.160	Establishment and maintenance of a quality program
1271.170	Organization and personnel
1271.180	Procedures
1271.190	Facilities
1271.195	Environmental control and monitoring
1271.200	Equipment
1271.210	Supplies and reagents
1271.220	Process controls
1271.225	Process changes
1271.230	Process validation
1271.250	Labeling controls
1271.260	Storage
1271.265	Receipt and distribution
1271.270	Records
1271.290	Tracking
1271.320	Complaint file

Source: Code of Federal Regulations. Current Good Tissue Practices for Manufacturers of Human Cellular and Tissue-Based Products; Inspection and Enforcement. 21 C.F.R. § 1271 (2004). Department of Health and Human Services: Food and Drug Administration.

addition to the medical and nursing care of the transplant patient, it has become essential to facilitate more efficient and timely international networking to expand knowledge and update the practice of transplantation. Exploration on the Internet may offer new possibilities for international communication through bulletins created for marrow/BSC transplantation. Transplant nurses and other disciplines must become familiar with the use of advanced communication technologies. Ultimately, use of computer-linked communication networks may facilitate the sharing of information, which could directly affect the care provided to transplant patients.

This chapter has discussed the networks and standards of care in transplantation available as of this writing. As new approaches to transplantation are introduced, it will become mandatory to continue to develop standards to assure appropriate and cost-effective use of new therapies. Interdisciplinary collaboration among academic research centers, community hospitals, outpatient clinics, home-care agencies, and other alternative sites must occur to coordinate care through the treatment process. Nationally recognized oncology organizations must jointly develop recommendations or guidelines for practice, which will serve as the basis for transplant program development, education of health-care providers caring for transplant patients, and clinical management of transplant recipients and donors.

References

American Association of Blood Banks. (1990). *Bone Marrow Transplantation: A Nursing Perspective*. Bethesda, MD: AABB.

American Society for Blood and Marrow Transplantation. (n.d.). What Is the ASBMT? Available from http://www.asbmt.org/whatis/whatis.html. Accessed January 17, 2006.

American Society for Blood and Marrow Transplantation. (2003, August 21). Joint Public Policy on Legislative and Regulatory Affairs. Available from http://www.asbmt.org/NR/rdonlyres/6D4007F5-9345-4A22-A43D-45E30DCAD6AF/0/PositionStatement224.pdf. Accessed January 17, 2006.

American Society of Clinical Oncology. (2003a). 2000 Update of Recommendations for the Use of Hematopoietic Colony-Stimulating Factors. Available from http://www.asco.org/ac/1,1003,_12-002032-00_18-0010944-00_19-0010945-00_20-001,00.asp. Accessed January 17, 2006.

American Society of Clinical Oncology. (2003b). Platelet Transfusion for Patients with Cancer. Available from http://www.asco.org/ac/1,1003,_12-002032-00_18-0011068-00_19-0011069-00_20-001,00.asp. Accessed January 17, 2006.

American Society of Clinical Oncology & American Society of Hematology. (1990a). The American Society of Clinical Oncology and American Society of Hematology recommended criteria for the performance of bone marrow transplantation. *J Clin Oncol, 8*, 563–564.

American Society of Clinical Oncology & American Society of Hematology. (1990b). ASCO/ASH recommended criteria for the performance of bone marrow transplantation. *Blood, 75*(5), 1209.

American Society of Clinical Oncology. (1994). American Society of Clinical Oncology recommendations for the use of hematopoietic colony-stimulating factors: evidence-based, clinical practice guidelines. *J Clin Oncol, 12*(11), 2471–2508.

Appelbaum, F., Fay, J., Herzig, G., et al. (1995). American Society for Blood and Marrow Transplantation guidelines for training. *Bio Blood & Marrow Transplant, 1*(1), 56.

Atkinson, K. (Ed.). (1994). *Clinical Bone Marrow Transplantation: A Reference Textbook*. New York: Cambridge University Press.

Barosi, G., Marchetti, M., Alessandrino, P., Locatelli, F., Casula, S., Lunghi, M., et al. (1999). A model for analyzing the cost of autologous peripheral blood progenitor cell (PBPC) transplantation. *Bone Marrow Transplant, 23*, 719–725.

Bennett, C.L., Waters, T.M., Stinson, T.J., Almagor, O., Pavletic, Z.S., Tarantolo, S.R., et al. (1999). Valuing clinical strategies early in development: a cost analysis of allogeneic peripheral blood stem cell transplantation. *Bone Marrow Transplant, 24*, 555–560.

Buchsel, P., & Kaputstay, P.M. (2000). *Stem Cell Transplantation: A Clinical Textbook*. Pittsburgh, PA: ONS Press.

Buchsel, P.C. (1993). Bone marrow transplantation. In S.L. Groenwald, M.H. Frogge, M. Goodman, & C.H. Yarbro (Eds.), *Cancer Nursing: Principles and Practice* (pp. 393–434). Sudbury, MA: Jones and Bartlett.

Buchsel, P.C., & Ford, R. (Eds.). (1988). Advances in bone marrow transplantation. *Semin Oncol Nurs, 4*(1), 1–78.

Buchsel, P.C., & Kelleher, J. (1989). Bone marrow transplantation. *Nurs Clin North Am, 24*(4), 907–938.

Buchsel, P.C., & Whedon, M.B. (Eds.). (1995). *Bone Marrow Transplantation: Administrative and Clinical Strategies*. Sudbury, MA: Jones & Bartlett.

Cheson, B.D. (1991). Clinical trials program. *Semin Oncol Nurs, 7*(4), 235–242.

Code of Federal Regulations. (2001). Chapter 21, Part 1271, Final Rule, Human Cells, Tissues, and Cellular and Tissue-Based Products; Establishment Registration and Listing. Washington, DC: Department of Health and Human Services, Food and Drug Administration.

Code of Federal Regulations. (2004a). Chapter 21, Part 1271, Final Rule, Current Good Tissue Practices for Manufacturers of Human Cellular and Tissue-Based Products; Inspection and Enforcement. Washington, DC: Department of Health and Human Services, Food and Drug Administration.

Code of Federal Regulations. (2004b). Chapter 21, Part 1271, Final Rule, Suitability Determination for Donors of Human Cellular and Tissue-Based Products. Washington, DC: Department of Health and Human Services Food and Drug Administration.

Couban, S., Dranitsaris, G., Andreou, P., Tinker, L., Foley, R., Walker, I.R., et al. (1998). Clinical and economic analysis of allogeneic peripheral blood progenitor cell transplants: a Canadian perspective. *Bone Marrow Transplant, 22*, 1199–1205.

Davis, B.V. (1991). Injury, potential for, related to graft versus host disease. In J.C. McNally, E. Somerville, C. Miaskowski, & M. Rostad (Eds.), *Guidelines for Oncology Nursing Practice* (pp. 223–230). Philadelphia, PA: Saunders.

Deeg, H.J., Klingemann, H.-G., & Gordon, P. (Eds.). (1992). *A Guide to Bone Marrow Transplantation.* New York: Springer-Verlag.

de la Montaigne, M., De Mao, J., Nuscher, R., & Stutzer, C. (1981). Standards of care for the patient with "graft versus host disease" post bone marrow transplant. *Canc Nurs, 4*, 191–198.

Dufoir, T., Saux, M.C., Terraza, B., et al. (1992). Comparative cost of allogeneic or autologous bone marrow transplantation and chemotherapy in patients with acute myeloid leukaemia in first remission. *BMT, 10*, 323–329.

Eddy, D.M. (1992). High dose chemotherapy with autologous bone marrow transplantation for the treatment of metastatic breast cancer. *J Clin Oncol, 10*(4), 657–670.

Ezzone, S. (Ed.). (1997). *Manual for Blood Stem Cell Transplantation: Recommendations for Nursing Education and Practice.* Pittsburgh, PA: ONS Press.

Ezzone, S. (Ed.). (2004). *Hematopoietic Stem Cell Transplant: A Manual for Nursing Practice.* Pittsburgh, PA: ONS Press.

Ezzone, S., & Camp-Sorrell, D. (Eds.). (1994). *The Manual for Bone Marrow Transplant Nursing: Recommendations for Education and Practice.* Pittsburgh, PA: ONS Press.

FACT. (2002). *Hematopoietic Progenitor Cell Collection, Processing, and Transplantation: Accreditation Manual* (2nd ed.). Omaha, NE: Author.

Flatau, A. (1995). BMT patients go online to tackle their disease: finding information on the Internet. *BMT Newsletter, 6*(2), 4.

Ford, R., & Eisenberg, S. (1990). Bone marrow transplant: recent advances and nursing implications. *Nurs Clin North Am, 25*(2), 405–422.

Forman, S.J., Blume, K.G., & Thomas, E.D. (1994). *Bone Marrow Transplantation.* Boston: Blackwell Scientific.

Frankel, W. (1995). To tackle their disease: getting support from cyperspace. *BMT Newsletter, 6*(2), 5.

Gratwohl, A., Baldomero, H., Schmid, O., Horisberger, B., Bargetzi, M., & Urbano-Ispizua, A. (2003). Change in stem cell source for hematopoietic stem cell transplantation (HSCT) in Europe: a report of the EBMT activity survey 2003 for the Joint Accreditation Committee of the International Society for Cellular Therapy ISCT and the European Group for Blood and Marrow Transplantation EBMT (JACIE). *Bone Marrow Transplantation,* 1–16.

Griffiths, R.I., Bass, E.B., Powe, N.R., et al. (1993). Factors influencing third-party payer costs for allogeneic BMT. *BMT, 12*, 43–48.

Hahn, T., Wingard, J.R., Anderson, K.C., Bensinger, W.I., Berenson, J.R., Brozeit, G., et al. (2003). The role of cytotoxic therapy with hematopoietic stem cell transplantation in the therapy of multiple myeloma: an evidence-based review. *Biol Blood Marrow Transplant, 9*, 4–37.

Hahn, T., Wolff, S.N., Czuczman, M., Fisher, R.I., Lazarus, H.M., Vose, J., et al. (2001). The role of cytotoxic therapy with hematopoietic stem cell transplantation in the therapy of diffuse large cell B-cell non-Hodgkins lymphoma: an evidence-based review. *Biol Blood Marrow Transplant, 7*, 308–331.

Hutchinson, M.Mc. (Ed.). (1983). Symposium on bone marrow transplantation. *Nurs Clin North Am, 18*(3), 509–610.

Hutchinson, M.Mc., & Itoh, K. (1982). Nursing care of the patient undergoing bone marrow transplantation for acute leukemia. *Nurs Clin North Am, 17*(4), 697–711.

International Bone Marrow Transplant Registry. (2003, November). Report on state of the art in blood and marrow transplantation—part 1 of the IBMTR/ABMTR summary slides with guide. *IBMTR/ABMTR Newsletter, 10*(1), 7–10. Available from http://ibmtr.org/about/news/2003Nov.pdf. Accessed May 5, 2005.

International Bone Marrow Transplant Registry. (2004, June). Report on state of the art in blood and marrow transplantation—part 2 of the IBMTR/ABMTR summary slides with guide. *IBMTR/ABMTR Newsletter, 10*(2), 6–9. Available from http://ibmtr.org/about/news/2004jun.pdf. Accessed January 17, 2005.

King, R.S., Wordell, C.J., & Haupt, B.A. (1994). Pharmaceutical services and inpatient drug costs in bone marrow transplantation. *Am J Hosp Pharmacists, 51*, 1339–1344.

Lee, S.J., Klar, N., Weeks, J.C., & Antin, J.H. (2000) Predicting costs of stem-cell transplantation. *J Clin Onc, 18*(1), 64–71.

Lonergan, J.N., Kelley, C.H., & McBride, L.H. (1994). *Homecare Management of the Bone Marrow Transplant Patient.* Northbrook, IL: Caremark.

Mitchell, S.V., Smallwood, R.A., Angus, P.W., & Lapsley, H.M. (1993). Can we afford to transplant? *Med J Australia, 158*(1), 190–194.

National Marrow Donor Program. (2004, June). National Marrow Donor Program 19th Edition Standards. Available from https://network.nmdp.org/PPP/STANDARDS/nmdp_standards_19.pdf. Accessed July 1, 2005.

Ohio BMT Consortium. (1992). *Ohio BMT Consortium Mission Statement*.

Ohio Department of Health. (2003). Ohio Administrative Code 3701-84, Certain Health Care Services' Standards.

Oncology Nursing Society. (2004). *Blood and Marrow Stem Cell Transplant Resource Directory*. Available from http://www.ons.org/clinical/Treatment/Directory.shtml. Accessed January 17, 2006.

Petros, W.P., & Peters, W.P. (1993). Cost implications of haematopoietic growth factors in the BMT setting. *BMT, 11*(suppl 2), 36–38

Phillips, G., Armitage, J., Bearman, S., et al. (1995). American Society for Blood and Marrow Transplantation guidelines for clinical centers. *Biology of Blood and Marrow Transplant, 1*(1), 54–55.

Rowe, J.M., Ciobanu, N., Ascensao, J., et al. (1994). Recommended guidelines for the management of autologous and allogeneic bone marrow transplantation: a report from the Eastern Cooperative Oncology Group. *Ann Intern Med, 120*, 143–158.

Shapiro, T.W., Davison D.B., & Rust, D.M. (1997). *A Clinical Guide to Stem Cell and Bone Marrow Transplantation*. Sudbury, MA: Jones and Bartlett.

Stewart, S. (1992). *Bone Marrow Transplants: A Book of Basics for Patients*. Highland Park, IL: Author.

Stream, P., Harrington, E., & Clark, M. (1980). Bone marrow transplantation: an option for children with leukemia. *Canc Nurs, 3*, 195–199.

Stroncek, D., Bartsch, G., Perkins, H.A., et al. (1993). The National Marrow Donor Program. *Transfusion, 33*(7), 567–577.

Sullivan, K.M., Dykewicz, C.A., Longworth, D.L., Boeckh, M., Baden, L.R., Rubin, R.H., et al. (2001). Preventing opportunistic infections after hematopoietic stem cell transplantation: the Centers for Disease Control and Prevention, Infectious Diseases Society of America, and American Society for Blood and Marrow Transplantation practice guidelines and beyond. *Hematology*, 392–421.

Warkentin, P.I., Nick, L., & Shpall, E.J. (2000). FACHT accreditation; common deficiencies during on-site visits. *Cytotherapy, 2*(3), 213–220.

Welte, K. (1994). Matched unrelated transplants. *Semin Oncol Nurs, 10*(1), 20–27.

Whedon, M.B. (Ed.). (1991). *Bone Marrow Transplantation: Principles, Practice, and Nursing Insights*. Sudbury, MA: Jones and Bartlett.

Whedon, M.B., & Wujcik, D. (Eds.). (1996). *Blood Cell and Marrow Transplantation: Principles, Practice, and Nursing Insights* (2nd ed.). Sudbury, MA: Jones and Bartlett.

Wikle, T. (1992). Implication of bone marrow transplantation. In J.C. Clark, & R.F. McGee (Eds.). *Oncology Nursing Society Core Curriculum for Oncology Nursing* (pp. 359–370). Philadelphia, PA: Saunders.

Wujcik, D. (Ed.). (1994). Advances in bone marrow transplant. *Semin Oncol Nurs, 10*(1).

Chapter 18

The Bone Marrow and Blood Stem Cell Transplant Marketplace

Rita Potter, RHIA

The boundaries between the business strategy of a health-care organization and the actual production of patient care are blurring. Cost reduction is a health-care management priority and clinicians find themselves practicing in a competitive and uncertain world.

This chapter provides an overview of the financial aspects of bone marrow transplantation (BMT) and blood cell transplantation (BCT). As the operating environment becomes more complex, a seamless integration of overall organizational strategy and transplantation-specific business strategy will be essential for success. This integration will require that clinicians have a working knowledge of the environmental factors that affect patient care. In this way, they will be able to participate in the formulation of strategy and will function to enact it. It is assumed that the era of operating programs as pure research endeavors without concern for the generation of revenue and patient volume is ending. As cost pressures force provider organizations to consider carefully the portfolio of services they provide, transplant programs will come under scrutiny as an area of potential savings. Several questions will be considered:

- How do reimbursement models affect the delivery of health care?
- What are the most important factors in the external environment that are influencing the direction of transplantation?
- What critical information should be gathered to decide whether to start a new transplant program?
- What opportunities exist for improvement of program performance?

Historical Perspectives

The 1940s to 1980s

As World War II (WWII) ended, health-care technology was developing rapidly. At the same time, many WWII veterans were reentering the workforce, and they began raising families. Memories of the Great Depression of the 1930s stimulated this generation of workers to explore ways to secure an income and their family's future. Because health-care costs could quickly deplete savings, systems to decrease economic risk due to illness were desired. Hospitals were also interested in developing a revenue system that would ensure a steady stream of income. Hospitals began to sponsor prepayment plans, which eventually became known as Blue Cross plans (Anderson, 1985). During the war years, the government had placed a freeze on wages but at the same time passed legislation which determined that health insurance coverage was a tax-exempt business expense. Providing health insurance as a fringe benefit became an economically sound investment for corporate America. It wasn't long before provisions for health-care insurance were identified as a desired component of corporate benefits packages. By 1952, more than 50% of the U.S. population was covered by some form of health insurance (Anderson, 1985).

In 1965, Medicare legislation was passed, along with Medicaid funding for the poor. Americans were beginning to believe that health insurance was no longer just a benefit, but a right. Insurers gave implicit support to cover all hospital and physician charges.

The National Cancer Act, signed by Richard Nixon in 1971 (Devita, 1993), provided researchers with funds to create new, sophisticated treatments. Many that were found to be beneficial also carried high price tags. Health-care costs rose at a rate greater than the rate of inflation, which caused the public and employers to complain bitterly about premiums for health insurance. Third-party payers looked for ways to control costs. At the same time, providers of cancer care were trying to demonstrate how much could be done for a person with cancer. Providers and payers were on a collision course.

The Late 1980s to Present

By the late 1980s, it could no longer be assumed that procedures such as transplantation would be paid for by insurers. Third-party pay-ers adopted the position that transplantation was an experimental procedure and had not been proved effective. Critics of BMT believed that bone marrow transplantation did not represent a cost-effective use of limited health-care dollars. Providers of care argued that it gave many patients their only chance for long-term survival.

As third-party payers began to deny coverage for high-cost treatment, individual patients were able to obtain media attention and public sympathy for their situations. Lawsuits were filed by patients denied coverage because transplantation was deemed experimental (Saver, 1992). As transplantation evolved into a treatment option for women with breast cancer, women activists worked to have payment for this treatment modality legislated (Wynstra, 1994). However, approvals for transplantation coverage continued to vary widely among insurance companies. Peters and Rogers (1994) examined the consistency of predetermination decisions by insurance companies for 533 patients enrolled in grant-supported clinical trials for transplantation for breast cancer. Requests for insurance coverage for transplantation was approved in 77% of cases. Patients who had payment denied were told the therapy was deemed experimental. The frequency of approval did not appear to be influenced by the patient's pretreatment clinical characteristics. There was substantial inconsistency in frequency of approval of coverage among insurers, and among decisions made by some individual insurers even for patients within the same study protocol. This type of variation has helped patients win large settlements and public attention. A California court awarded $89 million in damages to the family of a woman who died after her health maintenance organization refused to pay for her BMT (Meyer and Muir, 1994).

Health-care reform became the centerpiece for the 1992 presidential campaign. President Bill Clinton's election set the stage to move this agenda forward. A legislative compromise was not reached at that time. But as Baird (1995) states, marketplace reform has gathered strength and influence.

In the mid-1990s, the country saw market forces change in the managed care industry. Reform was already occurring at the state level when the federal government enacted the Health Insurance Portability and Accountability Act (HIPAA). Thirty-seven states, for instance, had already enacted guaranteed issue and renewal in the small group market; 33 states enacted restrictions on the use of preexisting condition limitations that were equal to or greater than the new law, and 20 states had enacted some form of legislation providing for the establishment of medical savings accounts (Kongstvedt, 1997). Another good example of managed care reform occurring at the state level first was the states' mandatory coverage of a minimum length of hospital maternity stay before the federal government took a similar stance in 1996. The forces of the market and the public backlash on HMOs and managed care plans that arose during the mid-1990s increased the movement of the states to take a more regulated approach and mandated more requirements for the industry to protect the patient and purchasers of care. With the increased legislation and regulatory requirements came a decrease in enrollment for HMOs. The first decline of HMO enrollment in 30 years came in 2000. Also in 2000, 37 states lost one or more HMOs. Choice and more freedom demanded by the public resulted in triple the enrollment in PPOs since 1990.

The reform of the private and public health-care markets will continue to be discussed among lawmakers, consumers, employers, providers, and regulators. The debate over network-based health-care systems versus the traditional individual practitioner will always be a component of the discussion. Additionally, the federal government is expected to focus on restructuring Medicare and Medicaid programs to keep them viable for taking care of their beneficiaries in the years to come. There has already been a shift by federal and state governments towards increased reliance on using managed care arrangements to meet budgetary spending targets (Kongstvedt, 1997). State Medicaid plans had $26 billion in budget shortfalls for FY02, and that amount increased to $69 billion in FY03 (Advisory Board Company, 2003). State Medicaid plans are using various cost-containment strategies, which include reducing covered prescriptions, increasing co-pays, and reducing eligibility or benefits. All of these reductions then shift impact to the members, and ultimately, the providers who are taking care of them. In a busy BMT program, these current changes could have a significant impact on Medicaid recipients coming to the program.

Reimbursement

The blending of the business and clinical domains in health-care delivery is very evident when the progression of change in reimbursement is examined. To meet the basic organizational objective of positive financial performance, managers and clinicians are working more closely to eliminate inefficient operations and identify the most appropriate therapeutic interventions in the proper clinical setting. Reimbursement is an excellent example of how market forces are influencing dramatic changes in the delivery of clinical care. It would be a gross oversimplification to suggest that reimbursement is the only factor forcing change. Issues beyond the scope of this chapter, such as cost-benefit-effectiveness analysis, quality-of-life issues, litigation by patients, analysis of clinical outcomes, and the definition of experimental treatments, are at the heart of a very difficult public policy debate. Reimbursement, however, provides an anchor for understanding a complex and volatile BMT/BCT operating environment.

Payers are reluctant to reimburse for procedures they consider experimental because such high-cost and potentially low-benefit procedures deplete their financial reserves and limit their ability to meet all the needs of their members. Providers are more convinced of the benefit of transplantation, and many are of the opinion that it is both a necessary and cost-effective therapy. As this debate continues, and a point on the continuum is determined, radical changes in the delivery of care will be needed in order to meet reimbursement levels and to maintain safe, effective patient care.

Fee for Service

Historically, third-party payers reimbursed hospitals retrospectively for services provided. A structure of charges was set by the hospital and often reviewed for appropriateness by a regulatory commission. No preauthorization or clearance for treatment from the payer was required prior to hospitalization. At the completion of the patient's encounter, a bill for physician and hospital services was submitted to the insurer. As long as the bill agreed with the approved charging structure, the payment was made. In this scenario, the provider organization was rewarded for long hospital stays and high use of ancillary services. The more tests ordered on a specific patient, the greater the potential revenue generated for the physician and hospital. This type of cost-plus (cost of the procedure plus some percentage for profit) has been a pivotal issue driving the restructure of health-care reimbursement. Here, all of the risk is assumed by the payer, who has minimal input into the process of care. Retrospective cost-reimbursement/fee-for-service systems still exist, but were thought to be becoming extinct.

The contracting strategies in the mid-1990s had one thought in mind—protect the volume of patients at any cost. This proved beneficial for the payers since they were able to shift more of the financial risk to the providers. As a result, many times, providers felt that any contract was better than none. However, the market forces shifted to the providers' position if they were at or near capacity, and providers began to manage their operating margins. In the late 1990s, hospitals and physicians proved they could walk away from bad deals. From 1998 to 2000 the market trend showed per diem rates increased by 10–20% (University Health System Consortium, 2002). Hospitals began to cover their operating margins and actually make some profits on the more high-cost outlier provisions, which usually cover the expensive, complex cases such as transplant. Thus, providers were actually taking a stance in negotiations that for high-cost procedures like transplant, they must cover the cost and the trend of signing contracts on a base rate without the financial protection of the complicated cases that go beyond that must be stopped. Instead of just a case rate with only outlier per diems, the market shift gave many centers that maintained quality programs with the required proven outcomes the ability to obtain a margin of cost plus the ability to protect them from taking a loss on too many of their cases.

Prospective Reimbursement and Package Case Rates

Many payers have developed prospective reimbursement systems. The first prospective reimbursement system was introduced by Medicare in 1983. This system was based on diagnosis related groups (DRGs) with pre-established reimbursement rates. In this scenario, payment for service is fixed, and providers of care are not rewarded for high use of services or long hospitalizations. In fact, the opposite is true. The system rewards efficient processes of care with early discharge and limited clinical intervention. This is the first example of a large payer forcing providers to think about how a service is provided. Overuse of services in this patient population erodes profitability.

Payers have also forced competition among health-care providers by negotiating discounts directly with hospitals and providers. For many high-cost, high-technology treatments such as BMT/BCT and solid organ transplantation, contractual agreements are made between the hospital and the payer for provision of services (Cleverly, 1986). Health-care providers compete for these contracts and winners are selected on the basis of service value (Arford and Allred, 1995). Service value is measured by using both cost and quality of outcomes. Bids are evaluated based on technical aspects, qualification of the personnel, and cost. If technical merits and personnel are deemed equal, the low bid will likely win the contract. This payment system was used more and more by health maintenance organizations and preferred provider organizations to fund bone marrow transplantation.

As BMT programs began to offer more treatment options for their patients, the larger programs could offer payers their unique ability to take care of their members for multiple types of BMT services. This differentiating ability to treat patients for treatment ranging from autologous to the very complicated unrelated allogeneic transplant programs became market leverage when the patients did not want to move from one center for their autologous transplant to another city across the country for the related or unrelated BMT. Many of the larger payers began to add this unique credentialing indication (the program must offer all types of BMT and meet their required outcomes), which would then move more of their members into "centers of excellence" types of agreements. The usual package case pricing driven by very low pricing (which could be below the operating margin) is now being replaced by the market trend of larger programs across the country being able to cover the cost of their operating margin and getting better package case pricing for the unique transplant services they offer.

Managed Care

In the managed care setting, primary care physicians (PCPs) direct how and when a population of patients will receive health-care services. Managed care organizations establish criteria to assist the PCP in the decision to use specialty and tertiary-care services. Systems such as case management are designed to monitor adherence to the criteria and limit overusage of more costly tertiary care. In this way, the risk-bearing organization (the managed care organization) can be managed.

Managed care systems have evolved as processes for managed care organizations to verify and participate in the care of their members. Again, financial risk plays an important role in a payer's desire to understand what it is purchasing, because the insurer is financially responsible for all of its members' health-care needs. Therefore, it is assuming the risk for providing services to all members. If an insurer has a high proportion of older, sicker members, it is exposed to high risk for associated hospitalization and physician costs. A small health maintenance organization (HMO) with limited financial reserves might be financially devastated by several transplantation patients who have complicated hospital courses with long lengths of stay and intensive care unit admissions.

Many HMOs have developed case management systems. Case management is a systematic, planned approach to patient care that emphasizes individual care planning and resource management to produce high-quality, cost-effective outcomes within and across settings. Case management personnel literally manage the care of the patient in concert with the transplantation program's staff to make certain there is agreement on the appropriateness of the care prior to allowing a patient to begin transplantation, as well as over the continuum of care. This hands-on process, combined with payment strategies that include discounted payments, helps to ensure that some risk is shifted to the provider organization.

Capitation

Capitation refers to the per capita payment a managed care organization or provider organization receives from a payer for the provision of specified clinical services to members (Grimaldi, 1995). The capitation payment is a per member per month (PMPM) rate: The provider will receive a rate for each month that each patient is a member (Grimaldi, 1995). For example, a hospital may negotiate with a payer to receive a payment of $50 PMPM for all of the lives that the payer covers. If the plan covers 95,000 lives, the hospital will receive $57 million (95,000 lives × $50 × 12 months) over the course of 1 year for provision of all services negotiated in the contract between the organizations. The health plan, in turn, determines a premium to charge its members that covers the cost of the PMPM and the health plan's administrative costs. In general, payers prefer capitation because most of the risk is shifted to the providers of care who are then rewarded for keeping patients healthy and out of the hospital or away from costly procedures. Contracts can be quite complex and involve the use of actuarial data to determine the types of services that will likely be required by the members of the health-care plan. In many instances, reimbursement for transplantation is a separately negotiated contract based on clinical, program, and price criteria.

At the present time, the BMT marketplace is a mixture of reimbursement methods. Many of the larger payers do not place transplants in capitation models for offering payments to providers. Many of the capitation models exclude high-cost cases that happen infrequently (like transplants), depending on the volume of members they bring to the negotiating table. Most large payers today place unique transplant services as one of those carve out services in a separate network of providers (centers of excellence) being paid a package case rate. Program managers for BMT need to communicate well with their respective managed care departments for a better understanding of the market forces in their community. Do the payers have the competitive edge to drive reimbursement below or at the current operating margins for current specialty services like transplant? It is always difficult to find the right balance between the payers and large self-insured employers wishing to reduce reimbursement and the providers needing to cover costs and not price below the margin for transplant business.

The Current Environment

Figure 18-1 illustrates that all products progress through a life cycle from introduction to decline (Wasson, 1978). Cues in the marketplace suggest that BMT is headed toward maturity. For example, Bennett and colleagues (1995) have documented a reduction of procedure cost from $96,000 to $55,000 over a period of 5 years as

experience has been gained treating Hodgkin's disease with transplantation. Proprietary companies are providing on-site stem cell collection and processing to organizations that do not have the capability or the capital to initiate such a service. This type of outsourcing places high-dose chemotherapy with stem cell rescue within the realm of many potential market entrants. Further, consider the work done by Duke University to move transplantation from the traditional inpatient setting to the outpatient setting (Peters et al., 1994). This type of procedural refinement could not have been considered without the experience of treating women with breast cancer in the traditional inpatient setting. Finally, new research efforts are suggesting that perhaps placental/umbilical cord blood can be used successfully in unrelated bone marrow transplantation (Beatty, 1995).

Figure 18-1 The product life cycle.

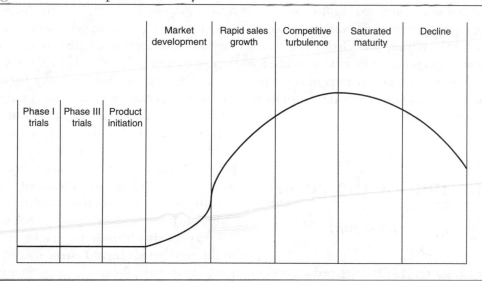

Source: Adapted with permission from Bonoma, T. and Kosnick, T., 1990. *Marketing management, text and cases.* Homewood, IL: Irwin, Ill.

These examples are in direct contrast to the transplantation market of 15 to 20 years ago, which was characterized by long hospitalizations, resource-intense delivery of care, high cost, and relatively few centers performing the treatment. There are now more than 250 BMT sites ranging from large academic programs to mobile (traveling) units (Beatty, 1995). Simply put, the research and design necessary to provide BMT has come to the point where market entrants have the potential to copy the technology, price the product to the market, and produce a process of care that may be as effective as that of entrenched providers. This type of external threat is characteristic of a maturing marketplace. It is also safe to assume that during this period of maturation, purchasers of transplantation have become more savvy about what they are paying for and are more demanding of documented high-quality outcomes. The proliferation of transplant centers has altered market forces and raised concern within the transplant community about defining self-imposed regulations to ensure appropriate program structure and function (Beatty, 1995). Within this volatile context, organizational and program effectiveness can only occur when the internal characteristics of an organization match and support the demands of the external marketplace.

Situation Analysis: Preparing for the Future

Analyzing the External Environment

Michael E. Porter (1979) developed a model to describe how competition in an industry can shape strategy. Porter's model (**Figure 18-2**) provides a good framework to contemplate the forces influencing BMT. The model considers five specific factors in the marketplace:

1. the bargaining power of buyers
2. the threat of substitute products
3. the bargaining power of suppliers
4. the threat of new entrants
5. rivalry among existing firms

By examining the current BMT/BCT operating environment using this framework, environmental opportunities and threats can be contemplated.

BARGAINING POWER OF BUYERS

Third-party payers are by far the largest purchasers of BMT. They have exerted significant influence in the health-care marketplace, and the transplantation community has not been immune to that influence.

A *center of excellence* is a transplant center that has been designated for use by a payer-based selection process. Generally, designation of centers is based on three hypotheses concerning the interrelationships among volume of cases, outcomes, and costs (Evans, 1992). Selection can also depend on other facets of program design and function, such as quality improvement programs, the experience of practitioners, a demonstration of user-friendly systems for communication with the payer and referring physician, the level of organizational commitment to transplantation measured by the amount and type of support allocated to the transplant effort, and the types of services available to patients who must travel long distances to the designated center. Patient-specific services may include, for example, discounts from airlines and lodging for patients and families forced to travel.

Figure 18-2 Competitive forces in an industry.

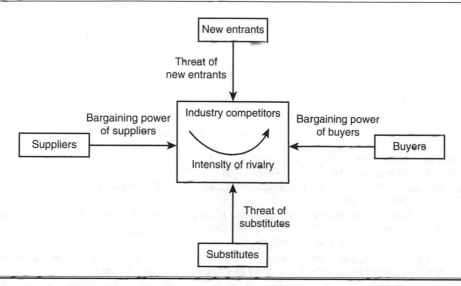

Source: Adapted from Mintzberg, B., and Quinn, J., 1996. *The strategy process, concepts, contexts, cases,* 2nd ed. Englewood Cliffs, NJ: Prentice-Hall, 62.

An important aspect of the selection process, and an area in which payers exert significant influence, is negotiation of a case rate or global price. A limited financial risk is shifted to the provider by pricing a bundled package of the services required to provide the process of transplant care, and determining a preset length of stay (LOS) for which the price will apply. **Figure** 18-3 shows an example of a typical contract that a health-care provider might negotiate with a health plan. The market now requires a minimum discount (ceiling), but providers can request a threshold (floor) to cover costs. This knowledge of where the hospital's costs are by transplant type is critical in negotiating a sound and financially viable contract.

The example in Figure 18-3 points to the need for appropriate patient selection, the need for a process of care that limits readmission rates, the need for an internal case management process that monitors use of services, and the benefit of such tools as critical pathways to provide consistency in practice. It also points to the benefits of creating good contracts and knowing the cost of producing the BMT process of care from referral through 100 days posttransplantation.

By forcing transplant centers to compete with each other with respect to price, program structure and function, and clinical outcomes, payers can create networks of preferred centers. Transplant centers participating in these networks are the beneficiaries of directed referrals.

Opportunity Seeking contracts with payers can increase the number of covered lives that a given transplant program can access. By becoming part of a transplant network, a type of directed referral system is established that places the transplant program in a corps of elite centers from which health plans can choose. An opportunity

Figure 18-3 Sample center of excellence pricing contract for hospitals and physicians.

	Case rate (1)	LOS outlier	Case rate outlier per diems (2)
AUTOLOGOUS BONE MARROW			
	$85,000	25	$1800 non-ICU
			$2400 ICU
ALLOGENEIC BONE MARROW	$130,000	40	$2000 non-ICU
			$3000 ICU

1. (A) Cost rate includes inpatient or outpatient maintenance that occurs from the transplant admission, organ acquisition (including repeat harvests, tissue typing, harvest hospitalization for live donors, marrow processing and storage), transplant stay, and all transplant-related readmission for 100 days following transplant infusion. The all-inclusive global rate covers hospital (inpatient and outpatient) and physcian services.

(B) Pretransplant outpatient evaluation and pretransplant hospitalization (excluding bone marrow harvest admission) will be paid at 75% of billed charges.

(C) Posttransplant care provided on an outpatient basis or an inpatient basis for services beyond 100 days posttransplant infusion to 1 year will be paid at 75% of billed charges.

(D) Retransplants will be considered a new procedure.

(E) In the event the patient dies during the transplant admission or discharge from the transplant admission occurs prior to the LOS cutoff, payment will be the lesser of the fixed fee or 75% of billed charges.

(F) Ceiling/floor: Hospital's global rate plus per diem shall provide compensation of not more than 75% of hospital and physician charges and not less than 55%.

2. If the cumulative inpatient stay, including inpatient days for entire transplant admission and all transplant-related readmissions within 100 days of transplant infusion, are greater than the LOS cutoff, then days beyond the cutoff shall be paid at per diems noted above. Per diems cover all hospital and physician services.

exists to develop internal case management systems that work in conjunction with managed care organizations. This type of willingness to collaborate on managing the care of transplant patients recognizes the inevitable future operating environment, and can be instrumental in winning contracts with payers.

Threat   Competitors for BMT service can come from any part of the country. Payers are willing to negotiate travel as part of a package price with a provider, and offer members the opportunity to obtain therapy at a center that meets their thresholds for price and clinical outcomes. Securing local access for a program's catchment area means, in many cases, securing local payer contracts. Price negotiation can have an adverse financial impact on an organization if the cost of treatment is not known. Meeting the market price may increase program volume but hurt the financial health of the organization when operating costs exceed revenues. The actual mix of payers that a transplant program attracts will have a profound impact on its financial performance. For example, a large pool of Medicare (prospective payment system) and uninsured patients would quickly create a poor financial picture. Conversely, a mixture of fee-for-service, minimal free care, and well-conceived managed care contracts could create a more positive financial performance. Organizations able to accurately determine the cost of providing BMT/BCT will be in a better position to negotiate financially sound contracts.

THREAT OF SUBSTITUTE PRODUCTS

The transplant community and the insurance community are moving past the issue of whether transplantation has a place in the care of cancer patients (Beatty, 1995). Progression to this point has not been without intense interaction between payers and providers. In many early cases, lawsuits were filed by patients denied coverage because transplantation was deemed experimental (Saver, 1992). Peters and Rogers (1994), in their examination of the consistency of predetermination decisions by insurance companies, found that only 77% of 533 patients enrolled in grant-supported clinical trials were approved for treatment. Analysis of cost-effectiveness provides systematic information about the consequences, both positive and negative, of allocating resources to perform a specific therapy (Arford and Allred, 1995). Research to evaluate cost-effectiveness has been attempted in BMT (Bennett et al., 1995; Faucher et al., 1994; Hillner et al., 1992; Uyl-de Groot et al., 1994). These studies demonstrate that evaluating economic outcomes is becoming just as important as evaluating clinical outcomes. These studies are a beginning attempt to match outcomes to cost. The use of this analytic methodology is now helping payers and providers to consider such issues as the timing and prognostic factors that will result in the best survival for a population of patients treated with BMT, and least use of this high-cost treatment in patients who would have no benefit (Beatty, 1995). However, while these issues are being debated, some patients who are eligible for transplantation may not be referred for consideration.

Opportunity Continuing medical education (CME) of referring providers can give providers the opportunity to make more informed referral decisions. CME has been documented as a marketing methodology that can improve referral rates (Van Harrison et al., 1990). Since many primary care providers now work in concert with managed care companies, marketing to the medical directors of health plans can augment participation in transplantation networks by highlighting the benefit of transplantation to an entire staff of primary care providers. An ongoing effort needs to be made to understand the cost-effectiveness of transplantation.

Threat Clinical trials were done to compare the effectiveness of standard therapy and autologous BMT or BCT for breast cancer. The findings of this research will have a profound impact on the transplantation community.

As the current process of care is refined, a new process that is substantively different may evolve. This type of change in production may make current facilities obsolete. Finally, without ongoing continuing medical education of referring physicians, referrals for transplantation can be lost to standard chemotherapy.

BARGAINING POWER OF SUPPLIERS

The transplant program must consider the payer, referring physician, and patient as a triad in the referral decision. In most cases, there is a relationship among the patient's insurance plan, the insurance company's negotiated contract with specific transplant centers, and the restrictions this negotiated contract places on the patient's physician concerning to which transplant center the patient can be referred. The structure of the transplant program must meet the needs of these stakeholders, especially in areas where competition offers an alternative choice to any member of this referral triad. As the process of care becomes more commonplace in a maturing marketplace, programs must focus on operational aspects other than direct clinical care (France and Grover, 1992). The concerns of the patient-payer-physician dynamic can exert significant influence on programmatic function by forcing competition among transplant centers. Some examples of the bargaining power of suppliers include:

- Payers can demand that hospitals and providers produce an invoice that incorporates all appropriate terms of the contract. This may seem like a small issue, but it usually means more administrative hours to individually track and calculate the patient's bill because the contract is complex and different from others the organization may have.
- Effective October 16, 2003, all entities (payers and providers) were required to be in compliance with the HIPAA Transactions and Code Sets, which were put in place for electronic simplification to make processing and paying claims easier than it was in the past. The new transactions and code sets for the 837 (replacing the UB92) and the 835 (electronic notification of the benefits being paid) are still being put into place by many providers and payers past the effective date. Contingency plans giving added time were granted to prevent materially impacted cash flow to all involved. As payers comply with the new HIPAA requirements, the demand for paper and invoice cover sheets for transplant claims will diminish from the various managed care organizations.

- Managed care organizations can demand prior authorization for all aspects of treatment from referral through post-transplantation, and they might insist on regular communication during the course of care to assess the appropriateness of care.
- Managed care organizations can assess a program's ability to measure effectiveness and document clinical outcomes through analysis of quality improvement activities.
- Referring providers can demand rapid turnaround time of written and oral follow-up communication, and base referrals on that criterion.
- Patients and referring physicians can demand rapid access to referral appointments and convenient hours of operation, especially if travel is involved.

Opportunity Developing systems for smooth interactions with payers and referring physicians can sometimes mean the difference between seeing an increase in referrals and losing market share. As the marketplace matures and outcomes begin to homogenize, suppliers will be drawn to transplant centers that make billing and communication easiest and most cost effective. Assessing patients' satisfaction and designing systems to meet and exceed the expectations of patients can influence the selection process of referring physicians and insurers. Anticipating payers' questions of quality and devising a well-conceived quality improvement program can demonstrate organizational commitment to transplantation.

Threat Clinical outcomes will always be the primary concern of providers. However, a lack of respect for a changed operating environment that is sensitive to all aspects of transplantation can limit the growth of a transplant center. If one considers the actual procedure as the center of the transplant product, referrals will be influenced by issues that are at the margins of the production process. In short, the many customers of transplantation must be satisfied. Additionally, because payers are negotiating with the competition, they are obtaining a database of comparative information that positions them to make informed decisions about which program offers patients the most value for their insurance premium.

THREAT OF NEW ENTRANTS

New entrants to an industry bring new capacity, the desire to gain market share, and often substantial resources (Porter, 1979). The motive of a potential entrant may be academic, such as a new research initiative of an academic cancer care effort. One cannot assume that the formidable barriers to entry, such as the volume thresholds of payers or capital-intense investment in transplant-trained physicians, will deter all interested parties. Constant assessment of the marketplace is required to remain certain that a program is current in its approach to clinical practice and to its many customers.

Opportunity   Careful assessment of developments in BMT on a national and local level can ensure that a BMT program remains well positioned in the marketplace. Working to force down the cost of BMT, for example, can create an insurmountable entry barrier for a new program. Constant assessment of the needs of the payer-referring physician–patient triad will help prevent loss of market share by ensuring that a program has a product that can be differentiated from that of the competition If your program

provides all forms of BMT for the population, this can be a great opportunity when negotiating with the payers.

Threat   As the available BMT cases are spread to more centers that do not participate in clinical trials, answers to overarching questions such as documentation of good outcomes in certain diseases and cost-effectiveness will be more difficult to research. Established programs that are not prepared for rivalry from new competition will be forced to react quickly. In most cases, the reaction will take the form of a reduction in price of service without a reduction of production cost, which may lead to poor financial performance.

RIVALRY AMONG EXISTING FIRMS

Porter (1979) suggests that rivalry among existing competitors takes the familiar form of tactics such as price competition, new product introduction, and advertising campaigns. The transplantation industry is no different. In the highly academic setting of transplantation, competition to write and manage groundbreaking clinical trials in which many centers will agree to participate is fierce. Academic medical centers and medical schools invest huge sums in research endeavors with the hope that significant grants will result. These same organizations recruit the brightest minds in transplantation to lead programs and attract research dollars and patients to their centers. Price competition comes in the form of aggressive price-cutting by competitors attempting to gain market share in new areas. The transplantation consumers (patients, payers, and referring physicians) are better informed about their options and are willing to look for the best care for the most reasonable price.

Transplantation is taking place in a very volatile setting. Offering a safe, effective clinical service no longer guarantees that patients will receive care. Marketing at the margins of the production process for transplantation, offering attractive packages to payers, and constant assessment of the actions of rival transplant programs are necessary to ensure that a program remains viable. Despite this complex situation and a sense that many of these obstacles are too great to overcome, opportunities abound for existing programs to take advantage of their experience.

Summary

Clinicians can no longer be concerned solely about the science and patient care aspects of transplantation. They must learn to blend these aspects of transplantation with the appropriate strategic thinking of senior leadership to develop a successful operating plan for the transplantation program. This chapter presented some of the global issues in the external marketplace that influence the direction of BMT/BCT. Certainly, many local influences exert pressure on the operations of a specific program. However, it should be stressed that the external environment was emphasized in the preceding pages. The key to success is matching or structuring the internal environment to meet the needs of stakeholders in the external environment.

An assessment of the strengths and weaknesses of the program in the context of a complex operating environment is a challenging endeavor, but is critical as a foundation for change. Some questions to consider might be:

- Do the management reports generated for the transplantation program allow management to accurately position the program in the marketplace?
- Does the financial reporting include accurate cost information?
- Can the management information system help to respond rapidly to managed care contracts by providing data to understand the impact of many pricing scenarios? Does the information system support both hospital and physician charge and cost data?
- Do the administrative, physician, and nursing leaders possess the skills and open communication channels necessary to lead in a complex and volatile environment?
- Do the staff of the BMT unit have the skills necessary to develop internal case management or continuous quality improvement efforts to reduce operating cost?

Once an understanding of how to structure a program to compete in a given marketplace is gained, it is critical to make certain that BMT/BCT is a product that is important to senior leadership of the organization. This can be accomplished by constantly assessing the external environment, making programmatic adjustments to meet the needs of customers, and keeping senior leaders informed of developments.

Acknowledgment

I would like to acknowledge and thank Marilyn Bedell and William Mroz for their contributions as authors for the second edition of this chapter.

References

Advisory Board Company. 2003. *The new margin imperative.* Washington, DC: Advisory Board Company.

Anderson, O.W. 1985. *Health services in the United States: A growth enterprise since 1875.* Ann Arbor, MI: Health Administration Press.

Arford, P., and Allred, CA. 1995. Value = quality + cost. *J Nurs Admin* 25(9):64–69.

Baird, S. 1995. The impact of changing health care delivery on oncology practice. In Hubbard, S.M., Goodman, M., and Knobf, T. (Eds.) *Oncology Nursing: Patient Treatment and Support*:1–13.

Beatty, P.G. 1995. Clinical and societal issues in blood and marrow transplantation for hematological diseases. *Biol Blood Marrow Transplant* 1:94–114. Cedar Knolls, NJ: Lippincott, Williams, and Wilkins.

Bennett, C.L., Armitage, J.L., Armitage, G.O., et al. 1995. Costs of care and outcomes for high-dose therapy and autologous transplantation for lymphoid malignancies: Results from the University of Nebraska 1987 through 1991. *J Clin Oncol* 13(4):969–973.

Bonoma, T., and Kosnik, T. 1990. *Marketing management, text and cases.* Homewood, IL: Irwin, 311.

Cleverly, W.O. 1986. *Essentials of health care reform,* 2nd ed. Rockville, MD: Aspen.

Devita, V.T. 1993. *Cancer principles and practice of oncology.* Philadelphia: Lippincott.

Evans, R.W. 1992. Public and private insurer designation of transplant programs. *Transplantation* 53(5):1041–1046.

Faucher, C., le Corroller, A.G., Blaise, D., et al. 1994. Comparison of G-CSF-primed peripheral blood progenitor cells and bone marrow auto transplantation: Clinical assessment and cost-effectiveness. *Bone Marrow Transplantation* 14:895–901.

France, K.R., and Grover, R. 1992. What is health care product? *JAMA* 12(2):31–38.

Grimaldi, M. 1995. Capitation savvy a must. *Nurs Manage* 23(2):33–34.

Hillner, B.E., Smith, T.J., and Desch, C.E. 1992. Efficacy and cost-effectiveness of autologous bone marrow transplantation in metastatic breast cancer. *JAMA* 267(15):2055–2061.

Kongstvedt, P.R. 1997. *Essentials of managed care.* 2nd ed. Gaithersburg, MD: Aspen Publishers.

Meyer, M., and Muir, A. 1994. Not my health care: Insurers beware, consumers are going to court to protect benefits. *Newsweek* January 10:36–38.

Mintzberg, H., and Quinn, J. 1996. *The strategy process, concepts, contexts, cases.* 2nd ed. Englewood Cliffs, NJ: Prentice-Hall, 62.

Peters, W.P., and Rogers, M.C. 1994. Variation in approval by insurance companies of coverage for autologous bone marrow transplantation for breast cancer. *N Engl J Med* 330(7):473–477.

Peters, W.P., Ross, M., Verdenburgh, J.J., et al. 1994. The use of intensive clinic support to permit outpatient autologous bone marrow transplantation for breast cancer. *Semin Oncol* 21(4 suppl 7):25–31.

Porter, M.E. 1979. How competitive forces shape strategy. *Harvard Bus Rev* (Mar–Apr):137–146.

Saver, R.S. 1992. Reimbursing new technologies: Why are the courts judging experimental medicine? *Stanford Law Rev* 44(1051):1095–1131.

University Health System Consortium. 2002. *Managed care contracting.* Oak Brook, IL: University Health System Consortium.

Uyl-de Groot, C.A., Richel, D.J., Rutten, F.F. 1994. Peripheral blood progenitor cell transplantation mobilized by r-metl-lug-CSF (Filgrastrim): A less costly alternative to autologous bone marrow transplantation. *Eur J Cancer* 30A(11):1631–1635.

Van Harrison, R., Gallay, L., McKay, N.E., et al. 1990. The association between community physician's attendance at a medical center's CME courses and their patients' referrals to the medical center. *J Contin Ed Health Prof* 10:315–320

Wasson, C.R. 1978. *Dynamic competitive strategy and product life cycles.* 3rd ed. Austin, TX: Austin Press.

Wynstra, N.A. 1994. Breast cancer: Selected legal issues. *Cancer Suppl* 74(1):491–511.

Chapter 19

Nursing Research in Blood Cell and Marrow Transplantation

Mel Haberman, PhD, RN, FAAN

The modern era of blood cell and marrow transplantation (BCMT) nursing research is typified by more sophisticated and clinically relevant studies than any time in history. The steady growth of BCMT nursing research during the past 2 decades can be attributed to several trends. One trend is the spirit of cooperation that exists among nurse clinicians and nurse scientists. Many practicing clinicians are conducting studies with the assistance of expert research mentors, and it is becoming commonplace for nurse investigators to ask clinicians for help in designing studies. Clinicians can evaluate studies for clinical feasibility and potential to fill existing gaps in practice knowledge.

Another trend is the tendency of clinical nurses to be critical consumers of research. BCMT nurses recognize the narrow range of outcomes generated by medical transplantation research and, subsequently, are turning to their own discipline for answers. Many of the most recent generation of nurse scientists entering BCMT research have come directly from clinical practice, resulting in a marked improvement in the clinical relevancy of studies.

Another reason for the emergence of BCMT nursing research as a leading field of oncology nursing research is the current popularity of quality-of-life research. Nurse scientists are leaders in this sophisticated field of inquiry, and many investigators have begun programs of research that address the quality of life of BCMT survivors.

Maintaining the momentum of progress will require new research initiatives and more sophisticated studies. Investigators will need to find new mechanisms for conducting large-scale, multi-institutional BCMT nursing research and be creative in securing funding for it. Moreover, a theoretical foundation for BCMT nursing therapies must be conceptualized and tested using intervention and outcome-oriented research designs. If BCMT therapy is to remain a viable treatment option in the future, nursing research must unravel the intricacies of care and link nursing actions with the biopsychosocial outcomes of BCMT therapy. We have yet to empirically answer the question, "What nursing therapeutics (interventions) actually make a difference (outcomes) in the lives of BCMT recipients and their families?"

Foundations for Nursing Research

Nurses researching and practicing BCMT nursing are fortunate to have a diverse and broad-based literature that is conceptually, if not empirically, strong. This body of nursing knowledge provides a beginning theoretical foundation for nursing therapeutics and future research. The literature gives us a snapshot of the developmental history of BCMT nursing. We are indebted to nurses who have taken the time to publish anecdotal, clinically based case histories; guidelines for practice; conceptual overviews; comprehensive reviews of the literature; teaching and documentation tools for nurses and caregivers; and research reports. Moreover, a milestone in the field occurred with the publication of two BCMT-related manuals, *Manual for Bone Marrow Transplant Nursing* (Ezzone and Camp-Sorrell, 1994), and *Peripheral Blood Stem Cell Transplantation* (Ezzone, 1997), that impressively attempted to identify and cite the research that supports practice guidelines.

The conceptual foundation that guides BCMT nursing practice is stronger than the existing empirical or research base for practice. Any review of the BCMT nursing literature will show that the number of research studies conducted by nurse investigators remains small when compared to the number of nursing publications in the field. It is a well-known fact that the current generation of BCMT nursing therapeutics is derived primarily from biomedical research or from other disciplines, such as nutrition sciences, psychology, and dentistry. Our reliance on other disciplines to lend guidance to nursing practice will continue until a sufficient cadre of BCMT nurse investigators is in place to design and test specifically tailored nursing therapies.

Research Foundations

A rudimentary research base for practice is emerging in several areas. An electronic search of the Cumulative Index for Nursing and Allied Health Literature (CINAHL) database yielded a total of 424 BCMT papers published in nursing journals since 1982. This number is conservative because many nurses are publishing BCMT articles in nonnursing journals indexed in CINAHL and other biomedical databases. Thirty-three papers from 1982 to 1994 and 46 from 1995 to December 2003 were empirical research reports representing 19% of the total number of published papers. **Table 19-1** lists the topic areas of these studies, the number of publications by topic, and the investigators.

As Table 19-1 shows, quality of life, pediatric issues, and right atrial/central venous catheters are the three most frequently studied topics. Fourteen of the 34 areas of practice (41%) have two or more published databased papers on the same topic. The remaining empirical papers consist of a wide compilation of single studies. No studies that represent direct replications of previous research were found. However, multiple studies on a single topic can be classified as conceptual replication, since the same concept is studied repeatedly from the different vantage points of several studies.

In general, the use of descriptive or correlational designs, small samples, and cross-sectional or single point-in-time measurement is the hallmark of two decades of BCMT nursing research. Advances in nursing research since 1996 are indicated by studies using prospective, repeated measures designs (Ben

Table 19-1 BCMT NURSING RESEARCH STUDIES BEFORE JANUARY 1, 2004, ORGANIZED BY TOPIC AREAS.

Topic Areas	Number of Studies	Citations
Quality of life	11	Belec, 1992; Ferrell et al., 1992a, 1992b; Haberman et al., 1993; Hacker and Ferrans, 2003; King et al., 1995; Molassiotis et al., 1995; Molassiotis, 1996; Molassiotis and Morris, 1998; So et al., 2003; Whedon et al., 1995
Pediatric issues: coping, pain, emesis, nutrition	10	DeSwarte-Wallace et al., 2001; Mardsen, 1988; McCarthy et al., 1996; Mehta et al., 1997; Pederson et al., 2000; Robb and Ebberts, 2003a, 2003b; Tomlinson et al., 1993; Tyc et al., 1998; Wood, 1990
Right atrial/central venous catheters	7	Brandt et al., 1996; Keller, 1994; Kelly et al., 1992; Larsen et al., 1996; Newman et al., 1984; Shivnan et al., 1991; Ulz et al., 1990
Hope	4	Artinian, 1984; Cohen and Ley, 2000; Ersek, 1992; Saleh and Brockopp, 2001a
Patient in isolation	4	Cohen et al., 2001; Collins et al., 1989; Gaskill et al., 1997; Zerbe et al., 1994
Mucositis/oral hygiene	4	Borbasi et al., 2002; Ezzone et al., 1993; McGuire et al., 1993; McGuire et al., 1998
Pain and psychological distress	3	Ben David and Musgrave, 1996; Gaston-Johannson et al., 1992; Pederson and Parran, 1999
Meaning of BCMT	3	Haberman, 1995; Shuster et al., 1996; Steeves, 1992
Infection prevention measures	2	Duquette-Petersen et al., 1999; Poe et al., 1994
Family caregivers	2	Foxall and Gaston-Johansson, 1996; Stetz et al., 1996
Maternal responses to a child's BCMT	2	Nelson et al., 1997; Nelson et al., 2003
Patient perception of needs	2	Campos de Carvalho et al., 2000; Tarzian et al., 1999
Research instrument development	2	Molassiotis, 1999; Saleh and Brockopp, 2001b
Symptom perception and management		Coleman et al., 2002; Larson et al., 1993

(continues)

Table 19-1 BCMT NURSING RESEARCH STUDIES BEFORE JANUARY 1, 2004,
ORGANIZED BY TOPIC AREAS *continued.*

Topic Areas	Number of Studies	Citations
Coping patterns and	2	Gaston-Johansson et al., 2000
strategies	1	
Cyclosporine regimens	1	Caudell and Adams, 1990
Dimensions of psychosocial	1	Winters et al., 1994
nursing		
Do-not-resuscitate orders	1	Kern et al., 1992
Graft-versus-host disease	1	Copel and Smith, 1989
Informed consent	1	Carney, 1987
IV immunoglobulin	1	Camp-Sorrell and Wujcik, 1994
administration		
Neurological complications	1	Furlong and Galluci, 1994
Patient acuity	1	Lovett and McMillan, 1993
Patient perception of	1	Thain and Gibbon, 1996
BCMT		
Nurses' attitudes toward	1	Pederson and Parran, 1997
pain management		
Palliative care	1	McDonnell and Morris, 1997
Nurses' burnout and job	1	Molassiotis and Haberman, 1996
satisfaction		
Pharmacologic pain	1	Pederson and Parran, 2000
management		
Music therapy as adjunct	1	Ezzone et al., 1998
therapy		
Marrow donation	1	Christopher, 2000
Granulocyte colony	1	Comley et al., 1999
stimulating factor		
Massage therapy and	1	Rexilious et al., 2002
healing touch		
Nursing diagnosis	1	Young et al., 2002
Patient decision making	1	Bywater and Atkins, 2001

David and Musgrave, 1996; Borbasi et al., 2002; Campos de Carvalho et al., 2000; Foxall and Gaston-Johansson, 1996; Hacker and Ferrans, 2003; Larsen et al., 1996; McGuire et al., 1998; Nelson et al., 1997; Nelson et al., 2003; Pederson and Parran, 1999; Pederson and Parran, 2000; Pederson et al., 2000; Shuster et al., 1996; Tarzian et al., 1999; Young et al., 2002) and intervention studies that ranged from true randomized controlled trials to studies using nonprobability samples with random assignment to groups (Brandt et al.,

1996; Comley et al., 1999; Duquette-Pedersen et al., 1999; Ezzone et al., 1998; Gaston-Johansson et al., 2000; Mehta et al., 1997; Rexilius et al., 2002).

In summary, there is a beginning research base for several areas of practice, and more studies in recent years are using prospective and randomized controlled clinical trial designs. Despite the cumulative evidence in several areas, new investigators should not be unduly worried about selecting a topic for study, because every facet of nursing knowledge needs further research and empirical development. Virtually any topic listed in Table 19-1 can serve as a launching point for further investigation.

Mechanisms for Conducting Nursing Research

Research Conducted by Clinical Nurses

Although several options exist for building a scientific base for BCMT nursing, the present cadre of BCMT nurse researchers is too small to accomplish the research mission of the specialty. More researchers are needed from the ranks of BCMT clinical nurses, new post-master's degree and postdoctorate nurses, as well as senior nurse scientists.

Mechanisms are needed so that more clinical nurses can become involved in research, receive paid release time for research, and obtain research consultation from nurse scientists. At this level of clinical research, staff nurses can either conduct their own independent studies or tag a nursing study onto an existing medical proto-col, often referred to as a companion study (Ferrell and Cohen, 1991). Because it is often unrealistic for clinicians to receive paid release time for research, it is advisable to conduct team projects, pool precious resources, and divide the workload. Each member of the team can write a different section of the research protocol or grant and be responsible for assembling the materials for that section (e.g., finding the instruments, preparing the consent form, and so forth). If members of the team are having trouble meeting their writing deadlines, a writing club can be started. Generally, writing clubs require each member to produce a few pages of text either every week or every other week. The members of the club set a realistic time line for meeting their goals, read and critique each others' work, and keep themselves motivated to finish the project.

Most studies conducted by staff nurses will be small-scale feasibility or pilot studies that may realistically take a couple of years to complete. Most, if not all of these studies, should be designed with the intent of sharing the findings through publication or presentation. Funding for these types of projects may be obtained from many sources, such as the nursing department, local representatives of the pharmaceutical industry, or local chapters of the Oncology Nursing Society or Sigma Theta Tau International. National funding is available from many nursing specialty organizations. The Oncology Nursing Foundation has an exceptional record of funding small grants and BCMT nursing studies. It is mandatory to begin a new program of BCMT research with some form of feasibility or pilot investigation. Funding agencies like the National Center for Nursing Research, National Cancer Institute, and American Cancer Society will rarely, if ever, fund large grants without first seeing the preliminary data that support a new line of inquiry or that demonstrate a new investigator's track record.

Research Conducted by Undergraduate and Graduate Students

Another mechanism for facilitating BCMT nursing research is to actively recruit bachelor's, master's, and doctoral students and to create an atmosphere of critical inquiry in your setting. Clinically based nurses can go to schools of nursing and invite students to conduct their research in BCMT, suggesting topics for study that have been identified by staff nurses. Clinical nurses can become involved in the development of these student projects, and many times, the projects end up providing staff nurses with the information they need for practice. Students and postdoctorate fellows can be asked to be guest members of the unit's nursing research committee, if such a committee exists.

Many schools of nursing are looking for clinical sites for their baccalaureate nursing students to conduct a feasibility study for their required nursing research course. To fulfill this requirement and to give students the opportunity to be involved in a clinical nursing study, students can be teamed with staff nurses who need additional help with their studies. At the Fred Hutchinson Cancer Research Center, 16 baccalaureate nursing students worked on a half dozen nursing studies over 2 years. They helped staff nurses with literature reviews, locating instruments, data collection, analysis of data, writing up the findings and preparing manuscripts, and preparing research presentations for local, regional, national, and international conferences. Graduate student research interns also provide an invalu-

able source of expertise to staff nurses and clinically based nurse investigators. Moreover, research assistance can be obtained from research nurses who are hired specifically to carry out clinical trials for physician investigators.

Research Conducted by Nurse Scientists

External investigators who import their projects to a BCMT unit are generally willing to mentor staff nurses in the research process. Staff nurses can be formally appointed as a clinical mentor to the external researcher, and the researcher can act as a research mentor in return. The clinical mentor can smooth the researcher's entry into the institution, teach the clinical realities of BCMT nursing, and critique the clinical feasibility of the researcher's proposed study. In return, staff nurses can negotiate a role in designing and implementing the research project, and many times, external researchers are willing to provide opportunities for staff to help with the preparation of manuscripts and to give presentations at conferences.

Expert Research Consultation

Blood cell and marrow transplantation nursing units should actively seek consultation from advanced nurse scientists by maintaining an ongoing recruitment campaign with local schools of nursing, other comprehensive and community cancer centers, and nursing specialty organizations or honorary societies.

Generally, most nurse investigators provide consultation gratis. However, when extensive work is needed to design a study, pull together a grant application, or provide long-term consultation, it is customary to pay an honorarium or consultation fee. The amount of the honorarium can be negotiated with the nurse investigator.

Additional sources of expertise are available to BCMT nurses. Many nurse scientists are in private practice and gladly consult with clinical nurses. Many new postdoctorate fellows and midcareer faculty members are looking for clinical sites to start or expand their research program. Nurse scientists working in other agencies are often looking for a comparison sample for their studies. At this level of advanced research preparation, nurses are capable of writing large proposals that include funding for staff nurses to become involved in the research project. The American Cancer Society's professors of oncology nursing are in many localities and are committed to advancing oncology nursing education and research in their communities. Moreover, it is easy to find out which nurse investigators in your community have received federal funding for oncology research by going online to the National Cancer Institute or National Center for Nursing Research. Federal funding agencies maintain listings of all publicly funded research on the World Wide Web. Medical libraries also can obtain this information for investigators who lack online access.

Multi-institutional Research

Research will progress slowly and in a haphazard manner unless a mechanism is developed for multi-institutional oncology nursing research. Many clinical nurses are familiar with the multisite clinical trials conducted by the National Cancer Institute's cooperative research groups, such as the Southwest Oncology Group (SWOG) or Eastern Cooperative Oncology Group (ECOG).

A cooperative BCMT nursing research group will help to focus what is currently a highly fragmented field of research. Clearly, studies conducted in an extensive network of sites can recruit large and diverse samples and obtain data that is generalizable to diverse populations of patients and nursing units. Implementing a multisite BCMT research project is expensive and will usually rely on a senior investigator obtaining federal funding.

Future Directions for Research

The Role of Oncology Nursing Research

Future research will be precipitated by breakthroughs in transplantation biology, immunology, and genetics. For instance, the advent of new conventional and biological agents, the potential benefits of gene therapy, advances in hematopoietic reconstitution and the mobilization of stem and progenitor cells, and the as-yet undiscovered frontiers of BCMT treatment all hold great promise.

Clinical nursing research focuses on the human experience of wellness and illness and on the clinical therapeutics that are under the control of nurses. Common problems that have faced transplant recipients from the earliest days of bone marrow transplantation will be with us for the foreseeable future and will need ongoing investigation by nurses; these include acute and chronic graft-versus-host disease, regimen-related toxicities and pancytopenia following intensive chemoradiotherapy, life-threatening infections, and impaired quality of life and long-term survival. **Table 19-2** lists some additional fruitful lines of inquiry for future research.

Medical advances in BCMT therapy that improve life expectancy and extend BCMT to a wider array of diseases will allow nurses to explore the biopsychosocial and spiritual implications of survivorship. A greater emphasis will be placed on quantifying nursing outcomes and linking these outcomes to the caring behaviors and interventions of nurses. CD-ROM, video streaming, handheld computer, and Internet technologies can now deliver tailored nursing interventions to rural and urban households.

Table 19-2 FUTURE DIRECTIONS FOR BCMT NURSING RESEARCH.

- Test new strategies to recruit women and ethnic minorities into BCMT clinical trials and to enhance compliance with aggressive therapeutic regimens.
- Design and test new models for research dissemination and utilization.
- Define nursing outcomes both conceptually and empirically at all phases of BCMT therapy and for different types of transplants (e.g., blood cell versus marrow, autologous versus allogeneic, single versus multiple, and related versus unrelated donor).
- Conduct methodological research to obtain reproducible outcome data across multiple research sites (e.g., data on regimen-related toxicities, infection rates, patient safety issues, quality of life, safety of early discharge, readmission rates, direct and out-of-pocket costs of care, and fatigue and pain intensity).
- Link models of nursing care delivery with clinical outcomes (e.g., models for critical pathways, case management, transition services, ambulatory care, home care, and palliative care).
- Test the ability of patient acuity systems to predict nursing outcomes, staff ratios and mix, staff satisfaction and retention, staff psychosocial morbidity, patient safety, cost-containment measures, and quality improvement practices.
- Develop instruments to standardize clinical assessment (e.g., fatigue and pain scales, quality of life questionnaires, demands of BCMT transplantation, and multiorgan/systems toxicity scales).
- Test models of long-term follow-up and the role of nurses in monitoring chronic symptoms and recurrences of cancer and in providing patient/family education and specialty referral.
- Identify caregiver issues (e.g., strategies for psychosocial support, educational needs, methods for monitoring the quality of care given by caregivers, and the long-range burden of the caregiver role).
- Explore ethical issues, the informed consent process, how information is given in family conferences, nurses' role in genetic counseling, the effect of advanced directives, and how treatment futility and end-of-life issues alter the delivery of care.
- Investigate the nursing therapeutics that support accelerated engraftment, graft failure, progenitor cell collection, and allogeneic stem cell donation.
- Investigate the biophysical and behavioral-psychosocial therapeutics that support new approaches to adoptive immunotherapy.
- Examine the nursing therapeutics associated with leukapheresis for blood cell transplants, improved antiemetic therapies, advances in prophylactic antibiotic therapy, the use of cytokines or growth factors and monoclonal antibodies, and protocols of single or multiple courses of high-dose therapy or sequential therapy followed by blood cell transplantation.
- Explore the nursing therapeutics for pediatric and elderly populations of BCMT recipients and for managing the lingering complications of long-range survivorship.
- Conduct research on the psychosocial morbidity of BCMT nursing practice and methods of providing effective support to nurses.

Although descriptive research is falling out of vogue in favor of intervention trials, there will remain a need to describe and explain the basic human responses to emerging BCMT therapies.

Rigorous, descriptive research is a prerequisite to the fundamental understanding of concepts that is needed for subsequent intervention trials and outcome-oriented research. Nurse investigators also will be challenged to use multiple and more sophisticated research methodologies to build a solid theoretical foundation for BCMT nursing and our parent specialty, oncology nursing.

Summary

As we move together to face an unforeseen future, nurses are confronted with the challenge of humanizing the technological breakthroughs that will undoubtedly occur in blood cell and marrow transplantation. Medical science will never provide nursing with the knowledge it needs for nursing therapeutics; it has enough challenges of its own. Our specialty must realize a philosophy of teamwork and a willingness of nurse clinicians, administrators, researchers, and educators to work together to achieve what remains an elusive goal. It is imperative that we anchor our BCMT nursing therapeutics in empirically derived knowledge, and that the best traditions of the art of nursing be embraced and given voice in the emerging science of nursing, while always keeping a clear vision of the ultimate goal—to improve the quality of life of persons with cancer and their families.

References

Artinian, B.M. 1984. Fostering hope in the bone marrow transplant child. *Matern-Child Nurs J* 13:57–71.

Belec, K. 1992. Quality of life: Perceptions of long-term survivors of bone marrow transplantation. *Oncol Nurs Forum* 19:31–37.

Ben David, Y., and Musgrave, C.F. 1996. Pain assessment: A pilot study in an Israeli bone marrow transplant unit. *Cancer Nurs* 19:93–97.

Borbasi, S., Cameron, K., Quested, B., et al. 2002. More than a sore mouth: Patients' experience of oral mucositis. *Oncol Nurs Forum* 29:1051–1057.

Brandt, B., DePalma, J. Irwin, M., et al. 1996. Comparison of central venous catheter dressings in bone marrow transplant recipients. *Oncol Nurs Forum* 23:829–836.

Bywater, L., and Atkins, S. 2001. A study of factors influencing patients' decisions to undergo bone marrow transplantation from a sibling or matched related donor. [Including commentary by Porter, H., and Clark, K.] *European J Oncol Nurs* 5:7–17.

Camp-Sorrell, D., and Wujcik, D. 1994. Intravenous immunoglobulin administration: An evaluation of vital sign monitoring. *Oncol Nurs Forum* 21(3):531–535.

Campos de Carvalho, E., Goncalves, P.G., Bontempo, A.P.M., et al. 2000. Interpersonal needs expressed by patients during bone marrow transplantation. *Cancer Nurs* 23:462–467.

Carney, B. 1987. Bone marrow transplantation: Nurses' and physicians' perceptions of informed consent. *Cancer Nurs* 10:252–259.

Caudell, K.A., and Adams, J. 1990. Cyclosporine administration practices on bone marrow transplant units: A national survey. *Oncol Nurs Forum* 17:563–568.

Christopher, K.A. 2000. The experience of donating bone marrow to a relative. *Oncol Nurs Forum* 27:693–700.

Cohen, M.Z., and Ley, C.D. 2000. Bone marrow transplantation: The battle for hope in the face of fear. *Oncol Nurs Forum* 27:473–480.

Cohen, M.Z., Ley, C., Tarzian, A.J. 2001. Isolation in blood and marrow transplantation. *Western J Nurs Research* 23:592–609.

Coleman, E.A., Coon, S.K., Mattox, S.G., et al. 2002. Symptom management and successful outpatient transplantation for patients with multiple myeloma. *Cancer Nurs* 25:452–460.

Collins, C., Upright, C., Aleksich, J. 1989. Reverse isolation: What patients perceive. *Oncol Nurs Forum* 16: 675–679.

Comley, A.L., DeMeyer, E., Adams, N., et al. 1999. Effect of subcutaneous granulocyte colony-stimulating factor injectate volume on drug efficacy, site complications, and client comfort. *Oncol Nurs Forum* 26:87–94.

Copel, L.C., and Smith, M.E. 1989. Oncology nurses' knowledge of graft-versus-host disease in bone marrow transplant patients. *Cancer Nurs* 12:243–249.

DeSwarte-Wallace, J., Firouzbakhsh, S., and Finklestein, J.Z. 2001. Using research to change practice: Enteral feedings for pediatric oncology patients. *J Pediatric Oncol Nurs* 18:217–223.

Duquette-Petersen, L., Francis, M.E., Dohnalek, L., et al. 1999. The role of protective clothing in infection prevention in patients undergoing autologous bone marrow transplantation. *Oncol Nurs Forum* 26:1319–1324.

Ersek, M. 1992. The process of maintaining hope in adults undergoing bone marrow transplantation for leukemia. *Oncol Nurs Forum* 19:883–889.

Ezzone, S., ed. 1997. *Peripheral blood stem cell transplantation: Recommendations for nursing education and practice.* Pittsburgh: Oncology Nursing Press.

Ezzone, S., Baker, C., Rosselet, R., et al. 1998. Music as an adjunct to antiemetic therapy. *Oncol Nurs Forum* 25: 1551–1556.

Ezzone, S., and Camp-Sorrell, D., eds. 1994. *Manual for bone marrow transplant nursing: Recommendations for practice and education.* Pittsburgh: Oncology Nursing Society.

Ezzone, S., Kapoor, N., Jolly, D., et al. 1993. Survey of oral hygiene regimens among bone marrow transplant centers. *Oncol Nurs Forum* 20:1375–1381.

Ferrell, B.R., and Cohen, M.Z. 1991. Companion studies. *Semin Oncol Nurs* 7:252–259.

Ferrell, B., Whitehead, C., Grant, M., et al. 1992a. The meaning of the quality of life for bone marrow transplant survivors: The impact of bone marrow transplant on the quality of life. Part 1. *Cancer Nurs* 15: 153–160.

Ferrell, B., Whitehead, C., Grant, M., et al. 1992b. The meaning of the quality of life for bone marrow transplant survivors: Improving quality of life for bone marrow transplant survivors. Part 2. *Cancer Nurs* 15: 247–253.

Foxall, M.J., and Gaston-Johansson, F. 1996. Burden and health outcomes of family caregivers of hospitalized bone marrow transplant patients. *J Advanced Nurs* 24: 915–923.

Furlong, T.G., and Gallucci, B.B. 1994. Pattern of occurrence and clinical presentation of neurological complications in bone marrow transplant patients. *Cancer Nurs* 17:27–36.

Gaskill, D., Henderson, A., and Fraser, M. 1997. Exploring the everyday world of the patient in isolation. *Oncol Nurs Forum* 24:695–700.

Gaston-Johansson, F., Fall-Dickson, J.M., Nanda, J., et al. 2000. The effectiveness of the comprehensive coping strategy program on clinical outcomes in breast cancer autologous bone marrow transplantation. *Cancer Nurs* 23:277–285.

Gaston-Johansson, F., Franco, T., and Zimmerman, L. 1992. Pain and psychological distress in patients undergoing autologous bone marrow transplant. *Oncol Nurs Forum* 19:41–47.

Haberman, M.R. 1995. The meaning of cancer therapy: Bone marrow transplantation as an exemplar of therapy. *Semin Oncol Nurs* 11:23–31.

Haberman, M., Young, K., Bush, N., et al. 1993. Quality of life of adult long-term survivors of bone marrow transplantation: A qualitative analysis of narrative data. *Oncol Nurs Forum* 10:1545–1553.

Hacker, E.D., and Ferrans, C.E. 2003. Quality of life immediately after peripheral blood stem cell transplantation. *Cancer Nurs* 26:312–322.

Keller, C.A. 1994. Methods of drawing blood samples through central venous catheters in pediatric patients undergoing bone marrow transplant: Results of a national survey. *Oncol Nurs Forum* 21:879–884.

Kelly, C., McGregor, S.E., Dumenko, L., et al. 1992. A change in flushing protocols of central venous catheters. *Oncol Nurs Forum* 19:599–605.

Kern, D., Albrizio, M., and Kettner, P. 1992. An exploration of the variables involved when instituting a do-not-resuscitate order for patients undergoing bone marrow transplantation. *Oncol Nurs Forum* 19:635–640.

King, C.R., Ferrell, B.R., Grant, M., et al. 1995. Nurses' perceptions of the meaning of quality of life for bone marrow transplant survivors. *Cancer Nurs* 18:118–129.

Larsen, J., Gardulf, A., Nordstrom, G., et al. 1996. Health-related quality of life in women with breast cancer undergoing autologous stem-cell transplantation. *Cancer Nurs* 19:368–375.

Larson, P.J., Dibble, S.L., Viele, C.S., et al. 1993. Comparison of perceived symptoms of patients undergoing bone marrow transplant and the nurses caring for them. [Including commentary by Ersek, M.] *Oncol Nurs Forum* 20:81–88.

Lovett, R.B., and McMillan, S.C. 1993. Validity and reliability of a bone marrow transplant acuity tool. *Oncol Nurs Forum* 20:1385–1392.

Marsden, C. 1988. Care giver fidelity in a pediatric bone marrow transplant team. *Heart & Lung* 17:617–625.

McCarthy, A.M., Cool, V.A., Petersen, M., et al. 1996. Cognitive behavioral pain and anxiety interventions in pediatric oncology centers and bone marrow transplant units. [Including commentary by Bowman, L.C.] *J Pediatric Oncol Nurs* 13:3–14.

McDonnell, T., and Morris, M. 1997. Pilot study reports. An exploratory study of palliative care in bone marrow transplant patients. *International J Palliative Nurs* 3:111–112, 114–117.

McGuire, D.B., Wingard, J.R., Altomonte, V., et al. 1993. Patterns of mucositis and pain in patients receiving chemotherapy and bone marrow transplantation. *Oncol Nurs Forum* 20:1493–1502.

McGuire, D., Yeager, K.A., Dudley, W.N., et al. 1998. Acute oral pain and mucositis in bone marrow transplant and leukemia patients: Data from a pilot study. *Cancer Nurs* 21:385–393.

Mehta, N.H., Reed, C.M., Kuhlman, C., et al. 1997. Controlling conditioning-related emesis in children undergoing bone marrow transplantation. *Oncol Nurs Forum* 24:1539–1544.

Molassiotis, A. 1996. Clinical late psychosocial effects of conditioning for BMT. *British J of Nurs* 5:1296, 1298–1302.

Molassiotis, A. 1999. Further evaluation of a scale to screen for risk of emotional difficulties in bone marrow transplant recipients. *J Advanced Nurs* 29:922–927.

Molassiotis, A., Boughton, B.J., Burgoyne, T., et al. 1995. Comparison of the overall quality of life in 50 long-term survivors of autologous and allogeneic bone marrow transplantation. *J Advanced Nurs* 22:509–516.

Molassiotis, A., and Haberman, M. 1996. Evaluation of burnout and job satisfaction in marrow transplant nurses. *Cancer Nurs* 19:360–367.

Molassiotis, A., and Morris, P.J. 1998. The meaning of quality of life and the effects of unrelated donor bone marrow transplants for chronic myeloid leukemia in adult long-term survivors. *Cancer Nurs* 21:205–211.

Nelson, A.E., Gleaves, L., and Nuss, S. 2003. Practice applications of research. Mothers' responses during the child's stem cell transplantation: Pilot study. *Pediatric Nurs* 29:219–223.

Nelson, A.E., Miles, M.S., and Belyea, M.J. 1997. Coping and support effects on mothers' stress responses to their child's hematopoietic stem cell transplantation. *J Pediatric Oncol Nurs* 14:202–212.

Newman, K.A., Schnaper, N., Reed, W.P., et al. 1984. Effect of Hickman catheters on the self-esteem of patients with leukemia. *Southern Medical J* 77:682–685.

Pederson, C., and Parran, L. 1997. Bone marrow transplant nurses' knowledge, beliefs, and attitudes regarding pain management. *Oncol Nurs Forum* 24:1563–1571.

Pederson, C., and Parran, L. 1999. Pain and distress in adults and children undergoing peripheral blood stem cell or bone marrow transplant. *Oncol Nurs Forum* 26:575–582.

Pederson, C., and Parran, L. 2000. Opioid tapering in hematopoietic progenitor cell transplant recipients. *Oncol Nurs Forum* 27:1371–1380.

Pederson, C., Parran, L., and Harbaugh, B. 2000. Children's perceptions of pain during 3 weeks of bone marrow transplant experience. *J Pediatric Oncol Nurs* 17:22–32.

Poe, S.S., Larson, E., McGuire, D., et al. 1994. A national survey of infection prevention practices on bone marrow transplant units. *Oncol Nurs Forum* 21:1687–1694.

Rexilius, S.J., Mundt, C.A., Megel, M.E., et al. 2002. Therapeutic effects of massage therapy and healing touch on caregivers of patients undergoing autologous hematopoietic stem cell transplant. *Oncol Nurs Forum* 29:E35–E44.

Robb, S.L., and Ebberts, A.G. 2003a. Songwriting and digital video production interventions for pediatric patients undergoing bone marrow transplantation, part I: An analysis of depression and anxiety levels according to phase of treatment. *J Pediatric Oncol Nurs* 20:2–15.

Robb, S.L., and Ebberts, A.G. 2003b. Songwriting and digital video production interventions for pediatric patients undergoing bone marrow transplantation, part II: An analysis of patient-generated songs and patient perceptions regarding intervention efficacy. *J Pediatric Oncol Nurs* 20:16–25.

Saleh, U.S., and Brockopp, D.Y. 2001a. Hope among patients with cancer hospitalized for bone marrow transplantation: A phenomenologic study. *Cancer Nurs* 24:308–314.

Saleh, U.S., and Brockopp, D.Y. 2001b. Quality of life one year following bone marrow transplantation: Psychometric evaluation of the quality of life in bone marrow transplant survivors tool. *Oncol Nurs Forum* 28:1457–1464.

Shivnan, J.C., McGuire, D., Freedman, S., et al. 1991. A comparison of transparent adherent and dry sterile gauze dressings for long-term central catheters in patients undergoing bone marrow transplant. *Oncol Nurs Forum* 18:1349–1356.

Shuster, G.F., Steeves, R.H., Onega, L., et al. 1996. Coping patterns among bone marrow transplant patients: A hermeneutical inquiry. *Cancer Nurs* 19:290–297.

So, W.K.W., Dodgson, J., and Tai, J.W.M. 2003. Fatigue and quality of life among Chinese patients with hematologic malignancy after bone marrow transplantation. *Cancer Nurs* 26:211–221.

Steeves, R.H. 1992. Patients who have undergone bone marrow transplantation: Their quest for meaning. *Oncol Nurs Forum* 19:899–905.

Stetz, K.M., McDonald, J.C., and Compton, K. 1996. Needs and experiences of family caregivers during marrow transplantation. *Oncol Nurs Forum* 23:1422–1427.

Tarzian, A.J., Iwata, P.A., and Cohen, M.Z. 1999. Autologous bone marrow transplantation: The patient's perspective of information needs. *Cancer Nurs* 22:103–110.

Thain, C.W., and Gibbon, B. 1996. An exploratory study of recipients' perceptions of bone marrow transplantation. *J Advanced Nurs* 23:528–535.

Tomlinson, P.S., Tomczyk, B., Kirshbaum, M., et al. 1993. The relationship of child acuity, maternal responses, nurse attitudes and contextual factors in the bone marrow transplant unit. *American J of Critical Care* 2:246–252.

Tyc, V.L., Bieberich, A.A., Hinds, P., et al. 1998. Survey of pain services for pediatric oncology patients: Their composition and function. *J Pediatric Oncol Nurs* 15:207–215.

Ulz, L., Peterson, F.B., Ford, R., et al. 1990. A prospective study of complications in Hickman right-atrial catheters in marrow transplant patients. *J of Parenteral & Enteral Nutr* 14:27–30.

Whedon, M., Stearns, D., and Mills, L.E. 1995. Quality of life of long-term adult survivors of autologous bone marrow transplantation. [Including commentary by Haberman, M.] *Oncol Nurs Forum* 22:1527–1537.

Winters, G., Miller, C., Maracich, L., et al. 1994. Provisional practice: The nature of psychosocial bone marrow transplant nursing. *Oncol Nurs Forum* 21:1147–1154.

Wood, R.M. 1990. Growth patterns in pediatric bone marrow transplant patients. *J of Pediatric Nurs* 5:252–258.

Young, L.K., Todd, S., and Simuncak, S.L. 2002. Validation of the nursing diagnosis anxiety in adult patients undergoing bone marrow transplant. *International J Nurs Terminologies and Classifications* 13:88–99.

Zerbe, M.B., Parkerson, S.G., and Spitzer, T. 1994. Laminar air flow versus isolation: Nurses' assessments of moods, behaviors, and activity levels in patients receiving bone marrow transplants. *Oncol Nurs Forum* 21:565–568.

Chapter 20

Patients' Perspectives

Susan Stewart

Surviving a bone marrow transplant is a challenging experience, both physically and emotionally. Patients leave the hospital physically changed, emotionally drained, and uncertain about whether they've bought a little more time or have actually been cured. Survivors ride an emotional roller coaster as days of improvement are often followed by complications that require the patient to be rehospitalized. For the first year following a BMT, survivors measure the "future" a day at a time, unable to commit with certainty to anything longer.

The following six survivors have written about various aspects of their transplants and survival experiences. They hope that these narratives will provide some insight into what it's like to undergo and survive a BMT.

Following a second relapse of acute lymphocytic leukemia in 1992, 27-year-old Lisa Powell underwent an allogeneic BMT with marrow from a matched unrelated donor. She is currently disease free.

Beating the Odds

—Lisa Powell

In 1977, when I was 11 years old, I was diagnosed with acute lymphocytic leukemia (ALL).

I achieved a remission and underwent 3 years of chemotherapy, looking forward to that magic 5-year mark when I would be considered cured. Four years and 9 months later I relapsed.

Fortunately, I was able to attain a good remission that lasted 9 years. During those years I attended college, earned a degree in finance and international business, married my husband, Rick, and began working as a claims adjuster at an insurance company. Life was great.

In the fall of 1991, I began getting excruciating headaches. I felt listless and sick all the time. The thought never crossed my mind that the cancer had returned. I thought leukemia was a thing of the past, something I had put behind me.

When my doctor told me I had relapsed, I was devastated and felt betrayed. But I told myself I had beaten leukemia twice and could do it again. At age 26, I underwent chemotherapy again and immediately went into remission. However, my doctor told me my only real chance for a cure was a bone marrow transplant.

Deciding to undergo a BMT was the hardest decision of my life. The odds of survival were not in my favor, and the fact that I would be infertile—could never bear a child of my own—following the transplant tore me apart. I finally decided I had too much to live for and too much more to accomplish to give up. I agreed to undergo a BMT.

Unfortunately, no one in my family matched my marrow type and could serve as my donor. One week after contacting the National Marrow Donor Program, an unrelated donor was found. On September 3, 1992, new life was transplanted into me. On October 19, my husband's birthday, I was released from the hospital and spent 3 months recuperating in an apartment close to the hospital.

Today I am considered cured of this dreadful disease, thanks to a wonderful man in California who donated his marrow to me, the transplant team at Shands Hospital, and my oncologist who gave me the strength and encouragement to proceed. Granted, life was not rosy during my hospitalization and recuperation—I had lots of ups and downs with infections and graft-versus-host disease. I still have some weakness in my legs and knees, but I hope to resolve that problem by working out every day.

I have been back to work for a year and am exuberant. My hair grew back thicker after the BMT and best of all, my new immune system is in peak condition. I hardly ever get sick. Other than minor skin rashes due to graft-versus-host disease, I feel as healthy as ever.

I believe the secret to my success was the support I received from my husband and parents—they were incredible. There wasn't a moment during the day when I was alone. They were always there to keep my spirits up.

I found it helpful to get ready emotionally for the BMT by reading books on imagery and visualization, developing a positive attitude, and praying. Each night before I retired, I would envision the radiation and chemotherapy attacking the cancer cells and then I would pray. I

tried not to dwell on the negative or the possibility of not having a successful BMT. Today, I take 1 day at a time, live for today, and appreciate life more than ever.

Margaret Steslicki underwent an allogeneic BMT for myelodysplasia in 1990. When she wrote this in 1996, she was disease free.

I'm Back on My Feet Again

—Margaret Steslicki

In 1990, my world fell apart. I was diagnosed with myelodysplastic syndrome (MDS) and was told that I needed a bone marrow transplant. Even though I'm a registered nurse, the only experience I'd had with BMTs was through a medical resident who had worked with me on a medical-surgical unit 9 to 10 years earlier. He had had leukemia, gone through chemotherapy, and then a BMT. He had made it through the BMT but died several weeks later. At age 33, I was told I, too, would need a BMT if I wanted to survive long term.

It took a while for everything to sink in—facing a life-threatening blood disorder that could only be cured with a medical procedure that was also life-threatening. I prayed a lot, and with the support of my husband, family, and friends, I developed a strong will to live. A BMT was my only chance for survival. I thought, "If 50 people out of 100 can survive a BMT, I can be one of those 50 people."

After researching BMT centers and their experience with MDS, I chose to have my BMT at Harper Hospital in Detroit. We were impressed with the BMT team, and being treated at Harper allowed me to remain close to my family, something I felt was very important.

The hardest part of the transplant was leaving my two small children. I remember thinking that if I died, 5-year-old David would remember me, but 2-year-old Rachel would not. My children gave me the strength and willpower to fight the disease. A quotation from one of Bernie Siegel's books stuck in my mind: "He who has a *why* to live can bear almost any *how*." I had every *why* in the world to live, and I was going to do just that.

Being an avid gardener, I and my husband explained the BMT process to our children using gardening metaphors. We compared the chemotherapy to a weed killer that would destroy my bad marrow or bad seeds. We then explained that new seeds in the bone marrow that Uncle Bill would give me would produce new blood cells and make my bone marrow and blood flower once again.

Before my hospitalization, I collected several small gifts for my children, including books, candy, balloons, small figurines, and toys. The gifts were not costly, just little things from the dime store. I also collected special cards and stationery. Each day in the hospital, I sent a letter or special card home to my children with a little surprise. It was a way that they could connect with me, and I with them.

On the morning of September 17, 1990, I left my in-laws' house to enter the hospital. It was one of the most difficult moments of my life. I said good-bye to my children and left the house with tears in my eyes. I had an overwhelming fear that I might never see them again.

The transplant wasn't easy. The 8 days of intensive chemotherapy were difficult for me. I was sedated most of the time and remember little except sleeping and vomiting. I remember that toward the end of my conditioning regimen I had awful feelings and hallucinations. I saw the room spinning and people melting into the floors and walls. A few days after my BMT, I figured out that the lorazepam was causing these feelings, and I refused to take it, preferring to control the nausea and vomiting with ice chips and crackers.

The day of transplant was an emotional, exciting day. This would be my new birthday, a day of new life. The actual transplant was anticlimactic. I tolerated the procedure well, although the nausea and vomiting persisted and I was started on total parenteral nutrition (TPN).

Days passed as I lay in protective isolation, listening to the hum of the large room filter. Being separated from my children was the most difficult thing at this point. My physician helped me cope with my loneliness by telling me, "These days and weeks away from your children may seem like a long time now, but it will mean a lifetime with them."

During my hospitalization I tried to phone my children daily, although sometimes I just wasn't up to it. My husband and family always made sure the children understood why I couldn't call, and gave them one of the presents I had collected for them. Sometimes my husband would bring the video camera into my hospital room so I could talk to the children and show them where I was. I'd read stories while my husband videotaped me. I was told that my daughter would carry the video around with her all day and watch it over and over. Videos of the kids were also done and brought to me in the hospital room.

On October 19, 1990, I was discharged to my in-laws' home. It was the happiest day of my life! I had survived the BMT! I knew there were potential complications and I wasn't yet free and clear, but I hoped and prayed that all would go well.

A day later I had a cerebral hemorrhage and ended up back in the hospital. I had been prepared for the BMT but not the stroke. I had survived one life-threatening disease and its treatment, only to face another. I had paralysis of my left arm, a left facial drop, weakness in my left leg, and difficulty with balance. "Why me?" I asked. My own little miracle was that if the hemorrhage had occurred 1 week earlier, I probably would have died, since my bone marrow had just started producing platelets.

As the days passed in the hospital, I saw a multitude of doctors and underwent a variety of tests. I developed symptoms of graft-versus-host disease and cytomegalovirus (CMV). After a few weeks, my abdomen was so swollen I looked like I was pregnant with twins. I developed a paralytic ileus and many high fevers. There were many days when I thought I wouldn't make it. I had hit an all-time low.

I needed to work on getting well, but didn't have much physical strength. I needed help with all my personal needs: dressing, bathing, going to the bathroom, walking, and preparing food. It was devastating and humiliating. I've always been the caregiver and very independent, and now my independence had been taken away.

With the help of physical therapy (PT) and occupational therapy (OT) I gradually learned to walk with a walker, then a four-pronged cane, and then a cane. Six weeks after entering the hospital for the stroke, I was discharged home, where I continued PT and OT for several weeks.

Post-BMT complications continued. I was admitted two more times with viral meningitis. The first time was 2 days after Christmas. After being admitted for observation, I had a grand mal seizure while undergoing a spinal tap. I had a respiratory arrest and had to be resuscitated. I

vividly remember going into the seizure; it is a feeling I will never forget. I woke up on a ventilator, the spinal tap was completed, and I was rushed to the intensive care unit.

In 1995, Steslicki provided a follow-up report: I'm doing very well and am considered cured. I still follow up with a neurologist regularly due to the stroke, and will probably be on phenytoin for the rest of my life. My mobility is about 95% normal; I occasionally get clumsy when I'm tired, but it's a manageable problem. I'm back to nursing and raising my two children, and am working on my master's degree in health promotion and health care management.

My BMT experience has changed my life forever. I have gained wisdom I never knew possible, both as a human being and as a nurse. I will never take life or people for granted, and I cherish my time with family and friends. I counsel patients who are about to go through a BMT to keep a positive attitude, and to be prepared for the ups and downs. With hope, they will find the end of the rainbow.

I found that emotional support, for both me and my family, was extremely important throughout my illness and treatment. While in the hospital, my mind was at ease knowing my children were well cared for, and my husband had the support of many family members and friends. Since recovering from my BMT, I have tried to support others facing a BMT or other life-threatening disease or treatment. I volunteer with groups such as the National Bone Marrow Transplant Link, the Red Cross and Saginaw Valley Blood Program, and the Central Michigan Gift of Life Bone Marrow Program. I believe that things happen for a reason.

The BMT experience has helped me find one of my purposes in life.

Judith Miller, at age 32, underwent an allogeneic BMT for acute myelogenous leukemia in 1993 and is disease free.

Living in the Post-BMT "Snake Pit"

—Judith A. Miller

A recent BMT survivor recently asked me, "Is it normal to feel as mean as a snake after a BMT?" I could only nod my head, remembering the first few months after my allogeneic BMT for AML in January 1993. "Oh, yes," I told her, "your feelings are normal. The drugs, stress, and emotional upheaval of a BMT can throw anyone into snakedom." I look back on the first few months after BMT with a mixture of wonder, sorrow, laughter, and enormous pity for anyone who had to put up with me.

My BMT at Emory University Hospital went smoothly; I was very lucky. My donor was my brother, and his marrow engrafted quickly. I had some graft-versus-host disease, and an infection or two, but no real trauma. My family and friends were terrific, caring for me throughout. To my great joy, I was released on day 32. And then, to my great shock, I crashed and entered full-blown "snakehood." Throughout the BMT I had operated on adrenaline. My experience before being diagnosed has colored my response to the disease; I had been sick for almost 2 years, but no physician had taken me seriously, and so there had even been some relief when I finally found out what was wrong. I embarked on treatment in a fairly aggressive frame of mind. I was 32, very independent, career oriented (I am a professor of French history at Emory), and liked a good challenge. I had a

deep, durable network of friends and incredible physicians and nurses.

My parents canceled a cruise to care for me after I was released from the hospital, and they pulled my cluttered apartment into shape. A dear friend, Melinda, arrived from Houston the following week to stay with me, and even planned a delayed birthday party for me with 30 people. So far, so good. Then I was on my own.

The first obstacle was to learn to ask for help and to accept it. I live alone, so that meant scheduling friends to help me with housekeeping, resisting the urge to entertain when they came to help, and most vexing, anticipating what I might need days in advance. On Mondays, one friend put laundry in the washer; on Tuesdays, another friend put it into the dryer; on Wednesdays, another friend folded it. (I couldn't bear to be around anyone, or to inflict myself on them, long enough to do a load from start to finish.) Often, I felt it was harder to schedule things than to do them myself. I had never realized how independent I had been used to being, and it was excruciating to have others helping me.

For months after my BMT, I was the "nausea queen." You name it, I could throw it up. My daily prayer became, "Let me make good choices." At first, that meant food; then, slowly, it expanded to cover the rest of my life. My selections were very odd, but finally some worked. For awhile, all I could handle was Carnation Instant Breakfast. Then, in the 4th and 5th months, it was Cap'n Crunch—box after box of it—then coffee and beer and finally, in the 8th month, a normal diet. I took lorazepam to relieve the nausea, but it didn't help too much and made me feel down. What a terrific choice: have a quieter stomach but feel blue, or keep throwing up and be slightly more cheerful. Now I can laugh about the situation, but at the time it really tested me.

I also experienced obsessive thoughts and irritability caused by the lorazepam and the cyclosporine I was taking to control graft-versus-host disease, and the general emotional trauma that comes with months of illness. One day, for example, I read that car timing belts need to be replaced at 60,000 miles. I thought I had replaced my belt the year before, but couldn't bring myself to check my car diary to confirm this. So I tooled around Atlanta for almost 6 months, worrying that the belt was going to snap and strand me, and feeling that the world was far too complicated.

Another day, I gazed at a construction site and realized I didn't understand what held up buildings. I became depressed every time I was in a tall building and felt it shake. I wasn't afraid it was going to collapse, but instead saw it as a further sign that the world was too complex.

After a while, almost every decision I had to make seemed too complicated. Even filling the gas tank or taking the cats to the vet was overwhelming. "How would I get them in the cat carrier?" I wondered, "How could I drive them to the vet and get the carrier back out to the car? What seat should I put the carrier in?" When I finally read the cyclosporine and lorazepam packaging and found irritability and depression listed as side effects, I felt much better about these crazed thoughts. When the drugs tapered off, the obsessions ended as well.

A few weeks after my release from the hospital, I simply decided I was tired of being sick and was ready to get on with life. On day 53, I signed up for a two-hour tennis lesson, suited up, scarf on my very bald head, mask on, and headed to the courts. I stayed until the very end

of the session on a bitterly cold March night, and trotted home, quite pleased that my backhand was still intact.

The next morning I could not move. Terrified, I called the hospital. I was sure I had relapsed. When I told them I had spent the prior night playing tennis, they read me the riot act. I was to depend more on friends, do less, and give my body a chance to recover, they said. I had no choice. My muscles were so sore I could only flop on the sofa for the next 3 weeks, playing with the TV remote control.

After the tennis debacle, depression hit hard. I hated sitting home alone, but was too cranky and tired to deal with people, even my family and dearest friends. And to make it even more frustrating, everyone was being wonderful. They were infinitely sympathetic, offering help, cassettes, videos, books, and visits, none of which I wanted in the least.

I couldn't concentrate. I couldn't read. I hated junk TV (but got hooked on *Wheel of Fortune* and MTV). I couldn't keep food down. I was tired of scheduling help and saying, "thank you." I hated being away from home, but hated being cooped up. I hated people who tried to cheer me up. I felt guilty that I wasn't radiantly happy to be in good health. "After all," everyone said, "think how terrific your blood counts look!" That argument left little leeway for whining. The days stretched endlessly into monotonous, more or less silent, self-pity. I even got to the point where I thought it might be easier to relapse than put my life back together. I feared the depression would continue, yet tried to take it on faith that it would ease as I became stronger and time passed.

There is, however, a cheerful ending to this tale. At about the 100-day mark, I began to improve, albeit haltingly, and by the 4th month I could feel week-by-week progress. My hair started to look like just a very bad styling choice. I kept down a bit of food and even, wonderfully, coffee, which gave me a bit more energy. Friends at the Leukemia Society support group helped me rediscover my sense of humor.

By the 5th month, I decided I was running a fun deficit and began going out a bit with friends. Slowly, reading came back, along with listening to music. I started working out, and by the 7th month was walking a brisk 3.5 miles per day, although I couldn't run until the 9th month.

I began teaching again in August. One of my happiest moments was the 1st day back teaching. I got to talk for 2 hours about French history—something, at last, that had nothing to do with leukemia. In the 10th month, I rushed back to France for a 2-week research trip and sat in my favorite cafe as if nothing had ever happened. On New Year's Day, 1994, I retackled my research, although concentration was very difficult. In the 14th month, I finally recovered my craving for chips and dip, a taste I thought had disappeared entirely (a terrific side benefit of the BMT, I had hoped!). And in the 18th month, I began to take stock, grieve some, and put things into perspective.

Putting my life back together has been a bit-by-bit process. I hadn't realized the various components that made it up: hair, fingernails, book chapters, my morning rhythm of coffee, the *New York Times* and National Public Radio, my niece, Garth Brooks played very loudly with my car windows rolled down, conference organizing, "my" seat in the French archives, dinner parties for 30 on the spur of the moment, pulling all-nighters, and driving very fast. New pleasures: a black leather jacket (paid for with the money I didn't spend on a wig); on the first anniversary of my transplant, skiing with my brother,

Robert (who was my donor) and his family; and my baby nephew. Of course, one has to add time for grieving about the years lost to illness, nearly overwhelming sadness for friends who didn't make it, frustration with colleagues who still can't understand what happened, and time for extra sleep, rebuilding, and letting go. I would not have guessed this would be the outcome during my "snake days."

I am thankful I survived the "snake days" and was able to return to my usual chaotic existence. And sometimes I crash, and sleep, and stare at a wall for a few hours when there is no adrenaline left, and I tire of proving I'm back.

I offer this story not to discourage anyone, but rather as a tale of what happened to one person, and as encouragement for both patients and caretakers to carry on. While the snakes are out there during the recovery period, so, too, are miracles, all part and parcel of returning to the life you love.

At age 39 Mike Eckhardt underwent an allogeneic BMT for chronic myelogenous leukemia in 1992. He wrote the following 2 years later. He is currently disease free.

Coming Out of the Fog

—Mike Eckhardt

It's been more than 2 years since my BMT for chronic myelogenous leukemia. I'm just now gaining some perspective on its repercussions on my life. I've wanted and needed to write about it for some time to sort it out. One thing's for sure—catastrophic illness is tremendously invasive and pervasive. It touches every facet of one's existence both in the short and long term. Though it may seem hard to believe, there are even some positive aspects of the experience.

I still find it almost bizarre that I would be the one to get so sick. I was very physically active. I rode my bike 2,000 miles a year, swam about 100 miles, and was active in my children's lives. Leukemia happens to people you read about in the newspaper during their appeals for donors or money for transplants. It doesn't strike enormously healthy, happy, and vital 39-year-old family men.

I had been having trouble with my hip. It was very stiff and painful and was absolute hell on my golf game. I was due for my biennial company physical and a colleague was going in for his, so I made an appointment with his doctor. I went in, the doctor walked me through the paces, and I then went on the road for a few days. When I got back, I found messages from the doctor waiting for me all over town. He told me I needed to repeat the blood test. I didn't think much of it until I saw his nurse running my blood sample over to the hospital across the street for testing. He told me that my white cell count was significantly elevated and suggested I see a hematologist.

There was never any cataclysmic moment when I discovered I had leukemia. I knew early on that leukemia was suspected. The genetic confirmation was almost an anticlimax. My wife, Karen, and I decided to be up front with our boys, so we told them that night. The fact that my 11-year-old son's appendix ruptured exactly at the moment we told them only makes the day more memorable. Gannon only paused from his pain long enough to ask me if he was going to lose his dad. I told him I didn't think so, and after he decided I was telling the truth, he went right back to clutching his stomach and groaning. At that moment, I learned something about unqualified love and acceptance. Our 14-year-old, Donovan, really didn't say much. Still

waters run pretty deep with Don, and I was a little concerned about how he would deal with this.

I mentioned there are some silver linings to this particular cloud. The best for me was the response by our two boys. They dealt with the situation in their own ways, and each contributed greatly to my recovery in different ways. Gannon is a real live wire. His natural enthusiasm for life energized me whenever I got to see him. Gannon's story was and is about unqualified love and support, which is exactly what a recovering cancer patient needs.

Our older son, Donovan, is a big strong kid. Now 16, at 6'4" and 210 football-playing pounds, I never felt more secure than when he had hold of me. He never hesitated to pitch in, even for an instant. He was a rock for both Karen and me. I think my illness robbed him of some of the innocence of youth, for which I am truly sorry. If I die tomorrow, I know he will grow up to be a good man because I've already seen that he is.

Karen and I have been married for 19 years. The vows read "in sickness and in health," but I'm not sure the author of those vows had this kind of sickness in mind. I have a lot of respect for Karen and her strength. Over the years, I've come to expect a lot from her. And she has never let me down. Karen really, really persevered, and I wouldn't have survived if it weren't for her. It never occurred to me that Karen wouldn't be there for me, which was probably unfair.

I have three bothers and two sisters. Fortunately, my younger brother, Bill, was a perfect six out of six antigen match. I had the BMT in April 1992. From then until March 1993, I was in and out of the hospital on seven occasions, including the initial 5-week stay. The remaining six were due to problems related to graft-versus-host disease. At one point, I was in for about 3 months.

Although I still deal with some GVHD, my family considers my leukemia a thing of the past, which is good. I'm not quite ready to give it up until I'm sure I've wrung everything I can out of the experience. Catastrophic illness and recovery offers a unique perspective on life that is too precious to waste. It's a physical and emotional roller coaster and I want and need to understand what it's done to me and how it has changed me.

I talk to as many patients as possible because cancer is very isolating. Although each person's cancer experience is different, it's important to know that one need not go through it alone. It's a pretty exclusive fraternity, even if I don't wish membership on anyone.

Brenda Herman, at age 52, underwent an autologous BMT for stage IV breast cancer in 1992. Three years later she relapsed. Her first essay was written 1 year after transplant. Her addendum was written 6 months after her relapse.

Inside This Patient There Is a Person

—Brenda J. Herman

I love to travel. Adventure travel. Leningrad by commuter train from Helsinki. Australia, snorkeling in the Great Barrier Reef. New Zealand, flying to the peak of Mount Cook in a three-passenger plane, landing on a glacier and stepping out into snow above my knees. Climbing inside an Egyptian pyramid. The Far East—Japan, Hong Kong, Thailand, and Singapore. Having just returned from the Galapagos Islands and the Amazon, I am in the process of

planning my next trip—China. My oncologist is clutching his chest. Mea culpa.

You see, I have breast cancer. By the time I was diagnosed in 1987, my disease had advanced to stage IV. Mammograms had revealed nothing, and breast exams every 3 or 4 months by competent physicians had revealed nothing. Caution was the watchword since my mother had had breast cancer 20 years earlier. A chance encounter with a new lump prompted me to have a biopsy. The lump was benign, but the surrounding tissue contained cancerous cells; there was cancer in both breasts.

There was no choice but to have a bilateral mastectomy. I agreed to it, along with immediate breast reconstruction. Twenty-five cancerous lymph nodes were removed. Breast cancer had spread to my bone marrow. The picture was bleak.

The disease took over my life. I was sick and bald from the chemotherapy for almost a year. Watching my red hair wash down the shower drain was a shock. But time and lots of TLC (tender loving care) heals. After a few years, I thought I was home free and began to relax. No such luck.

In 1991, I started having painful stomach problems. I was told I had ulcers caused by stomach cancer. Those breast cancer cells had spread once again. This was a warning. Next it could be a major organ. Drastic action was required. After much soul-searching and hand-holding, I decided on high-dose chemotherapy and an autologous bone marrow transplant.

Where to go? Rejected by several hospitals because of my advanced condition, I was finally accepted for treatment by the University Hospital in Denver, Colorado. They had a young, brilliant team of doctors and nurses, and a specially designed, high-tech environment.

What more could I ask for? I just wanted another chance at life, to be myself again.

I will never forget the summer of 1992. My husband and I moved to Denver—he to an apartment and I into the hospital. I spent half my time there in isolation. My oncologist had told me that this treatment would probably be the closest experience to death that I would ever encounter without dying. He was right. After leaving the hospital, there were lots of problems over the next 8 months—fevers, infections, anemia, scarred lungs, and neurological damage.

Was it worth it? I don't know yet, but I am grateful that 1 year later, against my doctor's best advice, I have just returned from a great adventure—a trip celebrating the renewal of life.

Inside this patient there is a person who wants to live life to the fullest according to her own rules. None of this would have been possible without a caring support team of family, friends, and physicians. I will be forever grateful to all of them. They will always receive my postcards from distant, exotic places.

Inside This Person There Is a Patient—Addendum

It has been 3 years since I had my BMT. During this time I have tried to resume my normal lifestyle, my piano, volunteering, traveling, and so on. In 1994, I had the opportunity to travel to Moscow and China. In Moscow, I was invited to perform in the International Music Festival. My family accompanied me. It was a wonderful experience.

We lived with families in the House of Composers. We met musicians, composers, artists, singers, and actors. We shared meals, communicating in Russian and English. Our hosts provided unique activities for us including a private outdoor concert on the banks of the Moscow River. A group of folk singers performed medieval songs a cappella. We all learned about a culture different but so much like our own.

Six weeks later, my husband and I toured China for nearly a month. Another group of interesting experiences—climbing the Great Wall, the hustle and bustle of Shanghai, the small towns, cruising the rivers, the ballet, opera, observing great artisans at work, Tiananmen Square. We learned about a completely different culture.

That was a lot of travel for a relatively brief period, so I decided to postpone any further travel for a while and enjoy my own home and beaches. A fortuitous decision. Things did not go exactly as planned.

Six months later my mother died unexpectedly. Shortly afterwards, my cancer recurred. My breast cancer had once again metastasized, but this time to my bones. My ribs, rampant with tumors, were continuously breaking. With almost every turn, pull, squeeze, and bend I could hear and feel them crack. Excruciating pain. Once again I was on chemotherapy and radiation. After about 30 radiation treatments, much of the pain was finally relieved.

How could this be happening? I have gone through so much treatment—surgery, chemotherapy, radiation, hormone drugs, and a BMT. It seems that every few years I am back to square one, back to 1987. How can I still survive mentally and physically?

What have I done wrong? Why does this keep happening? Intellectually, I know the answer. Emotionally, I do not. These experiences are not unique. Breast cancer is a chronic disease. It almost always returns.

Even though my current treatment is working, survival seems to become more and more difficult. I am trying to help myself in every way. I see a psycho-oncologist and participate in art therapy. Although I have not painted in 30 years, vivid images are exploding on my canvasses. I am engrossed in my music and learning the most difficult compositions I have ever attempted.

I don't know why all this is happening, but I feel there is a deadline. The privilege of old age has been revoked. I am a young woman in my sunset years. I have accepted that but there is much to do, much to see.

My perspective on life is clear. I am grateful to my family, friends, and doctors for their ongoing support. It is difficult for them as well. Every moment with my dear husband and daughters is precious. We will be traveling together again soon to Alaska. I will be involved in every detail, knowing it is important for me to plan for the future.

When my quality of life is no longer acceptable and no other treatment is appropriate, it will be time for me to let go. I hope I will be strong enough to realize that. I want my family and friends to remember me as the person they have grown with, not the patient they watched disintegrate. Meanwhile, I still remain optimistic and hopeful. My body will not leave here without a struggle. My soul will remain forever.

At age 33 Jim King underwent an allogeneic BMT for primary myelofibrosis in 1994. As of this writing in 1995, he was disease free.

It's a Marathon, Not a 10K

—Jim King

On March 17, 1994, I saw a physician for a simple ear infection. After noticing that my left abdomen was enlarged, he ran a few tests. Ten days later I was diagnosed with primary myelofibrosis. An oncologist told me I probably would not survive. My only hope was a bone marrow transplant, which had been successful in a few isolated cases.

I was in shock. I felt fine. I had completed the Chicago marathon only 4 months earlier. I couldn't be that sick. The denial phase lasted only a couple of days. Then I entered a state of despair. I was angry and confused. I had a wonderful wife and three small children whom I adored. I was going to die and leave them alone. I felt like my family was being cheated. I had dreamed of seeing my sons graduate from college, but now kindergarten was a stretch.

After a week of despair I roared into action. I knew I was in for the fight of my life and I needed a plan and support team. The first thing I did was take a 2-week vacation with my family and trade in my conservative Volvo for a Miata. Now was as good a time as any to have a midlife crisis. I read every book I could on survival and support. One of the books talked about building a support team. My wife was the coach (a Lou Holtz type). My brothers and sister were the dependable line, my old college roommates were the running backs, and a few great friends who had endured personal tragedies were the defense. As my transplant day grew closer, many other people joined the support team and were crucial to my ability to maintain a positive attitude.

I planned for the worst. I finalized a will, set up educational trusts for my children, finalized a buy/sell agreement with my business partner, and even picked out the songs and prayers for my funeral. I didn't actually expect them to be used, but wanted to get all the prudent planning out of the way so I could focus on winning. I was scared, but anxious to get on with it. My motto was "Bring it on"—false bravado, probably, but I wanted others to catch my optimism.

I was amazed at the number of people who flocked to help my family. Friends would ask what they could give me. I asked for platelets, and for them to put a collection of their favorite songs together on a cassette tape to remind me of them and keep me fired up during the transplant. I got a lot of great tapes but not a lot of platelets.

On June 28 my 8-pound spleen was removed. I recovered in a couple of weeks and felt ready for the transplant. I felt lucky—lucky to have had such a great life so far, lucky to have a wife who loved me, lucky to have my sons, and lucky to have an interesting career. I was mentally prepared for the transplant and ready to go.

I entered the BMT unit on a sunny day in August, full of optimism. The first thing I did was shave my head. It was my way of establishing who was in charge of this contest. I wasn't going to let radiation take my hair, I took it first. I decorated my hospital room with pictures of family and friends, a stereo, CD player, VCR, a small basketball hoop, Nintendo, and some books. The books proved to be worthless because I quickly lost my ability to concentrate, but the tunes really helped. Whenever I was down or a new drug or procedure was to start, I would crank REM's song "Superman" as loud as possible. Great songs helped keep me pumped.

After I got my room set up, the nurses introduced themselves. They were great. Nurses are a pretty special breed to begin with, but the BMT nurses were incredible. They bent over backwards to help me, comfort me, and educate me.

The first procedure was an intraspinal injection of methotrexate. It didn't hurt, especially when compared to a bone marrow biopsy, but I had to lie flat on my back for 6 hours. It was pretty boring so I counted all the dots on the ceiling.

The next morning the real fun began. At 7:30 AM I went for my first round of radiation and then had a Hickman catheter installed. I developed a love–hate relationship with my Hickman. I loved it because I was no longer stuck with needles all the time, but hated having it stick out of my body.

After 5 days of radiation therapy, I was given a chemotherapy drug called VP-16. I tolerated it well with few side effects. A week later my brother Kevin's marrow was transplanted into me. It was an emotional day, but the process itself was a yawner. It took 3 hours to infuse the new marrow, and I felt great. I started to think that the stories I'd heard about how tough it is to undergo a BMT were exaggerations. I felt a little weak, but was doing fine. I went to sleep that night feeling on top of the world.

The hammer came down the next morning. It was not gradual. I woke up feeling sicker than I had ever felt in my life. My hair was all over the sheets and my own spit made me nauseous. I had a fever, diarrhea, and could barely hold my head up. The next 10 days were terrible. I had trouble eating because of the nausea and sores in my stomach and mouth. I lost 30 pounds, got several rashes and infections, and had continuous fevers. This was the crucial period. I was getting packed red cells, TPN, antibiotics, filgrastim, fluids, and steroids. At one point I counted 15 bags on my IV pole. I was also given a wonderful little button that allowed me to self-dispense morphine every 5 minutes. I pushed it a lot. I don't remember much more about that week—I've blocked it out. It's a fog and I'm glad.

I began to feel better about 10 days after the transplant and was anxious to go home. I asked the doctor what I had to do to get out of there. He said my blood counts had to improve and I had to have solid stools. I couldn't control my counts, but I could control my eating and stools. That night I ate a ham sandwich—bad choice. It hurt a lot, but I was determined to hold it down no matter what. It came up a few times but I closed my mouth and swallowed—gross, but effective. My superstar nurses gave me hot packs to put on my stomach and encouraged me to keep fighting. I did, and soon I was eating regularly. Eating wasn't pleasant, but I was doing it. Finally, a solid stool. I still can't believe how excited I got when it happened.

At last the head of the transplant team said the four words I thought I'd never hear, "You can go home." I was ecstatic. I packed up my "war room," hugged any nurse I could find, and was wheeled out of the hospital. The air outside smelled wonderfully dirty and I took in all the sights. I was discharged just in time to get stuck in Chicago's rush-hour traffic and I enjoyed every minute of it.

My family had decorated our house with balloons and a big sign that said "Welcome Home Daddy." I felt like a grade-school kid whose long year had just ended and whose summer vacation was just beginning. I thought the tough part was over. Now I would rest a bit and then resume a normal life.

I had never been so wrong. The inpatient stay was the easiest part of the BMT process. I was focused and fired up for the inpatient phase of the battle. All the worldly things, such as my role as a husband and father were secondary to winning my inpatient battle. Other routine things such as house payments, medical bills, career, and church weren't even on my mind. Nurses and doctors took care of me. It wasn't easy, but I felt I was making significant progress toward beating my disease.

The clarity of purpose and sense of progress was lost when I came home. Instead of feeling like a successful patient, I felt like a failed person. All those worldly things that I had ignored in the hospital, such as my role as husband and father, came roaring back. They were once again important and I felt I was woefully inadequate in those roles. We had three children, a 4-year-old and a set of 8-month-old twins, and I couldn't help at all with their care. I wasn't allowed to change a diaper, and didn't have the strength to carry any of my boys upstairs. All my self-esteem and self-confidence were gone. I couldn't imagine ever functioning like a normal person again.

The steroids and cyclosporine made me extremely emotional and irrational. I would cry because I had too much milk on my cereal. I couldn't sleep (steroids), couldn't shower (Hickman), couldn't read (no concentration), couldn't drink coffee in the morning (nausea), couldn't exercise (no strength), and couldn't get close to my children (might get an infection). Even taking my medicine was confusing and overwhelming. I spent a lot of time worrying about things I couldn't control. I was convinced I was going to run out of money, lose my house, my dog, and so on. There was no measured progress anymore. I felt I was regressing.

To get out of my emotional rut, I began setting myself up for small victories, and treating myself to tastes of normal life. I would see how fast and accurately I could flush my Hickman catheter and change my dressing. If I did it in record time or could safely eliminate a step, I'd reward myself with a nap. I added an additional lap to my walk around the neighborhood every other day and felt like a winner. I'd drive my car to Burger King, get a drive-through breakfast, and cheer when I didn't throw up.

Not a big achievement, but it seemed huge then. I shampooed and conditioned my bald head so that I'd feel normal. I forced myself to read a whole section of the newspaper without giving up in frustration. I even called a restaurant and had them set up a table in an empty banquet section for me and my wife. I couldn't eat much but the fact that we were going out for dinner made me feel normal again, at least for an evening.

The number of small victories increased as the doses of steroids and cyclosporine tapered off. I began to feel normal around Christmas, 120 days after transplant.

Currently, I'm 14 months posttransplant. I celebrated my 1-year transplant anniversary by climbing a mountain in Colorado and getting second row, center section seats for a Jimmy Buffet concert. Lots of people celebrated with me and gave me inspirational messages, gifts, and support. My favorite gift came from Dr. Daugherty of the BMT unit—an interpretation of my latest bone marrow biopsy report. The interpretation pretty much describes my life today—normal.

Index

A

Abdominal cramping, after transplantation, 99

Abdominal distension, in liver failure, 287

ABMTR (Autologous Blood and Marrow Transplant Registry-North and South America), 82, 445

ABMTs (autologous bone marrow transplants). *See* Stem cell transplants

ABO-incompatible transfusion reaction, minimizing risk for, 11

ABO titers, 196

Acetretin, for GVHD, 167, 169

Acute myelogenous leukemia (AML)
  busulfan for, 120
    TBI conditioning regimen dosing, 114

Acute nonlymphocytic leukemia (ANLL), 7

Acute renal failure (ARF), 265–266

Acute respiratory distress syndrome (ARDS), 251

Acute tubular necrosis (ATN), 268–269

Advance care planning/advance directives, 380–383

Age, outpatient care and, 426–427

Agglutination, 46

Airway disease, 246

Alemtuzumab (CamPath), 126

Alkylating agents, neurotoxicity of, 315

Alloimmunity, 150

Alloreactions, engraftment/rejection process, 65–66

Ambulatory setting. *See* Outpatient setting

American Nurses Association, professional practice standards, 369–370

American Society for Blood and Marrow Transplantation (ASBMT), 445, 450

American Society of Clinical Oncology (ASCO), 444, 450–451

American Society of Hematology (ASH), 450–451

AML. *See* Acute myelogenous leukemia

Ammonia, serum, 299

Amphotericin B, 13, 186–187

Anaphylactic reaction, after transplantation, 99

Anemia, 37, 192–193. *See also* Aplastic anemia

Anesthesia risk, for marrow donation, 71

ANLL (acute nonlymphocytic leukemia), 7

Anorexia, 208, 212. *See also* Emetic response

Anthropometric measurements, in nutritional assessment, 229–230

Antibiotic resistant bacteria, 12

Antibiotics, 184–185

Antidepressants, neurotoxicity of, 315

Antidiarrheals, 135, 225

Antiemetics, 135, 315

Antiemetic therapy, 215–217

Antifungals, 169, 186–188

Antigen-antibody reactions, complement and, 46–47

Antigens (immunogens), 46

Antigen specificity, 46

Antileukemic effect. *See* Graft-versus-leukemia; Graft-versus-tumor

Antileukemic reaction, allorecognition in, 60

Antimicrobial agents, 11–14, 315

Antioxidant therapy, for VOD, 282

Antithrombin III, for VOD, 282

Antithymocyte globulins (ATGs)
  adverse effects, 169
  equine or Atgam, 127
  for GVHD, 165, 169
  rabbit or thymoglobulin, 127
  toxicities, 132–133

Anti-TNF, neurotoxicity of, 315

Antiviral agents, neurotoxicity of, 315

Anxiety, posttransplant, 311–312

Apheresis
  area, in transplant center, 430–431
  large-volume procedures, 93
  machine, for PBSCT, 92–93
  for peripheral stem cell harvest, 70

Aplastic anemia
  bone marrow transplants for, 2, 3, 19
  conditioning regimen, 8

Apoptosis (programmed cell death), 36

Aprepitant, 216

ARDS (acute respiratory distress syndrome), 251

Area under the curve (AUC), 281–282

ARF (acute renal failure), 265–266

Arrhythmias, 258

ASBMT (American Society for Blood and Marrow Transplantation), 445, 450

Ascites, minimizing effects of, 290

ASCO (American Society of Clinical Oncology), 444, 450–451

ASH (American Society of Hematology), 450–451

505